Springer
Tokyo
Berlin
Heidelberg
New York
Hong Kong
London
Milan
Paris

N. Hayashi
D.W. Dietrich

Brain Hypothermia Treatment

With 119 Figures

Springer

Nariyuki Hayashi, M.D., Ph.D.
Chair, Nihon University Emergency Medical Center
Professor, Department of Emergency and Critical Care Medicine
Nihon University School of Medicine
30-1 Oyaguchi-kamicho, Itabashi-ku, Tokyo 173-8610, Japan

Dalton W. Dietrich, Ph.D.
Distinguished Chair in Neurosurgery, Kinetic Concepts
Professor, Department of Neurological Surgery, Neurology
and Cell Biology and Anatomy
University of Miami School of Medicine
17641 SW 75 Ave., Miami, Florida 33157, U.S.A.
Scientific Director, The Miami Project to Cure Paralysis
1095 NW 14th Terrace (R-48), Miami, Florida 33136, U.S.A.

ISBN 4-431-40446-5 Springer-Verlag Tokyo Berlin Heidelberg New York

Library of Congress Cataloging-in-Publication Data

Hayashi, N. (Nariyuki)
Brain hypothermia treatment / N. Hayashi, D.W. Dietrich.
p. cm.
Includes bibliographical references and index.
ISBN 4-431-40446-5 (alk. paper)
1. Brain damage--Treatment. 2. Cold--Therapeutic use. I. Dietrich, D. W. (Dalton W.), 1952- II. Title.

RC387.5.H39 2003
617.4′810446--dc22

2003057114

Printed on acid-free paper

Second printing 2004
Printed in Japan

Typesetting: SNP Best-set Typesetter Ltd., Hong Kong
Printing and binding: Nikkei Printing Inc., Japan
SPIN: 11008361

Foreword

This tome heralds the renaissance of interest in and study of hypothermia. It was some 50 years ago that basic research began to address this subject, starting with the simplistic measurement of oxygen consumption during cooling and rewarming with the lowering of body temperature. This was the prelude to the introduction of surface cooling hypothermia as an adjunct to anesthesia for open heart surgery. The heart–lung machine had not been perfected, so the reduction of metabolism of the brain by cooling became the only means of excluding arterial circulation to the brain that would allow a prolongation of surgical time to correct cardiac abnormalities.

I was a young medical student then, 1950, and was an assistant to the cardiac surgeon, Charles Bailey, at an open-heart operation for repair of a transposition of the aorta in an infant. When Dr. Bailey explained this concept for the rationale of the operation, with my budding interest in the nervous system, I was bold enough to ask how he knew his calculation of exclusion time was correct based only on oxygen consumption measurements. After all, oxygen consumption was an arithmetic mean of all respiratory systems. Why couldn't the brain respire at a different rate, higher or lower as the case might be? If higher, miscalculation could lead to possible ischemia. Dr. Bailey was, of course, disturbed by this upstart intrusion and assumed "This is for a young whipper-snapper like you to figure out!" And I did!

A few years later, early in my neurosurgical residency, I embarked on a decade of research, starting with the effect of lowering body temperature on cerebral blood flow and oxygen consumption. The references to this work and others that followed are to be found in the appropriate chapters of this book, so I will not repeat them here. Of course, my personal interest and training led me to apply this thinking to neuroscience and neurosurgical applications, particularly for the surgery of cerebral aneurysms and vascular anomalies, as well as anoxia, brain injury, stroke, and allied conditions.

Of historical note, it should be remembered that the French, headed by Laborit , had been employing lowered body temperature for massive injuries during the French Indo-China wars preceding this era, but civilian application began with cardiac surgery, followed by neurosurgery and others. Those crude efforts pale by comparison with the techniques described herein by Professors Hayashi and Dietrich. Their work has kept alive the germination and maturation of this body of neuroscience with the promise of discovery of information well beyond the vista of early investigations. Clinicians have only barely begun to push the envelope of basic research and clinical application. Clearly, temperature control or manipulation is a basic parameter of biological systems unlocking the door for discovery.

It would be presumptuous of me to compare the elemental research of the 1950s to the sophistication of the modern neuroscientist and scientifically based clinician. The intricacy of the mechanisms of brain injury, brain edema, ischemia, cerebral perfusion, and intracranial pressure (ICP) now coming to be understood better in neurobiology and neurochemistry at the molecular level are overwhelmingly complicated and difficult to master. Yet, their importance to basic knowledge and the mapping of neuroprotective strategies are keystones to survival.

As pointed out so succinctly by Professors Hayashi and Dietrich, newly discovered brain injury mechanisms associated with neurohormonal release, blood–brain barrier dysfunction, thermo-pooling, and cardiopulmonary stabilization are all important to brain tissue survival and restoration. Neuronal function goes well beyond the light microscope and histochemical observations of yore, advancing toward higher brain function and cognition that identify the signature, and perhaps the genotype, of man.

The original concept of brain hypothermia treatment incorporated cerebral circulatory protection, so that the immediate concern was to create the lowest temperature/metabolic rate possible, thus allowing longer exclusion times of the circulation to facilitate anatomical repairs. This unifocal concept may still be appropriate for that purpose, but is quite limited. The "new concept" to control brain temperature to between 32°C and 34°C so as to maintain systemic circulation and metabolism, neurohormonal control, and stabilization of immune function for the restoration of injured neurons is panoramic and goes beyond the restoration of injured tissue; hypothermia alone is not sufficient. Added are the administration of oxygen, stabilization of metabolism with adequate substrates, and the prevention of excess neurohormonal and cellular reactions. Therefore, the proper function of cortical neurons, avoidance of prolonged neuroexeitation, and prevention of selective radical damage are important and now achievable, so as to provide recovery from disturbances of personality, memory loss, and vegetation with higher brain functions. Reduction of oxygen consumption and control of ICP and brain edema are no longer the major targets of hypothermia treatment.

Quite frankly, I am humbled with respect for the perseverance of Professors Hayashi and Dietrich and colleagues, their newly acquired funds of knowledge, and translation of that knowledge to the clinic. My admiration is boundless. I am honored to be asked to write this foreword, which I take to be out of respect for my early efforts in this field. I have traveled far since those days and am no longer conversant with this science and practice. I fully believe, however, as I did early on, that hypothermia has the potential for providing major insights into basic mechanisms with even greater discoveries for man's center of function, his brain.

Hubert L. Rosomoff, M.D., D.Med.Sc.
Professor Emeritus, Chairman Emeritus
Department of Neurological Surgery
University of Miami School of Medicine
Medical Director
The Rosomoff Comprehensive Pain and Rehabilitation Center
at South Shore Hospital
Miami, Florida, U.S.A.

Foreword

"Neuroscience" is a key word in neurosurgery, trauma and critical care medicine, and intensive care medicine. In the field of neuroscience, brain hypothermia treatment is both an old and a new strategic intervention.

Professor Nariyuki Hayashi, Chairman of the Department of Emergency and Critical Care Medicine at Nihon University School of Medicine, is a pioneer in brain hypothermia treatment, in Japan and throughout the world. The focus of his research work in brain hypothermia treatment has been to clarify not only the mechanism and outcome but the intracranial pathophysiology of severe brain damage, affecting cardiopulmonary deterioration, and also the pathophysiology of acute and chronic stages, as in vegetative states.

This book is a compilation of Dr. Hayashi's lifelong research work in brain hypothermia, and fully integrates basic neuropathophysiology along with practical techniques and current knowledge in the field.

One of the many fine attributes of the book is the high degree of scientific expertise that has gone into its preparation. Thus, not only neurosurgeons but critical care physicians, emergency physicians, and trauma specialists as well will benefit greatly from the practical approach presented here for universal problems in the management of severe brain damage.

Shuji Shimazaki, M.D., Ph.D.
President, Japanese Association of Acute Medicine
Chairman and Professor
Department of Trauma and Critical Care Medicine
Kyorin University School of Medicine
Tokyo, Japan

Preface

It is difficult for primary injured brain tissue to survive; therefore, secondary brain-injury mechanisms such as brain edema, brain ischemia, reduced cerebral perfusion pressure (CPP), and elevation of intracranial pressure (ICP) have been considered targets of initial treatment. Free radicals, blood brain barrier (BBB) dysfunction, toxic excitatory amino acid, and an increase of intracellular Ca^{++}—which are contributing factors of pathophysiology—also have been considered targets of treatment. Application of this management concept to severely brain-injured patients has long been supported by many animal studies, and various neuroprotection methods have been developed.

Recent experimental animal studies have suggested that hypothermia is very successful in preventing secondary brain damage in trauma, ischemia, and brain hypoxia. There have been many clinical experiences in the past in which hypothermia for severely brain-injured patients has been tried. However, successful clinical results are not recorded as animal studies are, and the evaluation of hypothermia in the management of severe brain trauma, stroke, and hypoxia remains controversial. How can the discrepancy between its effectiveness in animal models and in clinical patients be explained?

The development of monitoring systems and procedures for use in the intensive care unit (ICU), such as computerized monitors; microdialysis techniques; biochemical analysis of blood, cerebrospinal fluid (CSF), and interstitial brain tissue; and monitoring of brain tissue temperature and oxygen tension, revealed many errors in previous ICU management. For a long time, control of ICP and brain edema by osmotic therapy with limited normal systemic circulation were tried as initial care management. Brain edema and ICP elevation occur as a result of development of pathophysiological changes in injured brain tissue, such as neuronal hypoxia, vasoactive neurohormonal BBB dysfunction, elevation of brain tissue temperature with brain thermopooling, and release of neurotoxic substances. Therefore, as an initial treatment of hypothermia, we must focus on controlling each of these. At the same time, in severely brain-injured patients, cerebral oxygenation with normal PaO_2 and normal oxygen delivery are insufficient because hemoglobin dysfunction prevents the release of oxygen from bound hemoglobin. Oxygen therapy is required for neuronal oxygenation in injured brain tissue. All of these specific pathophysiological changes develop in clinical patients within 3h not only as a result of direct brain injury but also due to stress-associated activation of hypothalamus–pituitary–adrenal (HPA)-axis neurohormonal endocrinological reactions. Unfortunately, however, the specific stress-associated neuroendocrinological reactions are not recorded in animal models by anesthesia. Therefore, previous concepts of hypothermia treatment that focused on control of ICP and brain edema, the peak time of which is between 12 and 48h, were not correct, and the delay was too long for neuronal restoration of primary brain damage. For successful treatment of severely brain-injured patients, we must understand the precise mechanism of neuroprotection by hypothermia, which is revealed in many animal studies. We must also understand the differences in pathophysiology in patients and in experimental animal models.

Recent clinical management studies in our ICU have demonstrated other, until now unknown, secondary brain-injury mechanisms such as brain thermo-pooling; masking of neuronal hypoxia even with normal control of ICP, PaO_2, and CPP; harmful stress-induced insulin-resistant hyperglycemia; vasopressin release associated with macro-nutrient feedback mechanism;, cytokines; encephalitis; and pneumonia associated with severe BBB dysfunction. In severely brain-injured patients, all of these brain-injury mechanisms progress rapidly within 3–6h. The brain-injury mechanisms associated with excess neurohormone release, such as catecholamine surge, vasopressin, and growth hormone, have been found to strongly affect the reversibility and prognosis of injured neurons. The elevation of brain tissue temperatures, to 40°–44°C, although the core temperature was at 38°–40°C, was recorded in severely brain-injured patients with trauma, subarachnoid hemorrhage (SAH), and post-resuscitation of cardiopulmonary arrest (CPA) in shock or with reduced systemic blood pressure. We called these phenomena brain thermo-pooling, which occurs in association with the elevation of blood temperature, combined with difficult washout of elevated brain-tissue temperature as a result of cardiopulmonary dysfunction. Brain tissue temperature is different from the core temperature, especially in severely brain-injured patients. Monitoring of brain tissue temperature in the ICU suggests that dynamic changes occur in brain tissue temperature.

However, the brain-injury mechanism obtained from animal studies was from experiments carried out at around 37°C. As coauthor Dalton Dietrich pointed out, because of the dangers of hyperthermia in injured neurons, we must control brain tissue temperature carefully and precisely and prevent the activation of HPA-axis neurohormonal reactions in the acute stage. From these new findings on the brain-injury mechanism and new targets of treatment, hypothermia management that reduces body temperature is insufficient to restore injured neurons. We want to introduce a concept of brain hypothermia treatment that includes the precise control of brain tissue temperature and management of secondary brain damage from activation of the HPA axis for the treatment of neuronal restoration in severely brain-injured patients. This new concept of brain-injury mechanisms is not obvious in experimental animal studies.

The prevention of a vegetative state is another important clinical issue in severely brain-injured patients. The low incidence of memory disturbance and vegetation in patients who received brain hypothermia treatment is interesting. For many years we have evaluated disturbed consciousness by responses to outside stimulation such as pain, speech, and touch. However, human consciousness is more complex, consisting of two main elements. One is response to outside stimulation as evaluated by the Glasgow Coma Score. The other, comprising such factors as thinking, emotion, volition, memory, anger, and laughter, requires no outside stimulation. Here, we refer to those factors not needing outer stimulation as "inner consciousness". If we cannot bring about a recovery of inner consciousness and emotional response, a patient still can open his or her eyes as a result of outside stimulation; the patient is evaluated as being in a vegetative state. We are interested in the mechanism of damage to the inner consciousness and how to prevent such damage. At the conclusion of this book, the mechanism of selective damage of the inner consciousness and why brain hypothermia treatment prevents this damage are discussed. The theory of preventing a vegetative state still includes much speculation at present. However, a high incidence of selective CT changes in the hippocampus and amygdala, and detailed analysis of changes of chemical neurotransmitters in CSF in response to cerebral dopamine replacement therapy with a combination of pharmacological, estrogen, and median nerve stimulation, and clinical results paradoxically supported the concept of the inner consciousness theory. Further studies are needed. Clinical results have advanced, however, in severe brain injury, cardiac-arrested brain ischemia, brain infarction, and some cases of severe subarachnoid hemorrhage.

We appreciate the opportunity to describe in this book the basic research on the effectiveness of hypothermia, clinical issues in earlier hypothermia treatment, development of a new concept of brain hypothermia treatment, techniques for controlling brain temperature, management of unavoidable complications associated with hypothermia, prevention of vegetative states, successful computed algorithm care-management systems, and excellent clinical results.

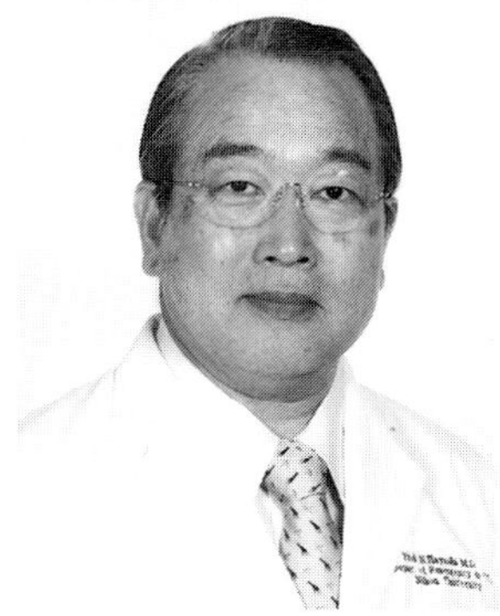

Nariyuki Hayashi, M.D., Ph.D.
Chair, Nihon University Emergency Medical Center
Professor, Department of Emergency and Critical Care Medicine
Nihon University School of Medicine
Tokyo, Japan

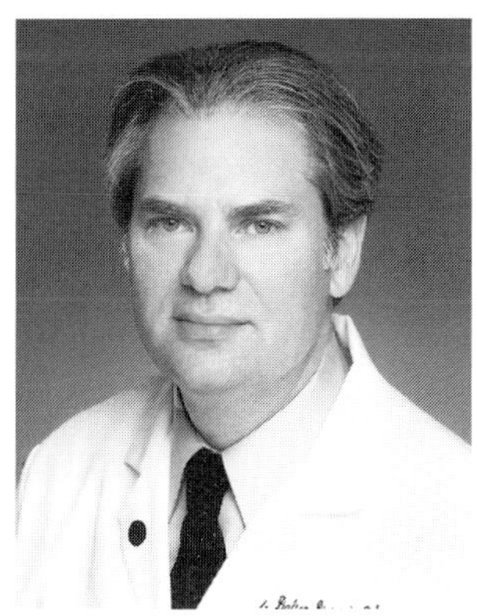

Dalton W. Dietrich, Ph.D.
Distinguished Chair in Neurosurgery, Kinetic Concepts
Professor, Department of Neurological Surgery, Neurology
and Cell Biology and Anatomy
University of Miami School of Medicine
Scientific Director, The Miami Project to Cure Paralysis, Florida, U.S.A.

Contents

Basic Research

Introduction

The beneficial effects of mild to moderate hypothermia in experimental models of brain [4–6,9,15,20,26] and spinal cord injury [1,18,21,22,24,27] have been reported in many laboratories. Using models of diffuse as well as focal injury, brain and spinal cord cooling have been shown to protect against neuronal damage and improve behavioral outcome. Recently, posttraumatic hypothermia has also been reported to protect against axonal damage [14,16,19]. In addition, the blood–brain barrier consequences of cerebral ischemia and traumatic brain injury are attenuated by moderate hypothermia [8,12,23]. Taken together, these investigations, using different animal models and various morphological and functional endpoints, emphasize how remarkably effective hypothermia can be in protecting central nervous system tissue [2]. Importantly, these experimental findings of therapeutic hypothermia have been supported by clinical data where hypothermic protection has been demonstrated in patients after cardiac arrest and brain trauma [7,10,13,17,25]. For example, a recent randomized clinical trial has shown that mild hypothermia improves outcome and reduces overall mortality in cases of cardiac arrest that occur outside of hospital [3,11].

This section reviews recent experimental data regarding the importance of temperature in models of brain and spinal cord injury. Specific mechanisms by which posttraumatic temperature alterations may affect the pathogenesis of brain injury and outcome are also reviewed.

References

1. Allen BT, Davis CG, Osborne D, Karl I (1994) Spinal cord ischemia and reperfusion metabolism: the effect of hypothermia. J Vasc Surg 19:332–339
2. Barone FC, Feuerstein GZ, White RF (1997) Brain cooling during transient focal ischemia provides complete neuroprotection. Neurosci Biobehav Rev 21:31–44
3. Bernard SA, Gray TW, Buist MD, Jones BM, Silvester W, Gutteridge G, Smith K (2002) Treatment of comatose survivors of out-of-hospital cardiac arrest with induced hypothermia. N Engl J Med 346:557–563
4. Bramlett H, Green EJ, Dietrich WD, Busto R, Globus MY-T, Ginsberg MD (1995) Post-traumatic brain hypothermia provides protection from sensorimotor and cognitive behavioral deficits. J Neurotrauma 12:289–298
5. Busto R, Dietrich WD, Globus MY-T, Valdes I, Scheinberg P, Ginsberg MD (1987) Small differences in intraischemic brain temperature critically determine the extent of ischemic neuronal injury. J Cereb Blood Flow Metab 7:729–738
6. Clark RSB, Robertson CL, Dixon CE, Alexander HL, Graham SH, Safar PJ, Kochanek PM (1999) Effect of hypothermia after severe traumatic brain injury with secondary hypoxemia in rats. J Neurotrauma 15:864 (Abstract)
7. Clifton GL (1995) Systemic hypothermia in treatment of severe brain injury: a review and update. J Neurotrauma 12:923–927
8. Dietrich WD, Busto R, Halley M, Valdes I (1990) The importance of brain temperature in alterations of the blood–brain barrier following cerebral ischemia. J Neuropathol Exp Neurol 49:486–497
9. Dietrich WD, Alonso O, Busto R, Globus MY-T, Ginsberg MD (1994) Post-traumatic brain hypothermia reduces histopathological damage following contusive brain injury in the rat. Acta Neuropathol 87:250–258
10. Hayashi N, Hirayama T, Utagawa A (1994) The cerebral thermo-pooling and hypothermia treatment of critical head injury patients. In: Nagai H (ed) Intracranial pressure IX. Springer, Berlin Heidelberg New York Tokyo, pp 589–599
11. Holzer M, Cerchiari E, Martens P, Roine R, Strez F (2002) Mild therapeutic hypothermia to improve the neurologic outcome after cardiac arrest. N Engl J Med 346:549–555
12. Jiang J-Y, Lyeth BG, Kapasi MZ, Jenkins LW, Povlishock JT (1992) Moderate hypothermia reduces blood–brain barrier disruption following traumatic brain injury in the rat. Acta Neuropathol 84:495–500
13. Jiang J-Y, Yu M-K, Zhu C (2000) Effect of long-term hypothermia therapy in patients with severe traumatic brain injury: 1-year follow-up review of 87 cases. J Neurosurg 93:546–549
14. Koizumi H, Povlishock JT (1998) Posttraumatic hypothermia in the treatment of axonal damage in an animal model of traumatic axonal injury. J Neurosurg 89:303–309
15. Lyeth BG, Jiang J-Y, Shanliang L (1993) Behavioral protection by moderate hypothermia initiated after experimental traumatic brain injury. J Neurotrauma 10:57–64

16. Marion DW, White MJ (1996) Treatment of experimental brain injury with moderate hypothermia and 21-aminosteroids. J Neurotrauma 13:139–147
17. Marion DW, Penrod LE, Kelsey SF, Obrist WD, Kochanek PM, Palmer AM, Wisniewki SR, DeKosky ST (1997) Treatment of traumatic brain injury with moderate hypothermia. N Eng J Med 336:540–546
18. Marsala M, Vanicky I, Yaksh TL (1994) Effect of graded hypothermia (27° to 34°C) on behavioral function, histopathology, and spinal cord blood flow after spinal ischemia in rat. Stroke 25:2038–2046
19. Maxwell WL, Donnelly S, Sun X, Fenton T, Pure N, Graham DI (1999) Axonal cytoskeletal response to nondisruptive axonal injury and the short-term effects of posttraumatic hypothermia. J Neurotrauma 16:1225–1234
20. Palmer AM, Marion DW, Botsceller ML, Redd EE (1993) Therapeutic hypothermia is cytoprotective without attenuating the traumatic brain injury-induced elevations in interstitial concentrations of aspartate and glutamate. J Neurotrauma 10:363–372
21. Robertson CS, Folz R, Grossman RG, Goodman JC (1986) Protection against experimental ischemic spinal cord injury. J Neurosurg 64:633–642
22. Rokkas CK, Cronin CS, Nitta T, Helfrich LR, Lobner DC, Choi DW, Kouchoukos NT (1995) Profound systemic hypothermia inhibits the release of neurotransmitter amino acids in spinal cord ischemia. J Thorac Cardiovasc Surg 110:27–35
23. Smith SL, Hall ED (1996) Mild pre- and posttraumatic hypothermia attenuates blood–brain barrier damage following controlled cortical impact injury in the rat. J Neurotrauma 13:1–9
24. Vacanti FX, Ames A (1984) Mild hypothermia and Mg^{++} protect against irreversible damage during CNS ischemia. Stroke 15:695–698
25. Wakamatsu H, Matsumoto M, Nakakimura K, Sakabe T (1999) The effects of moderate hypothermia and intrathecal tetracaine on glutamate concentrations of intrathecal dialysate and neurologic and histopathologic outcome in transient spinal cord ischemia in rabbits. Anesth Analg 88:56–62
26. Yamamoto M, Marmarou CR, Stiefel MF, Beaumont A, Marmarou A (1999) Neuroprotective effect of hypothermia on neuronal injury in diffuse traumatic brain injury coupled with hypoxia and hypotension. J Neurotrauma 16:487–500
27. Yu CG, Marcillo AE, Dietrich WD, Fairbanks CA, Wilcox GL, Yezierski RP (1999) Beneficial effects of hypothermia and/or agmatine on locomotor outcome following contusion spinal cord injury. Soc Neurosci Abstr 29:268

I. Basic Science of Brain Hypothermia

1. Global and Focal Cerebral Ischemia

The importance of small variations in brain temperature on ischemic outcome was first investigated in models of transient forebrain global ischemia [2]. These controlled studies followed preliminary observations in experiments in which only core (rectal) temperature was monitored and maintained (36.5°C) indicating that 1) ischemic CA1 hippocampal pathology commonly varied from one study to the next, 2) that rectal (core) and intraischemic brain temperature differed significantly, and 3) that in anesthetized rats, intraischemic brain temperature was commonly hypothermic. Thus, selectively decreasing intraischemic brain temperature to 30°–34°C protected the CA1 hippocampus and dorsolateral striatum [2,4]. In gerbils, a 2°C drop in body temperature provided 100% protection in the CA1 hippocampus [6]. Brain cooling during prolonged (30 min) global ischemia also protected the cerebral cortex from histopathological damage [12]. In models of cardiac arrest and cardiopulmonary bypass (CPB), hypothermic protection has also been reported [9,13–15,22]. For example, in a pig model of CPB, moderate hypothermia (27°C) prevented neuronal degeneration and astrocytic swelling after 2 h [13].

In addition to histopathological protection, the effects of moderate hypothermia on the behavioral and functional consequences of global ischemia and cardiac arrest have been investigated [8,14,15,19]. Green and colleagues reported that intraischemic hypothermia (30°C) during a 12.5-min ischemic period attenuated the cognitive and sensory motor consequences of global ischemia [8]. In dogs, mild hypothermia (34°C) resulted in significant improvement of neurologic function 96 h after cardiac arrest [14,15,22]. Okada and colleagues [19] reported that the period of oxygen and glucose deprivation during which neurons recovered function was extended by hypothermia (21°–28°C). In a functional study following global ischemia, accelerated recovery of glucose utilization after ischemia with intraischemic hypothermia was reported [7].

Focal ischemia models are commonly used to investigate the pathophysiology of stroke and the effects of moderate temperature reductions on histopathological outcome have been investigated [1,5,10,16,17,20,21,23]. Although no significant difference in infarct volume between hypothermic (30°C) and normothermic (36°C) rats was first reported after permanent middle cerebral artery (MCA) occlusion [20], significant protection was observed when brain temperature reduced to 24°C for 1 h after MCA occlusion [20]. Extended periods of mild hypothermia (31°C) are also reported to reduce infarct volume [23]. Thus, in conditions of permanent focal ischemia, profound degrees of hypothermia and/or extended hypothermic periods may be necessary to significantly protect the injured brain.

In models of transient MCA occlusion (TMCAO), more dramatic degrees of neuroprotection with moderate hypothermia have been reported [1,5,10,17,23]. Selective brain hypothermia (30°C) during a 2-h period of TMCAO significantly reduced infarct volume [17]. Whole body hypothermia (30°C) induced prior to ischemia and maintained for 2 h also decreased histopathological injury [1,3,4]. Recently, brain temperature reductions of 3°C and 8°C have been reported to provide dramatic and complete neuroprotection, respectively, following 80 min of TMCAO [1]. Mild hypothermia (33°C) during the 1-h ischemic period and first hour of reperfusion reduced infarct volume by 48% [23]. In clinical settings of postischemic reperfusion (i.e., spontaneous or thrombolysis), hypothermia may be most beneficial.

In addition to the degree and duration of cooling being critical factors in hypothermic treatment, rewarming conditions are of major consideration. In one study, rapid rewarming failed to provide the neuroprotective effect of hypothermia that was observed with slow rewarming [18]. Interestingly, gradual rewarming after controlled hypothermia has also been reported to produce axonal protection after traumatic brain injury [11]. Thus, although the detrimental consequences of rapid postinjury rewarming in the clinical arena are routinely appreciated, the importance of rewarming conditions in experimental models of brain injury requires additional investigation.

References

1. Barone FC, Feuerstein GZ, White RF (1997) Brain cooling during transient focal ischemia provides complete neuroprotection. Neurosci Biobehav Rev 21:31–44
2. Busto R, Dietrich WD, Globus MY-T, Valdes I, Scheinberg P, Ginsberg MD (1987) Small differences in intraischemic brain temperature critically determine the extent of ischemic neuronal injury. J Cereb Blood Flow Metab 7:729–738
3. Chen H, Chopp M, Vande Linde AMQ, Dereski MO, Garcia JH, Welch KMA (1992) The effects of post-ischemic hypothermia on the neuronal injury and brain metabolism after forebrain ischemia in the rat. J Neurol Sci 107:191–198
4. Chen H, Chopp M, Jiang Q, Garcia JH (1992) Neuronal damage, glial response and cerebral metabolism after hypothermic forebrain ischemia in the rat. Acta Neuropathol 84:184–189
5. Chen H, Chopp M, Zhang ZG, Garcia JH (1992) The effect of hypothermia on transient middle cerebral artery occlusion in the rat. J Cereb Blood Flow Metab 12: 621–628
6. Clifton GL, Jiang JY, Lyeth BG, Jenkins LW, Hamm RJ, Hayes RL (1991) Marked protection by moderate hypothermia after experimental traumatic brain injury. J Cereb Blood Flow Metab 11:114–121
7. Dietrich WD, Busto R, Alonso O, Pita-Loor Y, Globus MY-T, Ginsberg MD (1991) Intraischemic brain hypothermia promotes postischemic metabolic recovery and somatosensory circuit activation. J Cereb Blood Flow Metab 11(Suppl) 11:S854
8. Green EJ, Dietrich WD, van Dijk F, Busto R, Markgraf CG, McCabe PM, Ginsberg MD, Schneiderman N (1992) Protective effects of neural hypothermia on behavior following global cerebral ischemia. Brain Res 580:197–204
9. Horn M, Schlote W, Henrich, HA (1991) Global cerebral ischemia and subsequent selective hypothermia. Acta Neuropathol 81:443–449
10. Karibe H, Chen J, Zarow GJ, Graham SH, Weinstein PR (1994) Delayed induction of mild hypothermia to reduce infarct volume after temporary middle cerebral artery occlusion in rats. J Neurosurg 80:112–119
11. Koizumi H, Povlishock JT (1998) Posttraumatic hypothermia in the treatment of axonal damage in an animal model of traumatic axonal injury. J Neurosurg 89:303–309
12. Kuluz JW, Gregory GA, Yu ACH, Chang Y (1992) Selective brain cooling during and after prolonged global ischemia reduces cortical damage in rats. Stroke 23: 1792–1797
13. Laursen H, Waaben J, Gefke K, Husum B, Anderson LI, Sorensen HR (1989) Brain histology, blood–brain barrier and brain water after normothermic and hypothermic cardiopulmonary bypass in pigs. Eur J Cardio-thorac Surg 3:539–543
14. Leonov Y, Sterz F, Safar P, Radovsky A (1990) Moderate hypothermia after cardiac arrest of 17 minutes in dogs. Stroke 21:1600–1606
15. Leonov Y, Sterz F, Safar P, Radovsky A, Ohu K-I, Tisherman S, Stezoski W (1990) Mild cerebral hypothermia during and after cardiac arrest improves neurologic outcome in dogs. J Cereb Blood Flow Metab 10:57–70
16. Lo EH, Steinberg GK (1992) Effects of hypothermia on evoked potentials, magnetic resonance imaging, and blood flow in focal ischemia in rabbits. Stroke 23:889–893
17. Morikawa E, Ginsberg MD, Dietrich WD, Duncan RC, Kraydieh S, Globus MY-T, Busto R (1992) The significance of brain temperature in focal cerebral ischemia: histopathological consequences of middle cerebral artery occlusion in the rat. J Cereb Blood Flow Metab 12: 380–389
18. Nakamura T, Miyamoto O, Yanagami S-I, Hayashida Y, Itano T, Nagao S (1999) Influence of rewarming conditions after hypothermia in gerbils with transient forebrain ischemia. J Neurosurg 91:114–120
19. Okada Y, Tanimoto M, Yoneda K (1988) The protective effect of hypothermia on reversibility in the neuronal function of the hippocampal slice during long lasting anoxia. Neurosci Lett 84:277–282
20. Onesti ST, Baker CJ, Sun PP, Solomon RA (1991) Transient hypothermia reduces focal ischemic brain injury in the rat. Neurosurgery 29:369–373
21. Ridenour TR, Warner DS, Todd MM, McAllister AC (1992) Mild hypothermia reduces infarct size resulting from temporary but not permanent focal ischemia in rats. Stroke 23:733–738
22. Safar P, Klain M, Tisherman S (1996) Selective brain cooling after cardiac arrest. Crit Care Med 24:911–914
23. Xue D, Huang Z-G, Smith KE, Buchan AM (1992) Immediate or delayed mild hypothermia prevents focal cerebral infarction. Brain Res 587:66–72

2. Limitations of Postischemic Hypothermia

From a clinical treatment perspective, the question of whether postischemic brain hypothermia can protect the brain is an important one. In 1989, Busto and colleagues [1] reported that immediate postischemic hypothermia (30°C/3 h) significantly protected the CA1 hippocampus from histopathological injury after 3 days of recirculation. Hypothermia (32°C) after ventricular fibrillation cardiac arrest also reduced overall brain histologic damage [9,10]. Subsequent experiments in which the importance of ischemic duration was addressed [4] indicated that the degree of protection was reduced with longer ischemic durations or no significant benefit was reported. Animal studies indicate that the therapeutic window for postischemic hypothermia may be narrow and related to ischemic duration and ischemic severity [5].

In addition to the clinical importance of neuroprotection with postischemic hypothermia, these data reinforce the view that processes active in the postischemic setting can play a major role in ischemic cell death. The duration of the postischemic hypothermic period is now known to be another critical factor in determining the degree of neuroprotection [2,3,6–8] and may help explain the negative findings of some studies that utilized restricted hypothermic periods.

References

1. Busto R, Dietrich WD, Globus MY-T, Ginsberg MD (1989) Postischemic moderate hypothermia inhibits CA1 hippocampal ischemic neuronal injury. Neurosci Lett 101:299–304
2. Carroll M, Beek O (1992) Protection against hippocampal CA1 cell loss by post-ischemic hypothermia is dependent on delay of initiation and duration. Metabol Brain Dis 7:45–50
3. Chen H, Chopp M, Vande Linde AMQ, Dereski MO, Garcia JH, Welch KMA (1992) The effects of post-ischemic hypothermia on the neuronal injury and brain metabolism after forebrain ischemia in the rat. J Neurol Sci 107:191–198
4. Chopp M, Chen H, Dereski MO, Garcia JH (1991) Mild hypothermic intervention after graded ischemic stress in rats. Stroke 22:37–43
5. Coimbra C, Wieloch T (1994) Moderate hypothermia mitigates neuronal damage in the rat brain when initiated several hours following transient cerebral ischemia. Acta Neuropathol 87:325–331
6. Colbourne F, Sutherland G, Corbett D (1997) Postischemic hypothermia. A critical appraisal with implications for clinical treatment. Molec Neurobiol 14:171–201
7. Colbourne F, Li H, Buchan AM (1999) Indefatigable CA1 sector neuroprotection with mild hypothermia induced 6 hours after severe forebrain ischemia in rats. J Cereb Blood Flow Metab 19:742–749
8. Dietrich WD, Busto R, Alonso O, Pita-Loor Y, Globus MY-T, Ginsberg MD (1991) Intraischemic brain hypothermia promotes postischemic metabolic recovery and somatosensory circuit activation. J Cereb Blood Flow Metab 11(Suppl) 11:S854
9. Leonov Y, Sterz F, Safar P, Radovsky A (1990) Moderate hypothermia after cardiac arrest of 17 minutes in dogs. Stroke 21:1600–1606
10. Leonov Y, Sterz F, Safar P, Radovsky A, Ohu K-I, Tisherman S, Stezoski W (1990) Mild cerebral hypothermia during and after cardiac arrest improves neurologic outcome in dogs. J Cereb Blood Flow Metab 10:57–70

3. The Importance of Chronic Outcome Measures in Assessing Neuroprotective Strategies

Although cooling during the ischemic period provides chronic histopathological and behavioral protection, the issue of whether long-lasting protection occurs with postischemic hypothermia has been raised [4,5]. A lack of chronic protection with postischemic hypothermia was first reported after transient global ischemia [5] in which case significant CA1 hippocampal protection was seen at postischemic day three but not at 2 months. A failure of postischemic hypothermia to provide chronic protection using behavioral strategies was also subsequently reported [11]. These data emphasized the important point that chronic outcome measures should be used to assess neuroprotective procedures or pharmacological agents prior to the initiation of clinical trials.

In gerbils, Colbourne and coworkers [3,4] assessed a 24-h cooling period (32°C) initiated 1 h after 5 min of ischemia. Their data demonstrated substantial CA1 protection at 1 month (94%) and 6 months (70%). These experiments demonstrated for the first time that postischemic hypothermia can provide some degree of chronic protection if the duration and degree of hypothermia are sufficient. However, because gerbils are known to be extremely sensitive to neuroprotective strategies, similar studies using other animal species were needed to evaluate the chronic benefits of extended postischemic cooling [4]. Nevertheless, the use of hypothermia in experimental and clinical investigations should be advantageous in extending the therapeutic window for pharmacotherapy as well as providing some degree of neuroprotection.

In the clinical practice of cerebral protection following stroke, the use of thrombolytic agents to recanalize cerebral blood vessels has the great potential of providing dramatic protection from tissue damage (National Institute of Neurological Diseases & Stroke 1995). However, when reperfusion of the ischemic core is not possible, more limited degrees of neuroprotection are expected with pharmacotherapy. In experimental models, the ischemic penumbra surrounding the ischemic core has been targeted as a possible site for therapeutic interventions [12]. The inability of postischemic hypothermia to chronically protect may involve secondary injury mechanisms including inflammation. In such a setting, the acute benefits of cooling may be compromised by delayed inflammatory reactions commonly characterized as "reperfusion injury." Secondary injury mechanisms including leukocyte, macrophage, or microglia infiltration, as well as blood–brain barrier dysfunction, are known to contribute to progressive damage [8,10].

Because inflammatory cells may generate and release potentially neurotoxic factors including excitatory amino acids or free radicals [1,15], experiments have been conducted in which postischemic hypothermia was combined with delayed treatments of the NMDA antagonist MK-801 (dizocilpine) and the free-radical spin-trap agent PBN (*N-tert*-phenylnitrone) [6,11,14]. Using strategies in which hypothermia is combined with delayed therapeutic strategies that target inflammatory processes, significant protection has been reported. In this regard, Coimbra and colleagues [2] have combined postischemic hypothermia (33°C/7 h) started at 2 h with the antipyretic/anti-inflammatory drug, dipyrone. Although postischemic hypothermia alone delayed neuronal damage, cooling followed by dipyrone markedly diminished neuronal damage at both 7 days and 2 months. Most recently, mild postischemic hypothermia (33°–34°C/4 h) combined with the anti-inflammatory cytokine, IL-10, was used to treat transient global ischemia [7]. In that study, the combination of hypothermia and IL-10 but not either treatment alone led to long-lasting protection of the CA1 hippocampus.

Taken together, these data indicate that although postischemic brain cooling confers significant neuroprotection, especially in the early postischemic period, secondary injury mechanisms associated with rewarming should be targeted for therapeutic intervention. The use of hypothermia in combination with pharmacotherapy has the potential benefit of providing more complete and longer-lasting protection compared to single therapeutic strategies. In a model of permanent bilateral carotid artery occlusion, Schwab and colleagues [16] showed that the notropic drug Cerebrolysin (Ebewe, Austria) enhanced the beneficial effects of mild hypothermia (35°C) on local cerebral blood flow reduction and the development of brain edema. In another study, hypothermia enhanced the beneficial effects of MK-801 against hypoxic–ischemic brain damage in infant rats [13]. Combined hypothermia with the NMDA antagonist dextromethorphan protected the cerebral cortex following transient global ischemia in excess of the protection conferred by either hypothermia or drug alone [9]. Thus, hypothermic clinical trials may have to include treatment strategies that enhance the protective effects of cooling and/or protect the brain against delayed injury processes.

References

1. Banati RB, Rothe G, Valet G, Kreutzberg GW (1991) Respiratory brust in brain macrophages; a flow cytometric study on cultured rat microglia. Neuropathol Appl Neurobiol 17:223–230
2. Coimbra C, Drake M, Boris-Moller F, Wieloch T (1996) Long-lasting neuroprotective effect of postischemic hypothermia and treatment with an anti-inflammatory/antipyretic drug. Effect for chronic encephalopathic processes following ischemia. Stroke 27:1578–1585
3. Colbourne F, Corbett D (1994) Delayed and prolonged post-ischemic hypothermia is neuroprotective in the gerbil. Brain Res 654:265–272
4. Colbourne F, Li H, Buchan AM (1999) Indefatigable CA1 sector neuroprotection with mild hypothermia induced 6 hours after severe forebrain ischemia in rats. J Cereb Blood Flow Metab 19:742–749
5. Dietrich WD, Busto R, Globus MY-T, Ginsberg MD (1993) Intraischemic but not postischemic brain hypothermia protects chronically following forebrain ischemia in rats. J Cereb Blood Flow Metab 13:541–549
6. Dietrich WD, Lin B, Globus MY-T, Green EJ, Ginsberg MD, Busto R (1995) Effect of delayed MK-801 (dizocilpine) treatment with or without immediate postischemic hypothermia on chronic neuronal survival after global forebrain ischemia in rats. J Cereb Blood Flow Metab 15:960–968
7. Dietrich WD, Busto R, Bethea JR (1999) Postischemic hypothermia and IL-10 treatment provide long-lasting neuroprotection of CA1 hippocampus following transient global ischemia in rats. Exp Neurol 158:444–450
8. Gehrmann J, Bonnekoh P, Miyazawa T, Hossmann K-A, Kreutzberg GW (1992) Immunocytochemical study of an early microglial activation in ischemia. J Cereb Blood Flow Metab 12:257–269
9. Ginsberg MD, Globus MY-T, Busto R, Dietrich WD (1990) The potential of combination pharmacotherapy in cerebral ischemia. In: Oberpichler H (eds) Pharmacology of cerebral ischemia. Stuttgart, Wissenschaftliche, pp 499–510
10. Giulian D, Vaca K, Noonan CA (1990) Secretion of neurotoxins by mononuclear phagocytes infected with HIV-1. Science 250:1593–1596
11. Green EJ, Pazos AJ, Dietrich WD, McCabe P, Schneiderman N, Lin B, Busto R, Globus MY-T, Ginsberg MD (1995) Combined postischemic hypothermia and delayed MK-801 treatment attenuates neurobehavioral deficits associated with transient global ischemia in rats. Brain Res 702:145–152
12. Hossmann K-A (1994) Viability thresholds and the penumbra of focal ischemia. Ann Neurol 36:557–565
13. Ikonomidou C, Mosinger JL, Olney JW (1989) Hypothermia enhances protective effect of MK-801 against hypoxic/ischemic brain damage in infant rats. Brain Res 487:184–187
14. Pazos AJ, Green EJ, Busto R, McCabe PM, Baena RC, Ginsberg MD, Globus MY-T, Schneiderman N, Dietrich WD (1999) Effects of combined postischemic hypothermia and delayed *N-tert*-butyl-alpha-phenylnitrone (PBN) administration on histological and behavioral deficits associated with transient global ischemia in rats. Brain Res 846:186–195
15. Piani D, Frei K, Do KQ, Cuenod M, Fontana A (1991) Murine brain macrophages induce NMDA receptor mediated neurotoxicity in vitro by secreting glutamate. Neurosci Lett 133:159–162
16. Schwab M, Bauer R, Zwiener U (1997) Physiological effects and brain protection by hypothermia and cerebrolysin after moderate forebrain ischemia in rats. Exp Toxicol Pathol 49:105–116

4. Traumatic Brain Injury

Quantitative strategies have been developed to evaluate the effects of posttraumatic temperature on patterns of neuronal vulnerability in models of traumatic brain injury (TBI) (Table 1). In a model of parasagittal fluid-percussion (F-P) brain injury in which brain temperature was selectively reduced (30°C) for 3 h starting 5 min after TBI, posttraumatic hypothermia (30°C) significantly decreased contusion volume and reduced the frequency of damaged cortical neurons [5]. In a controlled cortical impact model in rats, mild hypothermia (32°–33°C) initiated 30 min before trauma and continued for 2 h decreased contusion volume at 14 days [2,8]. In a model of diffuse TBI coupled with hypoxia and hypotension, Yamamoto and colleagues [9] reported that moderate hypothermia (30°C) initiated 15 min after injury and maintained for 60 min provided almost complete protection against secondary insults. In contrast, posttraumatic hypothermia (32°C/2 h) failed to reduce volumes of necrotic tissue cavitation after cortical impact injury [6].

Recently, the progressive nature of histopathological damage after TBI was emphasized [1,9]. In one study, progressive atrophy was reported up to 1 year after F-P brain injury [9]. Based on data from the cerebral ischemia field describing the limitations of restricted periods of postinjury hypothermia [3,4], these findings raised the possibility that posttraumatic hypothermia provided temporary but not long-lasting protection. Thus, the long-term effects of posttraumatic hypothermia have been recently evaluated in a parasagittal F-P model [1]. Posttraumatic hypothermia (30°C/3 h) significantly attenuated the degree of cortical atrophy and inhibited the increase in ventricular enlargement at 2 months after trauma. Thus, restricted periods of moderate hypothermia immediately after TBI appear to provide some degree of acute and long-term histopathological protection in specific injury models.

References

1. Bramlett HM, Dietrich WD, Green EJ, Busto R (1997) Chronic histopathological consequences of fluid-percussion brain injury: effects of posttraumatic hypothermia. Acta Neuropath 93:190–199
2. Clark RSB, Kochanek PM, Marion DW, Schiding JK, White M, Palmer AM, DeKosky ST (1996) Mild posttraumatic hypothermia reduces mortality after severe controlled cortical impact in rats. J Cereb Blood Flow Metab 16:253–261
3. Colbourne F, Sutherland G, Corbett D (1997) Postischemic hypothermia. A critical appraisal with implications for clinical treatment. Molec Neurobiol 14:171–201
4. Dietrich WD, Busto R, Globus MY-T, Ginsberg MD (1993) Intraischemic but not postischemic brain hypothermia protects chronically following forebrain ischemia in rats. J Cereb Blood Flow Metab 13:541–549

Table 1. Studies of the effects of posttraumatic temperature on patterns of neuronal vulnerability in models of traumatic brain injury

Study	Year	Species	Delay	EC, duration	Outcome, measures
Dixon et al.	1998	Rat	5-min delay	32°C, 2 h	Behavior, pathology, 16 days
Yamamoto et al.	1999	Rat	15-min delay	30°C, 1 h	Pathology, 24 h
Maxwell et al.	1999	Rat	Immediately after	32–32.5°C, 2 or 4 h	Axonal damage, 4 h
Yamamoto et al.	1999	Rat	15-min delay	30°C, 1 h	Pathology, 4 and 24 h
Chatzipanteli et al.	1999	Rat	Before or 2 h after	32–33°C, 2 h	cNOS, iNOS activity, 5 min, 3 and 7 days
Zhao et al.	1999	Rat	5-min delay	30°C, 3 h	lCBF, glucose metabolism, 3 h
Chatzipanteli et al.	2000	Rat	5-min delay	32°C, 4 h	PMNL, MPO, 3 h; 1, 3, and 7 days
Markgraf et al.	2001	Rat	Immediately, 60 or 90 min after	30°C, 3 h	Edema, Behavior, 7 days

BBB, blood–brain barrier; PMNL, polymorphonuclear leukocyte; MPO, myeloperoxidase; 2,3 DHBA, dihydroxybenzoic acid; lCBF, local cerebral blood flow metabolism; iNOS, inducible nitric oxide synthase; cNOS, constitutive nitric oxide synthase

5. Dietrich WD, Alonso O, Busto R, Globus MY-T, Ginsberg MD (1994) Post-traumatic brain hypothermia reduces histopathological damage following contusive brain injury in the rat. Acta Neuropathol 87:250–258
6. Dixon CE, Markgraf CG, Angileri F, Pike BP, Wolfson B, Newcomb JK, Bismar MM, Blanco AJ, Clifton GL, Hayes RL (1998) Protective effects of moderate hypothermia on behavioral deficits but not necrotic cavitation following cortical impact injury in the rat. J Neurotrauma 15:95–103
7. Markgraf CG, Glifton GL, Moody MR (2001) Treatment window for hypothermia in brain injury. J Neurosurg 95:979–983
8. Palmer AM, Marion DW, Botsceller ML, Redd EE (1993) Therapeutic hypothermia is cytoprotective without attenuating the traumatic brain injury-induced elevations in interstitial concentrations of aspartate and glutamate. J Neurotrauma 10:363–372
9. Smith DG, Chen X-H, Pierce ES, McIntosh TK (1997) Progressive atrophy and neuronal death for one year following brain trauma in the rat. J Neurotrauma 14:715–727
10. Yamamoto M, Marmarou CR, Stiefel MF, Beaumont A, Marmarou A (1999) Neuroprotective effect of hypothermia on neuronal injury in diffuse traumatic brain injury coupled with hypoxia and hypotension. J Neurotrauma 16:487–500

5. Traumatic Axonal Injury

Diffuse axonal injury (DAI) leads to disconnection of various brain regions, a condition which translates into much of the morbidity seen with head injury [1–3,7,8]. Following spinal cord injury (Table 2), damage to major white matter tracts disrupts sensory and motor circuits. Moderate hypothermia has recently been reported to reduce axonal injury after experimental traumatic brain injury (TBI) [4,5]. Marion and White [5] first reported that posttraumatic hypothermia delayed up to 24 min after cortical impact injury significantly decreased the frequency of immunoreactive damaged axons. Using an impact acceleration rat model, Koizumi and Povlishock [4] reported that postinjury hypothermia delayed for 1 h (32°C/1 h) reduced beta-amyloid precursor protein (beta-APP) damaged axons at 24 h compared to non-treated controls. Reduced axonal swelling and abnormal beta-APP immunoreactivity was also reported with hypothermia treatment after severe spinal cord compression [10].

A recent study using a stretch injury model to optic nerve axons reported that hypothermia also reduced the number of axons labeled with antibodies against beta-APP [6]. This study also provided quantitative, morphometric evidence that posttraumatic hypothermia ameliorates the loss of axonal microtubules and compaction of neurofilaments in the acute stages of injury. Thus, hypothermia may improve outcome following brain and spinal cord injury by reducing the degree of cytoskeletal pathology generally observed after axonal injury. In this regard, Taft and colleagues [9] have reported that posttraumatic hypothermia (30°C) inhibits trauma-induced reductions in hippocampal microtubule-associated protein 2 (MAP-2) after TBI. Taken together, these histopathological and immunocytochemical studies clearly demonstrate that a brief duration of moderate hypothermia following TBI improves neuronal survival and protects against cytoskeletal damage.

References

1. Adams JH, Graham DI, Murray LS, Scott G (1982) Diffuse axonal injury due to non-missile head injury in humans: an analysis of 45 cases. Ann Neurol 12:557–563
2. Adams JH, Doyle D, Ford I, Graham DI, McLellan D (1989) Diffuse axonal injury in head injury: definition, diagnosis and grading. Histopathology 15:49–59
3. Gennarelli TA, Thibault LE, Adams JH, Graham DI, Thompson CJ, Marcincin RP (1982) Diffuse axonal injury and traumatic coma in the primate. Ann Neurol 12:564–574
4. Koizumi H, Povlishock JT (1998) Posttraumatic hypothermia in the treatment of axonal damage in an animal

Table 2. Hypothermia in experimental spinal cord trauma

Study	Year	Species	Cooling	EC, duration	Outcome Measures
Albin et al.	1965	Dog	Before and after	12°C, 25 h	Behavior, 2 min
Kelly et al.	1970	Dog	Before and 4-h delay	12–13°C, 2.5–3 h	Behavior, pathology, 3 min
Black and Marowitz	1971	Monkey	1-h delay	4–8°C, 5 h	Behavior, 2 weeks
Green et al.	1973	Cat	1- and 5-h delay	6–18°C, 3 h	Pathology, 3 h
Tator and Deecke	1973	Monkey	3-h delay	5°C, 3 h	Behavior/pathology, 3 months
Hansebout et al.	1975	Dog	Before and after	4°C, 4 h	Behavior, 7 weeks
Wells and Hansebout	1978	Dog	4-h delay	6°C, 1–8 h	Behavior, 48 days
Martinez and Green	1992	Rat	Before and after	31–32°C, 4 h	Pathology, 3 days
Yu et al.	1999a	Rat	Immediate postinjury	32°C, 20 min	Vascular permeability, 24 h
Yu et al.	1999b	Rat	30-min delay	32–33°C, 4 h	Behavior/pathology, 44 days
Chatzipanteli et al.	2000	Rat	5-min delay	32°C, 4 h	PMNP, MPO, 24 h

PMNL, polymorphonuclear leukocyte; MPO, myeloperoxidase; 2,3 DHBA, dihydroxybenzoic acid; lCBF, local cerebral blood flow metabolism; iNOS, inducible nitric oxide synthase; cNOS, constitutive nitric oxide synthase

model of traumatic axonal injury. J Neurosurg 89:303–309
5. Marion DW, White MJ (1996) Treatment of experimental brain injury with moderate hypothermia and 21-aminosteroids. J Neurotrauma 13:139–147
6. Maxwell WL, Donnelly S, Sun X, Fenton T, Pure N, Graham DI (1999) Axonal cytoskeletal response to nondisruptive axonal injury and the short-term effects of posttraumatic hypothermia. J Neurotrauma 16:1225–1234
7. Povlishock JT (1992) Traumatically induced axonal injury: pathogenesis and pathobiological implications. Brain Pathol 2:1–12
8. Povlishock JT, Becker DP, Cheng CLY, Vaughan GW (1983) Axonal changes in minor head injury. J Neuropathol Exp Neurol 42:225–242
9. Taft WC, Yang K, Dixon CE, Clifton GL, Hayes RL (1993) Hypothermia attenuates the loss of hippocampal microtubule-associated protein 2 (MAP2) following traumatic brain injury. J Cereb Blood Flow Metab 13:796–802
10. Westergren H, Yu WR, Farooque M, Holtz A, Olsson Y (1999) Systemic hypothermia following spinal cord compression injury in the rat: axonal changes studied by beta-APP, ubiquitin, and PGP 9.5 immunohistochemistry. Spinal Cord 37:696–704

6. Behavioral Improvements with Posttraumatic Hypothermia

The histopathological assessment of the injured brain is considered to be an important endpoint for evaluating neuroprotective strategies. Nevertheless, from a clinical perspective, it is critical to determine whether histopathological protection correlates with improved functional and behavioral performance. Clifton and colleagues [4] first reported that posttraumatic hypothermia (30° and 33°C) improved beam balance and beam walking tasks compared to normothermic rats (38°C) after midline F-P brain injury (2.10–2.25 atm). Subsequent studies using the F-P model demonstrated that posttraumatic hypothermia (30°C/3 h) improved both sensorimotor and cognitive behavioral deficits compared to normothermic rats [2,14]. In one study, the protective effect of hypothermia was not seen if the onset of hypothermia was delayed by 30 min [14]. In a cortical impact model, postischemic hypothermia treatment improved beam balance and spatial memory performance [6]. Cognitive deficits including memory impairments are commonly observed in humans suffering brain injury. Thus, the ability to improve cognitive function after traumatic brain injury (TBI) by hypothermic strategies appears to be an exciting direction for treating the postinjured patient [2].

In clinical studies, posttraumatic hypothermia has also been reported to be beneficial [3,10,15,16,21,23–25]. Recently, Marion and colleagues [16] demonstrated that posttraumatic hypothermia (32°–33°C/24 h) in patients with severe TBI and coma scores of 5 to 7 on admission hastened neurologic recovery and may have improved outcome. In a more recent study, Jiang and colleagues [10] reported that therapeutic hypothermia (33°–35°C) for a period of 3 to 14 days significantly improved outcome in patients with severe TBI (Glasgow Coma Score ≤8). One year after TBI, mortality rate and rate of favorable outcome were improved by hypothermic group. Also, mild hypothermia reduced intracranial pressure (ICP) and inhibited hyperglycemia while not significantly altering complication rate. These clinical findings are important in that they indicate that preclinical data are relevant to the clinical condition of TBI and that the selective application of hypothermia in severe TBI has promise. However, results from a recent multicenter TBI study [5] failed to demonstrate a beneficial effect of therapeutic hypothermia. It is therefore critical that more research be conducted to determine specific patient populations that may benefit from this therapy and the best ways to administer hypothermic treatment.

As previously discussed, hypothermia has also been reported to improve behavioral outcome after experimental spinal cord injury (SCI) [8,12,13,17–19,27,29,30]. Clinically, hypothermia has been reported to have beneficial effects by reducing the incidence of neurological deficits [19,26]. In early studies by Albin and colleagues [1] using profound hypothermia, selective spinal cord cooling (12°C) resulted in marked neurological and functional recovery up to 2 months after injury. In animal models of transient spinal cord ischemia, mild (34°C) and moderate (30°C) hypothermia have been reported to protect hindlimb function in rabbits [20]. Vanick and colleagues [28] used deep spinal cord hypothermia by epidural perfusion cooling (15°C) and found effective protection against spinal cord ischemia. Regional hypothermia (6°–18°C) initiated at 1 h after cat spinal cord contusion decreased edema formation and hemorrhage [7].

Previous studies on systemic hypothermia (30°C) reported improved neurological outcome, recovery of somatosensory evoked potentials and normal motor function up to 48 h following spinal cord ischemia [9,22]. Recent studies by Kakinohana and colleagues [11] demonstrated that immediate postischemic profound hypothermia (27°C/2 h) decreased motor dysfunction after spinal cord ischemia. However, a delay of 5 min failed to provide protection against spinal neuronal degeneration. Thus, the therapeutic window for postischemic hypothermia appears to be relatively brief in this injury model. Finally, Yu and colleagues [30] reported that posttraumatic hypothermia (32°–33°C/4 h) delayed 30 min after contusion SCI improved locomotor deficits and decreased tissue damage.

References

1. Albin MS, White RJ, Locke GE (1965) Treatment of spinal cord trauma by selective hypothermic perfusion. Surg Forum 16:423–424
2. Bramlett H, Green EJ, Dietrich WD, Busto R, Globus MY-T, Ginsberg MD (1995) Post-traumatic brain hypothermia provides protection from sensorimotor and cognitive behavioral deficits. J Neurotrauma 12:289–298
3. Clifton GL (1995) Systemic hypothermia in treatment of severe brain injury: a review and update. J Neurotrauma 12:923–927
4. Clifton G, Jiang JY, Lyeth BG, et al (1991) Marked protection by moderate hypothermia after experimental traumatic brain injury. J Cereb Blood Flow Metals 11:114–121
5. Clifton GL, Miller ER, Choi SC, Levin HS, McCauley S, Smith KR Jr, Muizelaar JP, Wagner FC, Marion DW, Luerssen TG, Chesnut RM, Schwartz M (2001) Lack of effect of induction of hypothermia after acute brain injury. N Eng J Med 344:556–563
6. Dixon CE, Markgraf CG, Angileri F, Pike BP, Wolfson B, Newcomb JK, Bismar MM, Blanco AJ, Clifton GL, Hayes RL (1998) Protective effects of moderate hypothermia on behavioral deficits but not necrotic cavitation following cortical impact injury in the rat. J Neurotrauma 15: 95–103
7. Green BA, Khan T, Raimondi AJ (1973) Local hypothermia as treatment of experimentally induced spinal cord contusion: quantitative analysis of beneficent effect. Surg Forum 24:436–438
8. Hansebout RR, Kuchner EF, Romero-Sierra C (1976) Effects of local hypothermia and of steroids upon recovery from experimental spinal cord compression injury. Surg Neurol 6:243–246
9. Herold JA, Kron IL, Langenburg SE, Blackbourne LH, Tribble CG (1994) Complete prevention of postischemic spinal cord injury by means of regional infusion with hypothermic saline and adenosine. J Thorac Cardiovasc Surg 107:536–541
10. Jiang J-Y, Yu M-K, Zhu C (2000) Effect of long-term hypothermia therapy in patients with severe traumatic brain injury: 1-year follow-up review of 87 cases. J Neurosurg 93:546–549
11. Kakinohama M, Taira Y, Marsala M (1999) The effect of graded postischemic spinal cord hypothermia on neurological outcome and histopathology after transient spinal ischemia in rat. Anesthesiology 90:789–798
12. Karibe H, Chen J, Zarow GJ, Graham SH, Weinstein PR (1994) Delayed induction of mild hypothermia to reduce infarct volume after temporary middle cerebral artery occlusion in rats. J Neurosurg 80:112–119
13. Kuchnor EF, Hansebout RR (1976) Combined steroid and hypothermia treatment of experimental spinal cord injury. Surg Neurol 7:371–376
14. Lyeth BG, Jiang JY, Shanliang L (1993) Behavioral protection by moderate hypothermia initiated after experimental traumatic brain injury. J Neurotrauma 10:57–64
15. Marion DW, Obrist WD, Carlier PM, Penrod LE, Darby JM (1993) The use of moderate therapeutic hypothermia for patients with severe head injuries: a preliminary report. J Neurosurg 79:354–362
16. Marion DW, Penrod LE, Kelsey SF, Obrist WD, Kochanek PM, Palmer AM, Wisniewki SR, DeKosky ST (1997) Treatment of traumatic brain injury with moderate hypothermia. N Eng J Med 336:540–546
17. Marsala M, Vanicky I, Yaksh TL (1994) Effect of graded hypothermia (27°–34°C) on behavioral function, histopathology, and spinal cord blood flow after spinal ischemia in rat. Stroke 25:2038–2046
18. Marsala M, Galik J, Ishikawa T, Yaksh TL (1997) Technique of selective spinal cord cooling in rat: methodology and application. J Neurosci Methods 74:97–106
19. Martinez-Arizala A, Green BA (1992) Hypothermia in spinal cord injury. J Neurotrauma 9:S497–S505
20. Matsumoto M, Iida Y, Sakabe T, Sano T, Ishikawa T, Nakakimura K (1997) Mild and moderate hypothermia provide better protection than a burst-suppression dose of thiopental against ischemic spinal cord injury in rabbits. Anesthesiology 86:1120–1127
21. Resnick DK, Marion DW, Darby JM (1994) The effect of hypothermia on the incidence of delayed traumatic intracerebral hemorrhage. J Neurosurg 34:252–256
22. Robertson CS, Folz R, Grossman RG, Goodman JC (1986) Protection against experimental ischemic spinal cord injury. J Neurosurg 64:633–642
23. Shiozaki T, Sugimoto H, Taneda M, Yoshida H, Iwai A, Yoshioka T, Sugimoto T (1993) Effect of mild hypothermia on uncontrollable intracranial hypertension after severe head injury. J Neurosurg 79:363–368
24. Shiozaki T, Sugimoto H, Taneda M, Oda J, Tanaka H, Hiraide A, Shimazu T (1998) Selection of severely head injured patients for mild hypothermia therapy. J Neurosurg 89:206–211
25. Shiozaki T, Hayakata T, Taneda M, Nakajima Y, Hashiguchi N, Fujimi S, Nakamori Y, Tanaka H, Shimazu T, Sugimoto H, Mild hypothermia study group in Japan (2001) A multi center prospective randomized controlled trial of the efficacy of mild hypothermia for severely head injured patients with low intracranial pressure. J Neurosurg 94:50–54
26. Svensson LG (1999) An approach to spinal cord protection during descending or thoracoabdominal aortic repairs. Ann Thorac 67:1935–1936
27. Tator CH, Deecke L (1973) Value of normothermic perfusion, hypothermic perfusion, and durotomy in the treatment of experimental acute spinal cord trauma. J Neurosurg 39:52–64
28. Vanicky I, Marsala M, Galik J, Marsala J (1993) Epidural perfusion cooling protection against protracted spinal cord ischemia in rabbits. J Neurosurg 79:736–741
29. Wells JD, Hansebout RR (1978) Local hypothermia in experimental spinal cord trauma. Surg Neurol 10:200–204
30. Yu CG, Marcillo AE, Dietrich WD, Fairbanks CA, Wilcox GL, Yezierski RP (1999) Beneficial effects of hypothermia and/or agmatine on locomotor outcome following contusion spinal cord injury. Soc Neurosci Abstr 29:268

7. Brain Tissue Temperature Measurements in Clinical Setting

Clinical data are available that indicate that body temperature and brain temperature can differ significantly and that there are temperature gradients within the injured brain. In head injured patients, brain temperature readings are commonly elevated compared with core temperature [1–6]. Sternau and colleagues [6] first directly measured brain temperature in head injured patients and reported transient periods of hyperthermia at variable periods after injury. Hayashi and colleagues [1] reported the elevation of brain tissue temperature up to 42°–44°C as brain thermo-pooling phenomenon after trauma. The mechanism underlying this brain thermo—pooling phenomenon is dependent upon several factors including core temperature, cerebral perfusion pressure, cerebral blood flow, and brain metabolism. Therefore, the elevation of brain temperature to levels greater than 38°C occurs with reduced systolic blood pressure (<90–100 mmHg), reduced cerebral perfusion pressure (<65–75 mmHg), and cerebral blood flow disturbances. The brain thermo—pooling phenomena that occur after trauma, stroke, and post—resuscitation following cardiac arrest represents a novel brain mechanism and an important target for hypothermic treatment. Because under normal physiological conditions brain tissue temperature is maintained very close to core temperature, brain temperature can be controlled by the precise management of systemic circulatory blood temperature under abnormal conditions. This new mechanism for altered brain tissue temperature after injury should allow for the accurate control of brain hypothermia in patients. These clinical issues regarding the control of brain temperature in the injured patient are described in detail in Chapter 2.

Recently, Schwab and colleagues [5] directly measured brain temperature in patients with severe middle cerebral artery (MCA) infarction. In that study, brain temperature was directly measured using the Spiegelberg intraparenchymatous probe fitted with a thermistor in the tip and a thermocouple that was introduced with the Licox system (CMS, Mielckendorff, Germany). These researchers reported that in 15 patients brain temperature exceeded body core temperature by up to 2°C. Temperature as measured in the jugular bulb using optimetric jugular bulb catheters showed values comparable with epidural temperature readings. In the brain tissue, regional perfusion is not similar with high flow in cortex and low flow in the white matter. The ability of washout of brain tissue temperature in the white matter is lower than in gray matter. Therefore, white matter brain tissue temperature is slightly higher than gray matter brain tissue temperature.

Systemic cooling was conducted by cooling blankets with cool air fanning the patient's body surface. Although effective lowering of brain temperature was accomplished with systemic cooling, brain temperature modulation was independent of pharmacologic treatments. Beneficial effects of hypothermia in the treatment of space-occupying MCA infarction have been reported [5], although the effects of hypothermic therapy on infarct volume and stroke outcome await future trials.

References

1. Hayashi N, Hirayama T, Ohata M (1993) The computed cerebral hypothermia management technique to the critical head injury patients. Adv Neurotrauma Res 5:61–64
2. Henker RA, Brown SD, Marion DW (1998) Comparison of brain temperature with bladder and rectal temperature in adults with severe head injury. Neurosurg 42:1071–1075
3. Ko K, Ghajar J, Harir RJ (1994) A method for monitoring intracranial temperature via tunneled ventricular catheter: technical note. Neurosurgery 34:927–930
4. Mellergard P, Nordstrom C-H (1991) Intracerebral temperature in neurosurgical patients. Neurosurgery 28:709–713
5. Schwab S, Spranger M, Aschoff A, Steiner T, Hacke W (1997) Brain temperature monitoring and modulation in patients with severe MCA infarction. Neurology 48: 762–767
6. Sternau L, Thompson C, Dietrich WD, Busto R, Globus MY-T, Ginsberg MD (1991) Intracranial temperature—observations in the human brain. J Cereb Blood Flow Metab 11:S123

8. Traumatic and Ischemic Hyperthermia

In contrast to hypothermia, periods of acute or delayed hyperthermia (>39°C) have been reported to worsen outcome in various animal models of brain injury [1,2,4–6]. Clinical data indicate that periods of core and brain hyperthermia occur in head-injured patients [3,8,9,11]. Many head-injured patients experience fever [10], and recent data indicate that bladder temperature and rectal temperature often underrepresent brain temperature after traumatic brain injury, particularly when the patient is hypo- or hyperthermic [7,9]. In an experimental study, artificially elevating brain temperature in rats to 39°C for a 3-h period 24 h after moderate parasagittal F-P injury increased mortality when compared with normothermic rats [6]. Delayed hyperthermia also significantly increased contusion volume and increased the frequency of myelinated axons of abnormal appearance and inflammatory cells. Thus, delayed elevations in brain temperature may represent a clinically important secondary injury mechanism. In the clinical setting, especially following severe brain trauma, fever should be aggressively treated. Recent studies have also determined the detrimental effects of hyperthermia on outcome after SCI [12]. Therapeutic hypothermia may improve outcome by attenuating the pathophysiological mechanisms associated with central nervous system injury as well as inhibiting transient elevations in temperature.

References

1. Baena RC, Busto R, Dietrich WD, Globus MY-T, Ginsberg MD (1997) Hyperthermia delayed by 24 hours aggravates neuronal damage in rat hippocampus following global ischemia. Neurology 48:768–773
2. Chen H, Chopp M, Welch KMA (1991) Effect of hyperthermia on the ischemic infarct volume after middle cerebral artery occlusion in the rat. Neurology 41:1133–1135
3. Corbett RJT, Laptook AR (1998) Failure of localized head cooling to reduce brain temperature in adult humans. Neuro Rep 9:2721–2725
4. Dietrich WD, Busto R, Halley M, Valdes I (1990) The importance of brain temperature in alterations of the blood–brain barrier following cerebral ischemia. J Neuropathol Exp Neurol 49:486–497
5. Dietrich WD, Busto R, Valdes I, Loor Y (1990) Effects of normothermic versus mild hyperthermic forebrain ischemia in rats. Stroke 21:1318–1325
6. Dietrich WD, Alonso O, Halley M, Busto R (1996) Delayed posttraumatic brain hyperthermia worsens outcome after fluid percussion brain injury: a light and electron microscopic study in rats. Neurosurgery 38:533–541
7. Hayashi N, Hirayama T, Ohata M (1993) The computed cerebral hypothermia management technique to the critical head injury patients. Adv Neurotrauma Res 5:61–64
8. Hayashi N, Hirayama T, Utagawa A (1994) The cerebral thermo-pooling and hypothermia treatment of critical head injury patients. In: Nagai H (ed) Intracranial pressure IX. Springer, Berlin Heidelberg New York Tokyo, pp 589–599
9. Henker RA, Brown SD, Marion DW (1998) Comparison of brain temperature with bladder and rectal temperature in adults with severe head injury. Neurosurg 42:1071–1075
10. Schwarz S, Häfner K, Aschoff A, Schwab S (2000) Incidence and prognostic significance of fever following intracerebral hemorrhage. Neurol 54:354–360
11. Sternau L, Thompson C, Dietrich WD, Busto R, Globus MY-T, Ginsberg MD (1991) Intracranial temperature—observations in the human brain. J Cereb Blood Flow Metab 11:S123
12. Yu C-G, Jagid J, Ruenes G, Dietrich WD, Marcillo AE, Yezierski RP (2001) Detrimental effects of systemic hyperthermia on locomotor function and histopathological outcome after traumatic spinal cord injury in the rat. Neurosurgery 49:152–159

9. Rewarming Phase

Recent investigations have emphasized the importance of the rewarming phase in determining whether brain cooling is protective. Slow but not rapid rewarming provides the benefit in terms of histopathological outcome. In clinical studies, slow rewarming after a period of induced hypothermia is used routinely because of the potential detrimental effects of rebound intracranial hypertension when temperature increases rapidly [1,2,4]. In experimental studies, several reports recently emphasized the importance of slow rewarming in injury models [5,7]. For example, in a transient forebrain ischemia study, rapid rewarming failed to provide the neuroprotective effect of hypothermia that was observed with slow rewarming [6]. In that study, rapid rewarming, after hypothermia resulted in poor recovery of mean arterial blood pressure and cortical blood flow. These investigators suggested that aggravated uncoupling between blood flow and metabolism with rapid rewarming might reduce its protection with hypothermia. In a model of traumatic brain injury (TBI), a gradual rewarming protocol after controlled hypothermia was reported to reduce axonal damage after experimental TBI [3]. Although the detrimental consequences of rapid postinjury rewarming in the clinical arena are appreciated, the importance of rewarming conditions in experimental models of brain injury require additional investigation. In this regard, recent data from our laboratory have shown that a slow rewarming following a hypothermic period is neuroprotective in a model of TBI complicated by secondary hypoxia [5]. These investigations emphasize another important factor determining whether hypothermia is neuroprotective.

References

1. Clifton GL, Miller ER, Choi SC, Levin HS, McCauley S, Smith KR Jr, Muizelaar JP, Wagner FC, Marion DW, Luerssen TG, Chesnut RM, Schwartz M (2001) Lack of effect of induction of hypothermia after acute brain injury. N Eng J Med 344:556–563
2. Enomoto S, Hindman BJ, Dexter F, Smith T, Cutkomp J (1996) Rapid rewarming causes an increase in the cerebral metabolic rate for oxygen that is temporarily unmatched by cerebral blood flow. Anesthesia 84:1392–1400
3. Koizumi H, Povlishock JT (1998) Posttraumatic hypothermia in the treatment of axonal damage in an animal model of traumatic axonal injury. J Neurosurg 89:303–309
4. Marion DW, Penrod LE, Kelsey SF, Obrist WD, Kochanek PM, Palmer AM, Wisniewki SR, DeKosky ST (1997) Treatment of traumatic brain injury with moderate hypothermia. N Eng J Med 336:540–546
5. Matsushita Y, Bramlett HM, Alonso OF, Dietrich WD (2001) Posttraumatic hypothermia is neuroprotective in a model of traumatic brain injury complicated by a secondary hypoxic insult. Crit Care Med 29:2060–2066
6. Nakamura T, Miyamoto O, Yanagami S-I, Hayashida Y, Itano T, Nagao S (1999) Influence of rewarming conditions after hypothermia in gerbils with transient forebrain ischemia. J Neurosurg 91:114–120
7. Suehiro E, Povlishock JT (2001) Rapid post hypothermic rewarming exacerbates traumatically induced axonal injury which is attenuated by cyclosporin A. J Neurosurg 94:493–498

10. Therapeutic Hypothermia in Complicated Models of Traumatic Brain Injury

Clinical and experimental data emphasize the importance of secondary injury mechanisms contributing to traumatic outcome [1–4,8]. Secondary injury mechanisms include a variety of systemic and intracranial processes including hypotension, hypoxia, ischemia, and hyperthermia, as well as intracranial pressure. Secondary hypoxia caused by respiratory distress is a common consequence of head injury. It has been reported to occur in 45.6% of severely head-injured patients.

Various neuroprotective strategies including therapeutic hypothermia have been tested in traumatic brain injury (TBI) animal models [7]. In these studies, relatively controlled injury models have been used to test the therapeutic efficacy of a drug or protocol. Because injury severity is a known factor in determining whether therapy is successful, an important question is whether a successful therapeutic strategy is also protective in more complicated models [9]. To date, few studies have critically evaluated normal therapies of brain injury complicated by secondary insults in animal models.

Recently, the potential benefits of posttraumatic hypothermia have been evaluated in diffused focal TBI models complicated by secondary hypoxia [5,10]. By using an impact acceleration model of diffuse TBI coupled with hypoxia and hypotension, Yamamoto and colleagues [10], reported that moderate hypothermia (30°C/1 h) significantly reduced neuronal damage at 4 in 24 h. In contrast, Clark et al. [5] reported no significant reduction in behavioral deficits or overall contusion volume with immediate posttraumatic hypothermia (32°C/4 h) after controlled cortical impact injury complicated by secondary hypoxia. Most recently, our laboratory reported the beneficial effects of posttraumatic hypothermia (33°C/4 h) in a fluid percussion model complicated by secondary hypoxia [6]. In that study, a period of hypothermia followed by slow (1.5 h), but not rapid (30 min), rewarming lead to a significant decrease in contusion volume compared with normothermic hypoxic animals. Taken together these results emphasized the importance of slow rewarming as well as the potential benefits of therapeutic hypothermia in complicated injury models.

References

1. Bramlett HM, Dietrich WD, Green E (1999) Secondary hypoxia following moderate fluid percussion brain injury in rats exacerbates sensorimotor and cognitive deficits. J Neurotrauma 16:1035–1047
2. Bramlett HM, Green EJ, Dietrich WD (1999) Exacerbation of cortical and hippocampal CA1 damage due to posttraumatic hypoxia following moderate fluid–percussion brain injury in rats. J Neurosurg 91:653–659
3. Chen M, Clark RSB, Kochanek PM, Chen J, Schiding JK, Stetler RA, Simon RP, Graham SH (1998) 72-kDa heat shock protein and mRNA expression after controlled cortical impact injury with hypoxemia in rats. J Neurotrauma 15:171–181
4. Chestnut RM (1995) Secondary brain insults after head injury: clinical perspectives. New Horiz 3:366–375
5. Clark RSB, Robertson CL, Dixon CE, Alexander HL, Graham SH, Safar PJ, Kochanek PM (1999) Effect of hypothermia after severe traumatic brain injury with secondary hypoxemia in rats. J Neurotrauma 15:864 (Abstract)
6. Matsushita Y, Bramlett HM, Alonso OF, Dietrich WD (2001) Posttraumatic hypothermia is neuroprotective in a model of traumatic brain injury complicated by a secondary hypoxic insult. Crit Care Med 29:2060–2066
7. McIntosh TK, Juhler M, Wieloch T (1998) Novel pharmacologic strategies in the treatment of experimental traumatic brain injury. J Neurotrauma 15:731–769
8. Nakamura T, Miyamoto O, Yanagami S-I, Hayashida Y, Itano T, Nagao S (1999) Influence of rewarming conditions after hypothermia in gerbils with transient forebrain ischemia. J Neurosurg 91:114–120
9. Statler KD, Jenkins LW, Dixon CE, Clark RS, Marion DW, Kochanek PM (2001) The simple model versus the super model: translating experimental traumatic brain injury to the bedside. J Neurotrauma 18:1195–1206
10. Yamamoto M, Marmarou CR, Stiefel MF, Beaumont A, Marmarou A (1999) Neuroprotective effect of hypothermia on neuronal injury in diffuse traumatic brain injury coupled with hypoxia and hypotension. J Neurotrauma 16:487–500

11. Mechanisms of Hypothermic Protection

The pathophysiology of brain and spinal cord injury is complex and many injury processes have been reported to be temperature-sensitive [1–4]. Indeed, it has become clear that a reason temperature is such an important factor in traumatic and ischemic outcome is that variations in temperature have dramatic effects on multiple pathophysiological mechanisms. The following sections therefore summarize the consequences of hypothermia on several injury mechanisms.

References

1. Colbourne F, Sutherland G, Corbett D (1997) Postischemic hypothermia. A critical appraisal with implications for clinical treatment. Molec Neurobiol 14:171–201
2. Dietrich WD, Busto R, Globus MY-T, Ginsberg MD (1996) Brain damage and temperature: cellular and molecular mechanisms. In: Siesjo B, Wieloch T (eds) Cellular and molecular mechanisms of ischemic brain damage. Advances in Neurology vol 71: Lippincott-Raven, Philadelphia, pp 177–198
3. Ginsberg MD (1998) Temperature influences on ischemic injury. In: Hsu CY (ed) Ischemic stroke: mechanisms to new development. Monpgr Clin Neurosci vol 16. Karger, Basel, pp 65–88
4. Kataoka K, Yanase H (1998) Mild hypothermia—a revived countermeasure against ischemic neuronal damages. Neurosci Res 32:103–117

12. Excitotoxicity

In addition to slowing oxygen consumption [5], posttraumatic and ischemic hypothermia has been reported to blunt the rise in extracellular levels of excitatory amino acids after parasagittal F-P injury [1–3]. However, in a model of controlled cortical impact, hypothermia failed to attenuate the rise in extracellular aspartate and glutamate although contusion volume was significantly reduced by cooling [4]. In a model of spinal cord ischemia, hypothermia effectively attenuated extracellular glutamate release [6]. Wakamatsu and colleagues [8] reported that intraischemic moderate hypothermia (32°C) significantly reduced glutamate concentrations of intrathecal dialysate and improved neurologic status and histopathology after spinal cord ischemia. In contrast, other reports have indicated that hypothermia did not attenuate extracellular accumulation of excitatory amino acids or improve energy metabolism. For example, hyperthermia (39°C) during middle cerebral artery occlusion led to increased levels of extracellular glutamate compared to normothermic animals [7]. Specific variables including injury models and severity may significantly affect neurochemical results of therapeutic hypothermia. The location of neurochemical sampling in relation to the contusion site (i.e., near, remote, gray vs white matter) is another important factor that may influence outcome.

References

1. Globus MY-T, Alonso O, Dietrich WD, Busto R, Ginsberg MD (1995) Glutamate release and free radical production following brain injury: effects of posttraumatic hypothermia. J Neurotrauma 65:1704–1711
2. Globus MY-T, Busto R, Lin B, Schnippering H, Ginsberg MD (1995) Detection of free radical activity during transient global ischemia and recirculation: effects of intraischemic brain temperature modulation. J Neurochem 65:1250–1256
3. Goss JR, Styren SD, Miller PD, Kochanek PM, Palmer AM, Graenen G, Jeftinija S, Grants I, Lucas JH (1996) The role of excitatory amino acids in hypothermic injury to mammalian spinal cord neurons. J Neurotrauma 13:809–818
4. Palmer AM, Marion DW, Botsceller ML, Redd EE (1993) Therapeutic hypothermia is cytoprotective without attenuating the traumatic brain injury-induced elevations in interstitial concentrations of aspartate and glutamate. J Neurotrauma 10:363–372
5. Rosomoff HL, Holaday S (1954) Cerebral blood flow and cerebral oxygen consumption during hypothermia. Am J Physiol 179:85–88
6. Saganova K, Marsala M (1994) Intrathecal administration of dizocilpine maleate (MK-801) attenuates ischemic damage in the rabbit spinal cord. Exp Neurol 130:337–343
7. Tagaki K, Ginsberg MD, Globus MY-T, Martinez E, Busto R (1994) Effect of hyperthermia on glutamate release in ischemic penumbra after middle cerebral artery occlusion in rats. Am Physiol Soc H1770–H1775
8. Wakamatsu H, Matsumoto M, Nakakimura K, Sakabe T (1999) The effects of moderate hypothermia and intrathecal tetracaine on glutamate concentrations of intrathecal dialysate and neurologic and histopathologic outcome in transient spinal cord ischemia in rabbits. Anesth Analg 88:56–62

13. Free Radical Production

Among the pathomechanisms involved with traumatic brain and spinal cord injury, reactive oxygen species and lipid peroxidation play an important role [3,4]. In a model of global cerebral ischemia, Baiping and colleagues [1] reported that moderate hypothermia (30°–32°C) attenuated lipid peroxidation. In a model of fluid–percussion brain injury, posttraumatic hypothermia (30°C) reduced the production of free radicals, as measured by the hydroxylation of salicylate by hydroxyl radicals to produce 2,5-dihydroxybenzoic acid, compared with normothermic trauma [2]. Interestingly, a significant correlation between the magnitude of glutamate release and the extent of hydroxyl radical production was demonstrated in that study, suggesting a link between the two responses. Posttraumatic hypothermia may therefore improve outcome by attenuating free radical formation and excitotoxicity. A current question is whether these relatively early posttraumatic events can be successfully targeted for treatment.

References

1. Baiping L, Xiujuan T, Hongwei C, Qiming X, Quling G (1994) Effect of moderate hypothermia on lipid peroxidation in canine brain tissue after cardiac arrest and resuscitation. Stroke 25:147–152
2. Globus MY-T, Alonso O, Dietrich WD, Busto R, Ginsberg MD (1995) Glutamate release and free radical production following brain injury: effects of posttraumatic hypothermia. J Neurotrauma 65:1704–1711
3. Hall ED, Andrus PK, Yonkers PA (1993) Brain hydroxyl radical generation in acute experimental head injury. J Neurochem 60:588–594
4. Kontos HA, Povlishock JT (1986) Oxygen radicals in brain injury. Cent Nerv Syst Trauma 3:257–263

14. Decrease of Vascular Permeability

Blood-brain barrier (BBB) dysfunction and cerebrovascular damage after neurotrauma are believed to participate in patterns of neuronal vulnerability [1,2,4,7,10,11]. Alteration in BBB permeability may contribute to the detrimental effects of traumatic injury through excitotoxic processes, as well as allowing abnormal passage of blood–borne exogenous neurotransmitters into the central nervous system and influencing injury processes [9]. Experimental data have demonstrated that postinjury temperature modulations significantly influence vascular permeability. For example, although moderate hypothermia after transient global ischemia attenuates the degree of postischemic horseradish peroxidase (HRP) extravasation compared to normothermia, hyperthermia aggravates permeability alterations [3]. In models of traumatic brain injury (TBI), the detrimental consequences of TBI on BBB damage have also been reported to be reduced by posttraumatic hypothermia [6,8]. In a model of spinal cord compression injury, systemic hypothermia (30°C/20 min) significantly reduced the degree of plasma protein extravasation compared to normothermic rats at 24 h. Finally, delayed posttraumatic hyperthermia induced 24 h after moderate F-P brain injury increased HRP extravasation compared to normothermia [5]. Posttraumatic temperature modifications may influence traumatic outcome by altering the vascular consequences of brain and spinal cord injury and the subsequent formation of vasogenic edema.

References

1. Chan PH, Schmidley JW, Fishman RA, Longar SM (1984) Brain injury, edema, and vascular permeability changes induced by oxygen-derived free radicals. Neurology 34:315–320
2. Cortez SC, McIntosh TK, Noble LJ (1989) Experimental fluid percussion brain injury: vascular disruption and neuronal and glial alterations. Brain Res 482:272–282
3. Dietrich WD, Busto R, Halley M, Valdes I (1990) The importance of brain temperature in alterations of the blood-brain barrier following cerebral ischemia. J Neuropathol Exp Neurol 49:486–497
4. Dietrich WD, Alonso O, Halley M (1994) Early microvascular and neuronal consequences of traumatic brain injury: a light and electron microscopic study in rats. J Neurotrauma 11:289–301
5. Dietrich WD, Alonso O, Halley M, Busto R (1996) Delayed posttraumatic brain hyperthermia worsens outcome after fluid percussion brain injury: a light and electron microscopic study in rats. Neurosurgery 38:533–541
6. Jiang JY, Lyeth BG, Kapasi MZ, Jenkins LW, Povlishock JT (1992) Moderate hypothermia reduces blood–brain barrier disruption following traumatic brain injury in the rat. Acta Neuropathol 84:495–500
7. Povlishock JT, Becker DP, Sullivan HG, Miller JD (1978) Vascular permeability alterations to horseradish peroxidase in experimental brain injury. Brain Res 153: 223–239
8. Smith SL, Hall ED (1996) Mild pre- and posttraumatic hypothermia attenuates blood–brain barrier damage following controlled cortical impact injury in the rat. J Neurotrauma 13:1–9
9. Povlishock JT, Dietrich WD (1992) The blood–brain barrier in brain injury: an overview. In: Globus MY-T, Dietrich WD (eds) The role of neurotransmitters in brain injury. Plenum, New York, pp 265–269
10. Tanno H, Nockels RP, Pitts LH, Noble LJ (1992) Breakdown of the blood–brain barrier after fluid percussion brain injury in the rat. part 2: effect of hypoxia on permeability to plasma proteins. J Neurotrauma 9:335–347
11. Yu WR, Westergren H, Farooque M, Holtz A, Olsson Y (1999) Systemic hypothermia following compression injury of rat spinal cord: reduction of plasma protein extravasation demonstrated by immunohistochemistry. Acta Neuropathol 98:15–21

15. Nitric Oxide

Recent data have implicated the importance of nitric oxide (NO) in the pathophysiology of traumatic brain injury (TBI) [2–5]. After controlled cortical impact injury, levels of neuronal nitric oxide synthase (nNOS), mRNA, and protein increased by 2 h after trauma [3]. Using a moderate F-P model, Wada and colleagues [4] reported the immediate but transient increase in constitutive nitric oxide synthase (cNOS) activity within the histopathologically injured cortical region. This increase in cNOS activity was followed by a sustained reduction in cNOS activity below control levels. Inducible NOS (iNOS) activity was also reported to increase at 7 days after TBI [5].

Recently, the effects of posttraumatic hypothermia on NOS activity have been reported [1]. Hypothermia (30°C) decreased the acute activation of cNOS, preserved cNOS activity during later posttraumatic periods, and prevented the delayed induction of iNOS compared with normothermic traumatized animals. Taken together, these studies indicate that therapeutic hypothermia may improve outcome after TBI by targeting the NO pathway.

References

1. Chatzipanteli K, Wada K, Busto R, Dietrich WD (1999) Effects of moderate hypothermia on constitutive and inducible nitric oxide synthase activities after traumatic brain injury. J Neurochem 72:2047–2052
2. Mesenge C, Verrecchia C, Allix M, Boulu RR, Plotkine M (1996) Reduction of the neurological deficits in mice with traumatic brain injury by nitric oxide synthase inhibitors. J Neurotrauma 13:209–214
3. Raghavendra Rao VL, Dogan A, Bowen K, Dempsey RJ (1999) Traumatic injury to rat brain upregulates neuronal nitric oxide synthase expression and L-[3H]nitroarginine binding. J Neurotrauma 16:865–877
4. Wada K, Chatzipantelli K, Busto R, Dietrich WD (1998) The role of nitric oxide on the pathophysiology of traumatic brain injury in the rat. J Neurosurg 89:807–818
5. Wada K, Chatzipantelli K, Busto R, Kraydieh S, Dietrich WD (1998) Inducible nitric oxide synthase activation after traumatic brain injury. Neurosurgery 43:1427–1436

16. Cerebral Blood Flow

The consequences of brain trauma on local cerebral blood flow (lCBF) have been documented clinically and in several experimental models [1–4,7]. Perfusion deficits and cerebral ischemia are believed to represent important secondary injury mechanisms after traumatic brain injury (TBI) [5,8]. Numerous studies have shown that systemic hypothermia decreased both CBF and $CMRO_2$ [6]. The consequences of early posttraumatic brain hypothermia on lCBF have been investigated after moderate F-P brain injury. Zhao and colleagues [9] reported that moderate hypothermia (30°C/3h) significantly lowered lCBF 6h after TBI when compared with normothermic animals. As a consequence, a state of mild metabolism-greater-than-blood-flow dissociation was demonstrated. Thus, posttraumatic brain hypothermia does not appear to improve outcome by increasing posttraumatic lCBF.

References

1. DeWitt DS, Prough DS, Tayor CT, Whitley JM (1992) Reduced cerebral blood flow, oxygen delivery, and electroencephalographic activity after traumatic brain injury and mild hemorrhage in cats. J Neurosurg 76:812–821
2. Dietrich WD, Alonso O, Busto R, Prado R, Dewanjee S, Dewanjee MK, Ginsberg MD (1996) Widespread hemodynamic depression and focal platelet accumulation after fluid percussion brain injury: a double-label autoradiographic study in rats. J Cereb Blood Flow Metab 16:481–489
3. Ginsberg MD, Zhao W, Alonso O, Loor-Estades JY, Dietrich WD, Busto R (1997) Uncoupling of local cerebral glucose metabolism and blood flow after acute fluid-percussion injury in rats. Am J Physiol 272:H2859–2868
4. Ishige N, Pitts LH, Berry I, Carlson SG, Nishimura MC, Moseley ME, Weinstein PR (1987) The effect of hypoxia on traumatic head injury in rats: alterations in neurologic function, brain edema, and cerebral blood flow. J Cereb Blood Flow Metab 7:759–767
5. Miller JD (1985) Head injury and brain ischemia: implication for therapy. Br J Anaesth 57:120–129
6. Rosomoff HL, Holaday S (1954) Cerebral blood flow and cerebral oxygen consumption during hypothermia. Am J Physiol 179:85–88
7. Steiger H-J, Asslid R, Stooss R, Seiler RW (1994) Transcranial doppler monitoring in head injury: relationship between type of injury, flow velocities, vasoreactivity and outcome. Neurosurgery 34:79–86
8. Young W (1988) Secondary Central Nervous System injury. J Neurotrauma 5:219–221
9. Zhao W, Alonso O, Loor J, Busto R, Ginsberg MD (1999) Influence of early posttraumatic hypothermia therapy on local cerebral blood flow and glucose metabolism after fluid-percussion brain injury. J Neurosurg 90:510–519

17. Inflammation

Inflammatory processes are believed to participate in the pathogenesis of traumatic brain and spinal cord injury (SCI) [4,9,11]. Strategies that target inflammation after neurotrauma have been reported to improve outcome. Of interest to the present discussion is the fact that therapeutic hypothermia has been reported to reduce the accumulation of polymorphonuclear leukocytes (PMNLs) after cerebral ischemia and trauma [10,12,13]. In a study of transient middle cerebral artery occlusion, postischemic hypothermia delayed neutrophil accumulation and microglial activation [6]. Following control cortical impact injury, Whalen and colleagues [12] reported that PMNL accumulation in the injured cortex after 4h was significantly decreased in rats maintained at 32°C vs 39°C. Chatzipanteli and colleagues [2] have demonstrated that hypothermia (32°C) after moderate F-P brain injury also reduces the degree of PMNL accumulation in damaged areas at 3h and 3 days after traumatic brain injury (TBI). In addition, posttraumatic brain hyperthermia (39°C/3h) elevated myeloperoxidase (MPO) activity when compared with normothermic values at both 3h and 3 days after TBI.

Acute and subacute inflammatory responses constitute a key component of secondary injury after SCI [8]. Activation of the transcription factor NF-kappaB which leads to activation of a variety of genes regulating inflammatory responses has been reported in macrophages/microglia as early as 30min after SCI [1]. Known critical inflammatory factors that are involved in the spread of secondary damage after SCI include the infiltration and accumulation of PMNLs [5,7]. In a recent SCI study, posttraumatic hypothermia (32°C/3h) reduced MPO activity at 24h when compared with normothermic rats [3]. Taken together, these findings indicate that temperature-dependent alterations in PMNL accumulation after brain and spinal cord injury may influence traumatic outcome.

References

1. Bethea JR, Castro M, Keane RW, Lee TT, Dietrich WD, Yezierski RP (1998) Traumatic spinal cord injury induces nuclear factor-kappaB activation. J Neurosci 18: 3251–3260
2. Chatzipanteli K, Alonso O, Kraydieh S, Dietrich WD (2000) The importance of posttraumatic brain temperature on the inflammatory response following parasagittal fluid percussion brain injury. J Cereb Blood Flow Metab 20:531–542
3. Chatzipanteli K, Yanagawa Y, Marcillo A, Kraydieh S, Yezierski RP, Dietrich WD (2000) Post-traumatic hypothermia reduces polymorphonuclear leukocyte accumulation following spinal cord injury in rats. J Neurotrauma 17:321–332
4. Clark RSB, Schiding JK, Kaczorowski SL, Marion DW, Kochanek PM (1994) Neutrophil accumulation after traumatic brain injury in rats: comparison of weight drop and controlled cortical impact models. J Neurotrauma 11:499–506
5. Hernandez LA, Grisham MB, Twohig B, Arfors KE, Harlan J, Granger DN (1987) Role of neutrophils in ischemia-reperfusion induced microvascular injury. Am J Physiol 253:H699–703
6. Inamasu J, Suga S, Sato S, Horigushi T, Akaji K, Manage K, Kawase T (2000) Post-ischemic hypothermia delayed neutrophil accumulation and microglial activation following transient focal ischemia in rats. J Neuroimmunol 109:66–74
7. Ishikawa T, Marsala M (1999) Hypothermia prevents biphasic glutamate release and corresponding neuronal degeneration after transient spinal cord ischemia in the rat. Cell Mol Neurobiol 19:199–208
8. Means ED, Anderson DK (1983) Neuronophagia by leukocytes in experimental spinal cord injury. J Neuropathol Exp Neurol 42:707–719
9. Schoettle RJ, Kochanek PM, Magargee MJ, Uhl MW, Nemoto EM (1990) Early polymorphonuclear leukocyte accumulation correlates with the development of posttraumatic cerebral edema in rats. J Neurotrauma 7: 207–217
10. Toyoda T, Suzuki S, Kaddell NF, Lee KS (1996) Intraischemic hypothermia attenuates neurophil infiltration in the rat neocortex after focal ischemia-reperfusion injury. Neurosurgery 39:1200–1205

11. Uhl MW, Biagas KV, Grundl PD, Barmada MA, Schiding JK, Nemoto EM, Kochanek PM (1994) Effects of neutropenia on edema, histology, and cerebral blood flow after traumatic brain injury in rats. J Neurotrauma 11:303–315
12. Whalen MJ, Carlos TM, Clarke RS, Marion DW, DeKosky ST, Heineman S, Schiding JK, Memarzadeh F, Dixon CE, Kochanek PM (1997) The relationship between brain temperature and neutrophil accumulation after traumatic brain injury in rats. Acta Neurochir 70:260–261
13. Whalen MJ, Carlos TM, Clarke RS, Marion DW, DeKosky ST, Heineman S, Schiding JK, Memarzadeh F, Kochanek PM (1997) The effect of brain temperature on acute inflammation after traumatic brain injury in rats. J Neurotrauma 14:561–572

18. Gene Expression and Apoptosis

Brain and spinal cord trauma have been reported to induce a variety of genes and proteins that would be expected to influence traumatic outcome [6,7,9–11,15,16,18]. Alterations in posttraumatic temperature may affect the induction of various genes in the injured tissue. Hypothermia was reported to attenuate the normal increase in interleukin-1beta RNA in traumatized rats [8]. In a model of transient global forebrain ischemia, Kamme and colleagues [12] reported that hypothermia altered the expression of specific genes. In regard to postischemic hyperthermia, Kim and colleagues [13] reported in a model of transient middle cerebral artery occlusion that c-fos and hsp70 mRNA expression were increased in heated rats when compared with normothermic animals. Because intraischemic hypothermia can significantly alter protein kinase C activity, temperature-sensitive intracellular mechanisms also participate in neuronal death [2]. Taken together, these results suggest that postinjury temperature modifications may alter outcome by influencing the expression of genes associated with cell death and/or by enhancing the expression of neuroprotective or repair genes.

Apoptosis has recently been implicated in the pathophysiology of brain and spinal cord injury [1,3,4,17,19]. In this regard, recent data indicate that hypothermia may also be neuroprotective by reducing neuronal apoptosis. In an experimental model of hypoxia–ischemia, moderate hypothermia reduced the fraction of apoptotic cells but not cells undergoing necrosis [5]. Currently it is unclear whether alterations in temperature after trauma also influence proapoptotic factors such as the respiratory chain component cytochrome C [14]. Thus, the consequences of therapeutic hypothermia on gene expression and apoptotic cell death represent an important direction in neurotrauma research [20].

References

1. Beattie MS, Shuman SL, Bresnahan JC (1998) Apoptosis and spinal cord injury. The Neuroscientist 4:163–171
2. Busto R, Globus MY-T, Neary JT, Ginsberg MD (1994) Regional alterations of protein kinase C activity following transient cerebral ischemia: effects of intraischemic brain temperature modulation. J Neurochem 63:1095–1103
3. Clark RSB, Kochanek PM, Dixon CE (1997) Early neuropathologic effects of mild or moderate hypoxemia after controlled cortical impact injury in rats. J Neurotrauma 14:179–189
4. Conti AC, Raghupati R, Trojanwski JQ, McIntosh TK (1998) Experimental brain injury induces regionally distinct apoptosis during the acute and delayed posttraumatic period. J Neurosci 18:5663–5672
5. Edwards AD, Uue X, Squier MV, Thoresen M, Cady EB, Penrice J, Cooper CE, Wyatt JS, Reynolds EOR, Mehmet H (1995) Specific inhibition of apoptosis after hypoxia-ischaemia by moderate post-insult hypothermia. Biochem Biophys Res Comm 217:1193–1199
6. Fan L, Young PR, Barone FC, Feuerstein GZ, Smith DH, McIntosh TK (1995) Experimental brain injury induces expression of interleukin-1B mRNA in the rat brain. Molec Brain Res 30:125–130
7. Fan L, Young PR, Barone FC, Feuerstein GZ, Smith DH, McIntosh TK (1996) Experimental brain injury induces differential expression of tumor necrosis factor-alpha mRNA in the CNS. Molec Brain Res 36:287–291
8. Goss JR, Styren PO, Miller PO, Kochanek PM, Palmer DW, Marion DW, DeKosky ST (1995) Hypothermia attenuates the normal increase in interleukin-1beta RNA and nerve growth factor following traumatic brain injury in the rat. J Neurotrauma 12:159–167
9. Goss JR, O'Malley ME, Zou L, Styren SD, Kochanek PM, DeKosky ST (1998) Astrocytes are the major source of nerve growth factor upregulation following traumatic brain injury in the rat. Exp Neurol 149:301–309
10. Hayes RL, Yang K, Raghupathi R, McIntosh TK (1995) Changes in gene expression following traumatic brain injury. J Neurotrauma 12:779–790
11. Hicks RR, Numan S, Dhillon HS, Prasad MR, Seroogy KB (1997) Alterations in BDNF and NT-3 mRNAs in rat hippocampus after experimental brain trauma. Molecular Brain Res 48:401–406
12. Kamme F, Campell K, Wieloch T (1995) Biphasic expression of the Fos and Jun families of transcription factors following transient forebrain ischaemia in the rat: effect of hypothermia. European J Neurosci 7:2007–2016

13. Kim Y, Truettner J, Zhao W, Busto R, Ginsberg MD (1998) The influence of delayed postischemic hyperthermia following transient focal ischemia: alterations of gene expression. J Neurological Sci 159:1–10
14. Perez-Pinzon MA, Xu GP, Born J, Lorenzo J, Busto R, Rosenthal M, Sick TJ (1999) Cytochrome c is released from mitochondria into the cytosol after cerebral anoxia or ischemia. J Cereb Blood Flow Metab 19:39–43
15. Raghupathi R, McIntosh TK (1996) Regionally and temporally distinct patterns of induction of c-fos, c-jun, and junB mRNA following experimental brain injury in the rat. Molec Brain Res 37:134–144
16. Raghupathi R, Welsh FA, Lowenstein DH, Gennarelli TA, McIntosh TK (1995) Regional induction of c-fos and heat shock protein 72 mRNA following fluid-percussion brain injury in the rat. J Cereb Blood Flow Metab 15:467–473
17. Rink A, Fung KM, Trojanowski JQ, Lee VM-Y, Neugbauer E, McIntosh TK (1995) Evidence of apoptotic cell death after experimental traumatic brain injury in the rat. Am J Pathol 147:1575–1583
18. Truettner J, Schmidt-Kastner R, Busto R, Alonso OF, Loor JY, Dietrich WD, Ginsberg MD (1999) Expression of brain-derived neurotrophic factor, nerve growth factor, and heat shock protein HSP70 following fluid percussion brain injury in rats. J Neurotrauma 16:471–486
19. Yakovlev AG, Knoblach SM, Fan L, Fox GB, Goodnight R, Faden AI (1997) Activation of CPT32-like caspases contribute to neuronal apoptosis and neurological dysfunction after traumatic brain injury. J Neurosci 17:7415–7424
20. Yenari MA, Iwayama S, Cheng D, Sun GH, Fujimura M, Morita-Fujimura Y, Chan PH, Steinberg GK (2002) Mild hypothermia attenuates cytochrome C release but does not alter Bcl-2 expression or caspase activation after experimental stroke. J Cereb Blood Flow Metals 22:29–38

19. Summary and Future Directions

Based on experimental data, mild to moderate hypothermia appears to be one of the most potent therapeutic approaches to treating neurotrauma. Clearly the ability of temperature to target multiple pathophysiological processes may help explain why hypothermia works in multiple trauma models. Nevertheless, the recent findings from the NIH-supported North American multicenter trial on the usage of hypothermia in head injury patients indicates that more work is required to systematically evaluate the beneficial and harmful effects of clinical hypothermia in different populations of injured patients [10]. In brain and spinal cord injury, the advantages of systemic cooling versus focal cooling must also be considered. The continued development of methods of imaging regional temperature gradients in patients should provide a powerful approach to assessing and treating patients.

In contrast to well-controlled animal models of neurotrauma, clinical trauma is frequently an extremely complicated insult to the central nervous system (CNS). Commonly, the patient undergoes both the primary insult as well as a variety of secondary injury mechanisms including hypotension, hypoxia, or hyperthermia. Each of these secondary insults has the potential to worsen outcome [5,6]. To date, hypothermic therapy has routinely been tested in relatively "clean" trauma models. It may therefore be important in future studies to assess the effects of hypothermia in animal models that are complicated by induced secondary insults [1,8]. By recognizing the strengths and weaknesses of animal models of CNS injury, researchers hope to move translational research forward for the development of new therapies for the acute stages after injury [4]. This approach could move our preclinical research closer to the clinical setting by indicating the limitations of hypothermic therapy alone.

Prolonged periods of hypothermia can create problems in terms of patient care including the increased risk of infection [9]. Thus, mild hypothermia combined with the administration of neuroprotective agents may allow restricted periods of hypothermia to confer more pronounced and long-term protection [3,7]. In addition, injury processes attenuated by the hypothermic period may become active once CNS temperatures have normalized. Because hypothermic temperatures have been reported to adversely affect locomotor recovery after spinal lesions [2], restricted periods of hypothermia may be best suited to cases in which reparative strategies are initiated. Combination therapy should continue to be tested in established models of brain and spinal cord injury.

The continued search for pharmacologic agents that reduce core and brain temperature when given systemically is also an exciting direction for research. The development of this class of drugs would allow emergency staff to administer agents at early periods after brain trauma. Finally, additional studies are required to establish the therapeutic window for hypothermia in the various neurotrauma models and the optimal methods of rewarming the patient after therapeutic hypothermia.

Acknowledgments. This work was supported by USPHS grants NS-30291, NS-05820, and NS-27127. The author thanks his colleagues in the Departments of Neurological Surgery, Neurology, Psychology, and the Miami Project at the University of Miami School of Medicine for helpful discussions regarding hypothermic research, the Charlaine Rowlette for expert editorial assistance and word processing.

References

1. Clark RSB, Robertson CL, Dixon CE, Alexander HL, Graham SH, Safar PJ, Kochanek PM (1999) Effect of hypothermia after severe traumatic brain injury with secondary hypoxemia in rats. J Neurotrauma 15: 864 (Abstract)
2. Cohen AH, Kiemel T, Pate V, Binder J, Guan L (1999) Temperature can alter the functional outcome of spinal cord regeneration in larval lampreys. Neuroscience 90:957–965
3. Dietrich WD, Busto R, Bethea JR (1999) Postischemic hypothermia and IL-10 treatment provide long-lasting

neuroprotection of CA1 hippocampus following transient global ischemia in rats. Exp Neurol 158:444–450
4. Gladstone DJ, Black SE, Hakim AM (2002) Toward wisdom from failure: lessons from neuroprotective stroke trials and new therapeutic directions. Stroke 33:2123–2136
5. Ishige N, Pitts LH, Berry I, Carlson SG, Nishimura MC, Moseley ME, Weinstein PR (1987) The effect of hypoxia on traumatic head injury in rats: alterations in neurologic function, brain edema, and cerebral blood flow. J Cereb Blood Flow Metab 7:759–767
6. Ishige N, Pitts LH, Hashimoto T, Nishimura MC, Bartkowski HM (1987) Effect of hypoxia on traumatic brain injury in rats: part 1. Changes in neurological function electroencephalograms, and histopathology. Neurosurgery 20:848–853
7. Marion DW, White MJ (1996) Treatment of experimental brain injury with moderate hypothermia and 21-aminosteroids. J Neurotrauma 13:139–147
8. Matsushita Y, Bramlett HM, Alonso O, Dietrich WD (2001) Posttraumatic hypothermia is neuroprotective in a model of traumatic brain injury complicated by a secondary hypoxic insult. Crit Care Med 29:2060–2066
9. Metz C, Holzschuh M, Bein T, Woertgen C, Frey A, Frey I, Taeger K, Brawanski A (1996) Moderate hypothermia in patients with severe head injury: cerebral and extra cerebral effects. J Neurosurg 85:533–541
10. Narayan RN (2001) Hypothermia for traumatic brain injury: a good idea proved ineffective. N Eng J Med 344:602–603
11. Yamamoto M, Marmarou CR, Stiefel MF, Beaumont A, Marmarou A (1999) Neuroprotective effect of hypothermia on neuronal injury in diffuse traumatic brain injury coupled with hypoxia and hypotension. J Neurotrauma 16:487–500

Clinical Management

Introduction

Secondary brain injuries such as brain edema, brain ischemia, and reduced cerebral perfusion pressure (CPP) caused by elevation of intracranial pressure (ICP) have been considered as important treatment targets, because survival rates after primary brain injuries are low. Therefore, factors that promote these pathophysiological changes such as the presence of free radicals, blood–brain barrier (BBB) dysfunction, excitatory amino acid levels, and high concentrations of intracellular Ca^{2+} have also been considered as treatment targets [1,16,17,19,20]. This concept of brain injury mechanism has long been supported by many animal studies and various neuroprotection strategies have been studied.

Experimental animal studies have suggested that hypothermia is the most successful method to prevent secondary brain damage in trauma, ischemia, and brain hypoxia, as described in Chapter 1. Although many clinical experiences of hypothermia treatment of severely brain-injured patients have been presented, very successful clinical results are not recorded in the same manner as animal studies [3].

In recent clinical studies, insufficient hypothermia management has been used because initial care focused on the prevention of ICP elevation [2,18]. ICP elevation caused by brain edema and brain swelling occurs as a result of many pathophysiological changes in the injured brain tissue [17]. Hypothermia treatment is indicated in cases of ICP elevation, the duration of which is limited to 48 h, because, in most cases of traumatic brain injury, the severity of brain edema peaks at 24–48 h after brain trauma [2,3]. Even with incorrect intensive care unit (ICU) management, the question remains: why is hypothermia management of clinical brain-injured patients not as effective as experimental animal studies? A major issue with hypothermia treatment is that it occurs too late to prevent ICP elevation and brain damage caused by stress-associated neurohoromonal systemic circulatory and metabolic changes [7,8,11,13,14].

Our recent clinical studies demonstrated previously unreported brain injury mechanisms. These include brain thermo-pooling [15] that masks neuronal hypoxia even with normal control of ICP, PaO_2, and CPP [11], increases in brain tissue lactate levels after insulin-resistant hyperglycemia [11], BBB dysfunction caused by excess release of vasopressin following stimulation of the hypothalamus–pituitary–adrenal axis (HPA), and acute elevation of serum glucose [11]. These new brain injury mechanisms, associated with excess neurohormone release, such as catecholamines, vasopressin, and growth hormone, have been found to exert a strong effect on the reversibility and prognosis of injured neurons [12]. Without management of these new brain injury mechanisms, hypothermia treatment is not effective.

The abovementioned brain injury mechanisms are difficult to monitor in anesthetized experimental animal models. The magnitude of neurohormonal reactions are related to the severity of harmful stress to clinical patients [4,11]. However, anesthesia conceals the severity of these stresses and makes monitoring of these brain injury mechanisms difficult in animal models. The brain injury mechanisms of anesthetized experimental animal models and clinical patients are dissimilar, especially in cases of severely brain-injured patients.

The brain thermo-pooling phenomenon also occurs with unstable cardiopulmonary dysfunction caused by stress-induced catecholamine surge [11,15]. The precise mechanism of brain thermo-pooling is described in Chap. 23. The elevation of brain tissue temperature to 40°–44°C is observed in severe brain-injured patients that suffer trauma, subarachnoid hemorrhage (SAH), and after resuscitation following cardiopulmonary arrest (CPA).

All experimental information using animal studies was obtained at 37°C or controlled body temperature (brain temperature about 37°–37.5°C). This new concept of brain injury mechanism is not demonstrated by experimental animal studies. The mechanism of brain injury derived from animal studies is not similar to clinical cases, especially those that include severe brain injury, severe SAH, and resuscitated cardiopulmonary arrested patients, and acute onset of cerebral occlusive disease. We have observed many cases of good recovery that are difficult to understand from the previous concept of management of severely brain-injured patients using brain hypothermia treatment [12,16]. All neurons in primary injured brain tissue do not die immediately, but rather, die gradually over time. Therefore, primary brain injury is also an initial treatment target for neuronal restoration in the acute stage.

To survive, severe brain-injured patients need a restoration therapy before neuroprotection therapy. Hypothermia is only one environmental factor to aid the success of restoration therapy and neuroprotection therapy. To promote the restoration of brain-injured patients, the management of brain edema, cerebral blood flow, ICP elevation, brain temperature, and also stress to the HPA-axis associated with hemoglobin dysfunction, insulin-resistant hyperglycemia, vasopressin-released BBB dysfunction, brain thermo-pooling, and systemic circulatory–metabolic changes, must be taken care of from the acute stage in ICU [10,11].

Recent clinical studies have found the mechanism of vegetation is related to damage of memory, volition, thinking, understanding, love, affection, and emotion. Laboratory diagnostic methods for these neuronal functions are also developed in our ICU [9,10,12]. Without recovery of higher brain functions, such as emotion, thinking, and volition, brain management in the ICU could not be regarded as successful. Neuroprotection and restoration of these higher brain functions are also important issues for brain hypothermia treatment [10,12,19].

In this chapter, all clinical issues of brain hypothermia treatment are discussed in detail.

Brain injury mechanism of severe brain injury based on experimental animal study
History of clinical trials of hypothermia
Clinical issues of previous hypothermia management
New findings of secondary brain injury mechanism by hypothalamus-pituitary-adrenal axis neurohormonal activation in severely brain injured patient
Difference between brain injury mechanism in experimental animal models and clinical patients
Basic concept of changing brain tissue temperature
Targets of treatment in the acute stage of severe brain injury
New concepts of brain hypothermia treatment
Indications for brain hypothermia treatment
Time limit for starting brain hypothermia
Pitfalls of brain hypothermia treatment
Improper management of brain hypothermia treatment
How to control brain tissue temperature
Technique for managing brain tissue temperature
Bed making
Design of ICU for brain hypothermia treatment
Nursing care for brain hypothermia
Preparation for the management of brain hypothermia treatment
Noninvasive monitoring of brain damage
Neuroprotection of injured brain tissue during surgery
Anesthesia for brain hypothermia treatment
Examination during brain hypothermia treatment
Induction of brain hypothermia treatment
Management of the cooling stage
When rewarming should begin
Preconditioning for rewarming
Management of rewarming
Posthypothermia resuscitation therapy
Clinical path of brain hypothermia treatment
Brain hypothermia after resuscitation from CPA
Brain hypothermia and occlusive cerebral stroke
Brain hypothermia and SAH
Clinical results of brain hypothermia treatment
Summary of brain hypothermia treatment for severely brain-injured patients

Much new information obtained from clinical studies of more than 400 cases will provide valuable support for clinical trials of brain hypothermia treatment.

References

1. Baker AJ, Zornow MH, Scheller MS, Yaksh TL, Skilling SR, Smullin DH, Larson AA, Kuczenski R (1991) Changes in extracellular concentrations of glutamate, aspartate, glycine, dopamine, serotonin, and dopamine metabolites after transient global ischemia in the rat. J Neurochem 57:1370–1379
2. Clifton GL, Allen S, Barrodale P, Plenger P, Berry J, Koch S, Fletcher J, Hayes RL, Choi SC (1993) A phase II study of moderate hypothermia in severe brain injury. J Neurotrauma 10:263–271
3. Clifton GL, Miller ER, Choi SC, Levin HS, McCauley S, Smith KP Jr, Muizelaar JP, Wagner FC Jr, Marion DW, Luerssen TG, Chesnut RM, Schwartz M (2001) Lack of effect of induction of hypothermia after acute brain injury. N Engl J Med 344:556–563
4. Corte FD, Mancini A, Valle D, Gallizzi F, Carducci P, Mignani V, De Marinis L (1998) Provocative hypothalamopituitary axis tests in severe head injury: correlations with severity and prognosis. Crit Care Med 26:1419–1426
5. Globus MYT, Ginsberg MD, Haris SI, Busto R, Dietrich WD (1987) Role of dopamine in ischemic striatal injury. Neurology 37:1712–1719
6. Globus MYT, Busto R, Dietrich WD, Martinez E, Valdes I, Ginsberg MD (1998) Effect of ischemia on the in vivo release of striatal dopamine, glutamate, and γ-aminobutyric acid studied by intracerebral microdialysis. J Neurochem 51:1455–1464
7. Hayashi N (1995) Cerebral hypothermia treatment. In: Hayashi N (ed) Cerebral hypothermia treatment. Sogo Igaku, Tokyo, pp 1–105

8. Hayashi N (1996) Advance of cerebral hypothermia treatment. J Critical Med 8:295–300
9. Hayashi N (1997) Combination therapy of cerebral hypothermia, pharmacological activation of the dopamine system, and hormonal replacement in severely brain damaged patients. J Jpn Soc Intensive Care Med 4: 191–197
10. Hayashi N (1997) Prevention of vegetation after severe head trauma and stroke by combination therapy of cerebral hypothermia and activation of immune-dopaminergic nervous system. Proceedings of the 6th annual meeting of Society for Treatment of Coma 6:133–145
11. Hayashi N (2000) Enhanced neuronal damage in severely brain injured patients by hypothalamus, pituitary, and adrenal axis neuro-hormonal changes. In: Hayashi N (ed) Brain hypothermia. Springer, Berlin Heidelberg New York Tokyo, pp 3–26
12. Hayashi N (2000) The clinical issue and effectiveness of brain hypothermia treatment for severe brain injured patients. In: Hayashi N (ed) Brain hypothermia. Springer, Berlin Heidelberg New York Tokyo, pp 121–151
13. Hayashi N, Hirayama T, Utagawa A (1994) The cerebral thermo-pooling and hypothermia treatment of critical head injury patients. In: Nagai H (ed) Intracranial pressure IX. Springer, Berlin Heidelberg New York Tokyo, pp 589–599
14. Hayashi N, Hirayama T, Utagawa T, Ohata M (1994) Systemic management of cerebral edema based on a new concept in severe head injury patients. Acta Neurochir [Suppl] 60:541–543
15. Hayashi N, Kinoshita K, Shibuya T (1997) The prevention of cerebral thermo-pooling, damage of A10 nervous system, and free radical reactions by control of brain tissue temperature in severely brain injured patients. In: Teelken AW (ed) Neurochemistry. Plenum New York, pp 97–103
16. Hayashi N, Nagao K, Utagawa A, Sakurai A (2001) The push back of life edge from cardiac death by combination therapy with percutaneous cardiopulmonary support and brain hypothermia treatment in cardiac arrested patients. Cardiovascular Med Surg 13:68–77
17. Maclntosh TK (1994) Neurological sequele of traumatic brain injury: therapeutic implications. Cerebrovasc Brain Metab Rev 6:109–162
18. Shiozaki T, Sugimoto H, Taneda M, Yoshida H, Iwai A, Yoshioka T, Sugimoto T (1993) Effects of mild hypothermia on uncontrollable intracranial hypertension after severe head injury. J Neurosurg 79:363–368
19. Silvka A, Coben G (1985) Hydroxyl radical attack on dopamine. J Biol Chem 260:15466–15472
20. Spuler A, Tan WKM, Meyer FB (1966) Molecular events in cerebral ischemia. In: Raffel C, Harsh GR (eds) The molecular basis of neurosurgical disease. Williams and Wilkins, Baltimore, pp 248–269

II. Overview of Clinical Development of Brain Hypothermia Treatment

20. Mechanism of Brain Damage and Management of Severe Brain Injury Based on Laboratory Studies

Primary brain-injured tissue is difficult to survive, therefore, secondary brain injury mechanisms such as brain edema, brain ischemia, and reduced cerebral perfusion pressure (CPP) caused by elevation of intracranial pressure (ICP) have been considered as treatment targets in the acute stage. The promoting factor of these pathophysiological changes, such as free radicals, blood–brain barrier (BBB) dysfunction, excitatory amino acid levels, and high concentrations of intracellular Ca^{2+} have also been considered as treatment targets. This concept of brain injury mechanism has long been supported by many animal studies [1,12,13,16–19,25].

Historical Concepts in the Mechanism of Brain Injury

Initial brain injury involves the destruction of brain tissue, damage to vasculature, and the release of potassium and vasoactive substances such as endogenous opiate [20], catecholamines [1], serotonin [1], and neurotoxic excitatory amino acids such as aspartate and glutamate [1]. These changes develop immediately in cerebral ischemia, which accompanies synaptic paralysis and temporary cardio-pulmonary dysfunction. In animal studies, the initial release of the excitatory amino acid glutamate, which is modulated by constitutive nitrous oxide (NO) radicals, has been reported to increase intracellular Ca^{2+} ion levels in injured brain tissue [25]. The release of glutamate, high intracellular Ca^{2+} levels, and the presence of constitutive free radicals impose severe damage on intracellular homeostasis and cause membrane dysfunction [20,25]. The relationship between these pathophysiological changes in injured brain tissue and neuroprotection reactions [2,15,23], and changes of systemic circulation and metabolism [28] are summarized in Fig. 1.

The cerebral neuroprotection reactions in injured brain tissue, such as neutralization of neuronal acidosis, metabolism of neurotoxic glutamate, scavenging of radicals, restoration by neurotrophic factors [2,27], and pH control by glial cells [11,27], is not enough in most cases. The brain tissue is rich in prothrombin and, in severely brain-injured tissue, disturbances of microcirculation and brain ischemia progress rapidly and are unavoidable following brain edema and ICP elevation. Therefore, brain ischemia, brain edema, and ICP elevation have long been counted as major pathophysiological changes in the acute stages of severe brain injury [6,13,16,18]. As a brain-specific pathophysiological change, ICP elevation itself results in a reduction of CPP [6] and brain ischemia with compartment syndrome [3]. The ICP at which reduction of CPP begins (20–25 mmHg) is higher than the cerebral capillary pressure. Therefore, in the intensive care unit (ICU), maintenance of CPP above 80 mmHg and ICP below 20 mmHg is fundamental in severely brain-injured patients. In recent animal studies, tissue destruction, vascular engorgement, brain edema, and cytokine inflammation with BBB dysfunction have been demonstrated as causes of brain edema and ICP elevation [8,20,25]. Before the elevation of ICP and progression of brain edema, functional changes in vascular permeability start between 2 and 15 h [6,11]. Before the progression of widespread brain edema, selective and specific neuronal damage of basal ganglia has also been reported [9]. Heterogenetic brain damage is understood to occur as a result of the vulnerability of brain tissue to non-homogeneous stress concentration and brain tissue rotation. One mechanism of brain vulnerability is the release of the neuroexcitatory amino acid glutamate, which has been nominated as a major contributing factor to delayed neuronal cell death [12,20,25]. In the management of severely brain-injured patients, prevention of neuroexcitation is understood to be an important care method.

After 24 h, brain edema and intracranial hypertension begin to progress, and are accompanied by further free radical reactions [24,25]. In this stage, intravascular release of thromboplastin, activation of intravascular coagulability, and consumption of thromboplastin fibrinolysis agents occur with changes in microcirculation of vascular permeability. Vascular engorgement, disturbances in microcirculation, ICP elevation, and inducible free radical reactions generate an ischemic malignant

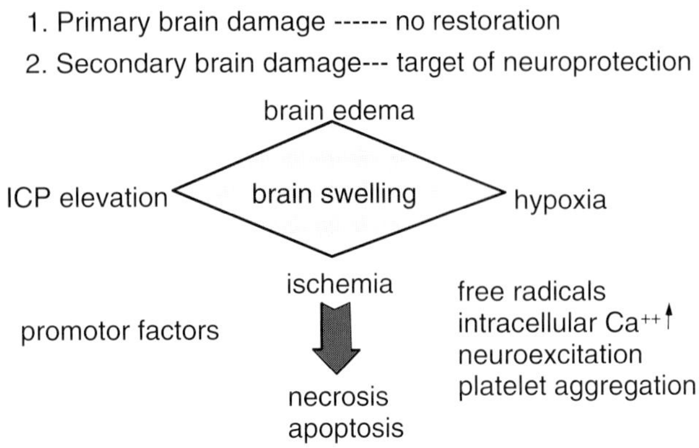

Fig. 1. Brain injury mechanism and promoter factors. *ICP*, intracranial pressure

circle and promote brain edema and intracranial hypertension (Fig. 1). As localized changes take place in injured brain tissue, infiltration of systemic immune-protective cells occurs, and neutrophils and microphages produce cytokines, inducible NO, and super oxide anion radicals [25]. The release of cytokines increases intravascular coagulation, activates adhesion molecules to the intima of vascular wall, and damages vascular permeability. The complication of systemic infection promotes these pathophysiological changes very easily and severely, and inducible free radicals cause more extensive brain damage.

Neuroprotection

It is considered that full recovery from primary brain injury is difficult. Therefore, the target of ICU management is neuroprotection from secondary brain damage caused by brain edema, ICP elevation, free radical reactions, changes of intravascular coagulability, BBB dysfunction, loss of vascular autoregulation, and cerebral blood flow (CBF) disturbances that occur from primary brain injury [1,6,12,13,16,18,19]. Neurons in the brain tissue consume more oxygen and metabolic substrates than other cells in the body and are much more sensitive to hypoxia and energy crisis than other cells. Because management of severely brain-injured patients in ICU is focused on neuroprotection rather than neuronal restoration therapy, ICU management is concentrated on maintaining oxygen delivery and CBF, and control of ICP and/or lowering of brain metabolism by barbiturate therapy or hypothermia. However, dying neurons in injured brain tissue require restoration therapy. Neuroprotection management is not enough for restoration of dying neurons. For restoration therapy to succeed, adequate neuronal oxygenation, administration of metabolic substrates, and control of secondary brain damage are required. This clinical issue is very important for the recovery of severely brain-injured patients as discussed in Chap. 26.

Brain Edema

Brain edema is morphologically divided into cellular edema and interstitial edema [13], while the mechanism of edema is divided into cytotoxic brain edema and vasogenic brain edema. For these two types of brain edema, the clinical cause and management methods are different. Cytotoxic cellular brain edema leads to interstitial edema with cell membrane dysfunction and disturbed intracellular homeostasis. In particular, glial cell swelling is very sensitive to ischemia and hypoxia for maintaining neuronal proton stability. To reverse cytotoxic cellular swelling, adequate administration of oxygen, control of serum glucose, and stabilization of cell membrane function are necessary to prevent interstitial edema, increased intravascular osmolarity, and intravascular normalization of pH and electrolytes. As a pharmacological treatment, steroid therapy is nominated. However, steroid therapy for the prevention of brain edema at the acute stage is still controversial. One disadvantage of steroid administration at the acute stage is that stress-associated hyperglycemia becomes much worse with increasing levels of brain tissue lactate, hemoglobin dysfunction, and increased vasopressin release and BBB dysfunction [8]. In our series of brain hypothermia treatments, steroid administration is contraindicated in the acute stage in cases of stress-associated hyperglycemia at levels above 180 mg/dl [9,10].

In most cases of brain trauma, brain edema progress is associated with vasogenic brain edema. The main pathophysiological change of brain edema is interstitial edema with BBB dysfunction. At a later stage, vasogenic brain edema promotes cellular edema. Progression of vasogenic brain edema is directly influenced by the severity of BBB dysfunction, serum osmolarity, and the presence of chemical substrates such as inflammatory cytokines [14]. Therefore, complication of systemic infection with BBB dysfunction causes rapid progression of vasogenic brain edema with cytokine encephalitis. BBB dysfunction reaches a critical level at a CSF albumin/serum albumin ratio above 0.01 [8,13]. Prevention of systemic infection, replacement of serum albumin, and infusion of manitol are recommended. In the directly injured brain tissue, however, vasogenic interstitial edema and cytotoxic brain edema progress simultaneously. Therefore, in injury management, we must take care of vasogenic brain edema and cytotoxic brain edema simultaneously. The peak times of vasogenic edema and cytotoxic cellular brain edema are 12–48h after insult.

Acute brain swelling associated with disturbed cerebral vascular autoregulation and or hypercapnea is a secondary brain injury mechanism [16,18]. The main pathophysiological change is increased cerebral blood volume with vascular engorgement and loss of vascular tone. A rapid increase of systemic blood pressure above 45mmHg $PaCO_2$, an increase of mediastinal pressure above 15mmHg, and abdominal hypertension above the range of 17–25mmHg are all critical conditions.

Management of Intracranial Pressure Elevation

The brain tissue is maintained in a floating condition in CSF within the closed cranium box. The volume of the cranial cavity is held constant by the brain tissue, blood volume, CSF, and meningens. Therefore, ICP elevation occurs in proportion to the total volume of brain tissue, blood volume, CSF, and meningens. Brain injury with brain edema involves an increasing volume of brain tissue after a similar reduction in blood volume or CSF [21]. Reduction of blood volume in the cranial cavity involves CBF disturbance and CSF reduction occurs as compensation for ICP elevation. Reported causes of ICP elevation include brain edema with increasing brain tissue volume, acute brain swelling with disturbed autoregulation, hypercapnea and mediastinal–abdomonal high pressure, and acute hydrocephalus with increasing of CSF volume that occurs via blockage of the subarachnoid space or the ventricular system. ICP elevation itself produces various CBF disturbances and worsens brain injury by the reduction of brain metabolism and oxygenation. However, the secondary brain damage caused by ICP elevation is not only highly correlated to ICP, but also to the speed of ICP elevation, because, ICP adaptation mechanism by CSF space and soft brain tissue are recorded. The basic pattern of CBF disturbance by elevation of ICP is summarized in the following discussion.

The initial pattern of CBF disturbance by ICP elevation is venous stasis (Table 3). The elevation of cerebral venous pressure reduces the waterfall pressure in intraparenchyma capillary vessels. The critical venous pressure to produce cerebral venous pressure is above 15–20mmHg. However, when ICP is elevated above 20–25mmHg, water filtration pressure between the interstitial space and the intravenous vascular system (WFcv) drops to −6mmHg that lowers 7mmHg of WFca as shown mathematically in Fig. 2. Therefore, control of ICP to below 20mmHg is recommended in ICU management. The typical pathophysiological changes that follow ICP elevation and the combination of these promoting factors are summarized in Table 3. The new finding of brain injury mechanism of brain thermo-pooling is described in Chap. 23. The fundamental pathophysiological changes in the brain tissue after elevation of ICP are described here. All of these pathophysiological changes become worse with various promoting factors. In the management of ICP elevation, two dangerous critical pressure levels must be diagnosed. One is elevation of ICP above the cerebral capillary pressure which results in CBF disturbance. The second is elevation of ICP until intercompartmental pressure differences occur, such as supratentorial and infratentorial pressure differences. Such intracranial compartment pressure differences can easily cause herniation and mechanical brain stem compression. With the cerebral capillary pressure in the range of 25–35mmHg, intercompartment pressure difference arises when ICP is elevated above 35–45mmHg. In ICU man-

Table 3. Intracranial pathophysiological changes and promotor factors of secondary brain damage in intracranial hypertension

Intracranial pathophysiology	Intracranial pressure (ICP) Cerebral perfusion pressure (CPP)	Promotor factors
1. Brain thermo-pooling	CPP <60mmHg	Fever and hypotension, elevation of mediastinal pressure and abdominal hypertension
2. Cerebral venous stasis	ICP 15–20mmHg	
3. CBF disturbances	ICP >25mmHg	Hypoalbuminemia
Brain edema[a]		Hypertension
4. Disturbance of autoregulation		Free radicals
5. Pressure wave		Systolic blood pressure >48mmHg
6. Nonfilling	ICP >70mmHg	Sleeping
		Shock and hypercapnea

[a]Water filtration (WF) at capillary by Staring's formula: WF = (capillary pressure-tissue pressure) − (serum osmotic pressure-brain tissue pressure); filtration pressure at arterial side is about 13mmHg; absorption pressure from venous side is −15mmHg

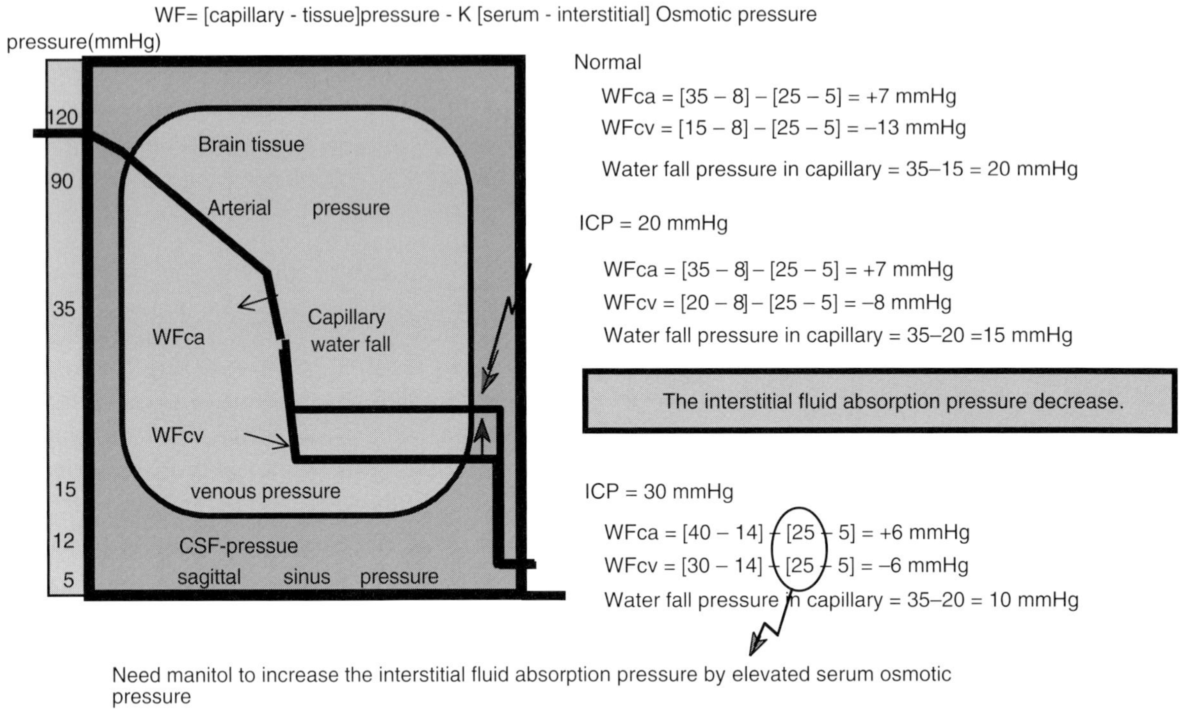

Fig. 2. ICP elevation with venous stasis and interstitial edema by capillary dysfunction. *WF*, water filtration; *K*, coefficient; *WFca*, water filtration at arterial side of cerebral capillary; *WFcv*, water filtration from brain tissue to venous side capillary

agement, ICP should be kept below the cerebral capillary pressure and preferably below 20 mmHg. When ICP is elevated above 45 mmHg and is difficult to manage with ventricular drainage and pharmacological treatment, surgical treatment such as external and/or internal decompressions may be required [22].

The management of ICP in patients with external decompression requires special consideration. The externally decompressed skull is not a closed box and therefore, the concept of ICP is not introduced. In such cases, changes in brain tissue pressure are localized and the brain tissue pressure is influenced not only by brain edema, but also by brain swelling, atmospheric pressure, and the weight of brain tissue which changes depending on head position.

Management of Acute Brain Swelling

Acute brain swelling occurs with a rapid increase in cerebral blood volume and vascular engorgement [16]. Under normal conditions, cerebral vessel walls are maintained with the same vasoconstrictive tension for consistent CBF [18].

CBF is maintained at a steady level by an autoregulation mechanism even with changes in arterial blood pressure across the range of 50–150 mmHg [18]. There are two types of autoregulation mechanism: localized metabolic control and compartment neurogenic control [16,17]. Severe brain injury and hypercapnea can easily disturb these autoregulation and cerebrovascular reactions. Levels of $PaCO_2$ above 45 mmHg are unsafe and produce relaxation of smooth muscle of the vascular walls. For ICU management of severely brain-injured patients, $PaCO_2$ should be kept below 40 mmHg.

Recently, the author reported elevation of brain tissue temperature (40°–44°C) as a new brain injury mechanism known as brain thermo-pooling which occurs under conditions of high fever (38.5°C and above) and systolic blood pressure below 90–100 mmHg, or with CPP below 60–70 mmHg. Especially at the reperfusion stage, the brain thermo-pooling phenomenon is recorded in high incidence [8,10]. It is likely that brain tissue temperature greater than 40°C caused by brain thermo-pooling also disturbs the autoregulation of cerebral circulation and results in acute brain swelling. Factors that promote acute brain swelling include hypercapnea, rapid elevation of systolic blood pressure, elevation of mediastinal pressure, abdominal hypertension, elevated bladder pressure caused by urinal obstruction, and the head down position.

For ICU management of ICP and CBF, the cerebral vascular disturbances of vascular engorgement and acute brain swelling are important clinical issues [16]. Recommendations for ICU management include maintenance of body temperature below 37°C, constant maintenance of systolic blood pressure above 100 mmHg, control of $PaCO_2$ within the range of 30–40 mmHg, management of mediastinal pressure below 5–7 mmHg, insertion of an ileum tube and urinary drainage to lower abdominal and bladder pressure to below 15 mmHg, and a head up position in bed of 5°–15°.

Brain explosion from craniotomy surgery is a different type of acute brain swelling and is another important treatment target [22]. Rapid opening of the duramater in a case of elevated ICP, can easily result in acute brain swelling. If brain explosion occurs during surgery, recovery is very difficult even with the subdural hematoma removed, because localized brain tissue laceration occurs in many areas of deep brain tissue in the closed craniotomy site. To prevent this serious complication, recommended measures include a head up position of 45° temporally, suction of the subdural hematoma through a small duramater incision until the subdural pressure is reduced, control of body temperature at 34°C, and application of elastic bandages to the extremities to prevent rapid changes in systolic blood pressure upon opening of the duramater.

Prevention of Brain Ischemia

CBF disturbance in severely brain-injured patients is a major issue for ICU management. Adequate administration of oxygen and metabolic substrates for restoration of injured neurons requires sufficient CBF (Fig. 3). In severely brain-injured patients, CBF disturbances occur as a result of many factors [14,15,18–20]. Reduced CPP caused by cardiogenic shock, peripheral vascular dilatation and/or hemorrhagic shock, shift of the systemic bloodstream to the abdominal side with dopamine-dominant circulation, and disturbance of microcirculation by reduced antithrombin have been observed [8]. The management of CPP above 80 mmHg, pharmacological treatment of cardiac function, fluid resuscitation and blood transfusion, and more than 100% of antithrombin-III (AT-III) are important [8,10].

Much clinical research has demonstrated that critical reversibility of CBF disturbance, the presence of a brain-specific ischemic pattern in the penumbra zone, and different time windows of pathophysiological changes (Fig. 4) must be considered in ICU management. The relationships between changes in CBF and the molecular changes in injured neurons are summarized in Fig. 5. However, in ICU management of severely brain-injured patients, it is very difficult to measure the quantitative changes of CBF in particular time windows. Therefore, many indirect parameters of

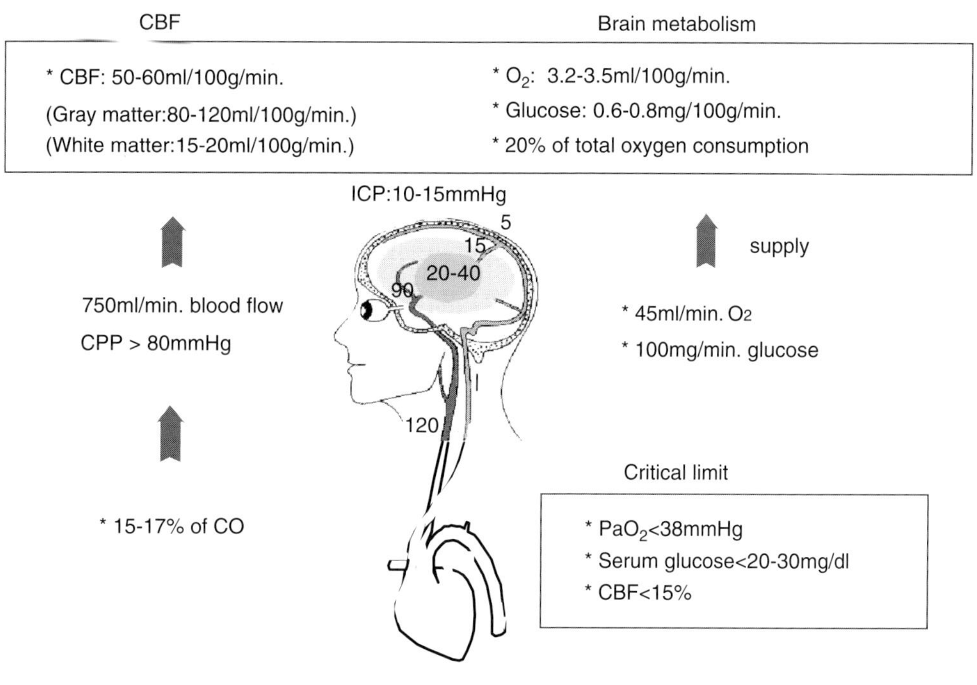

Fig. 3. Cerebral blood flow (CBF) and metabolism for neuronal restoration

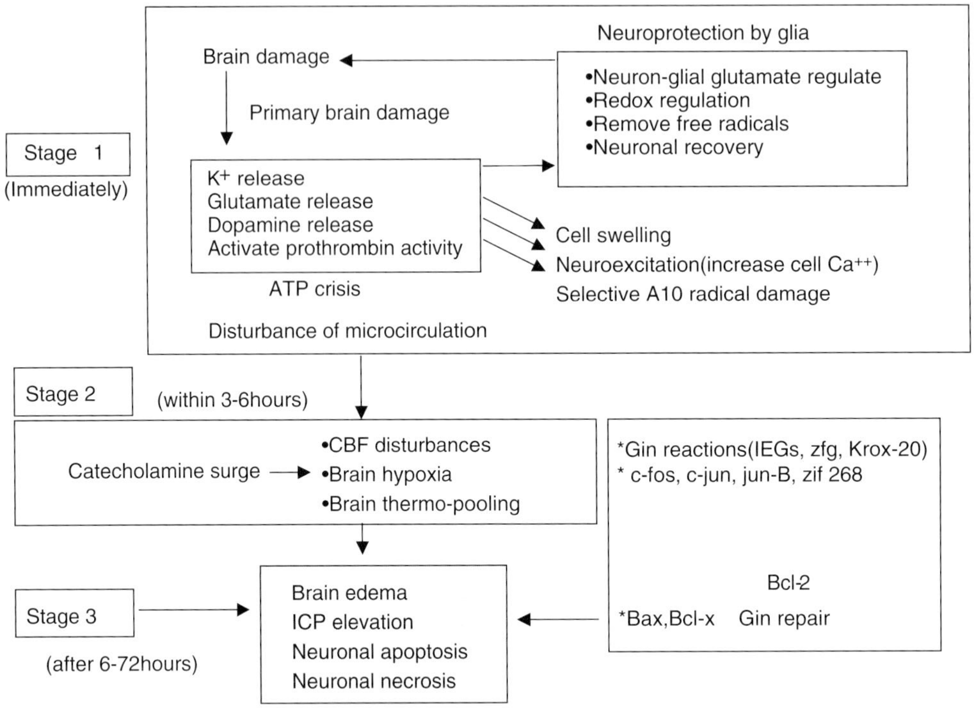

Fig. 4. Changes in brain injury mechanism after severe brain damage. *ATP*, adenosine triphosphate

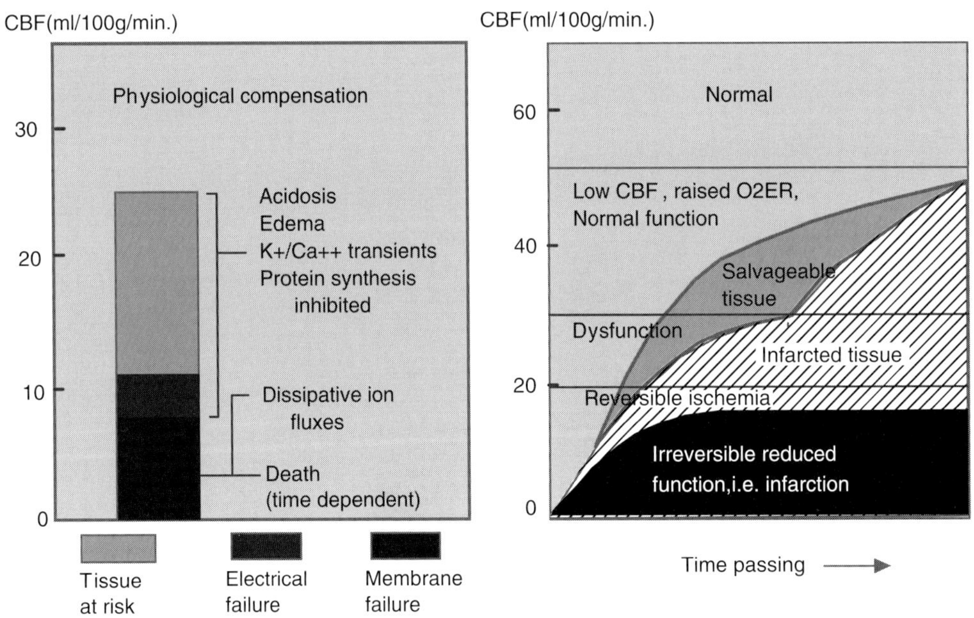

Fig. 5. The CBF thresholds for cell function and relationships between CBF levels, neuronal function, time, and the evolution of ischemic penumbra to infarction

CBF disturbance are monitored. As indirect parameters of CBF disturbance, reduction of tympanic membrane temperature/core temperature (or bladder temperature) ratio to less than 1.0, and less than 50% of jugular venous O_2 saturation are useful.

Brain Temperature

In experimental animal models of brain trauma, brain ischemia, and hypoxia, hypothermia management is very successful for neuroprotection [5,7]. The beneficial mechanism of hypothermia is multifaceted as described in detail in Chap. 1. However, clinical results of hypothermia management are still controversial [4]. Several factors may explain why hypothermia management is useful in experimental animal models and not for clinical patients. The concept of neuroprotection by hypothermia management alone, is probably not enough for clinical patients, and brain injury mechanism in experimental animal models and clinical patients are different [8,10]. The neuroprotection mechanism of hypothermia is reviewed in detail in Chap. 1. The clinical issues of hypothermia management are described in Chap. 22. New findings of brain injury mechanism that were not recorded in studies of experimental brain-injured animal models, such as hemoglobin dysfunction, ineffective oxygen inhalation, insulin-resistant hyperglycemia, increasing levels of brain tissue glucose, and vasopressin release of macronutrient neural reaction associated with BBB dysfunction were not successfully prevented after applying previous concepts in hypothermia treatment [8,10]. From this background, a new concept of brain hypothermia treatment has developed in our ICU. The concept of brain hypothermia treatment, technique and management methods, complications, management of severe infections associated with immune crisis, pitfalls of brain hypothermia treatment, indications and contraindications, clinical development for resuscitation of cardiopulmonary-arrested patients, and development of clinical results are described in the following chapters.

References

1. Baker AJ, Zornow MH, Scheller MS, Yaksh TL, Skilling SR, Smullin DH, Larson AA, Kuczenski R (1991) Changes in extracellular concentrations of glutamate, aspartate, glycine, dopamine, serotonin, and dopamine metabolites after transient global ischemia in the rat. J Neurochem 57:1370–1379
2. Boise LH, Gottschalk AR, Quintans J, Thompson CB (1995) Bcl-2 and Bcl-2-related proteins in apoptosis regulation. Curr Top Microbiol Immunol 200:107–121
3. Brock M, Beck J, Markakis E, Dietz H (1972) Intracranial pressure gradients associated with experimental cerebral embolism. Stroke 3:123–130
4. Clifton GL, Miller ER, Choi SC, Levin HS, McCauley S, Smith KR Jr, Muizelaar JP, Wagner FC Jr, Marion DW, Luerssen TG, Chesnut RM, Schwartz M (2001) Lack of effect of induction of hypothermia after acute brain injury. N Engl J Med 344:556–563
5. Dietrich WD, Busto R, Valdes I, Loor Y (1990) Effects of normothermic versus mild hypothermic forebrain ischemia in rats. Stroke 21:1318–1325
6. Feng H, Huang G, Gao L, Tan H, Liao X (2000) Effect of intracranial pressure and cerebral perfusion pressure on outcome prediction of severe traumatic brain injury. Chin J Traumatol 3:226–230
7. Globus MYT, Busto R, Martinez E, Valdes I, Dietrich WD, Ginsberg MD (1991) Early moderate postischemic hypothermia attenuates the rise in excitotoxic index in the hippocampus. A possible mechanism underlying the beneficial effects of early postischemic moderate cooling. J Cereb Blood Flow Metab 11 (suppl): S10
8. Hayashi N (2000) Enhanced neuronal damage in severely brain injured patients by hypothalamus, pituitary, and adrenal axis neuro-hormonal changes. In: Hayashi N (ed) Brain hypothermia. Springer, Berlin Heidelberg New York Tokyo, pp 3–26
9. Hayashi N, Hirayama T, Utagawa A, Ohata M (1993) Complete cerebral ischemia-induced circuit damage of the basal ganglia, substantia nigra and deep cerebellar nucleus in clinical cases. In: Tomita M, Mchedlishvili G, Rosenblum W, Heiss W-D, Fukuchi Y (eds) Microcirculatory stasis in the brain. Excepta Medica, Amsterdam, pp 555–562
10. Hayashi N, Kinoshita K, Shibuya T (1997) The prevention of cerebral thermo-pooling, damage of A10 nervous system, and free radical reactions by control of brain tissue temperature in severely brain injured patients. In: Teelken AW (ed) Neurochemistry. Plenum, New York, pp 97–103
11. Hertz L (1982) Astrocyte. In: Lajtha A (ed) Handbook of neurochemistry. Plenum, New York, pp 319–348
12. Kirino T (1982) Delayed neuronal death in the gerbil hippocampus following ischemia. Brain Res 239:57–69
13. Klatzo I (1967) Neuropathological aspects of brain edema. J Neuropath Exp Neurol 26:1–14
14. Kossmann T, Hans V, Lenzlinger PM, Csuka E, Stsahel PF, Trentz O, Morgani-Kossmann MC (1996) Analysis of immune mediator production following traumatic brain injury. In: Schlag G, Redel H, Traber D (eds) Shock, sepsis and organ failure. Springer, Berlin Heidelberg New York, pp 263–297
15. Krajewski S, Mai JK, Krajewaska M, Sikorska M, Massakowski MJ, Reed JC (1995) Upregulation of bax proteins in neurons following cerebral ischemia. J Neurosci 15:6364–6376
16. Langfitt TW (1969) Intracranial pressure. Clin Neurosurg 16:436–471
17. Lassen NA (1968) Brain extracellular pH: the main factor controlling cerebral blood flow. Scand J Clin Lab Invest 22:247–251

18. Mayer JS, Shimazu K, Fukuchi Y (1973) Cerebral dysautoregulation in central neurogenic orthostatic hypotension. Neurology 23:262–273
19. McIntosh TK, Hayes R, DeWitt D, Agura V, Faden AI (1987) Endogenous opioids may mediate secondary damage after experimental brain injury. Am J Physiol 258:E565–E574
20. MacIntosh TK (1994) Neurological sequele of traumatic brain injury: therapeutic implications. Cerebrovasc Brain Metab Rev 6:109–162
21. March K (2000) Intracranial pressure monitoring and assessing intracranial compliance in brain injury. Crit Care Nurs Clin North Am 12:429–436
22. Meier U, Zeilinger FS, Henzka O (2000) The use of decompressive craniectomy for the management of severe head injuries. Acta Neurochir Suppl 76:475–478
23. Oppenheim RW, Houenou LJ, Johnson JE, Lin LF, Li L, Lo AC, Newsome AL, Prevette DM, Wang S (1995) Developing motor neurons rescued from programmed and axtonomy-induced cell death by GDNF. Nature 373:344–346
24. Silvka A, Coben G (1985) Hydroxyl radical attack on dopamine. J Biol Chem 260:15466–15472
25. Spuler A, Tan WKM, Meyer FB (1966) Molecular events in cerebral ischemia. In: Raffel C, Harsh GR (eds) The molecular basis of neurosurgical disease. Williams and Wilkins, Baltimore, pp 248–269
26. Symon L, Branston NM, Strong AJ (1976) Autoregulation in acute focal ischemia. Stroke 7:547–554
27. Wang Y, Chang CF, Morales M, Chiang YH, Hoffer J (2002) Protective effects of glial cell line-derived neurotrophic factor in ischemic brain injury. Ann NY Acad Sci 962:423–437
28. Wong FW (2000) Prevention of secondary brain injury. Crit Care Nurse 20:18–27

21. History of Clinical Trials of Hypothermia Treatment of Severe Brain Injury

In 1943, Fay [14] reported the positive effect of hypothermia for brain trauma. However, the patient number was few and scientific data of effective hypothermia were not presented. In 1954, Rosomoff [32,35] measured the changes in cerebral blood flow (CBF) during hypothermia treatment and initiated clinical trials of the procedure. Subsequently, many clinical trials of hypothermia have been undertaken over a period of decades, and deep global hypothermia has been established as a principal cerebral protective technique for circulatory arrest procedures [1,2,28,37]. Hypothermia anesthesia was only successful for the prevention of brain damage during surgical accidents or in cases of temporary circulatory arrest. The classical mechanism proposed for the neuronal protection afforded by hypothermia is a reduction of oxygen and glucose consumption caused by lowering the rates of enzymatic reactions and metabolism. Brain hypothermia has thus been recommended to effect neuronal protection during anesthesia [2,28].

Between 1954 and 1970, many clinical trials were applied to cases of severe brain trauma and cerebral stroke [26,28,32,34,36]. However, the use of hypothermia in neurosurgical procedures has been restricted by postoperative complications such as severe pulmonary infection, cardiac dysfunction, and thrombocytopenia-induced microcirculatory disturbance. Numerous hazards of hypothermia have disturbed its clinical application to the management of brain injury patients.

In 1988 and 1989, Busto et al. [3–5] demonstrated that mild and moderate degrees of hypothermia (2°–4°C temperature reduction) are also associated with substantial effects involving histologic damage caused by reducing levels of excitatory neurotransmitters [3–5,25,34]. Several other animal studies have shown that mild hypothermia can stabilize ion homeostasis [31], membrane permeability [37], protein synthesis [6], acid–base balance, down regulation of protein kinase [6], the arachidonic acid cascade [10], membrane lipid peroxidation [27], free radical reactions, and permeability of the blood-brain barrier (BBB) [11,24]. However, intraischemic rather than postischemic brain hypothermia can protect after chronic global forebrain ischemia in rats [7,10,12,13,32].

From 1989, two pioneer's of hypothermia treatment, Guy Clifton and Don Marion, used mild-to-moderate hypothermia for management of severe brain trauma expecting few complications and good results comparable to animal studies [9,29,30]. Mild-to-moderate hypothermia may be expected to offer safer treatment than the previously used deep hypothermia treatment. Recently, details of two controlled, randomized clinical studies on the use of therapeutic moderate hypothermia for severe closed head injuries have been published [9]. Marion et al. [29,30] randomly assigned 40 patients with severe closed head injury (Glasgow Coma Scale scores 3–7) to either a hypothermia group or a normothermia group. The hypothermia patients were cooled to 32°–33°C (as BTT) within 10h after injury, maintained at that temperature for 24h, and rewarmed to 37°C over a period of 12h. Hypothermia significantly reduced the intracranial pressure (ICP) (40%) and CBF (26%) during the cooling period, and neither parameter exhibited a significant rebound increase after rewarming of the patients. At 3 months after injury, 12 patients in the hypothermia group had moderate, mild, or no disabilities, in contrast to 8 patients in the normothermia group. Systemic complications were similar in both groups. The authors concluded that therapeutic hypothermia (32°C) following severe closed head injury represents a safe procedure, and that the tendency toward a better outcome with hypothermia indicates limitation of secondary brain injury.

Clifton et al. [8] randomized 46 patients with severe nonpenetrating brain injury (Glasgow Coma Scores 4–7) into groups undergoing either standard management at 37°C ($n = 22$) or standard management with systemic hypothermia at 32°–33°C ($n = 24$). Surface cooling was initiated within 6h of injury, and maintained for 48h. There were no cardiac or coagulopathy-related complications, and the incidence of seizures was significantly lower in the hypothermia group. The mean Glasgow Outcome Score at 3 months after injury showed an absolute increase of 16% in terms of the number of patients in the good recovery/moderate disability category as compared with the severe disability/vegetative/dead categories. The evidence of an improved neurologic outcome suggested that phase III testing of moderate systemic hypothermia in patients with severe head injury is warranted. Although the effectiveness of neuroprotection by prolonged cerebral hypothermia has been clearly demonstrated in animal studies and clinical trials, such hypothermia treatment is still limited to within a 48-h period of cooling in order to avoid severe pulmonary infection and sepsis.

Clifton et al. [9] reported a randomized trial at 32°C, of 48-h duration, and moderate brain hypothermia to the severe brain injury. No clear beneficial results were obtained. Some clinical results are controversial, such as the observation of good results in large medical centers and poor prognosis in small medical centers. The quality of intensive care unit (ICU) management was suggested as one of factors that determines the prognosis. However, clear reasons for unsuccessful hypothermia treatment (32°C hypothermia, 48-h duration) were not confirmed. The prevention of secondary brain damage by reducing oxygen demand, prevention of brain edema, reduced release of neurotoxic amino acid, and prevention of free radical reactions was not as effective in severely brain-injured patients as in experimental animal models.

On the other hand, different views of hypothermia treatment developed after new findings of brain injury mechanism in 1994. In 1994, Hayashi et al. [20,21] reported the elevation of brain tissue temperature up to 42°C without elevation of ICP in severely brain-injured patients. This new brain injury mechanism known as the brain thermo-pooling phenomenon, required the precise management of brain tissue temperature. Identification of the regulation mechanism of brain tissue temperature allowed development of a suitable technique for the precise control of brain tissue hypothermia in clinical patients [15–18,22]. In 1997, another brain injury mechanism known as hemoglobin dysfunction that related to ineffective oxygen inhalation was reported to mask brain hypoxia in clinical studies [17–19]. Masking neuronal hypoxia in injured brain tissue is recorded even with normal values of cerebral perfusion pressure (CPP), PaO_2, and ICP because of slow release of bound oxygen from hemoglobin. Without management of hemoglobin dysfunction at the acute stage, brain hypothermia management and other ICU strategies cannot expect successful results in severely brain-injured patients with a Glasgow Coma Scale (GCS) score lower than 6. Recently, additional brain injury mechanisms that directly worsen primary brain injury, but were not recorded in experimental animal studies, were reported by the Hayashi group [18]. Insulin-resistant hyperglycemia associated with catecholamine surge, rapid increases in brain tissue glucose and lactate levels, excess release of vasopressin by macronutrient neural reaction to severe hyperglycemia that change BBB function, and pulmonary vascular changes are unavoidable in severely brain-injured patients. All of these pathophysiological changes are produced by hypothalamus–pituitary–adrenal (HPA) axis stimulation and increase neurohormonal release by 10–200 times. Catecholamines (epinephrine, norepinephrine, dopamine), vasopressin, and growth hormone are the major neuroendoclinological hormones [16–19,22]. However, in experimental animal models of severe brain injury, these new brain injury mechanisms were not recorded under anesthesia. To prevent the harmful effects of the newly reported brain injury mechanisms, special considerations are necessary for brain hypothermia treatment. For instance, early induction of brain hypothermia to give a brain tissue temperature of 34°C is very successful for the prevention of catecholamine surge, insulin-resistant hyperglycemia, and hemoglobin dysfunction; however, more rapid induction of brain hypothermia to 32°C can markedly reduce glucose consumption systemically and induce a shift to a lipid-dominant metabolism. As a result, brain tissue glucose levels increase more than at 34°C, brain tissue lactate levels increase, BBB dysfunction is activated by released vasopressin, and unstable cardiopulmonary function results from low serum catecholamine levels. These clinical issues were discussed at the first international symposium of brain hypothermia in Tokyo in 1998. However, to prevent nitrous oxide radical reaction in severely brain-injured patients, a brain tissue temperature of 34°C is not sufficient and evidence of the benefits of a brain tissue temperature of 32°–33°C was also presented. From 1993 to 2000, the primary purpose of brain hypothermia treatment in Japan changed from neuroprotection therapy to neurorestoration therapy. Hayashi summarized the major targets of brain hypothermia treatment in the acute stage in three points: sufficient neuronal oxygenation and suitable control of metabolic substrate, prevention of excess release of HPA axis hormones, and prevention of selective radical damage to the dopamine A10 nervous system [18,19]. The clinical issues of immune dysfunction and the pitfalls of hypothermia treatment were also clarified in clinical studies. The new concept of brain hypothermia treatment produced much improved clinical results compared with previous neuroprotection hypothermia therapy. However, the differences between previous hypothermia treatment and the new concept of brain hypothermia treatment are not clear.

It is hoped that this book may aid further advances in brain hypothermia treatment, improve survival rates of brain-injured patients, and lessen the number of cases that fall into vegetation.

References

1. Bigelow WG, Lindsay WK, Greenwood WF (1950) Hypothermia. Its possible role in cardiac surgery: an investigation of factors governing survival in dogs at low body temperatures. Ann Surg 132:849–866
2. Bottrerell EH, Lougheed WM, Scott JW, Vanderwater SL (1956) Hypothermia and interruption of carotid, or carotid vertebral circulation, in the surgical management of intracranial aneurysm. J Neurosurg 13:1–42
3. Busto R, Globus MY-T, Dietrich WD, Valdes I, Martines E, Watson DB, Ginsberg MD (1988) Reduction of extracellular glutamate release during ischemia does not ameliorate ischemic striatal damage. Soc Neurosci Abstr 14:301
4. Busto R, Dietrich WD, Globus MY-T, Ginsberg MD (1989) Postischemic moderate hypothermia inhibits CA1 hippocampal ischemic neuronal injury. Neurosci Lett 101:299–304
5. Busto R, Globus MY-T, Dietrich WD, Martines E, Valdes I, Watson DB, Ginsberg MD (1989) Effect of mild hypothermia on ischemia-induced release of neurotransmitters and free fatty acids in rat brain. Stroke 20:904–910
6. Cardell M, Boris MF, Wieloch T (1991) Hypothermia prevents the ischemia-induced trans-location and inhibition of protein kinase C in the rat striatum. J Neurochem 57:1814–1817
7. Chopp M, Chen H, Dereski MO, Garcia JH (1991) Mild hypothermic intervention after graded ischemic stress in rats. Stroke 22:37–43
8. Clifton GL, Allen S, Barrodale P, Plenger P, Berry J, Koch S, Fletcher J, Hayes RL, Choi SC (1993) A phase II study of moderate hypothermia in severe brain injury. J Neurotrauma 10:263–271
9. Clifton GL, Miller ER, Choi SC, Levin HS, McCauley S, Smith KR Jr, Muizelaar JP, Wagner FC Jr, Marion DW, Luerssen TG, Chesnut RM, Schwartz M (2001) Lack of effect of induction of hypothermia after acute brain injury. N Engl J Med 344:556–563
10. Dempsey IRJ, Combs DJ, Maley ME, Cowen DE, Roy MW, Donaldson DL (1987) Moderate hypothermia reduces postischemic edema development and leukotriene production. Neurosurgery 21:177–181
11. Dietrich WD, Busto R, Halley M, Valdes I (1990) The importance of brain temperature in alterations of the blood–brain barrier following cerebral ischemia. J Neuropathol Exp Neurol 49:486–497
12. Dietrich WD, Busto R, Valdes I, Loor Y (1990) Effects of normothermic versus mild hypothermic forebrain ischemia in rats. Stroke 21:1318–1325
13. Dietrich WD, Busto R, Alonse O, Pita-Loor Y, Globus MY-T, Ginsberg MD (1991) Intraischemic brain hypothermia promotes postischemic metabolic recovery and somatosensory circuit activation. J Cereb Blood Flow Metab 11:S846
14. Fay T (1945) Observations on generalized refrigeration in cases of severe cerebral trauma. Res Publ Ass Nerv Dis 24:611–619
15. Hayashi N (1995) Cerebral hypothermia treatment. In: Hayashi N (ed) Cerebral hypothermia treatment. Sogo Igaku, Tokyo, pp 1–105
16. Hayashi N (1996) Advance of cerebral hypothermia treatment. J Critical Med 8:295–300
17. Hayashi N (1997) Prevention of vegetation after severe head trauma and stroke by combination therapy of cerebral hypothermia and activation of immune-dopaminergic nervous system. Proceedings of the 6th annual meeting of Society for Treatment of Coma 6:133–145
18. Hayashi N (2000) Enhanced neuronal damage in severely brain injured patients by hypothalamus, pituitary, and adrenal axis neuro-hormonal changes. In: Hayashi N (ed) Brain hypothermia. Springer, Berlin Heidelberg New York Tokyo, pp 3–26
19. Hayashi N (2000) The clinical issue and effectiveness of brain hypothermia treatment for severe brain injured patients. In: Hayashi N (ed) Brain hypothermia. Springer, Berlin Heidelberg New York Tokyo, pp 121–151
20. Hayashi N, Hirayama T, Utagawa A (1994) The cerebral thermo-pooling and hypothermia treatment of critical head injury patients. In: Nagai H (ed) Intracranial pressure IX. Springer, Berlin Heidelberg New York Tokyo, pp 589–599
21. Hayashi N, Hirayama T, Utagawa T, Ohata M (1994) Systemic management of cerebral edema based on a new concept in severe head injury patients. Acts Neurochir [Suppl] 60:541–543
22. Hayashi N, Kinoshita K, Shibuya T (1997) The prevention of cerebral thermo-pooling, damage of A10 nervous system, and free radical reactions by control of brain tissue temperature in severely brain injured patients. In: Teelken AW (ed) Neurochemistry. Plenum, New York, pp 97–103
23. Jiang JY, Lyeth BG, Kapasi MZ, Jenkins LW, Povlishock JT (1992) Moderate hypothermia reduces blood–brain barrier disruption following traumatic brain injury in the rat. Acta Neuropathol Berl 84:495–500
24. Kristian T, Katsura K, Siesjo BK (1992) The influence of moderate hypothermia on cellular calcium uptake in complete ischaemia: implications for the excitotoxic hypothesis. Acta Physiol Scand 146:531–532
25. Kuroiwa T, Bonnekoh P, Hossmann K-A (1990) Prevention of postischemic hypothermia prevents ischemic injury of CA1 neurons in gerbils. J Cereb Blood Flow Metab 10:550–556
26. Lazoethes G, Campan L (1958) Hypothermia in the treatment of craniocerebral traumatism. J Neurosurg 15:162–167
27. Lel B, Tan X, Cai H, Xu Q, Guo Q (1994) Effect of moderate hypothermia on lipid peroxidation in canine brain tissue after cardiac arrest and resuscitation. Stroke 25:147–152
28. Longhead WM, Sweet WH, White JC, Brewster WR (1955) The use of hypothermia in surgical treatment of cerebral vascular lesions. J Neurosurg 12:240–255
29. Marion DW, Obrist WD, Carlier PM, Penrod LE, Darby JM (1993) The uses of moderate therapeutic hypothermia

for patients with severe head injuries: a preliminary report. J Neurosurg 79:354–362
30. Marion DW, Penrod LE, Kelsey SF, Obrist WD, Kochanek PM, Palmer AM, Wisniewski SR, Dekosky ST (1997) Treatment of traumatic brain injury with moderate hypothermia. N Engl J Med 336:540–546
31. Mitani A, Kadoya F, Kataoka K (1991) Temperature dependence of hypoxia-induced calcium accumulation in gerbil hippocampal slices. Brain Res 562:159–163
32. Rosomoff HL (1957) Hypothermia and cerebral vascular lesions. II. Experimental interruption followed by induction of hypothermia. AMA Arch Neurol Psychiatr 78: 454–464
33. Rosomoff HL (1959) Protective effects of hypothermia against pathological processes of the nervous system. Ann NY Acad Sci 80:475–486
34. Rosomoff HL (1983) Synaptic activity mediates death of hypoxic neurons. Science 220:236–237
35. Rosomoff HL, Holaday DA (1954) Cerebral blood flow and cerebral oxygen consumption during hypothermia. Am J Physiol 179:85–88
36. Swan H, Zeavin I, Blount SG (1953) Surgery by direct vision in the open heart during hypothermia. JAMA 153:1081–1086
37. Widmann R, Miyazawa T, Hossmann KA (1993) Protective effect of hypothermia on hippocampal injury after 30 minutes of forebrain ischemia in rats is mediated by postischemic recovery of protein synthesis. J Neurochem 61:200–206

22. Secondary Brain Injury Mechanism of Hypothalamus–Pituitary–Adrenal Axis Neurohormonal Activation in Severely Brain-Injured Patients

As a brain injury mechanism, direct modes of brain damage such as tissue laceration, ischemia, and hypoxia grouped as primary brain injuries, and secondary brain injuries such as brain edema [18], cerebral blood flow (CBF) disturbances [20,25], reduced cerebral perfusion pressure (CPP) [10], and elevation of intracranial pressure (ICP) [20] have been discussed. Formation of free radicals, blood–brain barrier (BBB) dysfunction [7,26], release of neurotoxic excitatory amino acids [1,3,11,19,22–24], and increased levels of intracellular Ca^{2+} [4] have been demonstrated as promoting factors of this brain injury mechanism. Therefore, these pathophysiological changes have been considered as initial targets of treatment in the intensive care unit (ICU). This management concept for treatment of severely brain-injured patients has long been supported by many animal studies. However, in recent clinical studies of severely brain-injured patients, a hypothalamus–pituitary–adrenal (HPA) axis neurohormonal brain injury mechanism was observed (Fig. 6) [5,6,8,13–15]. The selective damage of the dopamine A10 nervous system associated with the occurrence of vegetation is also another new topic [12–15,17]. However, these brain injury mechanisms have only been recorded in severely brain-injured patients, and have not been recorded in experimental animal brain injury models because stress to the HPA axis is reduced by anesthesia in experimental animal studies. Thus, the nature of brain damage that in cases in which occurs excess neurohormonal endoclinological reactions exert stress upon the HPA axis is of interest.

In this section, new findings of secondary brain injury mechanism and promoting factors such as cardiopulmonary dysfunction caused by catecholamine surge [14], stress to HPA axis [6,14,15], elevation of brain tissue temperature by brain thermo-pooling [12,16,17], increased brain tissue lactate levels caused by insulin-resistant hyperglycemia [14,15], masking of neuronal hypoxia even with normal control of CBF, PaO_2, oxygen delivery, and CPP [14,15], and hyperglycemia–vasopressin-associated BBB dysfunction [14] are discussed.

Catecholamine Surge and Cardiopulmonary Dysfunction

Under emergency conditions and with severe brain damage, the human body responds automatically to minimize brain damage by neurohormone release from the HPA axis (Fig. 7). The catecholamines such as norepinephrine, epinephrine, and dopamine are released to maintain cardiopulmonary function and neuronal oxygenation. Adequate release of catecholamines should maintain sufficient CBF and coronary circulation, and can minimize brain damage caused by trauma, cerebral occlusive stroke, brain hypoxia, and cardiac arrest. The same neuroprotection responses occur even in cases of severe brain damage.

However, in cases of severe brain injury, the catecholamine surge occurs at 50 to 200 times higher than the normal level (Fig. 8) [14]. These excess releases of catecholamines lead to various secondary brain injury mechanisms rather than neuroprotection. Unstable cardiopulmonary function, elevation of brain tissue temperature by brain thermo-pooling, insulin-resistant hyperglycemia, ineffective oxygen inhalation caused by hemoglobin dysfunction, increased levels of brain tissue glucose and lactate, and BBB dysfunction with vasopressin release are the main new findings of these brain injury mechanisms [12,14,15]. These various brain injury mechanisms are initially triggered by excess release of catecholamines after stimulation of the HPA axis. The severity of these brain injury mechanisms is in proportion to the severity of the stress to the HPA axis (Fig. 9). To design a management strategy for these brain injury mechanisms, consideration must be given to the severity and the time-window pattern of catecholamine surge. However, based on medical ethics, it is very difficult to study changes in the time window of catecholamine surge. We have collected information about changes in the time window of catecholamine surge in comatose patients that were admitted to the emergency medical center at different postinjury times (Fig. 8).

The changes in time window of each catecholamine surge do not follow the same pattern. Epinephrine

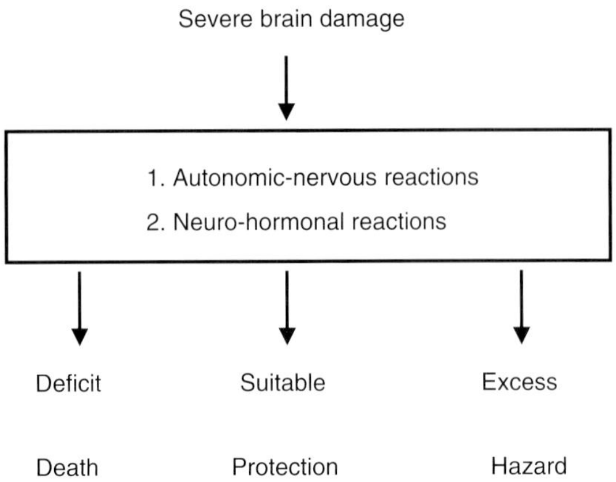

Fig. 6. The three stress reactions after severe brain damage throughout hypothalamus-pituitary-adrenal axis

increased within 3 h of injury, nor epinephrine increased within 1 h, dopamine increased after more than 3 h, and vasopressin was increased within 2 h. Therefore, at 3 h after accident or cerebral ischemic insults, a dopamine-dominant system maintains systemic circulation that includes brain circulation [14]. One of the hazards of dopamine-dominant systemic circulation is blood shift into the intra-abdominal cavity caused by visceral vascular dilatation. These blood shifts in systemic circulation caused by excess release of dopamine mask brain ischemia even at normal blood pressure and normal CPP.

Reported undesirable effects arising from excess release of catecholamines include cardiac dysfunction caused by coronary vasoconstriction, and myocytolysis [9]. On the electrocardiogram (Ecg), temporary down-

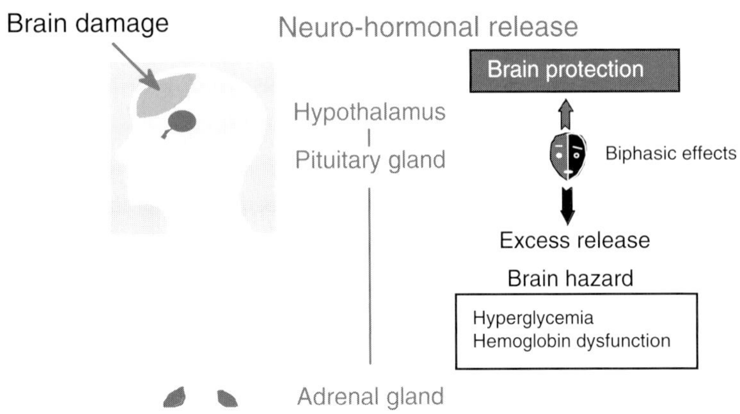

Fig. 7. Biphasic effects of hypothalamus-pituitary-adrenal (HPA) axis neurohormonal reactions after severe brain damage. The suitable release of catecholamines minimizes the brain injury. However, excess release of catecholamines and vasopressin produces insulin-resistant hyperglycemia, increased brain tissue lactate, and slow release of bound oxygen from hemoglobin caused by reduced levels of 2,3-diphosphoglycerate (DPG)

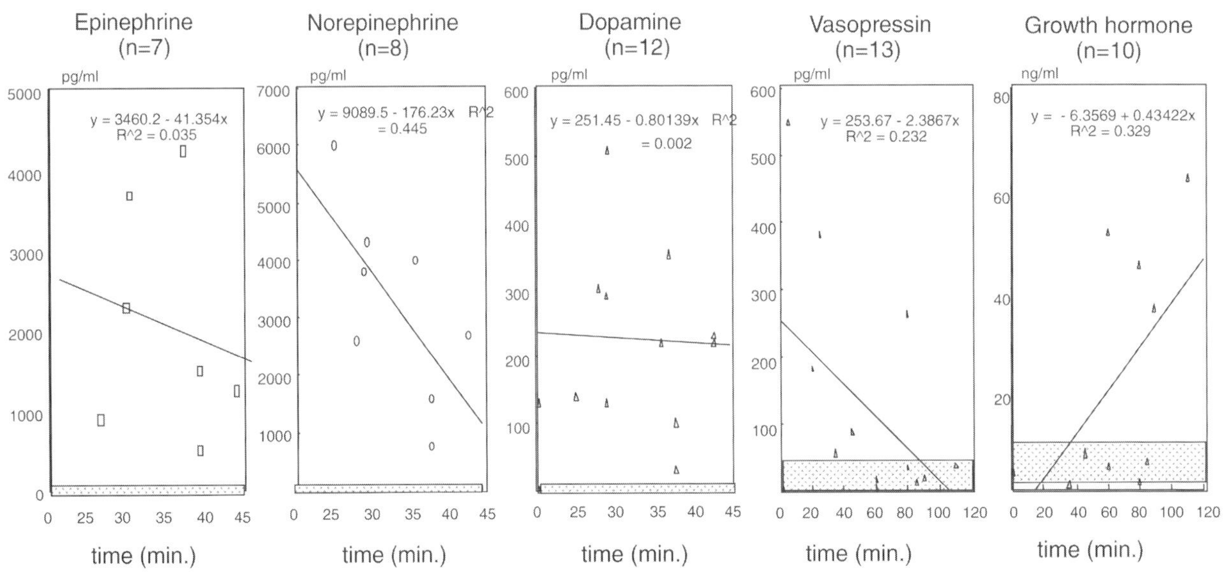

Fig. 8. The changes of serum catecholamines, vasopressin, and growth hormone in coma patients at time after severe brain damage. *Shaded area*, standard values

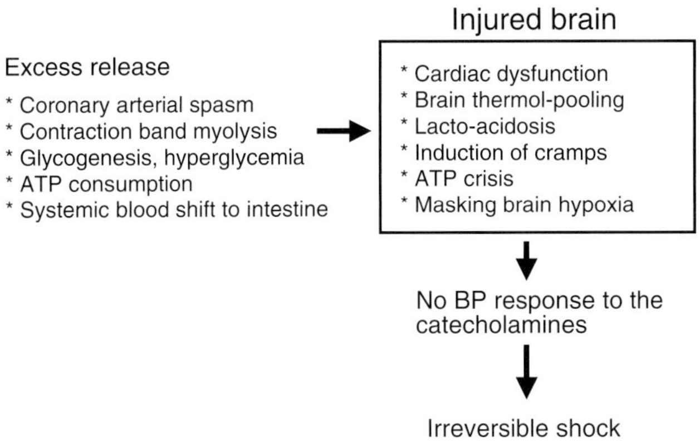

Fig. 9. The negative effects of hypothalamus-pituitary-adrenal axis neurohormonal reactions to the injured brain tissue

ward shift of the ST-junction indicative of cardiac ischemia, and elevation of the ST-junction indicative of cardiac infarction and tachycardia were recorded within 1 h after accident. Contraction band myonecrosis is another mechanism of cardiac dysfunction caused by catecholamine surge, and has been reported previously [9]. These clinical issues that are associated with catecholamine surge are not only limited to unstable cardiopulmonary dysfunction, but are also related to lower CPP, increased brain tissue temperature caused by brain thermo-pooling [8,12,14,17], insulin-resistant hyperglycemia, masked neuronal hypoxia even with normal PaO_2, ICP, and CPP, and activated release of vasopressin. The brain damage associated with catecholamine surge develops soon after brain injury and continues for a long time. The time limit for management of catecholamine surge is approximately 3 h. However, at later than 3–6 h after severe brain damage, the effectiveness of management of catecholamine surge will be reduced.

All these data suggest that the neurohormonal protective system of systemic circulation was limited to within 1–3 h and that the possibility of hazardous excess release of vasoactive neurohormones in severely brain injured patients occurs 3–6 h after insult.

The Alteration of Brain Tissue Temperature and Brain Thermo-pooling

Change in brain tissue temperature is dynamically influenced by the body temperature (core temperature), CPP which carries the core temperature into the brain tissue, brain metabolism, and CBF which is the final regulator to wash out elevated brain tissue temperature [14]. Under physiological conditions, brain tissue temperature was recorded as the highest in the body at 37.0° ±0.29°C, while the core temperature was 36.3° ±0.23°C, the tympanic membrane temperature was 36.7° ± 0.27°C, and the bladder temperature was 36.6° ±0.25°C. Normal brain tissue temperature is 0.2°–0.6°C higher than the core temperature (blood temperature). In most cases, brain tissue temperature is consistently maintained very close to the body core temperature. This means that brain tissue temperature is mainly determined by the blood temperature. Increases in brain tissue temperature are prevented by the CBF washout mechanism. CBF works as a bifunctional regulator of brain tissue temperature: one function is as a carrier of thermal energy into the brain, while the other is to wash out excess brain tissue temperature to prevent the accumulation of thermal energy (Fig. 10).

The carotid blood temperature is usually very similar to the brain tissue temperature; however, if the brain tissue temperature becomes elevated because of a reduction in the CBF washout mechanism, a discrepancy between the carotid blood temperature and blood tissue temperature arises. In such cases, jugular venous blood temperature becomes very close to the brain tissue temperature (Fig. 11). As a clinical monitor of brain tissue temperature, tympanic membrane temperature is monitored at the bedside. However, in cases of elevated brain tissue temperature caused by CBF disturbance, tympanic membrane temperature is not a good indicator of brain tissue temperature because the tympanic membrane temperature is a good indirect measure of carotid blood temperature.

For indirect monitoring of brain tissue temperature, measurement of jugular venous blood temperature (JvBT) is recommended because mean values of the two temperatures almost always coincide, except under special conditions in which internal jugular venous blood is lost to external circulation. A positive correlation was observed between changes in brain tissue temperature and tympanic membrane temperature and JvBT, although changes in brain tissue temperature more highly correlate to changes in JvBT than changes in tympanic membrane temperature (Fig. 11). During brain hypothermia treatment of treatable brain injuries, JvBT is very useful as a monitor of changes in brain tissue temperature. Under conditions in which JvBT does not accurately reflect brain tissue temperature, sensor position in the lower jugular venous vessels and terminal stages of poor or nonfilling of brain circulation may be recorded. In cases of terminal stage, severely elevated ICP markedly reduces the internal jugular venous circulation and causes blood contamination with extracranial venous blood by shunting.

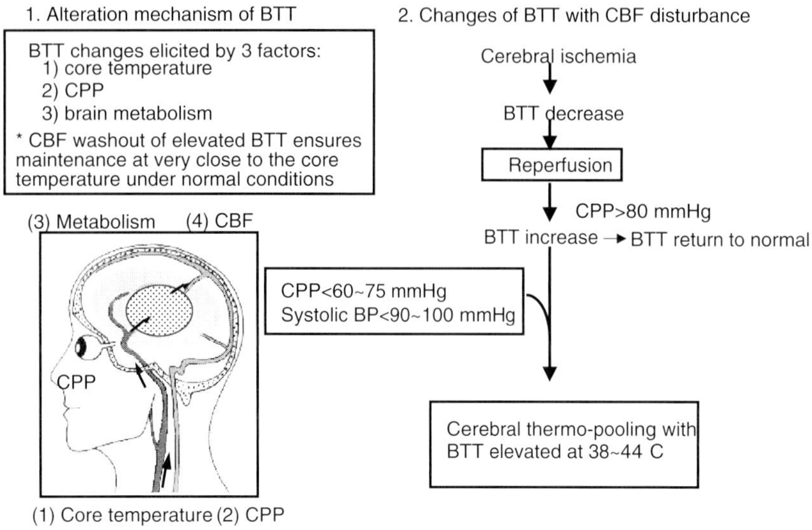

Fig. 10. The regulation mechanism of brain tissue temperature. *BTT*, brain tissue temperature; *CBF*, cerebral blood flow; *CPP*, cerebral perfusion pressure, *BP*, blood pressure

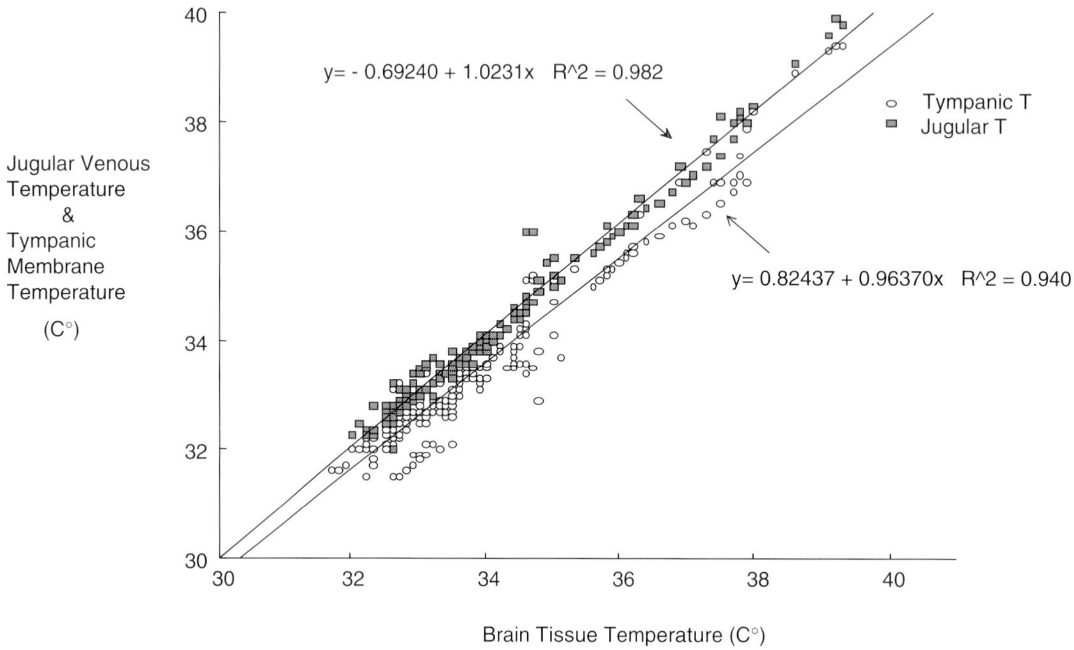

Fig. 11. The relationships between changes of brain tissue temperature, tympanic membrane temperature, and internal jugular venous blood temperature. The brain tissue temperature changes correlated to the internal jugular venous blood temperature more strongly than tympanic membrane temperature

In complete cerebral ischemia, lower brain tissue temperature can be monitored initially because transport of the core temperature is limited. However, incomplete brain ischemia elevates local brain tissue temperature by brain thermo-pooling. Causes of brain thermo-pooling have been found to be fever above 38°C, reperfusion, systolic blood pressure lower than 90–100 mmHg in adults (<60–90 mmHg in children), and CPP less than 60–75 mmHg. Brain tissue temperature changes dynamically at the acute stage of severe brain injury.

Figure 12 shows a typical case of brain thermo-pooling after severe brain injury without elevation of ICP. The brain tissue temperature was elevated to 42°C because of insufficient CPP. The patient was a 56-year-old man. After a traffic accident, he presented immedi-

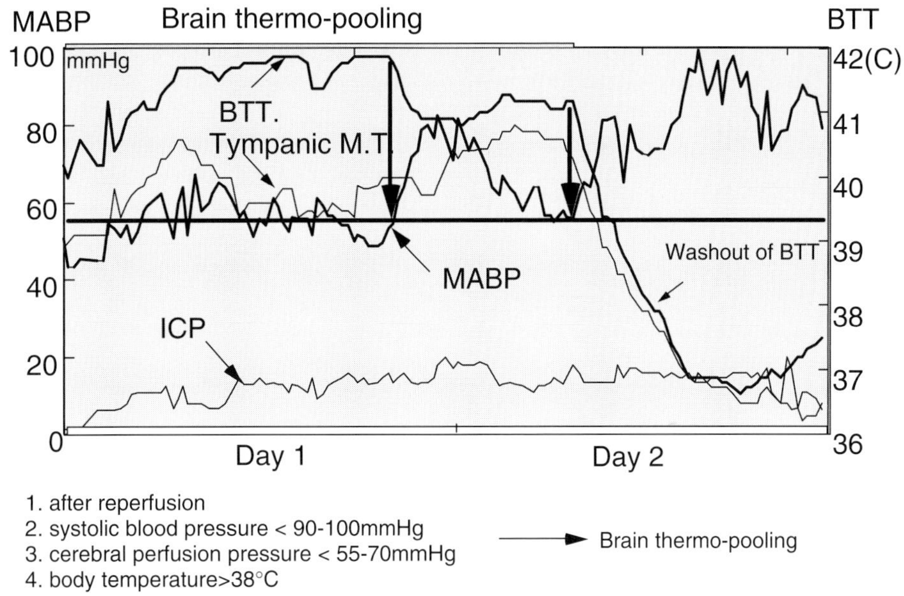

Fig. 12. The tissue temperature increased to 42°C by brain thermo-pooling for 35 h after brain injury. *ICP*, intracranial pressure; *MABP*, mean arterial blood pressure; *BTT*, brain tissue temperature; *MT*, membrane temperature

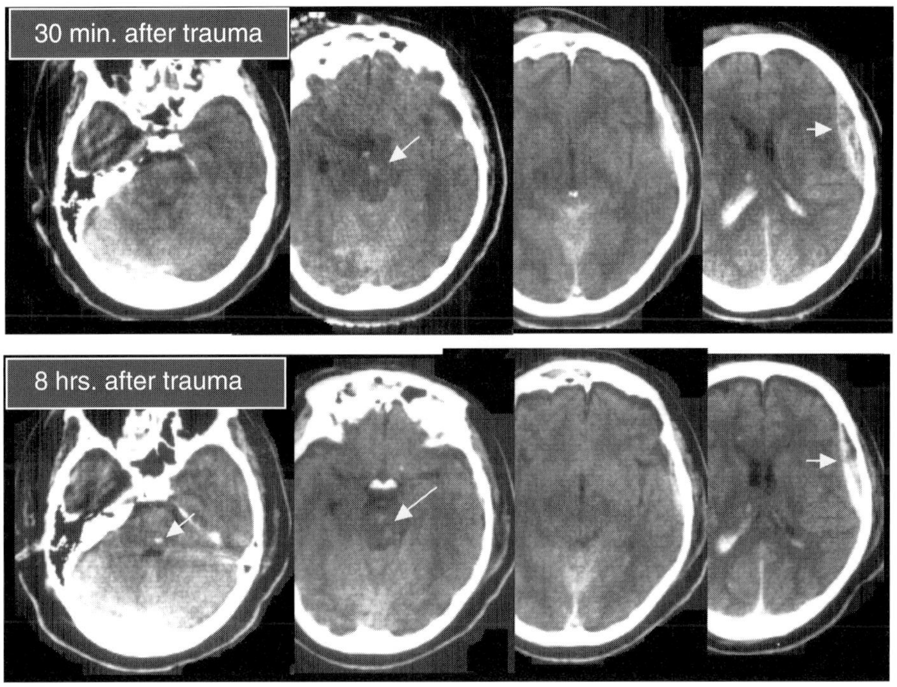

Fig. 13. Changes in the computed tomography scan after a traffic accident in a 56-year-old man. The diagnosis is epidural hematoma, diffuse brain injury, and brain stem hemorrhage (*arrows*).

ately in shock with multiple traumas, pulmonary contusion, diffuse brain injury, and small epidural hematoma (Fig. 13). ICP was controlled to below 20 mmHg; however, control of hypotension caused by low cardiac output after 6 h was difficult, and mean arterial blood pressure (MABP) below 55 mmHg produced typical brain thermo-pooling for 24 h. In this patient, the critical level of MABP required to wash out the elevated brain tissue temperature was 55 mmHg.

We started the management of brain tissue temperature and brain hypothermia treatment after identifying brain thermo-pooling as a secondary brain injury mechanism. Previous neuroprotective treatment such as administration of steroid, mannitol, anti-Ca^{2+} reagent, and radical scavengers was not expected to have any effect on the elevated brain tissue temperature of 42°C (Fig. 12).

Insulin-Resistant Hyperglycemia

Catecholamine surge increases systemic circulation and blood pressure by promoting the metabolic change of adenosine triphosphate (ATP) to cyclic adenosine monophosphate (AMP) and increases the metabolic source of brain serum glucose (Fig. 14). These metabolic changes help maintain neuronal function and minimize the neuronal damage in severely brain-injured patients. However, severe hyperglycemia is a drastic metabolic change, and introduces negative factors for neuronal recovery [14]. A mechanism for the production of stress-associated hyperglycemia is given in Fig. 15. Cyclic AMP (cAMP) is metabolized and finally glucose is produced after consumption of ATP and glycogen in major organs. Epinephrine is a major factor in the production of hyperglycemia after catecholamine

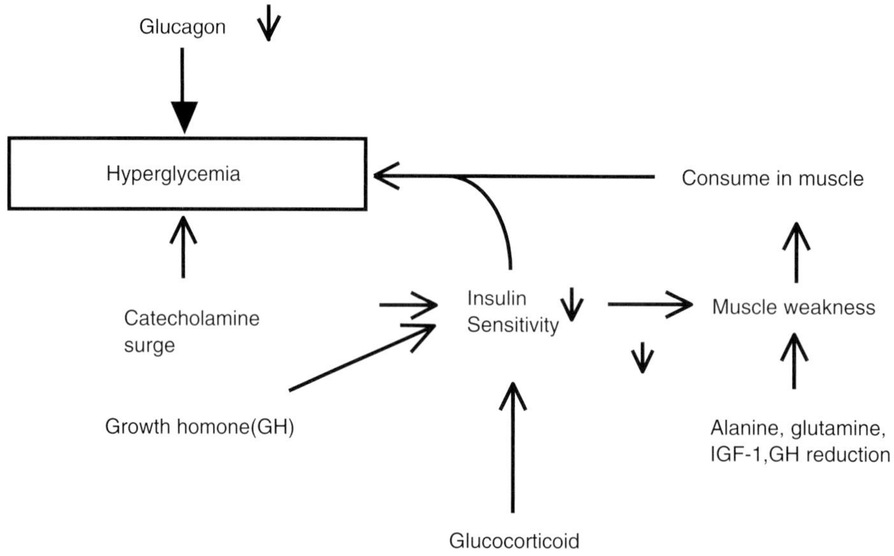

Fig. 14. Mechanism of hyperglycemia after severe brain damage. *IGF-1*, insulin-like growth factor

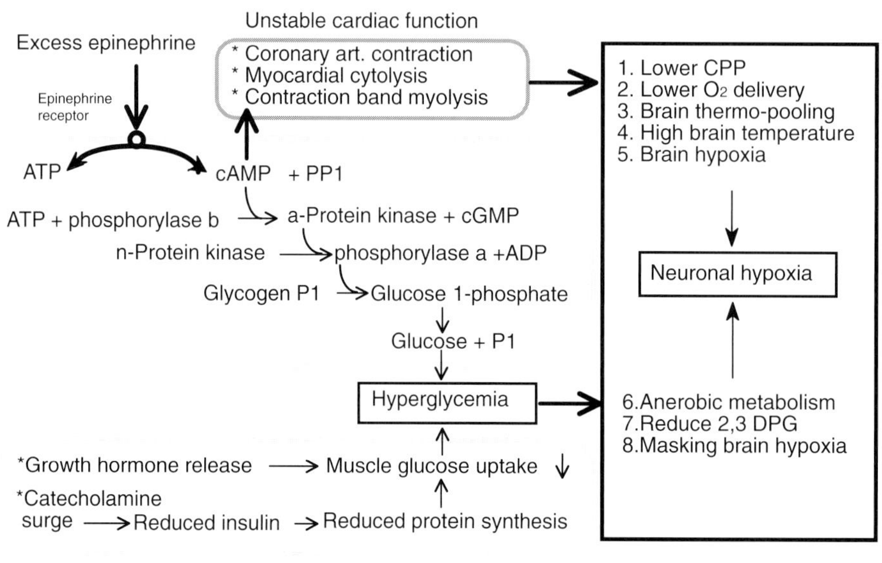

Fig. 15. The cardiopulmonary and metabolic changes following excess release of epinephrine after severe brain injury

surge. Therefore, serum hyperglycemia could be evaluated as an indirect parameter of the severity of catecholamine surge and stress to the HPA neurohormonal system.

Hyperglycemia after harmful stress is an unavoidable metabolic change in severely brain-injured patients (Fig. 16). On the other hand, absence of hyperglycemia after severe brain injury means harmful stress may not be so serious even with unconsciousness or no time to make a physical protective response by rapid cardiac arrest. Because hyperglycemia is unavoidable except in cases of sudden death within 3–5 min, monitoring of hyperglycemia severity is very useful to diagnose the presence of hypothalamus stress and other hyperglycemia-associated pathophysiological changes.

Reported hyperglycemia-related pathophysiological changes include increased brain tissue glucose and lactate levels, increased lactate in systemic circulation, activated anaerobic metabolism, low hemoglobin-2,3-diphosphoglycerate (Hb-DPG) level, ineffective oxygen administration, increased vasopressin release with BBB dysfunction, increased proinflammatory cytokine levels, and susceptibility to infection [12,14,16,17]. These clinical issues are discussed in other sections of this book.

Hyperglycemia in the acute stage of severe brain injury suggests the presence of damage to the HPA axis, catecholamine surge, and low levels of ATP in the liver and heart. The ATP crisis with hyperglycemia in the liver and heart, however, causes an unstable cardiopulmonary circulation with lower CPP, blood shift into the intestine, and reduced reactivity to anti-shock drugs. Serum glucose levels above 230 mg/dl at the acute stage is indicative of hyperglycemia and, in our clinical studies, was closely related to the deterioration of consciousness into coma (Fig. 17). Young children and old-age patients are more strongly correlated to clinical worsening than adults as shown in Fig. 16.

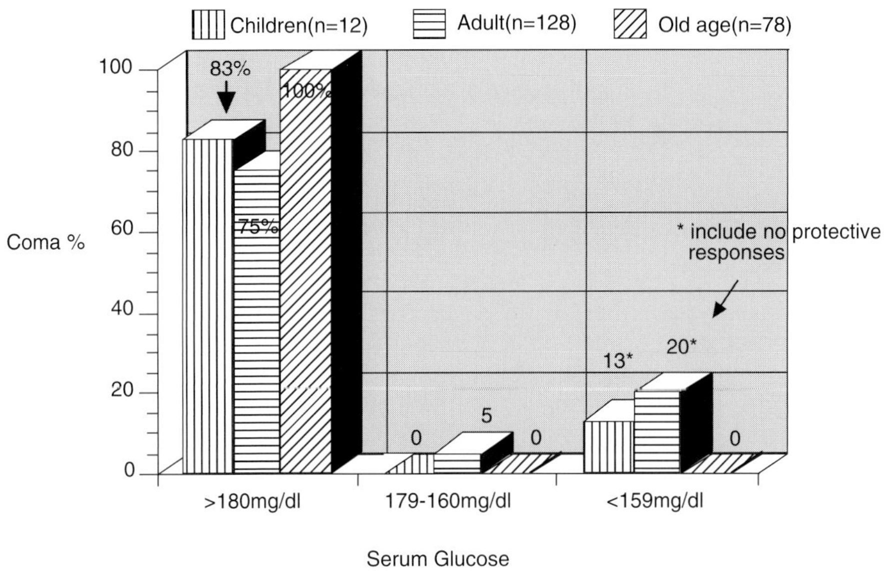

Fig. 16. The relationships between changes of stress-associated hyperglycemia and occurrence of coma after severe brain injury

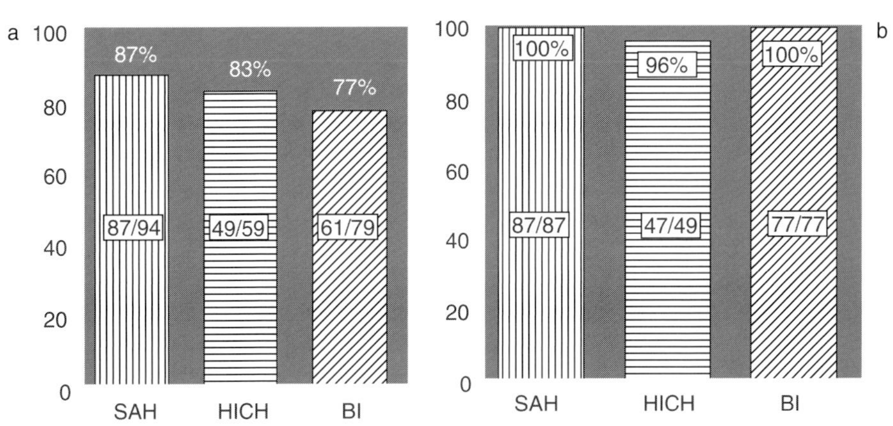

Fig. 17. Stress-associated hyperglycemia in severely brain-injured patients. **a** The incidence of hyperglycemia in cases of GCS 3–9 (n=232). **b** The percentage of coma in stress-associated hyperglycemia (>180 mg/dl)

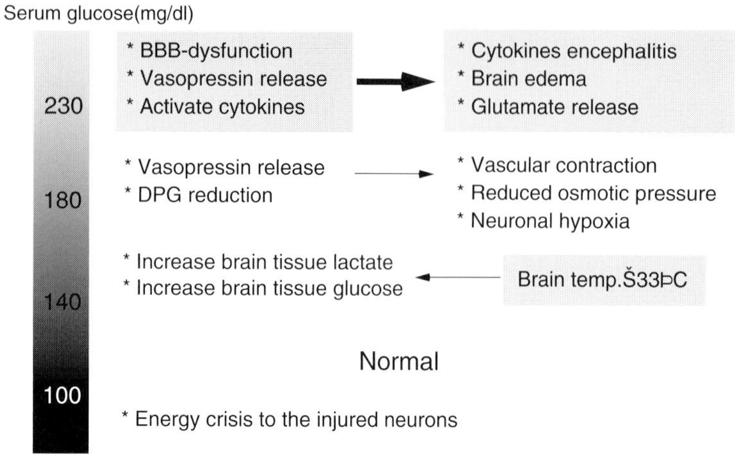

Fig. 18. Brain damage caused by hyperglycemia at acute stage in severe brain injury

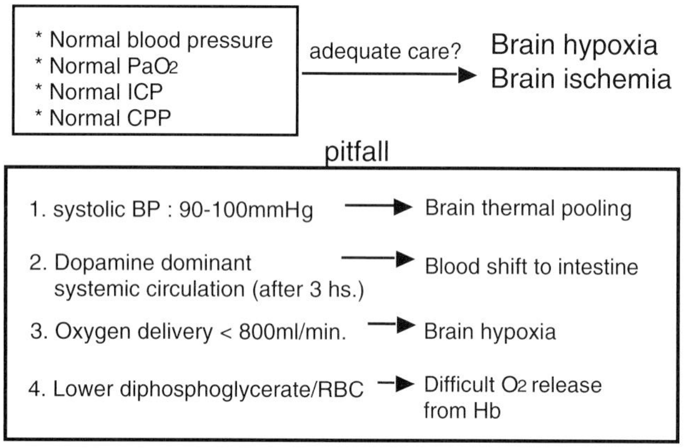

Fig. 19. The pitfall of management of brain hypoxia and ischemia. *ICP*, inracranial pressure; *SBP*, systolic blood pressure; *CPP*, cerebral perfusion pressure

The evaluation of serum glucose levels to determine worsening of various neuronal pathophysiologic changes in injured brain tissue is summarized in Fig. 18. During brain hypothermia treatment, the serum glucose level must be maintained between 120 and 140 mg/dl. At glucose serum levels above 180 mg/dl, hyperglycemia directly affects the level of consciousness, and at levels above 230 mg/dl, hyperglycemia promotes BBB dysfunction, brain edema, and cytokine encephalitis [14,15]. If pulmonary or systemic infections complicate severe hyperglycemia, increased proinflamatory cytokines in the peripheral blood can easily penetrate the BBB and promote cytokine encephalitis with uncontrollable increases in glutamate in injured brain tissue. In this situation, we have never observed good recovery even with moderate brain hypothermia treatment at 32–34°C.

The correct management of hyperglycemia, prevention of inflammation of vascular endothelial cells, and control of BBB dysfunction must all occur simultaneously. Administration of insulin is fundamental to the treatment of hyperglycemia. However, hyperglycemia that occurs by stimulation of the HPA axis is resistant to insulin in severely brain-injured patients. The detailed mechanism of the insulin resistance of hyperglycemia associated with HPA stimulation is not clear.

Excess release of epinephrine, reduced sensitivity to insulin caused by adrenocorticotropic hormone (ACTH) release, reduced consumption of serum glucose by weakened skeletal muscle and liver dysfunction all act to worsen hyperglycemia. Special considerations for ICU management of insulin-resistant hyperglycemia are necessary. Management strategies are discussed in Chap. 44.

Masking Neuronal Hypoxia in Brain Injury

In severely brain-injured patients, brain hypoxia occurs in the primary injured tissue and is accompanied by abrupt cell swelling with K^+ ion release causing Na^+ channels to open, synaptic paralysis leading to respiratory arrest, and low cerebral perfusion elicited by cardiac dysfunction with a 50–200-fold increase in catecholamine surge. ICU management to maintain normal PaO_2, normal ICP, and normal CPP has long been considered as reasonable treatment. However, this management is not correct, especially in severe cases (Fig. 19) because neuronal hypoxia can also occur because of slow release of oxygen from hemoglobin. Our recent clinical studies confirmed causes of neuronal hypoxia in injured brain tissue as elevation of brain tissue temperature by brain thermo-pooling (Figs. 10, 12), systemic circulation shift into the intestinal organs, lower oxygen delivery by reduced cardiac output, and hemoglobin dysfunction caused by reduced Hb-DPG levels (Fig. 20). All of these new mechanisms of neuronal hypoxia are associated with stress to the HPA axis [14]. However, in experimental animal brain injury models, stress to the HPA axis, catecholamine surge, release of vasopressin, and hemoglobin dysfunction are not apparent or are limited by anesthesia. Because this neuronal hypoxia in injured brain tissue occurs even with normal control of PaO_2, ICP, CPP, and CBF, these neuronal hypoxia are known as "masking brain hypoxia" and are understood as a one of the inadequacies of ICU management of severe brain damage caused by trauma, stroke, hypoxia, or cardiac arrest.

As previously described in this book, after reperfusion, an elevated body temperature of more than 38°C combined with a systolic blood pressure less than 90–100 mmHg is a cause of brain thermo-pooling. Also, activation of the dopamine-dominant systemic circulation is a cause of systemic circulation shift into the abdominal intestinal organs. Although dopamine increases cardiac output, it causes selective vasodilatation of intestinal vasculature and renal blood vessels. This specific dopamine-dominant catecholamine imbalance makes possible a blood shift into the intestine rather than the brain even with normal CPP and normal oxygen delivery. Clinically, this phenomenon is recorded by elevated rectal temperature rather than brain tissue temperature or tympanic membrane temperature [17]. Under normal conditions, brain tissue temperature is always higher than rectal or bladder temperature. It is very difficult for brain-injured patients to survive when the brain tissue temperature/rectal temperature ratio (or tympanic membrane temperature/rectal temperature ratio) becomes less than 0.96 [17].

To avoid masking brain hypoxia, management of these parameters is important in ICU. The critical level of oxygen delivery for successful ICU management of brain hypoxia is more than 700–800 ml/min [15]. This criteria applies during brain hypothermia and also at normothermic brain tissue temperature. In our clinical studies, differences in oxygen consumption between the nonsurvival and survival groups were not observed, although management of oxygen delivery above 700 ml/min was more successful than a rate below 600 ml/min, as shown in Fig. 21. Maintenance of oxygen delivery at the acute stage of severe brain injury is not easy because of reduced cardiac output and/or lower hemoglobin values in systemic circulation. Many factors have been nominated as causes of reductions in cardiac output, such as damage of cardiac muscles by excess release of catecholamines (associated with coronary arterial spasm), contraction myocytolysis, difficult

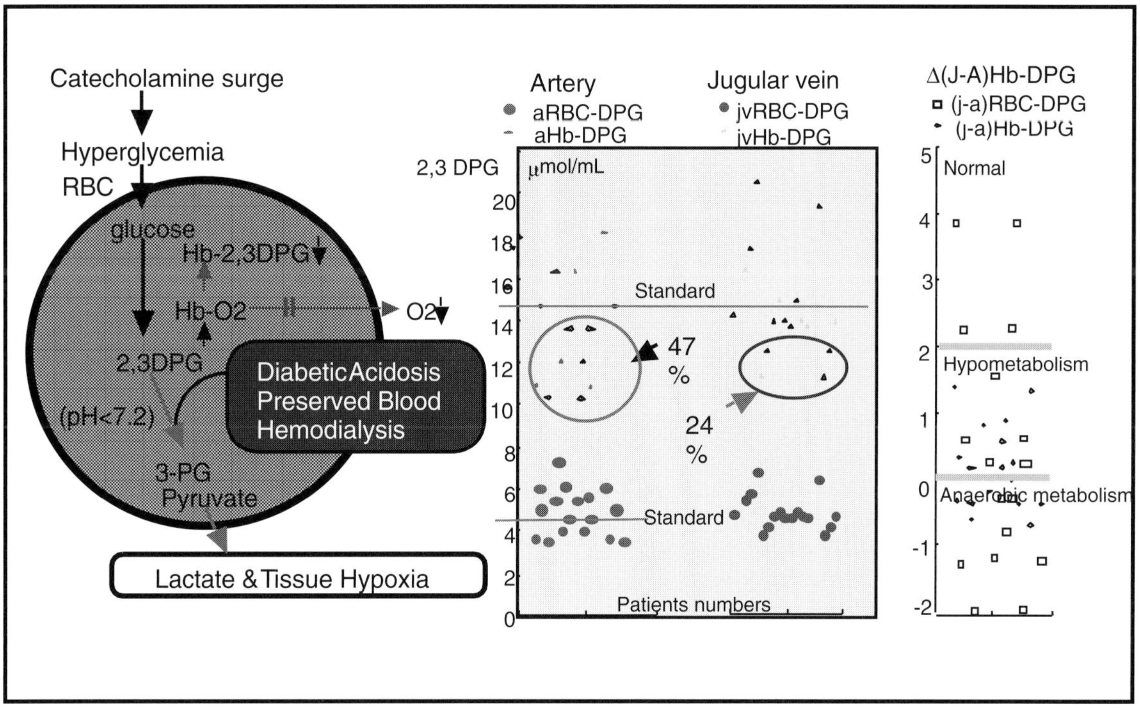

Fig. 20. The reduction of DPG after severe brain injury. DPG is a regulator for the release of bound oxygen from hemoglobin. Diabetic acidosis, blood transfusion, and hemodialysis are causes of reduction of DPG in RBC

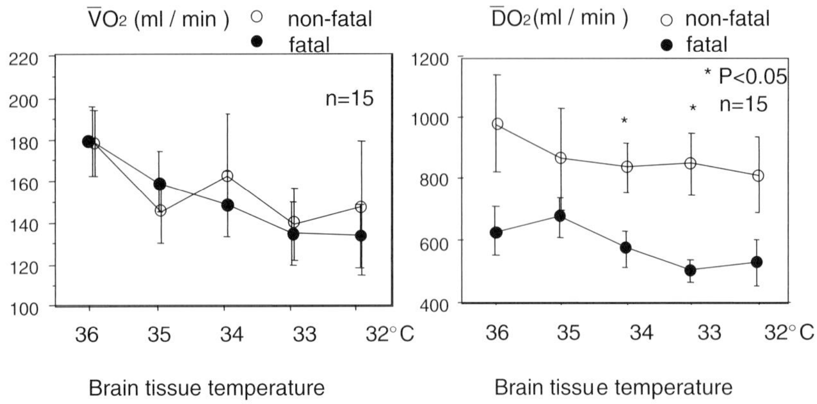

Fig. 21. The difference of oxygen consumption ($\bar{V}O_2$) and oxygen delivery ($\bar{D}O_2$) in fatal and non-fatal groups following various brain hypothermia

expansion of the heart caused by cardiac muscle contraction, and metabolic changes to cardiac muscles. Excess release of catecholamines produces two metabolic disturbances: markedly increased cyclic AMP levels, and hyperglycemia with consumption of ATP and glycogen in major organs, heart, and liver (Fig. 15). Increased levels of cyclic AMP immediately produces vascular contraction and cardiac ischemia due to coronary spasm and contraction myocytolysis. A similar pattern of ST-junction elevation caused by cardiac infarction and prolongation of the QT interval to 450 mm/sec are recorded on the ECG.

Hemoglobin dysfunction is a major issue for management of severely brain-injured patients. Slow release of oxygen from hemoglobin causes ineffective oxygen inhalation and respiratory management. In our recent clinical studies with injuries on the GCS less than 6, hemoglobin dysfunction was recorded in 41% of patients as shown by low arterial blood Hb-DPG. In 24% of these patients, markedly reduced jugular venous Hb-DPG was recorded (Fig. 20).

Our preliminary studies suggested that reductions in Hb-DPG are caused by severe ketoacidosis (pH < 7.2), hyperglycemia with serum glucose levels above 230 mg/dl, massive blood transfusion, and continuous hemodiafiltration therapy. In most cases of reduced Hb-DPG, the complication of increased serum lactate level was recorded [14]. This harmful stress-induced hyperglycemia with reduced DPG must be considered as an important cause of masking neuronal hypoxia in initial ICU management.

From studies of stress-induced catecholamine surge, we must appreciate that control of ICP, CPP, and PaO_2 to normal levels is not always the correct management for the survival of severely injured neurons. The control of brain tissue temperature to 32°–34°C can only prevent excess release of catecholamines and improve management of masking neuronal hypoxia.

The main purpose of brain hypothermia treatment is to halt or retard these pathophysiological changes by precise lowering of brain tissue temperature and to make available sufficient oxygen and metabolic substrates. Previous procedures used to control ICP and prevent brain edema are inadequate for handling masking neuronal hypoxia and pathophysiological changes that are related to brain thermo-pooling.

Blood-Brain Barrier Dysfunction from Vasopressin Release

As causes of BBB dysfunction, many factors have been postulated as contributors. Clearly, the shear and tensile strains of trauma may act directly upon the cerebral vessels and elicit both structural and functional changes. The traumatic events in the brain accompany catecholamine surge with accelerated metabolism of arachidonate and increased production of prostaglandin [23,25]. With the increased production of prostaglandin, there is concomitant production of oxygen radicals of which the super oxide anions figure prominently [26]. The super oxide anion has been clearly linked to many vascular abnormalities. With regard to the endothelium, the associated radical production has been linked to altered endothelial-dependent responses, alteration of BBB status, overt endothelial changes, and the potential for enhanced platelet aggregation [26]. All of these BBB dysfunction mechanisms were demonstrated on experimental animal models. In recent clinical studies using microdialysis, another neurohormonal BBB dysfunction mechanism was recorded.

Severe hyperglycemia occurs with catecholamine surge, and stimulates the feedback mechanism of macronutrient intake with increasing brain tissue glucose levels. This macronutrient feedback mechanism includes the release of vasopressin to reduce the elevated serum osmolarity, and the release of insulin to activate the consumption of serum glucose by skeletal muscles as shown in Fig. 22.

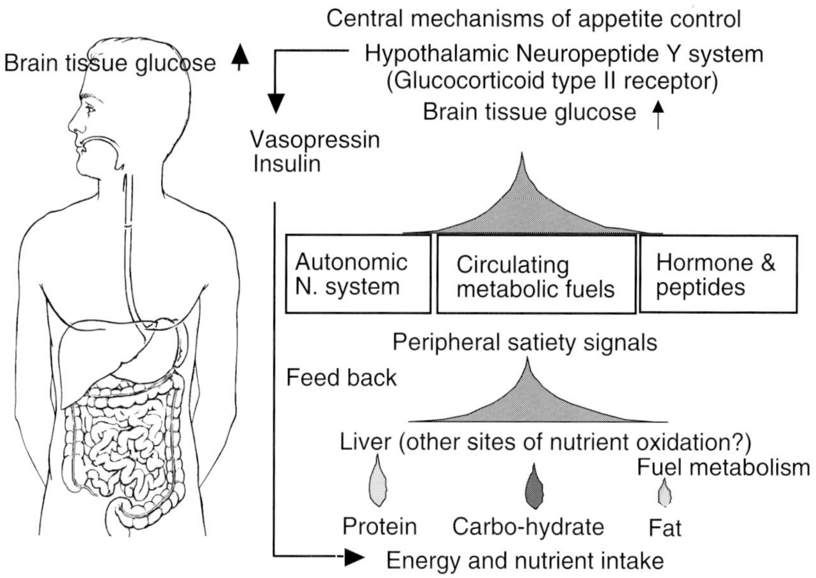

Fig. 22. The macronutrient feedback mechanism after nutrient intake and hyperglycemia

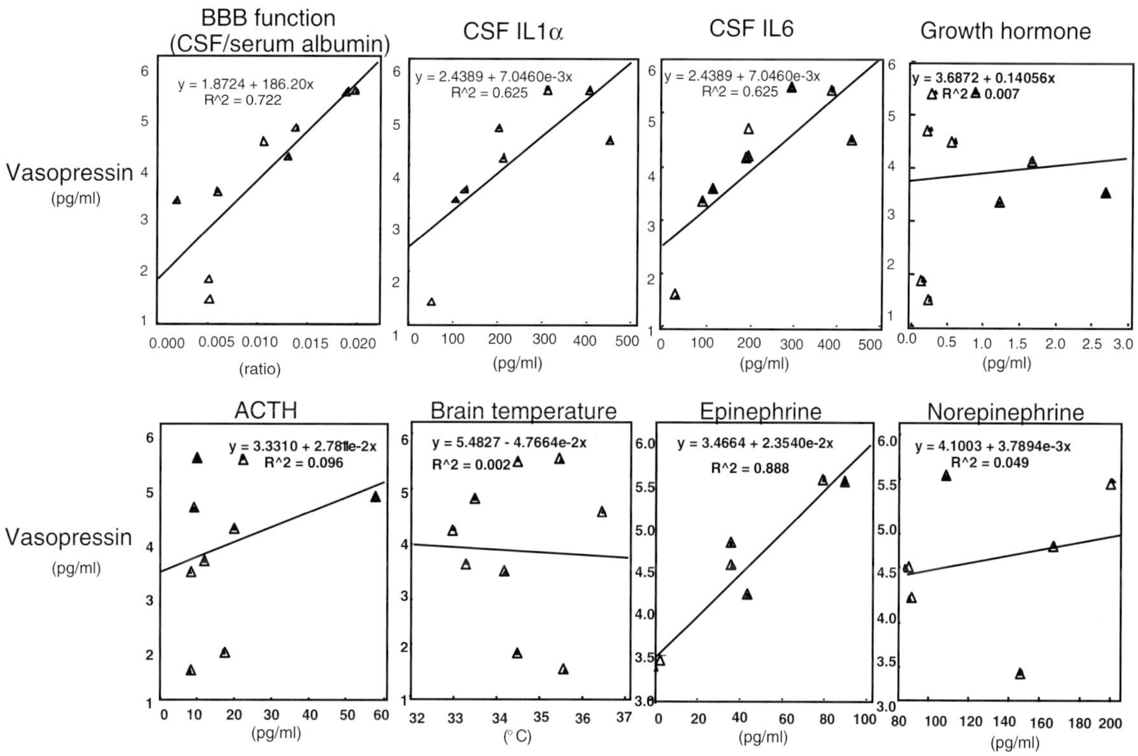

Fig. 23. The effect of excess release of vasopressin on blood–brain barrier (BBB) dysfunction, activation of cytokines, stress hormones, and brain tissue temperature. *CSF*, cerebrospinal fluid; *ACTH*, adrenocorticotropic hormone; *IL1*, interleukin 1; *IL6*, interleukin 6

The hypothalamus neuron endoclinological hormone, vasopressin, works not only as an antidiuretic hormone, but also causes vasoconstriction, stimulates proinflamatory cytokines [6], and changes the BBB function [14]. Our recent clinical studies using microdialysis suggested that the changes in brain tissue glucose level, CSF-IL6 IL-1, and BBB dysfunction are highly correlated with vasopressin release as shown in Fig. 23.

Abnormalities that were demonstrated in experimental animal studies and clinical studies include the profound irregularities in the course of vessels and the vascular basement membrane, changes in specific proteins and receptors associated with the cerebral endothelium, and increases in perivascular infiltration and brain edema.

To avoid the BBB dysfunction caused by vasopressin, control of the brain tissue glucose level is necessary. However, increases in the brain tissue glucose level are associated with many causes such as hyperglycemia, reduced consumption of brain tissue glucose in injured tissue, hypothermia, and changes to metabolic enzymes by acidosis ($pH < 7.2$). For the management of BBB dysfunction, all of these abnormal mechanisms of BBB dysfunction must be carefully controled.

Clinical studies have suggested that for the prevention of BBB dysfunction and related vasopressin release, the serum glucose level should be less than 230 mg/dl and the brain tissue glucose level should be less than 0.8 mmol/l (Fig. 23). The adequate serum glucose level for the prevention of brain tissue lactate accumulation is between 120 and 140 mg/dl.

The management of hyperglycemia is very important not only under the conditions of normothermia but also during hypothermia at the acute stage within 6 h of insult. Without good management of serum hyperglycemia and prevention of excess release of vasopressin, brain edema will be promoted by BBB dysfunction.

References

1. Baker AJ, Zornow MH, Scheller MS, Yaksh TL, Skilling SR, Smullin DH, Larson AA, Kuczenski R (1991) Changes in extracellular concentrations of glutamate, aspartate, glycine, dopamine, serotonin, and dopamine metabolites after transient global ischemia in the rat. J Neurochem 57:1370–1379
2. Beck B (2000) Quantitative and macronutrient-related regulation of hypothalamic neuropeptide Y, galanin and neurotensin. In: Berthoud HR, Seeley RJ (eds) Neural and metabolic control of macronutrient intake. CRC, Boca Raton, pp 455–464
3. Benveniste H, Drejer J, Schousboe A, Diemer NH (1984) Elevation of the extracellular concentrations of glutamate and aspartate in rat hippocampus during transient cerebral ischemia monitored by intracerebral microdialysis. J Neurochem 43:1369–1374
4. Benveniste H, Jorgensen MB, Sandberg M, Christensen T, Hagberg H, Diemer NH (1989) Ischemic damage in hippocampal CA1 is dependent on glutamate release and intact innervation from CA3. J Cereb Blood Flow Metab 9:629–639
5. Billiau A, Vankelecom H (1992) Interferon-g: general biological properties and effects on the neuro-endocrine axis. In: Bartfai T, Ottoson D (eds) Neuro-immunology of fever. Pergamon, Oxford, pp 65–77
6. Corte FD, Mancini A, Valle D, Gallizzi F, Carducci P, Mignani V, De Marinis L (1998) Provocative hypothalamopituitary axis tests in severe head injury: correlations with severity and prognosis. Crit Care Med 26:1419–1426
7. Dietrich WD, Busto R, Halley M, Valdes I (1990) The importance of brain temperature in alterations of the blood–brain barrier following cerebral ischemia. J Neuropathol Exp Neurol 49:486–497
8. Dudariev VP, Lanovenko II (1999). Changes in the oxygen-binding properties of the blood in white rats under the influence of hypoxia and its pharmacological correction. Fiziol Zh 45:97–103
9. Elizari MV (1999) Chagasic myocardiopathy: historical perspective. Medicina (B Aires). 59 Suppl 2:25–40
10. Feng H, Huang G, Gao L, Tan H, Liao X (2000) Effect of intracranial pressure and cerebral perfusion pressure on outcome prediction of severe traumatic brain injury. Chin J Traumatol 3:226–230
11. Globus MY-T, Ginsberg MD, Haris SI, Busto R, Dietrich WD (1987) Role of dopamine in ischemic striatal injury. Neurology 37:1712–1719
12. Hayashi N (1997) Prevention of vegetation after severe head trauma and stroke by combination therapy of cerebral hypothermia and activation of immune-dopaminergic nervous system. Proceedings of the 6th annual meeting of Society for Treatment of Coma 6:133–145
13. Hayashi N (1998) Brain hypothermia treatment to the neurosurgical disease; prevention of interigency. Dementia and Aging 12:71–78
14. Hayashi N (2000) Enhanced neuronal damage in severely brain injured patients by hypothalamus, pituitary, and adrenal axis neuro-hormonal changes. In: Hayashi N (ed) Brain hypothermia. Springer, Berlin Heidelberg New York Tokyo, pp 3–26
15. Hayashi N (2000) The clinical issue and effectiveness of brain hypothermia treatment for severe brain injured patients. In: Hayashi N (ed) Brain hypothermia. Springer, Berlin Heidelberg New York Tokyo, pp 121–151
16. Hayashi N, Hirayama T, Utagawa A (1994) The cerebral thermo-pooling and hypothermia treatment of critical head injury patients. In: Nagai H (ed) Intracranial pressure IX. Springer, Tokyo, pp 589–599
17. Hayashi N, Kinoshita K, Shibuya T (1997) The prevention of cerebral thermo-pooling, damage of A10 nervous system, and free radical reactions by control of brain tissue temperature in severely brain injured patients. In: Teelken AW (ed) Neurochemistry. Plenum, New York, pp 97–103
18. Klatzo I (1967) Neuropathological aspects of brain edema. J Neuropath Exp Neurol 26:1–14
19. Kontos HA, Wei EP, Povlishock JT, Christman CW (1984) Oxygen radicals mediate the cerebral arteriolar dilatation from arachidonate and bradykinin in cats. Circ Res 55:295–303
20. Langfitt TW (1969) Intracranial pressure. Clin Neurosurg 16:436–471
21. MacIntosh TK (1994) Neurological sequele of traumatic brain injury: therapeutic implications. Cerebrovasc Brain Metab Rev 6:109–162

22. Rothman SM (1984) Synaptic release of excitatory amino acid neurotransmitter mediates anoxic neuronal death. J Neurosci 4:1884–1891
23. Rothman SM, Olney JW (1986) Glutamate and the pathophysiology of hypoxic–ischemic brain damage. Ann Neurol 19:105–111
24. Silvka A, Coben G (1985) Hydroxyl radical attack on dopamine. J Biol Chem 260:15466–15472
25. Wei EP, Dietrich WD, Povlishock JT, Navari RM, Kontos HA (1980) Functional morphologic, metabolic abnormalities of the cerebral microcirculation after concussive brain injury in cats. Circ Res 46:37–47
26. Wei EP, Kontos HA, Ellison MD, Povlishock JT (1986) Oxygen radicals in arachidonate induced increased blood–brain barrier permeability to proteins. Am J Physiol 251:693–699

23. Clinical Failures of Previous Hypothermia Management

Clinical issues of unsuccessful hypothermia treatment have not been elucidated at previously. Without understanding the clinical issues of hypothermia management, it is difficult to successfully treat severely injured patients with hypothermia management. Five reasons for unsuccessful treatment in previous Hypothermia management are discussed here.

Management of Secondary Brain Damage by Hypothalamus–Pituitary–Adrenal Neurohormonal Excess Reactions not Included in Previous Hypothermia Treatment

Release of catecholamines such as epinephrine, norepinephrine, and dopamine, vasopressin, and growth hormone occurs within 3 min of brain trauma and cerebral ischemic insult by stimulation of the hypothalamus–pituitary–adrenal (HPA) axis [1,8,9,11,12,17,21]. Therefore, without early induction of hypothermia management, the brain damage by HPS neurohormonal excess reactions cannot be prevented at the acute stage [9–11,13]. Only the early induction of hypothermia can minimize these stress-associated brain hazards. At the acute stage of severe brain injury, sufficient neuronal oxygenation, suitable control of metabolic substrates, prevention of excess release of HPA axis hormones, and prevention of selective radical damage of the dopamine A10 nervous system are basic intensive care unit (ICU) management strategies [12]. In particular, ineffective oxygen administration caused by hemoglobin dysfunction, rapid progress of cerebral anaerobic metabolism by complication of insulin-resistant hyperglycemia, and prolonged cytokine attack to the brain by blood-brain barrier (BBB) dysfunction associated with vasopressin release are prime treatment targets of ICU management [9–11,13]. However, previous hypothermia treatment did not include care management for these pathophysiological brain injury mechanisms. Actual ICU management methods are described in Chaps. 44–46.

Short Duration of Hypothermia Worsens the Rewarming Stage

Previous hypothermia treatments have focused on the prevention of brain edema, intracranial pressure (ICP) elevation, free radical attack, and neuroexcitation. These pathophysiological changes are most severe within 48 h of brain damage. Therefore, many previous cases of hypothermia treatment were limited to a 48–72 h duration. However, in cases of severely brain-injured patients with Glasgow Coma Scale (GCS) score of less than 6, a short duration of brain hypothermia does not aid recovery or stop pathophysiological changes. Without the control of pathophysiological changes before the rewarming stage, the elevation of brain tissue temperature by rewarming promotes the progression of pathophysiological changes and worsens the outcome [2,12]. Therefore, before rewarming is commenced, we must diagnose whether the injured brain is on the way to recovery. If the injured brain shows signs of recovery, rewarming can be commenced. However, if pathophysiological changes have not recovered or are not on the way to recovery, then rewarming can worsen the condition and result in unsuccessful hypothermia treatment [12].

Many doctors believe that the rewarming technique is difficult, although this is not true. There are many misunderstandings concerning rewarming timing and indications [12]. The concept of hypothermia treatment is based on restoration therapy rather than neuroprotection therapy. Following this concept, the maintenance of sufficient cerebral oxygenation for injured neurons in injured brain tissue, maintenance of metabolic substrate levels, maintenance of stable systemic circulation and neuron hormonal functions rather than reducing brain metabolism, neuron protection from brain edema, prevention of brain ischemia, and control of ICP elevation throughout brain cooling are all important [12]. Brain hypothermia treatment of 24–48 h for the prevention of brain edema and control of ICP elevation is too short for restoration in severely brain-injured patients. In cases of severe brain damage with GCS less than 5, patients need more prolonged brain hypothermia treatment for restoration. The adequate duration of brain hypothermia is theoretically variable depending on the severity and cause of brain damage.

However, prolonged brain hypothermia ICU management can lead to an immune crisis and complication of severe pulmonary infection with reduced growth hormone production [2,6,7,12,18]. Therefore, to keep an adequate duration of brain hypothermia, much skill is required to control an immune crisis and deal with a high incidence of systemic severe infections [12]. As a result, the duration of hypothermia treatment must be changed in accordance with the severity of brain damage.

Prolonged Moderate Hypothermia: Unavoidable Complication of Immune Crisis

The immune function in the human body is maintained by various factors such as lymphocytes (T-cells and B-cells, neutrophils, monocyte immune phagocytes), immune opsonin, and neurohormonal regulation by growth hormone [5,11,14,15,18]. Because a low pituitary gland temperature is unavoidable during brain hypothermia, reduction of serum growth hormone is highly correlated with the severity of brain hypothermia (Fig. 24). As a result, lymphocytopenia can occur depending on the reduction in growth hormone level (Fig. 25). The critical temperature in the brain tissue for lymphocytopenia to occur is below 32°C. However, brain tissue temperature less than 33°C can result in lymphocytopenia (Fig. 25).

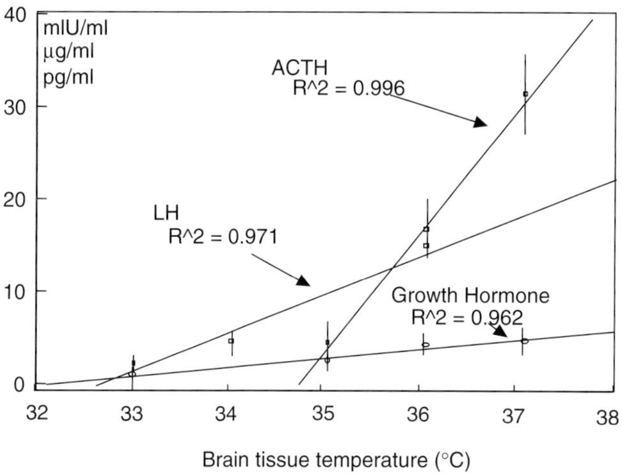

Fig. 24. Effects of cerebral hypothermia on pituitary hormones (n=10). Pituitary hormone levels decrease with brain tissue hypothermia. *ACTH*, adrenocorticotropic hormone; *LH*, luteinizing hormone

Recent clinical studies of immune function demonstrated that growth hormone activates cellular CD4 immune functions and increases levels of the proinflammatory cytokines interleukin 1 (IL1) and IL6; however, CD8 immune function is suppressed and levels of the anti-inflammatory cytokines IL8 and IL10 are reduced (Fig. 26) [8]. Brain hypothermia management with any kind of cooling method, including selected blood cooling, cannot avoid the reduction of immune function caused by low pituitary gland temperature and reduced levels of growth hormone in systemic circulation. Put simply, cellular immune dysfunction or reduction of immune activity is difficult to avoid during brain hypothermia treatment.

In summary, prolonged brain hypothermia below 33°C can allow systemic infections complicated with immune crisis. The severity of immune crisis can be diagnosed by lymphocytopenia and reduced levels of CD4. The management technique for such a condition is described in Chap. 44.

Complication of Severe Pulmonary Infection Means Unsuccessful Hypothermia Treatment

The complication of systemic infection on the management of severe brain damage is very serious. With pulmonary infections, increased levels of proinflammatory cytokines in systemic circulation can easily permeate the BBB and worsen edema by cytokine encephalitis [12]. Our clinical studies suggest that the severe damage of BBB function with an elevated CSF/serum albumin ratio higher than 0.01–0.02 is a serious condition of complicated pulmonary infection. The microdialysis monitor suggested that uncontrollable increases in brain tissue glutamate levels occur in most cases of complicated severe pulmonary infection during the management of brain trauma patients with GCS score less than 6. These specific pathophysiological conditions cannot be controlled by mild brain hypothermia or even with moderate (32°C) brain hypothermia treatment. This phenomenon is observed with CSF/serum albumin ratio above 0.02 and is evidenced by worsening brain edema despite administration of brain hypothermia (Figs. 27, 54, 55).

The complication of systemic infection itself produces dysfunction of major important organs, inadequate neu-

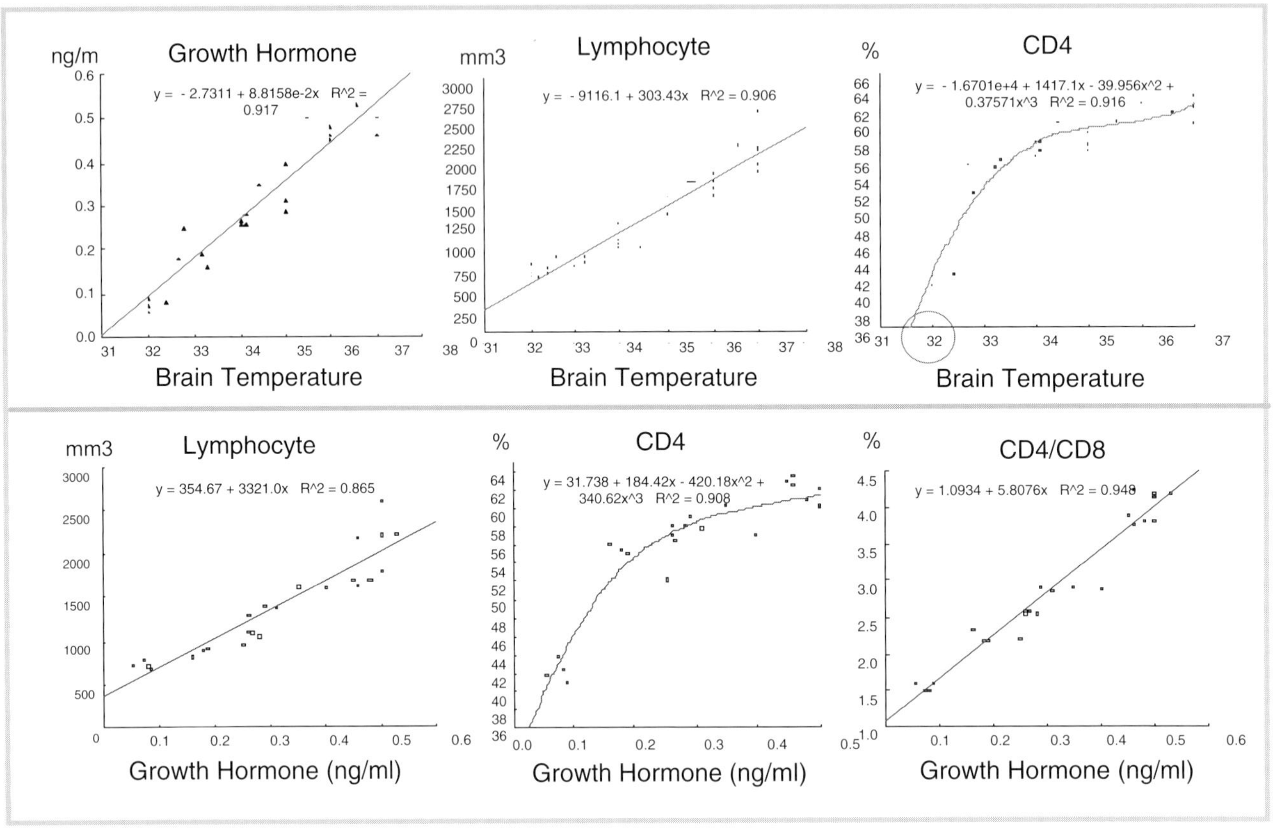

Fig. 25. The changes of growth hormone, lymphocyte, and CD4 following brain hypothermia, and relationships growth hormone and immune functions. *CD4*, CD4 T cell; *CD8*, CD8 T cell

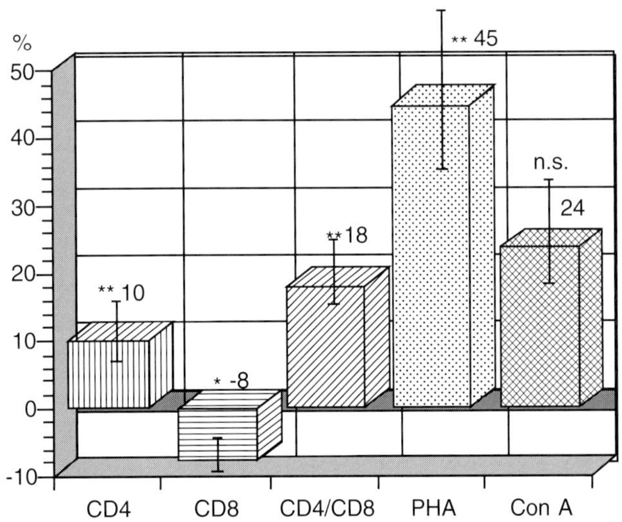

Fig. 26. Percentage changes in T-cell markers after administration of growth hormone ($n=7$). *PHA*, phytohemagglutinin; *Con A*, concanavalin *A*; *n.s.*, not significant; ★, $p < 0.05$; ★★, $p < 0.01$: Significant difference between before (base line: 0%) and after administration of growth hormone

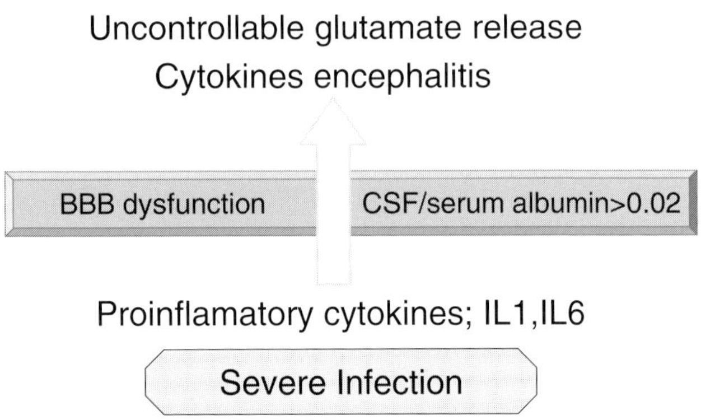

Fig. 27. Severe infection during dysfunction of the blood-brain barrier (BBB; CSF/serum albumin ratio >0.02) produces cytokine encephalitis with uncontrollable glutamate release

ronal oxygenation via pulmonary infection, activates brain edema by hypo-albuminemia, and cytokine encephalitis. The worsening of brain injury by complicated infection includes many considerations, some of which are not simple and do not directly affect the prognosis. Uncontrollable increasing levels of neurotoxic glutamate in the injured brain, even with 32°–33°C moderate brain hypothermia management, results in unsuccessful treatment. In a recent controversial clinical study by Clifton et al. [3], a high incidence (44%–70%) of complications from infection were recorded. Unsuccessful management of infection during hypothermia treatment suggests insufficient application of brain hypothermia. The ICU technique of infectious control is one of the very important factors that decides the effectiveness of brain hypothermia treatment. In our clinical series of about 300 cases of brain hypothermia treatment, a high incidence of 64% systemic infection was also recorded at the initial stage. However, when infectious control was based on the causes of immune crisis and macronutrient neural dysregulation following brain damage, systemic infection was less than 10% during the 7–10 days of prolonged brain hypothermia treatment.

For brain hypothermia to succeed, although infections must be prevented, care must also be applied to vascular inflammation, vascular permeability, hypo-albuminemia, and BBB dysfunction. To control these pathophysiological changes, early management of AT-III above 100% to prevent vascular inflammation and microembolus formation, followed by administration of albumin are useful to maintain BBB function. The CSF/serum albumin ratio should be maintained below 0.01 to prevent cytokine encephalitis and to manage systemic infection.

The management of hyperglycemia and AT-III to prevent increased vascular permeability, and the control of serum albumin level above 3.5 mg/dl to maintain BBB function are also very useful to prevent the complication of disseminated intravascular coagulability (DIC). However, in severely brain-injured patients, hypo-albuminemia progresses rapidly. The mechanism of hypo-albuminemia in severely brain-injured patients is not clear, although it is speculated that it occurs after damage of messenger RNA by cytokines. The replacement of albumin is very important to prevent intestinal mucous edema, obstructive pancreatic dysfunction, free bacteria, and free pharmacology. Unsuccessful management of immune crisis, hyperglycemia associated with catecholamine surge, hypo-albuminemia, intestinal pressure, and BBB dysfunction at the acute stage are major causes of severe pulmonary infection and ineffective hypothermia treatment of the injured brain. The details of ICU infectious control during brain hypothermia treatment is described in Chap. 44.

Worsening Condition Caused by Inadequate Brain Temperature and High Serum Glucose

In severely brain-injured patients, hyperglycemia associated with catecholamine surge is unavoidable [4,7,9,11]. Catecholamine surge can be reduced by early induction of brain hypothermia but cannot be stopped completely. The rapid excess release of epinephrine in catecholamine surge produces severe metabolic hyperglycemia by consuming ATP and glycogen in the liver and muscles. This HPA axis stress-associated hyperglycemia is recorded in very high incidence. Delayed induction of hypothermia, especially later than 3 h after severe brain injury, has difficulty with the control of catetholamine surge-associated hyperglycemia and lactic acidosis in the injured brain tissue. This is because hyperglycemia associated with catecholamine surge is resistant to insulin caused by reduced insulin sensitivity, disturbed muscle protein synthesis, and suppressed release of insulin. Therefore, early induction of brain hypothermia treatment is necessary to prevent these complications [11,12].

On the other hand, rapid induction of hypothermia and excess hypothermia also produce hyperglycemia by reduced consumption of serum glucose [12]. It has long been believed that hypothermia reduces the systemic metabolism; however, this concept is not correct. Following hypothermia, the metabolism shifts from a glucose-based cycle to a lipid-based cycle. The glucose metabolism reduces in accordance with the applied hypothermia; however, lipid metabolism increases at the low body temperature. The ratio of glucose to lipid metabolism is essentially the same during brain tissue hypothermia at 34°C [10–12]. Therefore, at the acute stage, two types of hyperglycemia must be considered. One is associated with epinephrine surge after slow induction of hypothermia at the acute stage, and the other is related to increased serum glucose levels caused by excess hypothermia in the cooling stage. This inadequate control of serum glucose level in the cooling stage causes an increase in brain tissue lactate, pyruvate, and glucose levels as shown in Fig. 28. In this case, brain tissue temperature should be controlled at 34°C rather than 33°C. Microdialysis suggests that critical levels of serum glucose to cause an increase in lactate concentration is above 140 mg/dl at 33°C in the cooling stage.

Uncontrolled hyperglycemia at the acute stage causes serious complications and is one of the main reasons for unsuccessful hypothermia treatment. Increased brain tissue glucose levels way also increase vasopressin release by a feedback mechanism of neural control of macronutrients [2,6,10,13,15,16,19,20].

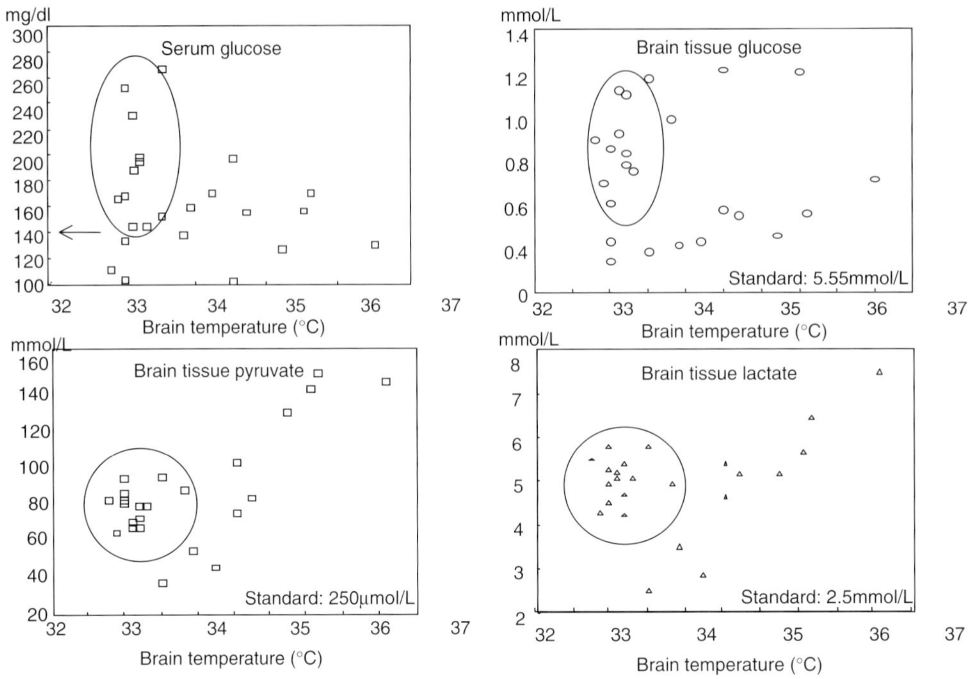

Fig. 28. The brain tissue pyruvate and lactate levels increased more markedly at 33°C than at 34°C by inadequate control of hyperglycemia

In previous animal studies, excess release of vasopressin changes the endothelial cell function and causes vascular contraction with cerebral blood flow disturbance. Our clinical studies using microdialysis studies suggested that hyperglycemia with serum glucose levels above 230 mg/ml produces an increase in brain tissue glucose level, vasopressin release, activates cytokines IL1 and IL6, and increases the permeability of the BBB [11]. This means that brain edema and BBB dysfunction cannot be successfully controlled by hypothermia without good management of hyperglycemia [12]. The careful management of serum glucose level to within the range of 120–140 mg/dl is recommended. Although the management of this insulin-resistant hyperglycemia is very important in hypothermia treatment, such control is not so easy to obtain. The management method in the induction and cooling stages are discussed in Chaps. 43 and 44.

References

1. Billiau A, Vankelecom H (1992) Interferon-g: general biological properties and effects on the neuro-endocrine axis. In: Bartfai T, Ottoson D (eds) Neuro-immunology of fever. Pergamon, Oxford, pp 65–77
2. Bioch M (1967) Cerebral effects of rewarming following prolonged hypothermia: significance for the management of severe cranio-cerebral injury and acute pyrexia. Brain 90:769–784
3. Clifton GL, Miller ER, Choi SC, Levin HS, McCauley S, Smith KR Jr, Muizelaar JP, Wagner FC Jr, Marion DW, Luerssen TG, Chesnut RM, Schwartz M (2001) Lack of effect of induction of hypothermia after acute brain injury. N Engl J Med 344:556–563
4. Corte FD, Mancini A, Valle D, Gallizzi F, Carducci P, Mignani V, De Marinis L (1998) Provocative hypothalamopituitary axis tests in severe head injury: correlations with severity and prognosis. Crit Care Med 26:1419–1426
5. Davila DR, Breif S, Simon J, Hammer RE, Brinster RL, Kelley KW (1987) Role of growth hormone in regulating T-dependant immune events in aged, nude, and transgenic rodents. J Neurosci Res 18:F108–116
6. Fedor EJ, Fisher ER, Lee SH, Weitzel WK, Fisher B (1956) Effect of hypothermia upon induced bacteremia. Proc Soc Exp Biol Med 93:510–512
7. Gadkary CS, Alderson P, Signorini DF (2002) Therapeutic hypothermia for head injury. Cochrane Rev 1:CD001048
8. Grundy PL, Harbuz MS, Jessop DS, Lightman SL, Sharples PM (2001) The hypothalamo-pituitary-adrenal axis response to experimental traumatic brain injury. J Neurotrauma 18:1373–1381
9. Hayashi N (1995) Cerebral hypothermia treatment. In: Hayashi N (ed) Cerebral hypothermia treatment. Sogo Igaku, Tokyo, pp 1–105
10. Hayashi N (1997) Prevention of vegetation after severe head trauma and stroke by combination therapy of cerebral hypothermia and activation of immune-

dopaminergic nervous system. Proceedings of the 6th annual meeting of Society for Treatment of Coma 6:133–145
11. Hayashi N (2000) Enhanced neuronal damage in severely brain injured patients by hypothalamus, pituitary, and adrenal axis neuro-hormonal changes. In: Hayashi N (ed) Brain hypothermia. Springer, Berlin Heidelberg New York Tokyo, pp 3–26
12. Hayashi N (2000) The clinical issue and effectiveness of brain hypothermia treatment for severe brain injured patients. In: Hayashi N (ed) Brain hypothermia. Springer, Berlin Heidelberg New York Tokyo, pp 121–151
13. Hayashi N, Kinoshita K, Shibuya T (1997) The prevention of cerebral thermo-pooling, damage of A10 nervous system, and free radical reactions by control of brain tissue temperature in severely brain injured patients. In: Teelken T (ed) Neurochemistry. Plenum New York, pp 97–103
14. Kossmann T, Hans V, Lenzlinger PM, Csuka E, Stsahel PF, Trentz O, Morgani-Kossmann MC (1996) Analysis of immune mediator production following traumatic brain injury. In: Schlag G, Redel H, Traber D (eds) Shock, sepsis and organ failure. Berlin Heidelberg New York Tokyo, pp 263–297
15. Leibowitz SF (1999) Macronutrients and brain peptides: what they do and how they respond. In: Berthoud HR, Seeley RJ (eds) Neural and metabolic control of macronutrient intake. CRC, Boca Raton, pp 389–406
16. Leibowiz SF, Sladek C, Spencer L, Temple D (1988) Neuropeptide Y, epinephrine and norepinephrine in the paraventricular nucleus: stimulation of feeding and the release of corticosterone, vasopressin and glucose. Brain Res Bull 21:905
17. Payne LC, Obal F Jr, Opp MR, Krueger JM (1992) Stimulation and inhibition of growth hormone secretion by IL1: the involvement of growth hormone. Neuroendocrinology. 56:118–123
18. Russwurm S, Stonans I, Schwerter K, Stonane E, Meissner W, Reinhart K (2002) Direct influence of mild hypothermia on cytokine expression and release in cultures of human peripheral blood mononuclear cells. J Interferon Cytokine Res 22:15–21
19. Stanley BG (1993) Neuropeptide Y in multiple hypothalamic sites controls eating behavior, endocrine, and autonomic system for body energy balance. In: Colmers WF, Wahlestedt C (eds) Biology of neuropeptide Y and related peptides. Humana Press, Totowa, NJ, 457–509
20. Temple DL (1994) The neuropeptide Y system (hypothalamus) has a dense concentration of glucocorticoide (type II) receptors that mediate carbon hydrate intake. J Neuroendocrinol 6:479–501
21. Woiciechowsky C, Schoning B, Daberkow N, Asche K, Stoltenburg G, Lanksch WR, Volk HD (1999) Brain-IL-1beta induces local inflammation but systemic anti-inflammatory response through stimulation of both hypothalamic-pituitary-adrenal axis and sympathetic nervous system. Brain Res 816:563–571

24. The Difference in Brain Injury Mechanism in Experimental Laboratory Models and Human Patients

The clinical treatment of brain-injured patients has been previously based on information derived from experimental animal studies concerning brain trauma, ischemia, infarction, hypoxia, and cardiac arrest [9]. However, the differences between species from animal to human, including differences in pathophysiology of severely brain-injured patients and experimental animal models, are not absolutely clear. One difference in brain injury mechanism is the effect of anesthesia. The direct brain injury mechanisms such as necrosis, ischemia, brain edema, intracranial pressure (ICP) elevation, and nonspecific brain damage caused by neuroexcitation apoptosis are not so different between clinical patients and experimental animal models [1,5,10,11]. However, systemic stress reaction is more severe in patients than in experimental animal models, because stress-associated neurohormonal reaction is limited under anesthesia. In experimental animal studies, harmful stress-associated neurohormonal reactions caused by stimulation of the hypothalamus-pituitary-adrenal (HPA) [2,3] and hypothalamus-pituitary-thyroid axis are prevented by anesthesia. Therefore, catecholamine surge-associated cardiac ischemia, contraction myocytolysis, changes in dynamic hemometabolism, insulin-resistant hyperglycemia, immune dysfunction, brain thermo-pooling, vasopressin-associated blood–brain barrier (BBB) dysfunction, and neuronal hypoxia-associated hemoglobin dysfunctions [6,7] are not observed in severe brain injury with anesthesia.

However, in clinical patients, and especially in severely injured patients, the stimulation of the HPA axis occurs by chemical mediators from injured tissue or by direct injury [9]. These stresses produce the release of many neuroendoclinological hormones, vasopressin, catecholamines, and pituitary hormones [2,5,7]. However, these stress-associated neurohormonal reactions are not the same in each patient and changes depend on severity, acuteness, age, and gender. These pathophysiological changes associated with HPA axis stimulation also produce neuronal hypoxia despite normal control of PaO_2, oxygen delivery, cerebral blood flow (CBF), and perfusion pressure because of slow release of bound oxygen from hemoglobin (masking neuronal hypoxia) [6,7]. These stress-associated neuronal injuries decide the clinical prognosis more directly than brain edema and ICP elevation in severely brain-injured patients. The precise brain injury mechanisms of HPA axis neuroendoclinological reactions are still under research. The injured brain tissue releases many proinflammatory cytokines, such as interleukin 1 (IL1), TNF, and IL6. These cytokines stimulate the HPA axis to release catecholamines to maintain the cardiopulmonary–cerebral circulation [9]. However, the control system for adequate volume of catecholamine release for various injury levels is not so accurate. Therefore, in severely brain-injured patients, overprotective neurohormonal reactions occur that produce an excess release of catecholamines and vasopressin. The excess catecholamine surge causes unstable cardiac function, brain thermo-pooling, insulin-resistant hyperglycemia, and slow release of oxygen from hemoglobin caused by low 2,3-diphosphoglycerate (DPG) in blood cells, as described previously. The excess release of vasopressin activates production of proinflammatory cytokines, BBB dysfunction, and promotes cytokine encephalitis. Therefore, in severely brain-injured patients, the brain injury mechanism is not as simple as that observed in animal studies. In experimental animal brain injury models, some HPA axis neurohormonal reactions that include catecholamine surge-associated myocytolysis, severe hyperglycemia, hemoglobin dysfunction, vasopressin-related BBB dysfunction, and cytokine encephalitis with uncontrollable glutamate release are not apparent under conditions of anesthesia.

Based on recent clinical studies, the brain injury mechanisms of severe brain damage are summarized by three main mechanisms: neuronal hypoxia and metabolic imbalance associated with hemoglobin dysfunction and insulin-resistant hyperglycemia, neurohormonal BBB dysfunction and immune crisis, and selective radical damage to the dopamine A10 nervous system. None of these brain damage mechanisms was recorded in experimental animal studies.

In studies of brain injury mechanism, the issues affecting the occurrence of vegetation in different species have not been discussed. It is likely that emotional reactions, quality of memory, and thinking level are not similar between humans and animals. Because the dopamine A10 nervous system has been demonstrated as an emotional center relating to the function of memory, volition, thinking, and excitation, massive damage to the cerebral hemisphere and selective damage to the A10 nervous system causes damage of emotion, volition, thinking, memory, and personality, and can lead to the vegetative state [6,7,8]. The release of dopamine from the dopamine nervous system after severe brain damage produces neurotoxic hydroxide radicals that are generated by the reaction of oxygen and released dopamine in the brain tissue [1,4,11]. These pathophysiological reactions cause selective radical damage of the dopamine central nervous system. The dopamine central nervous system, that includes dopamine A10 nervous system, functions as a center of emotion and affects personality, interagency ability, emotion, memory, and consciousness. In humans, this function is more sensitive than in experimental animals. However, the precise mechanism of damage to emotion and memory in experimental animal models is unknown.

Recent clinical studies suggest that a brain tissue temperature below 34°C may prevent the release of cerebral dopamine [8]. The management of brain tissue temperature in the range of 32–34°C with sufficient neuronal oxygenation is very successful for the prevention of damage to emotion and memory in severely brain-injured patients with a Glasgow Coma Scale (GCS) score of 4–6. To make a recovery from the vegetative state, restoration therapy for nonfunctioning neurons in the dopamine A10 nervous system is necessary. The responsiveness of the dopamine A10 nervous system in various treatments for recovery from the vegetative state can be diagnosed by monitoring the increase in CSF dopamine, the decline of ploractin, or the increase in the CSF dopamine/CSF ploractin ratio. The actual management technique and diagnostic method is discussed later in this book.

References

1. Baker AJ, Zornow MH, Scheller MS, Yaksh TL, Skilling SR, Smullin DH, Larson AA, Kuczenski R (1991) Changes in extracellular concentrations of glutamate, aspartate, glycine, dopamine, serotonin, and dopamine metabolites after transient global ischemia in the rat. J Neurochem 57:1370–1379
2. Chiolero R, Lemarchand TH, Schutz Y, de Tribolet N, Felber JP, Freeman J, Jequier E (1988) Plasma pituitary hormone levels in severe trauma with or without head injury. J Trauma 28:1368–1374
3. Corte FD, Mancini A, Valle D, Gallizzi F, Carducci P, Mignani V, De Marinis L (1998) Provocative hypothalamopituitary axis tests in severe head injury: correlations with severity and prognosis. Crit Care Med 26:1419–1426
4. Globus MY-T, Ginsberg MD, Haris SI, Busto R, Dietrich WD (1987) Role of dopamine in ischemic striatal injury. Neurology 37:1712–1719
5. Globus MY-T, Busto R, Dietrich WD, Martinez E, Valdes I, Ginsberg MD (1998) Effect on ischemia on the in vivo release of striatal dopamine, glutamate, and γ-aminobutyric acid studied by intracerebral microdialysis. J Neurochem 51:1455–1464
6. Hayashi N (1997) Prevention of vegetation after severe head trauma and stroke by combination therapy of cerebral hypothermia and activation of immune-dopaminergic nervous system. Proceedings of the 6th annual meeting of Society for Treatment of Coma 6:133–145
7. Hayashi N (2000) Enhanced neuronal damage in severely brain injured patients by hypothalamus, pituitary, and adrenal axis neuro-hormonal changes. In: Hayashi N (ed) Brain hypothermia. Springer, Berlin Heidelberg New York Tokyo pp 3–26
8. Hayashi N (2000) The clinical issue and effectiveness of brain hypothermia treatment for severe brain injured patients. In: Hayashi N (ed) Brain hypothermia. Springer Berlin Heidelberg New York Tokyo, pp 121–151
9. Kossmann T, Hans V, Lenzlinger PM, Csuka E, Stsahel PF, Trentz O, Morgani-Kossmann MC (1996) Analysis of immune mediator production following traumatic brain injury. In: Schlag G, Redel H, Traber D (eds) Shock, sepsis and organ failure. Springer Berlin Heidelberg New York Tokyo, pp 263–297
10. MacIntosh TK (1994) Neurological sequele of traumatic brain injury: therapeutic implications. Cerebrovasc Brain Metab Rev 6:109–162
11. Silvka A, Coben G (1985) Hydroxyl radical attack on dopamine. J Biol Chem 260:15466–15472

25. The Regulatory Mechanism of Brain Tissue Temperature and Brain Thermo-pooling

The management of severely brain-injured patients in the intensive care unit (ICU) has been carried out without considering changes in brain tissue temperature. However, brain tissue temperature in severely brain-injured patients does change dynamically over time. Previous scientific information concerning brain injury in experimental animal studies was obtained at 37°C in most cases, because consistent data cannot be obtained at variable body temperature. Put simply, the effect of temperature on the brain injury is considerable. We have directly monitored the brain tissue temperature in more than 100 cases in many types of brain injury and brain diseases in ICU.

We studied the defense and control mechanism of brain tissue temperature in humans. The brain tissue temperature is usually maintained relatively constant. The four defense and control factors were recorded under physiological conditions [4]. The main factor that decides the baseline for brain tissue temperature is core blood temperature. This baseline brain tissue tempera-

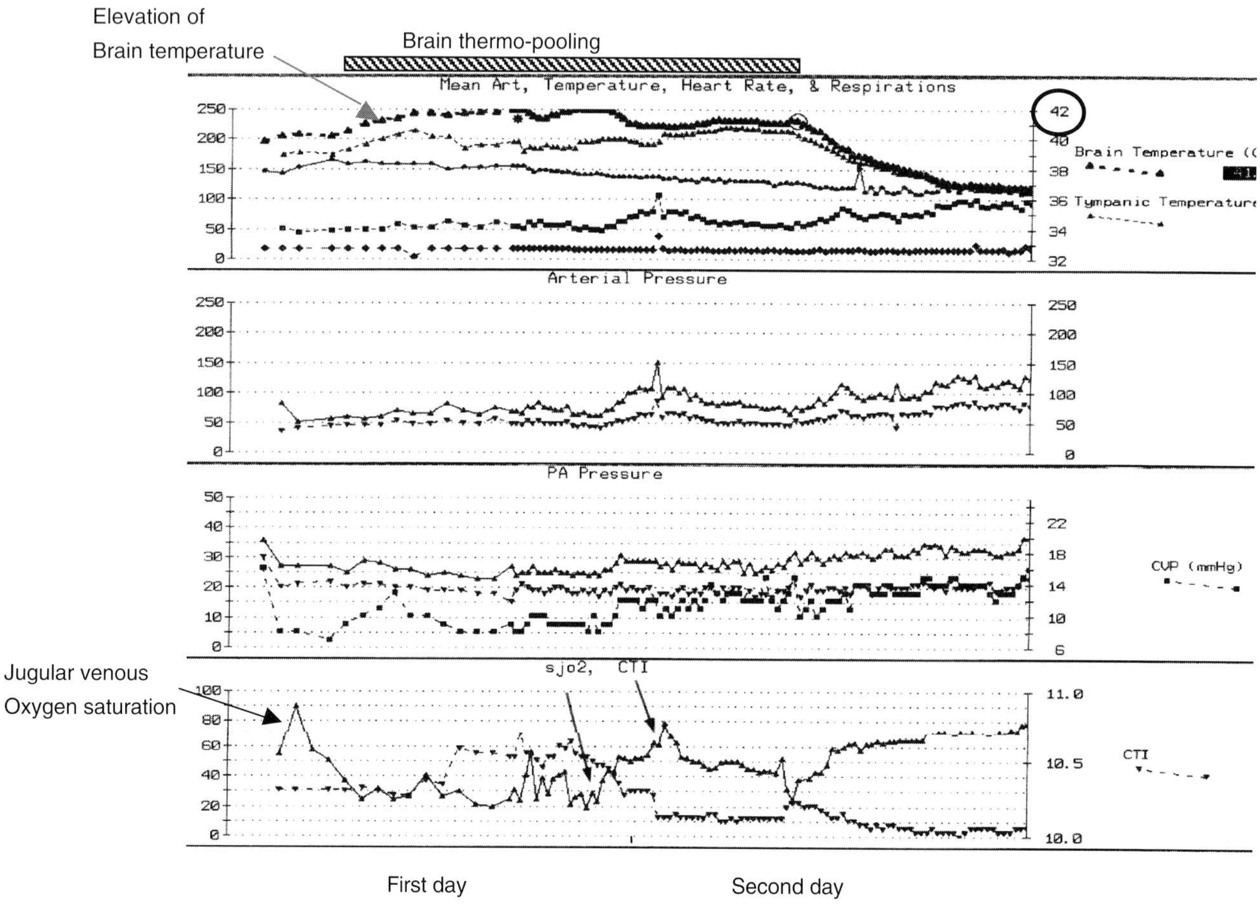

Fig. 29. Typical case of brain thermo-pooling after severe brain injury. *PA*, pulmonary arterial pressure; *sjo2*, jugular venous oxygen saturation; *CTI*, cerebral thermal index (brain tissue temperature ÷ tympanic membrane temperature)

ture changes dynamically by alteration of cerebral perfusion pressure (CPP) (or blood pressure), brain metabolism, and cerebral blood flow (CBF). The effect of brain metabolism on the brain tissue temperature is small (0.4°–0.8°C) under physiological conditions. The CPP carries the blood temperature into the brain tissue and CBF removes the elevated brain tissue temperature by venous circulation. The imbalance of CPP and CBF produce brain thermo-pooling with elevation of brain tissue temperature up to 44°C. Figure 29 is a typical case of complicated elevation of brain tissue temperature up to 42°C caused by brain thermo-pooling. A 56-year-old male patient was admitted to a medical center after a traffic accident. His blood pressure was 65/42 mmHg, tachycardia 105/min, tachypnea 24/min, and the Glasgow Coma Scale score was 6. The clinical diagnosis was diffuse brain injury with a small epidural hematoma in the left hemisphere, and a small hemorrhage of the brain stem. Although the management of systolic blood pressure was very difficult, ICP was easy to control to below 20 mmHg. The brain tissue temperature increased to 42°C as shown in Fig. 29. After cerebral reperfusion, brain tissue temperature was difficult to wash out with mean arterial blood pressure lower than 55 mmHg. This brain thermo-pooling phenomenon was relieved by control of mean arterial blood pressure above 55 mmHg (systolic blood pressure 96 mmHg). However, effective management of brain injury failed after prolonged brain thermo-pooling despite control of ICP to normal levels, and the patient died 48 h after the accident.

The CBF is the main mechanism by which elevated brain tissue temperature can be washed out [1–4]. Therefore, internal jugular venous blood temperature shows the mean value of the whole brain tissue temperature except in cases of contamination of internal jugular venous blood with external cerebral circulation (Fig. 11, Chap. 22). The continuous monitoring of jugular venous blood temperature could be useful as an indirect monitor of mean values of brain tissue temperature in ICU. The simultaneous continuous monitoring of jugular venous blood temperature and tympanic membrane temperature is very effective to evaluate not only changes in brain tissue temperature but also for detecting imbalance between inflow and outflow in brain tissue caused by CBF disturbances. The details of monitoring and diagnostic techniques are discussed in Chap. 42.

The brain tissue temperature is maintained at near the blood core temperature by a simple control mechanism. The brain tissue temperature is determined by core temperature, CPP that carries the core temperature into the brain tissue, and brain metabolism (Fig. 10, Chap. 22). Elevated brain tissue temperature is lowered by the washout mechanism of CBF. In the brain tissue, regional CBF is high flow in the cortex and low flow in the white matter. Therefore, the ability of CBF to washout brain tissue temperature in the white matter is lower than in the gray matter such that white matter brain tissue temperature is slightly higher than gray matter brain tissue temperature.

The techniques for management of brain tissue hypothermia are described in Chap. 35.

References

1. Hayashi N (1995) Cerebral hypothermia treatment. In: Hayashi N (ed) Cerebral hypothermia treatment. Sogo Igaku, Tokyo, pp 1–105
2. Hayashi N (1996) Advance of cerebral hypothermia treatment. J Critical Med 8:295–300
3. Hayashi N (2000) Enhanced neuronal damage in severely brain injured patients by hypothalamus, pituitary, and adrenal axis neuro-hormonal changes. In: Hayashi N (ed) Brain hypothermia. Springer, Berlin Heidelberg New York Tokyo, pp 3–26
4. Hayashi N, Hirayama T, Utagawa A (1994) The cerebral thermo-pooling and hypothermia treatment of critical head injury patients. In: Nagai H (ed). Intracranial pressure IX. Springer, Berlin Heidelberg New York Tokyo, pp 589–599

26. The Target of Treatment of Severe Brain Injury in the Acute Stage

The target of treatment of brain injury in the acute stage is variable and depends on severity, time after injury, and presence or not of hypothalamus–pituitary–adrenal (HPA) axis neurohormonal reactions. This section focuses on severe brain injury cases that require brain hypothermia treatment. Three major targets of intensive care unit (ICU) management in the acute stage are summarized: neuronal oxygenation and adequate administration of metabolic substrates for injured neurons, management of HPA axis neurohormonal dysfunction, and prevention of selective radical attack of the dopamine A10 nervous system.

Adequate Oxygenation and Administration of Metabolic Substrates for Injured Neurons

Many neurons in primary injured brain tissue do not die immediately. However, restoration of these dying neurons has long been considered to be difficult or impossible. Therefore, neuroprotection therapy to prevent the progression of secondary brain damage has been the main goal of ICU management [18]. The maintenance of cerebral blood flow (CBF), prevention of brain edema, and control of intracranial pressure (ICP) and cerebral perfusion pressure (CPP) with stabilized vital signs were initial ICU management strategies [1,7,17,18,22]. However, recent clinical studies demonstrated that this management concept is not sufficient for severely brain-injured patients. More precise management of neuronal oxygenation and control of brain metabolic substrates could assist neuron restoration even with respiratory arrest and the presence of no light reflex [11,13,14]. To control the oxygenation of injured neurons, the management of hemoglobin function to allow release of bound oxygen from hemoglobin, sufficient PaO_2 and oxygen delivery, stabilized cardiopulmonary function, adequate CPP, control of catecholamine surge, prevention of blood shift to the intestine by dopamine dominant circulation, control of brain thermo-pooling, and maintenance of CBF are required, at least in the acute stage [11,13,14]. However, without adequate administration of metabolic substrates, control of severe insulin-resistant hyperglycemia that is produced by stress-associated catecholamine surge is impossible and neuronal oxygenation therapy is not effective [11–13]. The careful management of excess release of HPA-axis neurohormones is also important. The management of hypothermia treatment at the acute stage is summarized in Fig. 30.

To maintain sufficient oxygenation and an adequate supply of metabolic substrates to injured neurons, control of ICP below 20 mmHg, PaO_2/FiO_2 ratio to over 300, antithrombin-III (AT-III) over 100%, and serum glucose between 120 and 140 mg/dl are fundamental. If the serum glucose level cannot be controlled between 120 and 140 mg/dl and increases above 140 mg/dl, hyperosmotic antibrain edema therapy with glycerol is contraindicated for the control of brain tissue glucose [13]. The administration of oxygen and glucose into the brain tissue is maintained throughout with a 10-mmHg waterfall pressure gradient in capillary vessels. To maintain this pressure difference in capillary vessels, the cerebral venous pressure should be controlled to less than 20 mmHg. Therefore, ICP elevation above 20 mmHg is in danger of reducing the waterfall pressure gradient and decreasing the transfer of metabolic substrates from vessel to brain tissue. The ICP should be controlled below 20 mmHg as part of basic ICU management (Table 3).

Brain edema, acute brain swelling with vascular engorgement, and mass lesion are the main causes of ICP elevation. However, brain edema and acute brain swelling occur as results of unsuccessful management of brain hypoxia, brain metabolism, systemic circulation and metabolism, immune dysfunction, and neurohormonal abnormality. The management of these pathophysiological changes should be scheduled before treatment of brain edema. Early administration of steroids can worsen the patient condition in cases of catecholamine surge-associated hyperglycemia by progressing hyperglycemia, wasting BBB function, promoting vasopressin release, and activating neuronal hypoxia because of slow release of bound oxygen from

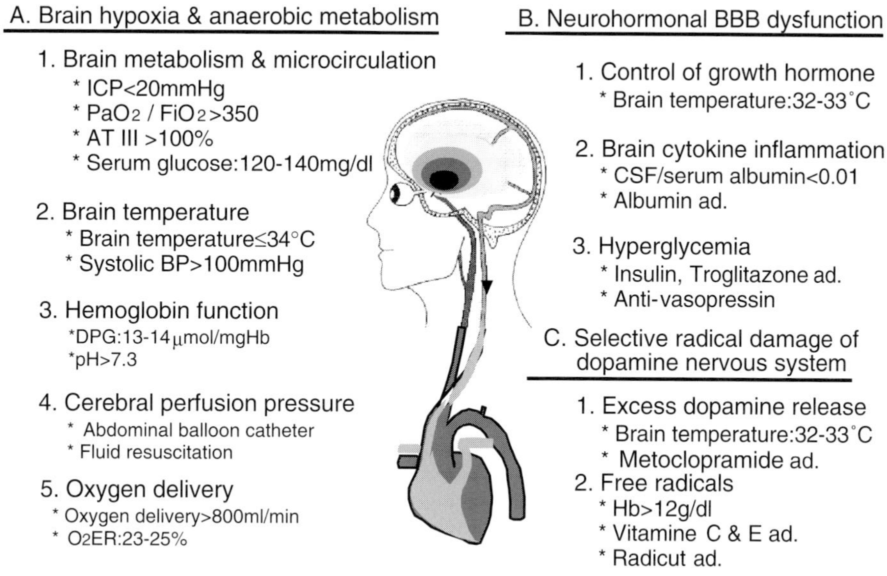

Fig. 30. The management of brain hypothermia treatment in the acute stage

hemoglobin [12]. Early administration of steroids is only recommended in cases with no signs of hyperglycemia. The head-up position for control of venous stasis ICP elevation is also recommend after stabilizing neuronal oxygenation, brain metabolism, and CBF. Management of hypercapnea to prevent acute brain swelling is also possible. $PaCO_2$ greater than 45 mmHg can trigger vascular engorgement, a reduction of 2,3-diphosphoglycerate (DPG) in hemoglobin, cellular acidosis, and lower cardiac output. Ideally, $PaCO_2$ should be controlled to within the range of 34 and 38 mmHg. Hypocapnea less than 24 mmHg produces vascular contraction and reduces the CBF.

The management of the PaO_2/FiO_2 ratio to greater than 300 suggests the balance of oxygen inhalation and pulmonary functions. PaO_2/FiO_2 ratio between 200 and 300 indicates the presence of lung injury, while lower than 200 indicates the possibility of adult respiratory distress syndrome. Cardiac dysfunction, pulmonary congestion, pulmonary edema complicated with hypo-albuminemia, Mendelson's syndrome with vomiting, pulmonary atelectasis, and increasing mediastinal pressure are important targets of ICU management. AT-III is a good indirect parameter of intravascular coagulability and disturbance of cerebral microcirculation. The microcirculation in intestinal mucous is also very sensitive to reductions in AT-III levels. The critical level of AT-III for production of microcirculation derangement in intestine is less than 100% under hypothermia conditions [12]. However, under normothermic conditions, management of AT-III above 130%–150% is advised to prevent disturbance of cerebral microcirculation.

For the management of brain tissue temperature, control of body (or core) temperature at 34°C for the prevention of catecholamine surge is recommended [10,11,13]. After stabilizing the cardiac functions and systolic blood pressure above 100 mmHg, the brain tissue temperature should be reduced to 33°–32°C over about 3–6 h. Two steps for the induction of brain hypothermia control are recommended [13]. The criteria and technique for managing brain tissue temperature are described in Chaps. 34–35.

The management of hemoglobin dysfunction [6,12,19] is very important in the initial management of neuronal oxygenation, although this task has not received sufficient attention, previously. The slow release of bound oxygen from hemoglobin in brain tissue is an unavoidable complication of neuronal hypoxia in injured brain tissue, despite normal control of PaO_2, oxygen delivery, and CBF. The main causes of hemoglobin dysfunction are reduced levels of 2,3-diphosphoglycerate (DPG), in stroke, brain hypoxia, and cardiac arrest. Hyperglycemia with glucose serum levels above 230 mg/dl, severe acidosis (pH < 7.3) in the bloodstream, blood transfusion, and deep hypothermia with temperatures below 30°C are known as causes of reduced DPG levels [12,13]. In our clinical studies, DPG was reduced in 44%, and reduced to critical levels in 24% of 17 severely brain-injured patients [Glasgow Coma Scale (GCS) <6]. In conditions with DPG concentration reduced to less than 10 μmol/ml, oxygen inhalation is not effective even with normal PaO_2. The control of serum pH above 7.3, serum glucose to within 120–140 mg/dl, serum inorganic phosphate at 3–5 mg/dl, serum magnesium at 1.4–1.8 mEq/l, and serum albumin above 3.5 mg/dl are useful to prevent hemoglobin dysfunction. Management of serum acidosis is particularly important for hemoglobin function [6,13,19] during brain hypothermia treatment [13].

For neuronal oxygenation, maintenance of oxygen delivery is also important in ICU management. In our series of brain hypothermia treatment for severe brain injury, the level of oxygen delivery directly affected the prognosis with or without brain hypothermia. Good prognosis was recorded in cases in which oxygen delivery was maintained above 800 ml/min. Poor prognosis was recorded in cases in which oxygen delivery was less than 600 ml/min (Fig. 21). Oxygen delivery can be computed as shown in the following equation.

$$\text{Oxygen delivery} = \text{cardiac output} \times \text{Hb} \times \text{SaO}_2 \times 1.39 \quad (1)$$

Therefore, maintenance of oxygen delivery above 800 ml/min is very difficult at Hb < 10 g/dl. In the management of oxygen delivery, increase in cardiac output, replacement of hemoglobin, and provision of sufficient oxygen are important. In conditions with hemoglobin concentration above 13 mg/dl it is much easier to maintain oxygen delivery above 800 ml/min. In severely brain-injured patients, it is very difficult to control cardiac output by coronary spasm and myocontraction with catecholamine surge, myorelaxant with hypercapnea, cardiac dysfunction by hyper- or hypokalkemia, cardiac ischemia complicated with hemorrhagic shock, and excess release of catecholamines by stimulation of hypothalamus in acute stage. To manage cardiac output, monitoring by electrocardiogram, cardiac echo, and directly with a Swan-Ganz catheter are essential.

The control of CPP is important not only to maintain CBF but also to wash out the elevated brain tissue temperature [13,14]. Management of CPP is recommended above 80 mmHg in adults with sufficient fluid resuscitation. In children, CPP should be maintained above 60–80 mmHg depending on age. If fluid resuscitation is not successful in maintaining the systolic blood pressure above 100 mmHg in adults, temporary blockage of the abdominal aorta using an abdominal balloon catheter (Fig. 31) is an alternative. The early administration of manitol to prevent brain edema is not recommended, because hypovolemia with dehydration produces disturbances of microcirculation in the brain and intestinal organs. Without maintaining stable systemic circulation, osmotic dehydration therapy is not indicated, especially during brain hypothermia treatment. As an initial fluid resuscitation, normalization of systemic circulation is very important rather than dehydration management. This is because brain tissue hypothermia below 34°C causes a reduction in serum catecholamines of about 50% and difficulty in maintaining blood pressure without adequate fluid replacement (Fig. 32). Oxygen therapy focused on the delivery of oxygen at rates higher than 700–800 ml/min kg^{-1} with an oxygen extraction ratio (O_2ER) of 0.22–0.25 is important for restoration of injured neurons [1,13,22].

Management of Hypothalamus-Pituitary-Adrenal (HPA) Axis Neurohormonal Dysfunction

HPA axis neurohormonal reaction is a physiological reaction that minimizes brain damage by increasing blood pressure and increasing serum glucose with catecholamine release. This reaction is very successful in cases of mild-to-moderate brain injury because of the release of serum catecholamines [4]. However, in severe brain damage caused by trauma, stroke, or hypoxia, uncontrolled excess neurohormonal reaction of the HPA axis introduces a hazard to injured neurons (Table 4) [9,13]. The excess release of catecholamines and vasopressin by stimulation of the HPA axis produces more negative effects for injured neurons than does neuroprotection. Direct neuronal stimulation of the hypothalamus and indirect chemical stimulation such as proinflammatory cytokines may contribute to the release of HPA-axis neurohormones [21].

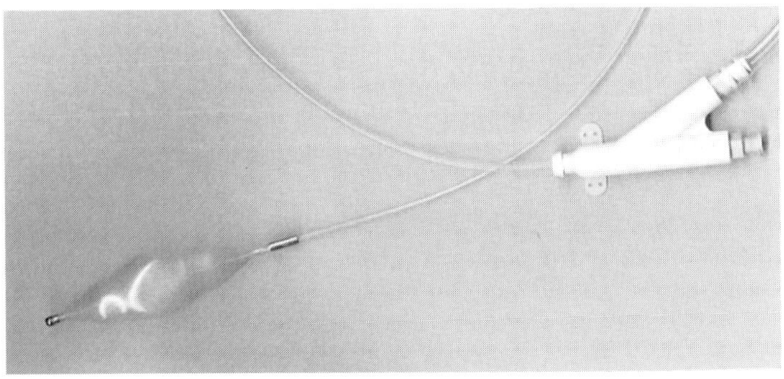

Fig. 31. Intra-abdominal balloon catheter for maintaining cerebral blood flow and cardiac coronary circulation

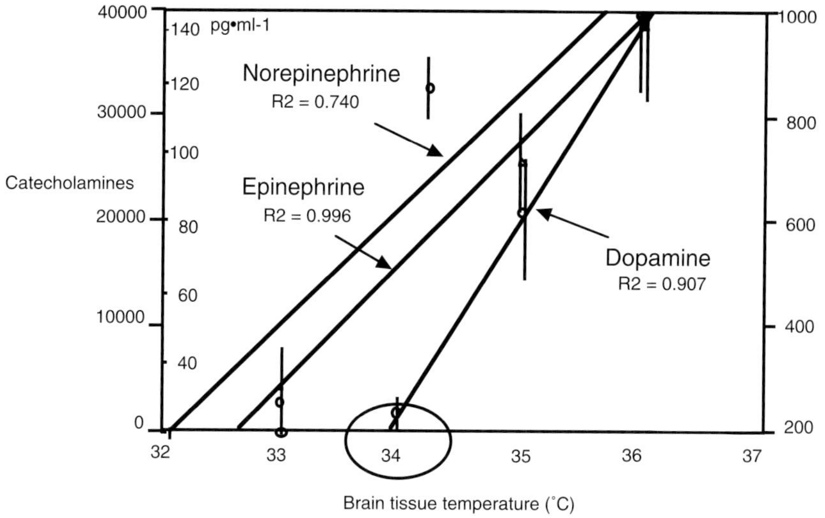

Fig. 32. Effects of brain hypothermia on jugular venous blood catecholamines (n= 10). Among the changes in jugular venous blood catecholamines, dopamine is the most sensitive to cooling of the brain tissue temperature. The dopamine release could be prevented by control of brain tissue temperature below 34°C

Table 4. The clinical issues of hypothalamus-pituitary-adrenal axis neurohormonal dysfunction

1. Insulin-resistant hyperglycemia	→	Anaerobic brain metabolism Activate glutamate toxicity Hemoglobin dysfunction and neuronal hypoxia
2. Vasopressin release	→	Hypoalbuminemia BBB dysfunction Cytokine encephalitis Brain edema
3. Glycogenesis of protein (Progressive hypoalbuminemia)	→	Progression of brain edema Hypo-phosphate and Mg^{++} Intestinal mucous edema and immune dysfunction Unsuccessful enteral nutrition Respiratory muscle weakness
4. Delayed HPA axis suppression by dopamine	→	Free bacteria Unstable antibiotics Reduced T3 and libido

Catecholamine surge of epinephrine, norepinephrine, and dopamine, multiphase release of vasopressin, and prolonged release of growth hormone were recorded in all severely brain-injured patients (Glasgow Coma Scale score of less than 6) [3,13]. The excess release of catecholamines produces coronary ischemia, cardiac muscle contraction, contraction myocytolysis, contraction band necrosis, unstable cardiopulmonary dysfunction, hemoglobin dysfunction with slow release of bound oxygen from hemoglobin, insulin-resistant severe hyperglycemia, metabolic acidosis, and brain thermo-pooling. The excess release of epinephrine and severe hyperglycemia stimulate the hypothalamus neuropeptide Y receptor [24] and release of vasopressin through a feedback mechanism of neural control of macronutrients (Fig. 22, Chap. 22) [13].

Release of vasopressin occurs within a few minutes of trauma by direct neural stimulation. This reaction was recorded for about 2h after trauma and insults in most cases. However, if stress-associated hyperglycemia with serum glucose levels above 230mg/dl is not controlled, vasopressin release will continue until the reserve vasopressin in the pituitary gland is consumed. The excess release of vasopressin produces renal dysfunction, oliguria and annuli with persistent cell-toxic metabolic substrates, reduced serum osmolarity with third-space interstitial edema, reduction of CBF with vasoconstriction, activation of CSF cytokines, and BBB dysfunction. The early diagnosis of these complications is important for the success of ICU management. Prolonged hyperglycemia-complicated oliguria with serum glucose levels above 230mg/dl suggests the possibility of these complications. The complication of severe pulmonary infection with severe BBB damage (CSF/serum albumin ratio >0.02) can promote the complication of cytokine encephalitis. Cytokine encephalitis is a serious complication for severely brain-injured patients because severe brain edema becomes uncontrollable even with brain hypothermia of 32°–34°C (see Chap. 39).

For management of secondary brain damage related to HPA axis neurohormone release, early induction of brain hypothermia of 32°–34°C, and control of serum glucose concentration to 120–140 mg/dl, serum phosphate at 3–5 mg/dl, serum magnesium to 1.6 ± 0.2 mEq/l, serum albumin above 3.0 mg/dl, control of BBB dysfunction [5,13,16], and activation of immune function are recommended. To avoid the progression of catecholamine surge and hyperglycemia, use of 7% acetic Ringer's solution followed by 4% saline fluid infusion is advised.

The Prevention of Selective Radical Attack of the Dopamine A10 Nervous System

The dopamine A10 nervous system is important for maintaining the neuronal functions of emotion, memory, volition, thinking, and love [8]. Whole brain damage of the brain mantle and selective damage of the A10 nervous system, especially hippocampus and amygdala nucleus in the deep brain produces the vegetative state from which the personality of the patient is difficult to maintain [9–11]. The release of many neurotransmitters that include glutamate, dopamine, opioids, and serotonin occurs in severely brain-injured patients [2,3,8,9,11,17]. The release of neurotoxic glutamate specifically produces delayed neuronal death in the short memory center (hippocampus). The release of dopamine from the dopamine central nervous system causes production of OH^- radicals by the reaction of oxygen with dopamine (Fig. 33) [1,23]. The selective OH^- attack of the dopamine nervous system is unavoidable in severe brain injury. Recently, concern over the formation of NO radicals caused by serotonin release has emerged. Selective radical attack of the hippocampus and amygdala in dopamine A10 nervous system produces a high degree of neuronal dysfunction and damage to memory, emotion, and thought (Fig. 34). Therefore, prevention of selective damage to the hippocumpus and amygdala in dopamine A10 nervous system is very important at the acute stage to prevent vegetation [9].

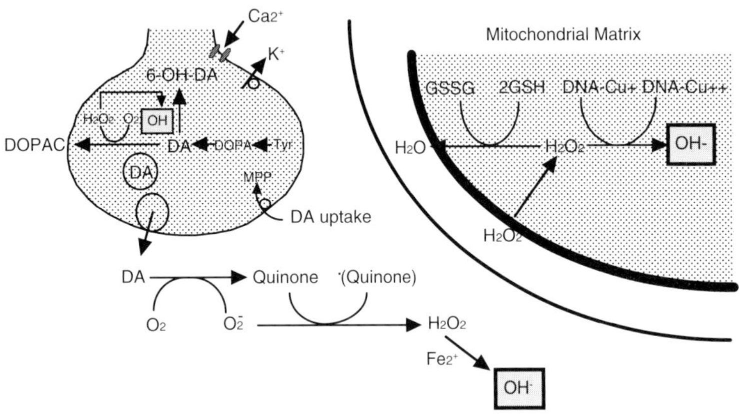

Fig. 33. The mechanism of radical formation by dopamine release after acute severe brain damage. This reaction produces selective radical attack of the dopamine central nervous system. *DOPAC*, 3,4-dihydroxyphenylacetic acid; *DA*, dopamine; *Tyr*, tyrosine; *MPP*, l-methyl-4-phenylpyridinium; *GSSG*, oxidized glutathione; *GSH*, reduced glutathione

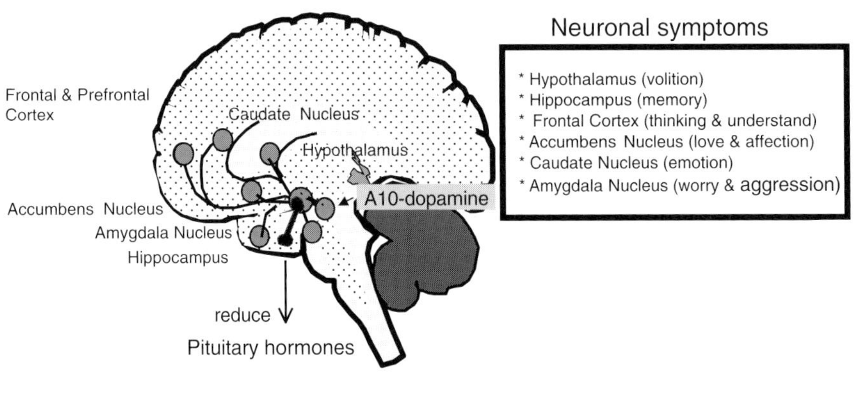

Fig. 34. The selective damage of dopamine A10 nervous system produces vegetation

Two treatments for the prevention of selective damage to the hippocumpus and amygdala in dopamine A10 nervous system are the use of brain hypothermia to minimize the release of neurotransmitters, glutamate, and serotonin [9–11,13,20,21], and the administration of radical scavengers. The use of anesthesia, hypothermia, and pharmacological blockers of neurotransmitter release have been investigated for the reduction of glutamate and dopamine release. Free radical reactions are not prevented by one method alone, but probably by a combination of anesthesia, hypothermia, administration of pharmacological blockers of dopamine release, and radical scavengers. Our preliminary clinical studies of the NO_2/NO_3 ratio [13,15] suggested that brain hypothermia at 34°C prevented about 50% of radical reactions; however, brain hypothermia at 32°C was very powerful in the prevention of free radical reactions. Because free radical reactions occur very rapidly, combination of early two-step induction of hypothermia under anesthesia and administration of metoclop-aramide (a dopamine-release blocker in the brain tissue) are useful for the prevention of selective damage to the dopamine A10 nervous system. There are many reports which describe additional treatments for the scavenging of radicals that include control of hemoglobin concentration above 11 mg/dl and administration of vitamins E and C. One of the advantages of brain hypothermia treatment that became apparent in our clinical studies, is the low incidence of vegetation and memory disturbance.

References

1. Almeida A, Delgado-Esteban M, Bolanos JP, Medina JM (2002) Oxygen and glucose deprivation induces mitochondrial dysfunction and oxidative stress in neurones but not in astrocytes in primary culture. Neurochem 81:207–217
2. Baker AJ, Zornow MH, Scheller MS, Yaksh TL, Skilling SR, Smullin DH, Larson AA, Kuczenski R (1991) Changes in extracellular concentrations of glutamate, aspartate, glycine, dopamine, serotonin, and dopamine metabolites after transient global ischemia in the rat. J Neurochem 57:1370–1379
3. Chiolero R, Lemarchand TH, Schutz Y, de Tribolet N, Felber JP, Freeman J, Jequier E (1988) Plasma pituitary hormone levels in severe trauma with or without head injury. J Trauma 28:1368–1374
4. Corte FD, Mancini A, Valle D, Gallizzi F, Carducci P, Mignani V, De Marinis L (1998) Provocative hypothalamopituitary axis tests in severe head injury: correlations with severity and prognosis. Crit Care Med 26:1419–1426
5. Dietrich WD, Busto R, Halley M, Valdes I (1990) The importance of brain temperature in alterations of the blood–brain barrier following cerebral ischemia. J Neuropathol Exp Neurol 49:486–497
6. Dudariev VP, Lanovenko II (1999) Changes in the oxygen-binding properties of the blood in white rats under the influence of hypoxia and its pharmacological correction. Fiziol Zh 45:97–103
7. Feng H, Huang G, Gao L, Tan H, Liao X (2000) Effect of intracranial pressure and cerebral perfusion pressure on outcome prediction of severe traumatic brain injury. Chin J Traumatol 3:226–230
8. Globus MY-T, Ginsberg MD, Haris SI, Busto R, Dietrich WD (1987) Role of dopamine in ischemic striatal injury. Neurology 37:1712–1719
9. Hackl JM, Gottardis M, Wieser C, Rumpl E, Standler C, Schwarz S, Monkayo R (1991) Endocrine abnormalities in severe traumatic brain injury—a cue to prognosis in severe craniocerebral trauma? Intensive Care Med 17:25–29
10. Hayashi N (1997) Combination therapy of cerebral hypothermia, pharmacological activation of the dopamine system, and hormonal replacement in severely brain damaged patients. J Jpn Soc Intensive Care Med 4:191–197
11. Hayashi N (1997) Prevention of vegetation after severe head trauma and stroke by combination therapy of cerebral hypothermia and activation of immune-dopaminergic nervous system. Proceedings of the 6th annual meeting of Society for Treatment of Coma 6:133–145
12. Hayashi N (2000) Enhanced neuronal damage in severely brain injured patients by hypothalamus, pituitary, and adrenal axis neuro-hormonal changes. In: Hayashi N (ed) Brain hypothermia. Springer, Berlin Heidelberg New York Tokyo, pp 3–26
13. Hayashi N (2000) The clinical issue and effectiveness of brain hypothermia treatment for severe brain injured patients. In: Hayashi N (ed) Brain hypothermia. Springer, Berlin Heidelberg New York Tokyo, pp 121–151
14. Hayashi N, Hirayama T, Utagawa A (1994) The cerebral thermo-pooling and hypothermia treatment of critical head injury patients. In: Nagai H (ed). Intracranial pressure IX. Springer, Berlin Heidelberg New York Tokyo, pp 589–599
15. Hayashi N, Utagawa A, Kinosita K, Izumi T (1999) Application of a novel technique for clinical evaluation of nitric oxide-induced free radical reactions in ICU patients. Cell Mol Neurobiol 19:3–17
16. Jiang JY, Lyeth BG, Kapasi MZ, Jenkins LW, Povlishock JT (1992) Moderate hypothermia reduces blood–brain barrier disruption following traumatic brain injury in the rat. Acta Neuropathol Berl 84:495–500
17. MacIntosh TK, Hayes R, DeWitt D, Agura V, Faden AI (1987) Endogenous opioids may mediate secondary damage after experimental brain injury. Am J Physiol 258:E565–574
18. MacIntosh TK (1994) Neurological sequele of traumatic brain injury: therapeutic implications. Cerebrovasc Brain Metab Rev 6:109–162
19. Morgan TJ, Koch D, Morris D, Clague A, Purdie DM (2001) Reduced red cell 2,3-diphosphoglycerate concen-

trations in critical illness without decreased in vivo P50. Anaesth Intensive Care 29:479–483
20. Okuda C, Saito A, Miyazaki M, Kuriyama K (1986) Alteration of the turnover of dopamine and 5-hydroxytryptamine in rat brain associated with hypothermia. Pharmacol Biochem Behav 25:79–83
21. Russwurm S, Stonans I, Schwerter K, Stonane E, Meissner W, Reinhart K (2002) Direct influence of mild hypothermia on cytokine expression and release in cultures of human peripheral blood mononuclear cells. J Interferon Cytokine Res 22:15–21
22. Shoemaker WC, Apple PL, Kram HB, Waxman K, Lee T (1988) Prospective trial of supernormal values of survivors as therapeutic goals in high-risk surgical patients. Chest 94:1176–1186
23. Silvka A, Coben G (1985) Hydroxyl radical attack on dopamine. J Biol Chem 260:15466–15472
24. Temple DL (1994) The neuropeptide Y system (hypothalamus) has a dense concentration of glucocorticoide (type II) receptors that mediate carbon hydrate intake. J Neuroendocrinol 6:479–501

27. New Concept of Brain Hypothermia Treatment

The basic concept of brain hypothermia treatment is the control of brain tissue temperature to between 32° and 34°C, maintenance of systemic circulation–metabolism, neurohormonal control, and stabilization of the immune function, for the restoration of injured neurons [14]. Reduced brain metabolism for neuroprotection from brain ischemia and the prevention of intracranial pressure (ICP) elevation are not initial goals. To restore dying neurons in injured brain tissue, hypothermia itself is not sufficient. Administration of oxygen, stabilization of brain metabolism with adequate metabolic substrates, and prevention of excess neurohormonal reactions of the hypothalamus–pituitary–adrenal (HPA) axis are the initial goals of brain hypothermia [13–15]. The early induction of mild to moderate brain hypothermia (32–34°C) is very successful in the prevention of hazardous excess neurohormonal reactions of HPA axis. Early anesthesia is also helpful in preventing excess stimulation of the HPA axis [9,10,14–16].

The recovery from disturbances of personality, memory loss, and vegetation are also important in brain hypothermia treatment [11,12,14,15]. Therefore, proper function of cortical neurons, avoiding prolonged neuroexcitation of the hippocampus, and prevention of selective radical damage to the dopamine A10 nervous system [5,21,27] in deep brain tissue are important goals of intensive care unit (ICU) management [9–12,14,15]. The prevention of brain edema and ICP elevation are essential during this treatment. The lowering of brain metabolism to reduce oxygen consumption, control of ICP, and management of brain edema are not major targets of brain hypothermia treatment.

Initial Management: Prevention of Neuronal Hypoxia, Metabolic Changes, Brain Thermo-pooling, and Cardiopulmonary Dysfunction in the Acute Stage

Most neurons in injured brain tissue do not die immediately and can be sustained until recovery. To allow recovery of these neurons in primary-injured brain tissue, maintenance of adequate oxygen supply [1,10,14] and a balanced glucose metabolism are necessary despite brain hypothermia treatment [13,14]. However, our recent clinical studies showed a high incidence of brain tissue hypoxia (neuronal hypoxia) even with normal management of PaO_2, oxygen delivery, systolick blood pressure (SBP), ICP, and cerebral perfusion pressure (CPP) within 6h of the acute stage [10,12–14]. Cases of neuronal hypoxia that occurred despite normal oxygen delivery were attributed to the slow release of bound oxygen from hemoglobin [13]. This specific hemoglobin dysfunction was produced by insulin-resistant hyperglycemia and excess neurohormonal reactions of the HPA axis. We call this phenomenon "masking brain hypoxia" [10,13,14]. Without understanding masking brain hypoxia, successful restoration therapy for injured neurons is difficult. The main cause of hemoglobin dysfunction is reduced levels of hemoglobin diphosphoglycerate (DPG) [6,13,22]. Slow release of oxygen from hemoglobin, massive blood transfusion, shifting of the blood flow to the intestine caused by changes of dopamine-dominant systemic circulation, elevation of brain tissue temperature above 40°C caused by brain thermo-pooling, and unstable cardiac output (CO) were recorded as causes of masking brain hypoxia [10,12–14].

The early induction of mild to moderate hypothermia is very successful to control catecholamine surge (Fig. 25, Chap. 23). One benefit of brain hypothermia is the prevention of masking brain hypoxia by control of catecholamine surge and serum hyperglycemia. The adequate release of catecholamines and neurohormones following brain damage is effective for maintaining cerebral blood flow (CBF) and brain metabolism [3,4,8]. However, excess release of catecholamines produces not only masking brain hyoxia [10,13,14], but also cardiac ischemia, insulin-resistant hyperglycemia [10,13], blood–brain barrier (BBB) dysfunction caused by vasopressin release [17], and acute pulmonary edema. Therefore, the question of how to diagnose the severity and critical conditions of catecholamine surge following brain damage is important. Direct monitoring of serum catecholamines is most reliable to diagnose the severity of catecholamine surge. However, this method is not practical because the measurement of serum catecholamines is time consuming. As an alternative method, the level of hyperglycemia can be evaluated as an indirect parameter of catecholamine (epinephrine) surge [10,12–14]. The dangerous level of catecholamine surge is regarded as hyperglycemia with serum glucose level over 180 mg/dl. The critical level is over 230 mg/dl.

The desirable brain temperature for the control of catecholamine surge is about 32°–34°C. Moderate brain hypothermia (32°–33°C) can sometimes reduce the levels of serum catecholamines (dopamine > epinephrine > norepinephrine) significantly and can cause unstable systemic circulation without appropriate fluid resuscitation [10,12,14]. Therefore, adequate fluid resuscitation and oxygenation are important throughout brain hypothermia management. Dehydration therapy for the prevention of brain edema, such as manitol and glycerol infusion, is not suitable under brain hypothermia, especially in the initial stage.

Neuronal recovery essentially requires appropriate oxygen–glucose metabolisms. However, it has long been considered that the suppression of brain metabolism allows brain ischemia to be tolerated by reducing oxygen and glucose demand. Part of this philosophy may be correct for the protection of patients who are not severely brain injured from future ischemic insults. However, for severely injured patients, this philosophy is not correct. Injured neurons in damaged brain tissue need sufficient production of adenosine triphosphate (ATP) to maintain cellular homeostasis with stable neuronal cell membrane functions [1,19]. These processes open the way for neuronal restoration in injured brain tissue. Our clinical studies of systemic metabolic changes during moderate hypothermia suggested that a systemic metabolic shift from glucose to lipid metabolism occurs at brain tissue temperatures below 35°C [10,12,14]. Therefore, the concept of reducing the brain metabolism of glucose, protein, and lipid is not correct. At brain tissue temperature of 34°C, equal balance of glucose and lipid metabolism was recorded systemically [14]. These metabolic changes are consid-

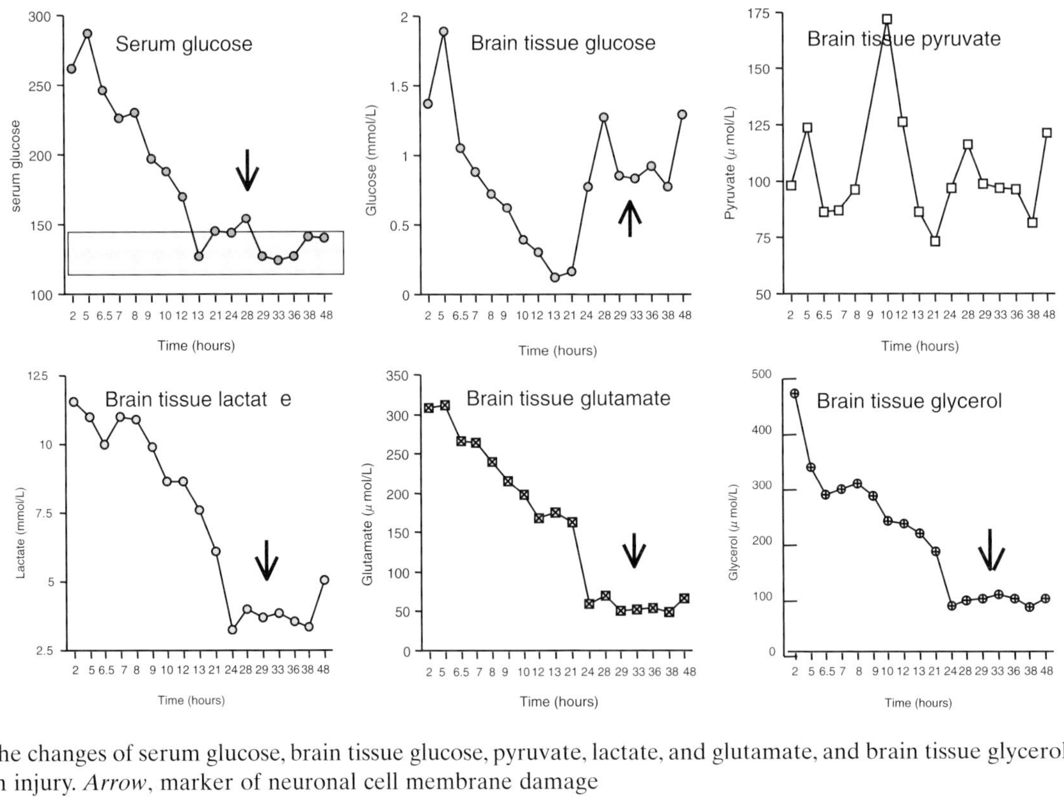

Fig. 35. The changes of serum glucose, brain tissue glucose, pyruvate, lactate, and glutamate, and brain tissue glycerol with time after brain injury. *Arrow*, marker of neuronal cell membrane damage

ered to occur in the brain metabolism during brain hypothermia.

Our clinical studies of brain metabolism during brain hypothermia treatment using a microdialysis monitor suggested that precise control of serum glucose concentration is especially important to maintain the brain metabolism (Fig. 35) and BBB dysfunction [10,14]. The degree of hyperglycemia that occurs initially depends on the severity of catecholamine surge (Figs. 8 and 15, Chap. 22), and, also, on the reduced systemic glucose utilization that occurs with rapid induction of brain hypothermia. In most cases, brain tissue temperature below 33°C can easily produce hyperglycemia by reducing the consumption of serum glucose [14]. In such cases, brain tissue pyruvate and lactate levels become higher than those at a brain tissue temperature of 34°C (Fig. 28, Chap. 23). The critical level of serum glucose to prevent brain tissue lactate accumulation is more than 140–160 mg/dl. From these results, it was suggested that brain hypothermia treatment requires sufficient neuronal oxygenation and adequate control of serum glucose to maintain metabolic balance as shown in Fig. 16 (Chap. 22). Therefore, the serum glucose level must be carefully monitored throughout brain hypothermia treatment. If rapid progression of hyperglycemia during brain hypothermia treatment is observed, hypothermia is not further indicated. When brain tissue temperature is lowered to between 33° and 34°C, changes in serum glucose concentration must be followed carefully.

Management Choice Depending on the Presence of HPA-Axis Abnormality, Cardiac–Respiratory Brain Damage, and Complication of Infections

The development of secondary brain damage after brain trauma, and the occurrence of occlusive cerebral–vascular stroke, hypoxia, shock, and cardiac arrest depend on the presence of HPA-axis abnormality [4,12–14,18]. The magnification of stress to the HPA axis is suppresed under anesthesia. Therefore, the mechanisms of secondary brain damage with and without anesthesia are not the same. The management of accidental brain damage during surgery should focus on stabilizing vital signs before attention is paid to brain ischemia, brain edema, neuroexcitaion, and ICP elevation, as previously discussed [19,25]. Administration of brain hypothermia is effective for the prevention of brain edema and ICP elevation [10,14]. Mild brain hypothermia (around 34°C) is sufficient for most of these brain-injured patients.

However, if brain damage occurs without anesthesia, ICU management must not only be watchful of the direct brain injury mechanism, but also of various pathophysiological changes that are associated with excess neurohormone release by stimulation of the HPA axis [3,4,8,13,14,18,20]. In such cases, the mechanism of brain damage is not as simple as that of experimental animal models. Recorded effects of stress reactions of the HPA axis include insulin-resistant hyperglycemia, neuronal hypoxia with slow release of oxygen from hemoglobin in injured brain tissue, lactic acidosis, excess release of vasopressin, pulmonary edema with vascular contraction, cardiac dysfunction that includes contraction myocytolysis, and brain thermo-pooling [13]. The detail of pathophysiological changes associated with stimulation of HPA axis are described previously in this book. To prevent HPA axis-related brain damage, control of excess catecholamine surge by early induction of brain hypothermia is recommended as a first step [10,14,23,24]. In severe cases at the acute onset of brain damage, a brain tissue temperature of 34°C is not sufficient to prevent NO radical reactions and brain edema, especially in cases of hyperglycemia with serum glucose levels above 230 mg/dl [10,14]. Severe hyperglycemia in the acute stage of brain damage indirectly suggests excess catecholamine surge and the presence of stress to the HPA axis. In these cases, two-step induction of brain hypothermia, initial control of brain tissue temperature at 34°C, followed by 32°–33°C brain tissue temperature, is recommended with careful management of serum glucose. Our recent clinical ICU studies using microdialysis suggested that increased levels of brain tissue glucose and lactate, and glutamate toxicity occur with unsuccessful management of hyperglycemia at 120–150 mmHg during brain hypothermia treatment [14].

Rapid induction of brain hypothermia to prevent brain edema also produces the increases in serum glucose levels by reduction of systemic glucose consumption. Therefore, at the induction stage of brain hypothermia, the cause of hyperglycemia must be carefully diagnosed as either unsuccessful management of catecholamine surge, or reduced systemic glucose consumption. The two-step induction of brain hypothermia to around 34°C initially, and then followed by the careful induction of 32°–33°C brain hypothermia allows easier diagnosis of hyperglycemia [10,14].

Recent nutritional studies revealed the mechanism of neural control for macronutrient intake. Our recent clinical studies of neural control of macronutrients in serum using microdialysis recorded the interactions between severe insulin-resistant hyperglycemia, excess

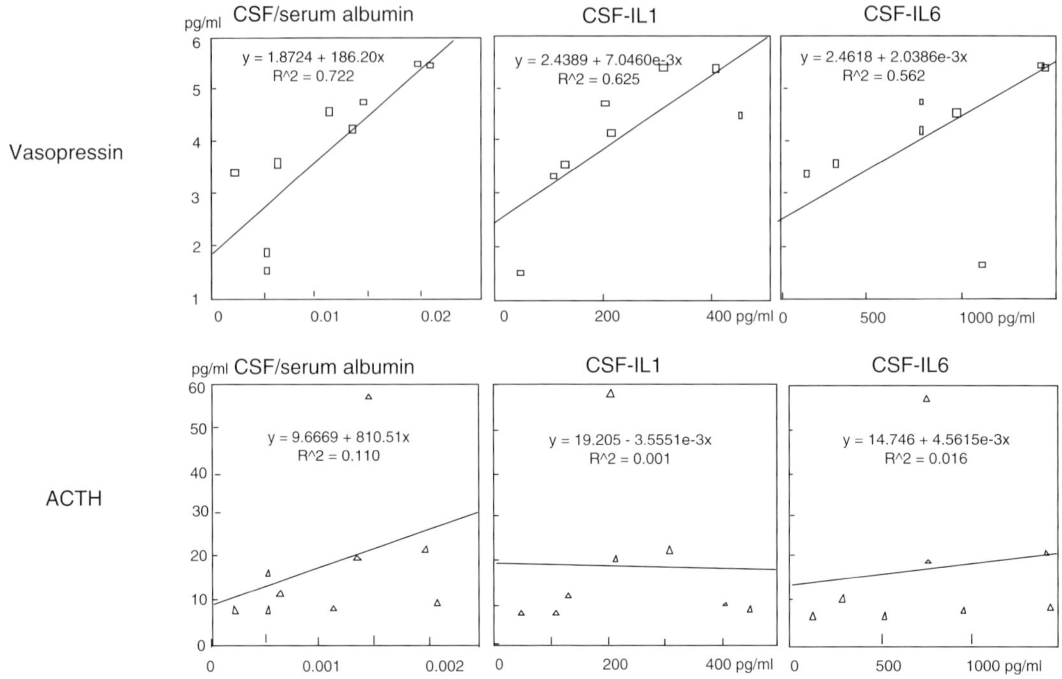

Fig. 36. The release of vasopressin activates proinflammatory cytokines IL1, IL6, and changes the blood–brain barrier (CSF/serum albumin ratio)

release of vasopressin, and BBB dysfunction [14]. The excess release of vasopressin promotes BBB dysfunction with cytokine activation (Fig. 36) [10,13,14]. The presence of severe BBB dysfunction, shown as a CSF/serum albumin ratio greater than 0.02, is a serious condition caused by systemic infection and pneumonia. Increased serum cytokines can easily permeate the BBB and promote cytokine inflammation in the injured brain tissue [13]. This serious complication is also modulated by the release of growth hormone (GH) from the pituitary gland. The prolonged release of GH was recorded after severe brain injury as a consequence of stress to the HPA axis [3,8,13]. Our clinical studies suggest that GH is one of the regulators of immune function by the activation of CD4 and suppression of CD8. Activating CD4 increases levels of interleukin 1 (IL1), IL6, and suppressing CD8 reduces the anti-inflammatory cytokine IL10 [13,14]. Therefore, excess release of GH results in complex and severe secondary brain damage caused by cytokine encephalitis and diminished anti-inflammatory mechanism.

Recent clinical studies of ICU management of critically ill patients also suggested poor prognosis with reduced GH levels [3,13,14]. The time of maximum release of GH is between 3 and 4 days. The management of brain hypothermia below 34°C is very effective for the prevention of excess release of GH. However, prolonged brain hypothermia below 34°C produces an immune crisis because of reduced GH release, especially in the late stages of brain hypothermia management. Excess release of GH promotes the activation of proinflammatory cytokines and worsens infections; however, excess suppression of GH release reduces the immune activity and allows easy infection. During brain hypothermia treatment, control of GH and hyperglycemia are very important to prevent complications and secondary brain damage. Combinations of severe pulmonary infection with GH imbalance and BBB dysfunction caused by brain damage and vasopressin-associated uncontrolled hyperglycemia promote cytokine encephalitis [13]. In our series of clinical studies, uncontrollable increases in cytotoxic glutamate levels were recorded even with brain hypothermia management at 32°–33°C [14]. Therefore, complication of severe pulmonary infection during brain hypothermia management means the hypothermia treatment is unsuccessful. Unfortunately, recent statistical clinical studies of hypothermia treatment recorded a high incidence of complication by pulmonary infections of 44%–65%. In our clinical studies, complication from severe pneumonia was limited to about 10% [14].

The precise mechanism of vasopressin release in severely brain-injured patient is not clear. The hypothalamus neuropeptide Y network stimulates the release of vasopressin for the control of macronutrient intake via a feedback mechanism and cerebral vascular reactions [13,14,17,18]. The hypothalamus neuropeptide Y network is stimulated by norepinephrine and increased brain tissue glucose levels. Therefore, excess release of vasopressin and GH are also associated with catecholamine surge that occurs as a neuroendocrinological hormonal reaction following harmful stress such as severe brain injury, stroke, or subarachnoid hemorrhage.

The management of excess release of vasopressin and GH is very important for the survival of severely brain-injured patients. The reduction of catecholamine surge by using mild to moderate brain hypothermia, control of hyperglycemia, suppression of inflammatory reactions by activating prostaglandin I (PGI) 2 with AT-III, and maintenance of the BBB function by replacement of hypo-albuminemia are summarized as the initial treatments for pathophysiological changes related to excess release of neurohormones [13,14].

The successful management of hyperglycemia, BBB dysfunction, hemoglobin dysfunction, and systemic infection during brain hypothermia management is important to determine the clinical prognosis. The practical management of hyperglycemia associated with catecholamine surge during brain hypothermia treatment is described in Chaps. 43 and 44.

Protection of Dopamine A10 Nervous System for Prevention of Disturbances to Memory, Emotion, and Personality

Prevention of vegetation is an important matter in the management of severely brain-injured patients. The precise mechanism of vegetation is still not clear. Massive cortical destruction of the brain mantle and selective neuronal damage of the dopamine A10 nervous system that includes the hippocampus and amygdala in the deep brain are considered as causes of vegetation [7,9–12,14]. Recovery from massive cortical brain destruction is very difficult. However, with selective localized neuronal damage of the hippocampus and amygdala in dopamine A10 nervous system, there is some possibility of restoration. The hippocampus is the short memory center for new information. The dopamine A10 nervous system consists of the hippocampus, hypothalamus, frontal cortex, accumbens nucleus, caudate nucleus, and amygdala nucleus [5, 21]. Selective neuronal damage of the hippocampus and the dopamine A10 nervous system causes loss of recent memory, loss of volition, lack of understanding, and loss of emotion and affection. A mechanism of selective damage to the hippocampus neurons is known to be prolonged neuroexcitation caused by release of the excitatory amino acid glutamate. On the other hand, selective free radical attack by $\cdot OH^-$ radicals derived from reaction of oxygen with released dopamine is considered to be a mechanism of damage to the dopamine A10 nervous system (Fig. 33, Chap. 26) [2,28].

In our clinical studies, brain tissue glutamate and CSF dopamine were recorded at very low levels during brain hypothermia at 33°C [13,14]. This implies that brain hypothermia at 32°–33°C prevents excess release of glutamate and dopamine from the injured brain. In addition, early induction of brain hypothermia protects against delayed neuronal death in the hippocampus and selective radical damage of the dopamine nervous system in the acute stage. This concept is supported by clinical evidence of good recovery of the dopamine A10 nervous system, as shown by the low incidence of disturbances to consciousness, thinking, memory, volition, and emotional expression in patients treated by brain hypothermia [10,14,23]. The effectiveness of hypothermia treatment of severe head injuries, with Glasgow Coma Scale (GCS) scores less than 7, is also supported by the hypothermia group recording lower incidence of vegetation [14] than the nonhypothermia group. The CT finding of selective low density of hippocampus and amygdala in vegetation is another support for importance of management of dopamine A10 nervous system. Therefore, we have hypothesized that excess release of dopamine causes selective radical damage to the dopaminergic central nervous system, which includes the A10 nervous system, and results in indifference, prolonged memory disturbances, reduced activity, and disturbed volition.

The severity and reversibility of damage to the dopamine A10 nervous system at the chronic stage are diagnosed by monitoring of responsiveness of the CSF dopamine/Prolactin ratio with varying cerebral dopamine replacement therapies. This diagnostic method of responsiveness of the dopamine A10 nervous system is useful to evaluate the reversibility of the vegetative state. As a treatment for the prevention of vegetation, reduction of excess release of dopamine at the acute stage is necessary to prevent radical attack of the dopamine A10 nervous system. Early induction of brain hypothermia (32°–33°C) or combination of Metoclopramide administration and hypothermia are very succesful in the prevention of dopamine release in the acute stage and easily reduce selective damage to the dopamine A10 nervous system. If prolonged neuronal damage to emotion, thinking, and responsiveness is observed at 2–3 weeks, cerebral dopamine replacement therapy (administration of Leodopa and Amantadine, Estrogen patch, and median nerve stimulation) is suggested for neuronal activation of the dopamine A10 nervous system [5,9,10,14].

Our two-step restoration therapy of the dopamine A10 nervous system that included neuroprotection of

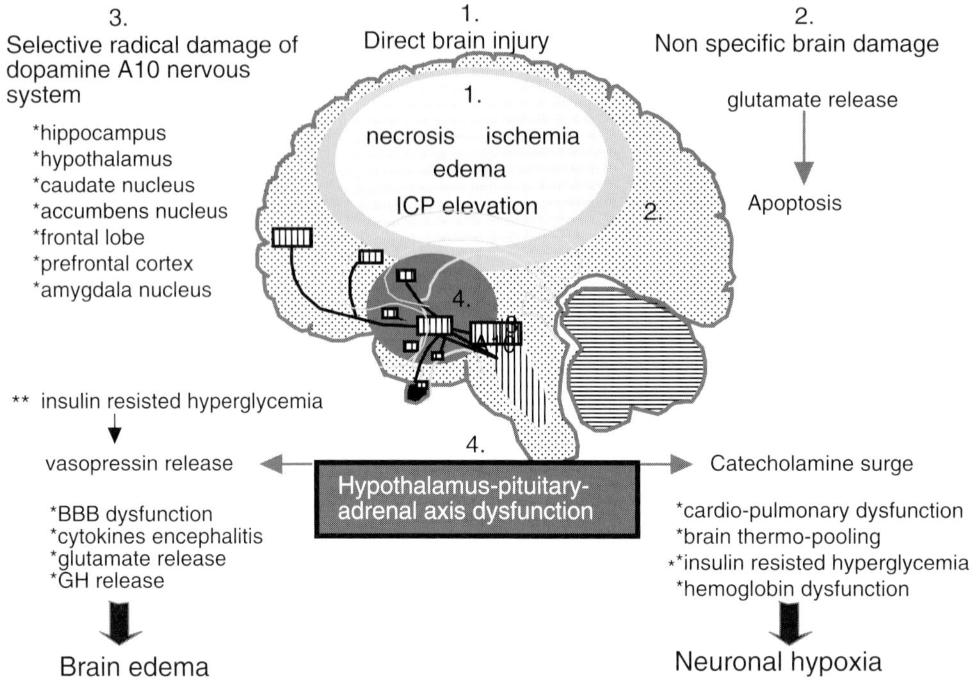

Fig. 37. The mechanism of brain damage after severe brain injury

the dopamine A10 nervous system from selective radical attack by combination of brain hypothermia and pharmacological treatment in the acute stage, and activation of dopamine A10 nervous system by dopamine replacement therapy, was very useful to prevent vegetation in severely brain-injured patients (GCS <6). Neuroprotection afforded by the prevention of excess neurotransmitter release in the acute stage and neuronal activation of the dopamine A10 nervous system with cortical neurons in the chronic stage is very important for the minimization of damage to neuronal functions, thought, emotion, intelligence, and maintenance of personality in the management of severely brain-injured patients. The timing and detailed technique of dopamine replacement therapy is dicussed in Chap. 49.

The new findings of brain injury mechanisms are summarized in Fig. 37 in four parts: direct brain injury mechanism, apoptosis nonspecific brain damage mechanism, selective radical damage of the dopamine A10 nervous system, and neuronal hypoxia and brain edema associated with HPA axis neurohormonal dysfunction. In the management of severe brain damage caused by brain trauma, cerebral stroke, brain hypoxia, or cardiac arrest, these four brain injury mechanisms are important targets. The reduction of brain tissue temperature, as reported in previous hypothermia studies, is not sufficient treatment for these four brain injury mechanisms. The management of neuronal oxygenation, suitable metabolic balance, and control of neurohormononal-immune function under brain hypothermia at 32°–34°C is standard treatment for neuronal restoration. The previously accepted procedure of neuroprotection by management of CBF, ICP, and brain edema is insufficient therapy for dying neurons in primary injured brain tissue.

References

1. Almeida A, Delgado-Esteban M, Bolanos JP, Medina JM (2002) Oxygen and glucose deprivation induces mitochondrial dysfunction and oxidative stress in neurones but not in astrocytes in primary culture. Neurochem 81: 207–217
2. Baker AJ, Zornow MH, Scheller MS, Yaksh TL, Skilling SR, Smullin DH, Larson AA, Kuczenski R (1991) Changes in extracellular concentrations of glutamate, aspartate, glycine, dopamine, serotonin, and dopamine metabolites after transient global ischemia in the rat. J Neurochem 57:1370–1379
3. Chiolero R, Lemarchand TH, Schutz Y, de Tribolet N, Felber JP, Freeman J (1988) Plasma pituitary hormone levels in severe trauma with or without head injury. J Trauma 28:1368–1374
4. Corte FD, Mancini A, Valle D, Gallizzi F, Carducci P, Mignani V, De Marinis L (1998) Provocative hypothalamopituitary axis tests in severe head injury: correlations with severity and prognosis. Crit Care Med 26:1419–1426

5. Creutz LM, Kritzer MF (2002) Estrogen receptor-beta immunoreactivity in the midbrain of adult rats: regional, subregional, and cellular localization in the A10, A9, and A8 dopamine cell groups. J Comp Neurol 446:288–300
6. Dudariev VP, Lanovenko II (1999) Changes in the oxygen-binding properties of the blood in white rats under the influence of hypoxia and its pharmacological correction. Fiziol Zh 45:97–103
7. Globus MY-T, Ginsberg MD, Haris SI, Busto R, Dietrich WD (1987) Role of dopamine in ischemic striatal injury. Neurology 37:1712–1719
8. Hackl JM, Gottardis M, Wieser C, Rumpl E, Stadler C, Schwarz S, Monkayo R (1991) Endocrine abnormalities in severe traumatic brain injury—a cue to prognosis in severe craniocerebral trauma? Intensive Care Med 17:25–29
9. Hayashi N (1997) Combination therapy of cerebral hypothermia, pharmacological activation of the dopamine system, and hormonal replacement in severely brain damaged patients. J Jpn Soc Intensive Care Med 4: 191–197
10. Hayashi N (1997) Prevention of vegetation after severe head trauma and stroke by combination therapy of cerebral hypothermia and activation of immune-dopaminergic nervous system. Proceedings of the 6th annual meeting of Society for Treatment of Coma 6:133–145
11. Hayashi N (1998) The control of brain tissue temperature and stimulation of dopamine-immune system to severe brain injury patients. Nippon Rinsho 56:1627–1635
12. Hayashi N (1999) Brain hypothermia therapy for prevention of vegetation after severe brain injury. Nippon Geka Gakkai Zasshi 100:443–448
13. Hayashi N (2000) Enhanced neuronal damage in severely brain injured patients by hypothalamus, pituitary, and adrenal axis neuro-hormonal changes. In: Hayashi N (ed) Brain hypothermia. Springer, Berlin Heidelberg New York Tokyo, pp 3–26
14. Hayashi N (2000) The clinical issue and effectiveness of brain hypothermia treatment for severe brain injured patients. In: Hayashi N (ed) Brain hypothermia. Springer, Berlin Heidelberg New York Tokyo, pp 121–151
15. Hayashi N (2000) Brain hypothermia treatment for the management of severe pediatric brain injury. No To Hattatsu 32:122–131
16. Hayashi N, Hirayama T, Utagawa A (1994) The cerebral thermo-pooling and hypothermia treatment of critical head injury patients. In: Nagai H (ed) Intracranial pressure IX. Springer, Berlin Heidelberg New York Tokyo, pp 589–599
17. Kagawa M, Nagao S, Bemana I (1996) Arginine vasopressin receptor antagonists for treatment of vasogenic brain edema: an experimental study. J Neurotrauma 13:273–279
18. Leibowitz SF, Sladek C, Spencer L, Temple D (1988) Neuropeptide Y, epinephrine and norepinephrine in the paraventricular nucleus: stimulation of feeding and the release of corticosterone, vasopressin and glucose. Brain Res Bull 21:905–912
19. MacIntosh TK (1994) Neurological sequele of traumatic brain injury: therapeutic implications. Cerebrovasc Brain Metab Rev 6:109–162
20. MacIntosh TK, Hayes R, DeWitt D, Agura V, Faden AI (1987) Endogenous opioids may mediate secondary damage after experimental brain injury. Am J Physiol 258:E565–E574
21. Moore RY, Bloom FE (1978) Central catecholamine neuron systems: anatomy and physiology of the dopamine system. Ann Rev Neurosci 1:129–169
22. Morgan TJ, Koch D, Morris D, Clague A, Purdie DM (2001) Reduced red cell 2,3-diphosphoglycerate concentrations in critical illness without decreased in vivo P50. Anaesth Intensive Care 29:479–483
23. Nagao K, Hayashi N, Kanmatsuse K, Arima K, Ohtsuki J, Kikushima K, Watanabe I (2000) Cardiopulmonary cerebral resuscitation using emergency cardiopulmonary bypass, coronary reperfusion therapy and mild hypothermia in patients with cardiac arrest outside the hospital. J Am Coll Cardiol 36:776–783
24. Russwurm S, Stonans I, Schwerter K, Stonane E, Meissner W, Reinhart K (2002) Direct influence of mild hypothermia on cytokine expression and release in cultures of human peripheral blood mononuclear cells. J Interferon Cytokine Res 22:15–21
25. Shoemaker WC, Apple PL, Kram HB, Waxman K, Lee T (1988) Prospective trial of supernormal values of survivors as therapeutic goals in high-risk surgical patients. Chest 94:1176–1186
26. Silvka A, Coben G (1985) Hydroxyl radical attack on dopamine. J Biol Chem 260:15466–15472
27. Simon H, Le Moal M, Stinus L, Calas A (1979) Anatomical relationships between the ventral mesencephalic tegmentum-A10 region and the locus coeruleus as demonstrated by anterograde and retrograde tracing technique. J Neural Trans 44:77–86

III. Approach to Brain Hypothermia Treatment

28. Contraindications

The prognosis of severe brain damage is decided by several factors such as severity, cause of brain damage, the hypothalamus–pituitary–adrenal (HPA) axis neurohormonal release [1], severity of circulatory metabolic changes [2] associated with catecholamine surge, stress-related hyperglycemia, time after the accident, age, and sex [3,4]. Therefore the indication of hypothermia includes several viewpoints as shown in Table 5 in chapter 29. The contraindications are as follow.

1. Shock
2. Severe dehydration
3. More than 450 mm/sec QT interval on electrocardiogram (ECG)
4. Uncontrollable hyperglycemia
5. Compromised patient
6. Glasgow Coma Score (GCS): 3

A positive response to brain hypothermia treatment cannot always be expected from the brain-injured patients because hypothermia is an unusual physiological condition for the human body. Hypothermia results in reduction of cardiac output and blood pressure, suppression of catecholamine release, metabolic shift from glucose to lipid, difficulty controlling hemorrhage with reduced platelets, and activated hyperglycemia [3,4]. These complications must be avoided in intensive care unit (ICU) management. If it is difficult to control such complications during brain hypothermia treatment, then brain hypothermia treatment is contraindicated.

The introduction of brain hypothermia to shocked patients is particularly difficult because hypothermia reduces serum catecholamines in accordance with lower body temperature (Fig. 32, Chap. 26). The cardiac output begins to decrease below a brain tissue temperature of 33°C (Fig. 38). Therefore, without management of blood volume in cases of hemorrhagic shock, dehydration with administration of manitol, and insufficient fluid resuscitation, brain hypothermia treatment is contraindicated. Before starting brain hypothermia treatment, fluid resuscitation and maintenance of stable blood pressure are necessary. Regarding effects of hypothermia on the heart, a J-wave on the ECG without cardiac dysfunction is recorded [4]. Critical cardiac condition following hypothermia treatment is observed as an abnormal QT interval on the ECG of more than 450 mm/s. This negative effect upon the cardiac function is probably caused by rapidly diminished catecholamine release in the bloodstream and rapid suppression of HPA axis function. Unless the blood pressure and cardiac output are stabilized, brain hypothermia is not indicated. Brain hypothermia management may be possible at a brain tissue temperature of 34°C after improvements in the shock condition and stabilized cardiac function.

Severely brain-injured patients with the complication of uncontrollable serum hyperglycemia are also contraindicated for brain hypothermia management, or at least theoretically so. Hypothermia accentuates hyperglycemia because of diminished glucose expenditure, and produces increased levels of brain tissue glucose, pyruvate, and lactate. The advantages of brain hypothermia to severely brain-injured patients are negated by these brain tissue reactions. Resultant complications include hyperglycemia with serum glucose levels above 230 mg/dl and hemoglobin dysfunction observed as slow release of bound oxygen from hemoglobin caused by diminished levels of 2,3-diphosphoglycerate (DPG) in hemoglobin metabolism [2,3,5]. Therefore, precise management of serum glucose throughout brain hypothermia management is one of the key points for success of hypothermia treatment. The complication of uncontrollable hyperglycemia is not an absolute contraindication for brain hypothermia because early induction of brain hypothermia can prevent excess release of catecholamines and minimize the occurrence of insulin-resistant hyperglycemia. In cases of early induction of brain hypothermia within 3 h after insult, hyperglycemia is not a contributor to contraindication. If brain hypothermia treatment is started between 3 and 6 h after insult, very careful management of hyperglycemia is recommended. However, at more than 6 h after insult brain hypothermia is likely to be contraindicated by hyperglycemia. In such cases, brain hypothermia treatment can be started after control of serum glucose levels to below 180 mg/dl. The control of serum glucose to within the range of 120–150 mg/dl throughout brain hypothermia is important.

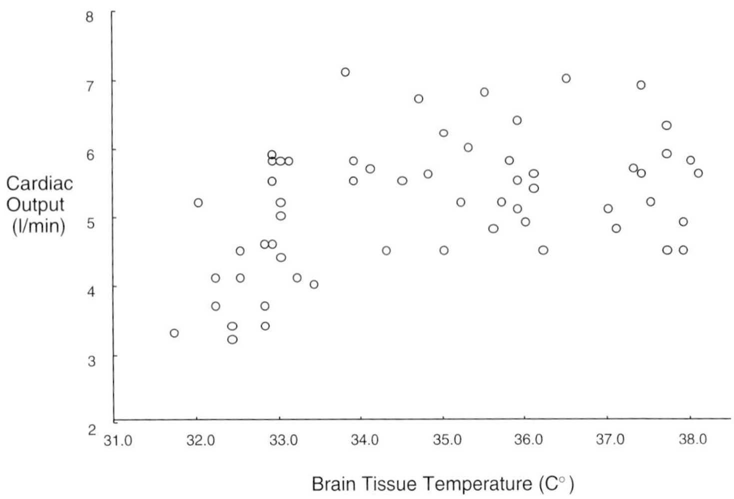

Fig. 38. The inter-relationship between brain tissue temperature and cardiac output ($n = 59$)

Compromised patients such as those with advanced carcinoma, acute myocardial infarction, acute respiratory distress syndrome, sepsis, or malnutrition, are not recommended for brain hypothermia treatment [3]. Cases of severe brain damage with multiple hemorrhage, diffuse brain injury, GCS of 3, and massive cerebral hemorrhage are not indicated for brain hypothermia treatment; however, in cases with a GCS of 3 caused by extracranial diseases such as brain hypoxia, cardiac arrest, or accidental hypothermia, brain hypothermia of 34°C is indicated. For cases involving cardiac arrest, special consideration of combination therapy with percutaneous cardiopulmonary support and brain hypothermia treatment is recommended. Details of this treatment are described in Chap. 54.

References

1. Corte FD, Mancini A, Valle D, Gallizzi F, Carducci P, Mignani V, De Marinis L (1998) Provocative hypothalamopituitary axis tests in severe head injury: correlations with severity and prognosis. Crit Care Med 26:1419–1426
2. Dudariev VP, Lanovenko II (1999) Changes in the oxygen-binding properties of the blood in white rats under the influence of hypoxia and its pharmacological correction. Fiziol Zh 45:97–103
3. Hayashi N (1997) Prevention of vegetation after severe head trauma and stroke by combination therapy of cerebral hypothermia and activation of immune-dopaminergic nervous system. Proceedings of the 6th annual meeting of Society for Treatment of Coma 6:133–145
4. Hayashi N (2000) The clinical issue and effectiveness of brain hypothermia treatment for severe brain injured patients. In: Hayashi N (ed) Brain hypothermia. Springer, Berlin Heidelberg New York Tokyo, pp 121–151
5. Morgan TJ, Koch D, Morris D, Clague A, Purdie DM (2001) Reduced red cell 2,3-diphosphoglycerate concentrations in critical illness without decreased in vivo P50. Anaesth Intensive Care 29:479–483

29. Indications

The effectiveness of brain hypothermia for severe brain injury is mainly determined by several factors as shown in Fig. 30 (Chap. 26). Coma with Glasgow Coma Scale (GCS) less than 4, uncontrollable hyperglycemia with serum glucose levels above 230 mg/dl, delayed induction of hypothermia, and low systolic blood pressure are negative factors for the success of brain hypothermia treatment [1]. Coma (GCS > 3), control of serum glucose levels to below 180 mg/dl, induction of brain hypothermia within 3 h after insult, and control of systolic blood pressure above 100 mmHg without catecholamines are good indications for the effectiveness of brain hypothermia treatment.

Conditions such as acute brain damage (GCS > 3) caused by diffuse brain injury, acute subdural hematoma, acute epidural hematoma, the acute onset of obstructive cerebral stroke, brain hypoxia, and after resuscitation from cardiac arrest all indicate brain hypothermia treatment. However, severe subarachnoid hemorrhage is still a controversial indication for brain hypothermia treatment. In cases of subarachnoid hemorrhage, hypothermia treatment cannot prevent vasospasm. Therefore, severe subarachnoid hemorrhage with vasospasm is not a good indication for brain hypothermia treatment. However, in our clinical studies, if the serum glucose was controlled below 180 mg/dl within 6 h, brain hypothermia management was successful even in cases complicated by cerebral vasospasm. However, obstructive cerebral stroke without recanalization does not respond to brain hypothermia treatment. To restore neuronal function in cases of cerebral ischemia, combination therapy consisting of cerebral angioplasty, thrombolysis, and brain hypothermia treatment is necessary as soon as possible [1]. If combination therapy is started within 3 h, brain hypothermia treatment is indicated for obstructive cerebral stroke because spontaneous recanalization by thrombolysis has been recorded in many cases. If brain hypothermia treatment can protect against necrosis in ischemic lesions until spontaneous recanalization, neuronal recovery can be expected. Although brain hypothermia is very effective with severly brain-injured patients, clinical results are not always as good as expected. Causes of ineffective brain hypothermia treatment are listed as coma (GCS < 5), serum glucose level greater than 230 mg/dl and delayed control of hyperglycemia, late induction of brain hypothermia treatment, unstable cardiopulmonary function, complication of pneumonia, and rapid brain tissue destruction by hypertensive intracerebral hemorrhage (Table 5).

References

1. Hayashi N (2000) The clinical issue and effectiveness of brain hypothermia treatment for severe brain injured patients. In: Hayashi N (ed) Brain hypothermia. Springer, Berlin Heidelberg New York Tokyo, pp 121–151.

Table 5. Indications for brain hypothermia treatment

	Good indication	Comparative indication	Contraindication
Severity	Coma (GCS < 8)	Coma (GCS < 5)	Shock, brain death
Pathophysiology	Control of serum glucose to 120–140 mg/dl	Control of serum glucose to <230 mg/dl	Blood pressure maintained by medication
Timing	Within 3 h after injury	Within 3–6 h after injury	After 6–12 h
Other conditions	Severe brain injury, cardiopulmonary arrest, cytokine encephalitis, brain hypoxia, obstructive cerebral stroke	Subarachnoid hemorrhage, control of serum glucose <180 mg/dl, hypertensive intracerebral hemorrhage	—

GCS, Glasgow Coma Scale

30. Beyond Indication and Contraindication

At the emergency medical center, management of severe brain damage caused by trauma, stroke, brain hypoxia, or cardiac arrest requires an assessment of the condition reversibility in addition to indications for treatment [1,2]. The reversibility of severe brain injury is decided not only by the severity of brain damage, age, time after insult, and original cause of brain damage, but also the level of medical management. For the success of brain hypothermia treatment beyond contraindication, advanced brain hypothermia intensive care unit (ICU) management techniques must be applied early on. Factors that decide the prognosis of severely brain-injured patients include the Glasgow Coma Scale (GCS), complicated trauma of major organs, age, sex, start of treatment time, type of original disease, immune activity, and cardiopulmonary function. To introduce the new concept of treatment beyond indication and contraindication, the treatment goal must be determined for each severely brain-injured patient. For instance, injury with a GCS of 3 is very difficult to recover from without neurological deficit or persistent vegetation [1]. The goal of treatment for such a case is survival, probably in a state of vegetation. In cases with GCS of 4–6, about 25% may expect good recovery if brain hypothermia treatment is started within 3–6h of brain injury [1]. However, poor prognosis is unavoidable if brain hypothermia treatment is initiated 6h after brain injury. The new criteria to determine the goal of brain hypothermia treatment must be considered beyond contraindication. Accurate criteria that can be used in combination with many factors can determine the prognosis. However, criteria that include multiple factors are not practical in the emergency room or emergency medical center. Simple and more effective criteria should be considered.

The GCS, induction time, causes of coma, and level of hyperglycemia are major factors in deciding the clinical prognosis. We have considered a new classification to provide more effective treatment beyond contraindication. The classification is divided into 5 levels that decide the goal of brain hypothermia treatment, with control of serum glucose below 180mg/dl.

Level I: GCS 6–8, brain hypothermia started within 3–6h of injury, original disease is brain trauma or hypoxia. The goal of treatment is good prognosis.

Level II: GCS 4–5, brain hypothermia is started within 3–6h of injury, and original disease is brain trauma or hypoxia. The goal of treatment is good to moderate (average–mild) recovery.

Level III: GCS 4–6, brain hypothermia started within 3–6h of injury, original disease is cardiopulmonary arrest (CPA), subarachnoid hemorrhage (SAH), or hypertensive intracerebral hemorrhage (HICH). Treatment is expected to result in mild to severe disability (average–moderate).

Level IV: GCS 4–6, brain hypothermia started later than 6h after injury, original disease is brain trauma or hypoxia. Treatment is expected to result in moderate disability or vegetative state (average–severe disability).

Level V: GCS 3, treatment is started within 3h of brain injury, original disease may be one or more of many. Treatment provides no expectation of recovery except for cardiac arrest during oxygen inhalation.

However, hyperglycemia cannot control at lower than 180mg/dl, the level of reversibility count increase one or two step (Tables 6 and 7).

Table 6. The level of effectiveness of brain hypothermia treatment with severe brain injury

Level	GCS	Time after injury (hours)	Disease
I	6–8	<3–6	Trauma or hypoxia
II	4–5	<3–6	Trauma or hypoxia
III	4–6	<3–6	CPA, SAH,HICH
IV	4–6	>6	Trauma or hypoxia
V	3	<3	

GCS, Glasgow Coma Scale; CPA, cardiopulmonary arrest; SAH, subarachnoid hemorrhage; HIGH, hypertensive intracerebral hemorrhage

Table 7. The level of effectiveness of combined brain hypothermia and recanalization therapy with ischemic brain insults

Level	GCS	Time after stroke (hours)	Clinical signs
I	~9	<3	Focal signs
II	4–8	<3	Brain stem
III	~9	3–6	Focal signs
IV	4–8	3–6	Brain stem
V	~4	>6	Focal and brain stem signs

References

1. Hayashi N (2000) The clinical issue and effectiveness of brain hypothermia treatment for severe brain injured patients. In: Hayashi N (ed) Brain hypothermia. Springer, Berlin Heidelberg New York Tokyo, pp 121–151
2. Nagao K, Hayashi N, Kanmatsuse K, Arima K, Ohtsuki J, Kikushima K, Watanabe I (2000) Cardiopulmonary cerebral resuscitation using emergency cardiopulmonary bypass, coronary reperfusion therapy and mild hypothermia in patients with cardiac arrest outside the hospital. J Am Coll Cardiol 36:776–783

IV. The Technique of Brain Hypothermia Treatment

31. Induction of Brain Hypothermia

Early Induction of Brain Hypothermia Within 3h of Insult

The state of neuronal damage after severe brain injury may progress with time. Similary, the target of management may also differ within the injury time window in severely brain-injured patients. In addressing this clinical issue, early management is much easier and simpler than delayed induction of hypothermia treatment. Accordingly, the main targets of treatment at early and late stages need to be defined. In some cases, control of brain edema and intracranial pressure (ICP) elevation have been the focus of initial treatment for neuroprotection in severely brain-injured patients [2,11,14]. However, this approach is not correct because brain edema and ICP elevation occur as a result of neuronal hypoxia, adequate metabolic supply to the injured neurons, cerebral blood flow (CBF) disturbances, unsuccessful management of cardiopulmonary dysfunction, and hemoglobin dysfunction [4]. For brain hypothermia management of severe brain injury, the starting time is important and the main target of management will change according to the time after insults and trauma [3,4].

There are two mechanisms of secondary brain damage. One is a neurohormonal dysfunction related to cardiopulmonary function, hemoglobin dysfunction, neuronal hypoxia, blood–brain barrier (BBB) dysfunction, and brain thermo-pooling [3,4,6]. The other is related to brain edema, ischemia, and ICP elevation [2,11,13]. Free radicals promote these pathophysiological changes [1,13]. The time limits to prevent these pathophysiological changes are summarized in Table 5. To prevent hypothalamus–pituitary–adrenal (HPA) axis neurohormonal dysfunction, catecholamine surge, vasopressin release, and growth hormone release, brain tissue temperature should be reduced to 34°C within 3h of severe brain damage [5]. The early induction of brain hypothermia, within 3h, is most effective against these pathophysiological changes because epinephrine, a trigger factor for these changes, is released in high concentration immediately after insult [3,4]. Brain damage caused by excess release of epinephrine is diagnosed by observation of hyperglycemia with serum glucose levels above 230mg/dl [3,4]. Therefore, in severely brain-injured patients that are admitted with severe hyperglycemia, early induction of brain hypothermia treatment (within 3h of insult) is indicated.

In cases with no recorded hyperglycemia, early induction of brain hypothermia is not necessary at all and priority should be given to stabilization of vital signs and brain-oriented neuroprotection management that include consideration of brain hypoxia, CBF disturbances, brain edema, and brain thermo-pooling [3–5].

The early induction of brain hypothermia (33°–34°C) within 3h of insult is effective in controlling secondary brain damage caused by HPA axis neurohormonal abnormality and helps to prevent development of brain edema and ICP elevation.

Delayed Induction of Brain Hypothermia Between 3 and 6h After Insult

For patients that are admitted to the medical center between 3 and 6h after brain damage, brain hypothermia treatment must address many brain injury mechanisms. In severely brain-injured patients, systemic circulation changes to dopamine-dominant circulation 3h after insult and trauma. If severe hyperglycemia is recorded with serum glucose levels above 230mg/dl after 3h, it is suggested that systemic circulation is maintained with not only dopamine but also vasopressin release [4]. Severe vasopressin release activates hyperglycemia, increases permeability of the BBB, and activates neurogenic pulmonary edema [3,4,8–10]. In most cases of severe brain injury, BBB function is severely damaged. In these cases of severe BBB dysfunction (CSF/serum albumin ratio >0.02), increased serum concentrations of dopamine and vasopressin can easily permeate into the brain tissue through the injured BBB [4]. These specific pathophysiological conditions produce dramatic increases in brain tissue dopamine and cytotoxic $\cdot OH^-$ radical concentrations. Dopamine reacts with oxygen to produce H_2O_2 and Quinone anion, and, in turn, H_2O_2 reacts with Fe^{++} to produce $\cdot OH^-$ [1,13]. To manage free radical attack of injured neurons, prevention of dopamine release from the central dopamine nervous system by combined hypothermia and pharmacological treatment, administration of free radical scavengers, and stabilization of the BBB function are important [4,12]. The brain tissue temperature for effective control of $\cdot NO$ radicals in the brain tissue is an important parameter. Our preliminary studies suggested that serum NO_2 and NO_2/NO_3 ratio were reduced by 50% at a brain tissue temperature of 34°C and by 80%–90% at 32°C [3,7]. Therefore, delayed induction of brain hypothermia later than 3h after insult requires a two-step induction. Delayed induction of brain hypothermia requires a lower brain tissue temperature (32°–33°C) than early induction of brain hypothermia (33°–34°C).

The prevention of dopamine release in the deep brain is very important to minimize damage to memory, volition, and emotion and to prevent vegetation [5,12]. Excessive increase of dopamine in the brain tissue produces selective radical attack of the dopamine A10 nervous system [1,5,13]. Early induction of brain hypothermia treatment provides control of dopamine release and is effective in minimizing the complication of vegetation. For brain hypothermia treatment to achieve social recovery, management of the dopamine A10 nervous system is important from the acute stage. Brain hypothermia treatment should be started within 6h of insult at the latest.

Late Induction of Brain Hypothermia More Than 6h After Insult

Brain damage progresses severely from 6h after brain insult. The main targets of treatment in this stage are stabilization of the vital signs, management of insulin-resistant hyperglycemia, maintenance of CBF, control of ICP, normalization of antithrombin-III (AT-III), prevention of brain edema, and control of brain thermo-pooling [3–6]. However, the negative effects of masking neuronal hypoxia and insulin-resistant hyperglycemia have already started at this stage [4]. In such cases, the effectiveness of brain hypothermia treatment is less successful than early induction to give a brain tissue temperature of around 34°C. To control ICP elevation and prevent free radical reactions, more severe brain hypothermia (around 32°–33°C) is necessary. The control of brain tissue temperature to around 32°–33°C cannot avoid pituitary hormonal dysfunction that includes immune suppression. The management technique becomes much more complicated than that of mild brain hypothermia (34°C) and the effectiveness of brain hypothermia becomes incomplete [5]. One of the difficulties in ICU management with late induction of brain hypothermia is the control of hyperglycemia. At times after 6h from insult, insulin-resistant hyperglycemia progresses severely. The management of brain hypothermia below 33°C produces a systemic reduction in glucose expenditure and increases serum glucose levels markedly [5]. The inability to control hyperglycemia produces dramatic increases in brain tissue glucose levels with excess release of vasopressin, increases in brain tissue lactate levels with activation of glutamate toxicity, and reduced 2,3-diphosphoglycerate (DPG) that results in ineffective oxygen inhalation [4]. As a resalt, induction of brain hypothermia itself may impose negative effects on injured brain tissue.

Although there is no time limit for the induction of brain hypothermia, the target of treatment will change depending on the time window, and the effectiveness of treatment will be reduced according to the delayed induction times. For late induction of brain hypothermia, careful diagnosis and excellent ICU management techniques are required.

References

1. Baker AJ, Zornow MH, Scheller MS, Yaksh TL, Skilling SR, Smullin DH, Larson AA, Kuczenski R (1991) Changes in extrascellular concentrations of glutamate, aspartate, glycine, dopamine, serotonin, and dopamine metabolites after transient global ischemia in the rat. J Neurochemistry 57:1370–1379
2. Feng H, Huang G, Gao L, Tan H, Liao X (2000) Effect of intracranial pressure and cerebral perfusion pressure on outcome prediction of severe traumatic brain injury. Chin J Traumatol 3:226–230
3. Hayashi N (1995) Cerebral hypothermia treatment. In: Hayashi N (ed) Cerebral hypothermia treatment. Sogo Igaku, Tokyo, pp 1–105
4. Hayashi N (2000) Enhanced neuronal damage in severely brain injured patients by hypothalamus, pituitary, and adrenal axis neuro-hormonal changes. In: Hayashi N (ed) Brain hypothermia. Springer, Berlin Heidelberg New York Tokyo, pp 3–26
5. Hayashi N (2000) The clinical issue and effectiveness of brain hypothermia treatment for severe brain injured patients. In: Hayashi N (ed) Brain hypothermia. Springer, Berlin Heidelberg New York Tokyo, pp 121–151
6. Hayashi N, Hirayama T, Utagawa A (1994) The cerebral thermo-pooling and hypothermia treatment of critical head injury patients. In: Nagai H (ed) Intracranial pres-

sure IX. Springer, Berlin Heidelberg New York Tokyo, pp 589–599

7. Hayashi N, Utagawa A, Kinosita K, Izumi T (1999) Application of a novel technique for clinical evaluation of nitric oxide-induced free radical reactions in ICU patients. Cell Mol Neurobiol 19:3–17
8. Kagawa M, Nagao S, Bemana I (1996) Arginine vasopressin receptor antagonists for treatment of vasogenic brain edema: an experimental study. J Neurotrauma 13:273–279
9. Kow LM, Pfaff DW (1986) Vasopressin excites ventromedial hypothalamus glucose-responsive neurons in vitro. Physiol Behav 37:153–158
10. Lin TW, Kuo YS (1996) Acute pulmonary oedema following administration of vasopressin for control of massive GI tract haemorrhage in a major burn patient. Burns 22:73–75
11. Maclntosh TK (1994) Neurological sequele of traumatic brain injury: therapeutic implications. Cerebrovasc Brain Metab Rev 6:109–162
12. Okuda C, Saito A, Miyazaki M, Kuriyama K (1986) Alteration of the turnover of dopamine and 5-hydroxytryptamine in rat brain associated with hypothermia. Pharmacol Biochem Behav 25:79–83
13. Silvka A, Coben G (1985) Hydroxyl radical attack on dopamine. J Biol Chem 260:15466–15472
14. Suarez JI (2001) Treatment of acute brain edema. Rev Neurol 32:275–281

32. The Protocol for Brain Hypothermia Treatment

The main targets of brain hypothermia treatment are the adequate administration of oxygen, control of metabolic substrates, prevention of hypothalamus–pituitary–adrenal (HPA) axis neurohormonal brain damage, and exclusion of selective neuronal damage to the dopamine A10 nervous system by controlling the brain tissue temperature to 32°–34°C [5–7]. The fundamental plan for brain hypothermia treatment is summarized in Fig. 39. After treatment, additional cerebral dopamine replacement therapy is followed to prevent memory disturbance and vegetation [4,5,7].

The Early Induction of Brain Hypothermia

Adequate Administration of Oxygen and Metabolic Substrates with Rapid Induction of Brain Hypothermia (34°C)

The management of intracellular homeostasis in injured brain tissue creates opportunity for restoration. The adequate administration of oxygen and metabolic substrates occurs under the control of microcirculation and is essential in initial intensive care unit (ICU) management. The early induction of brain hypothermia after stabilizing vital signs allows effective control of intra cranial pressure (ICP) below 20 mmHg, PaO_2/FiO_2 ratio above 300, antithrombin-III (AT-III) greater than 100%, and serum glucose to between 120 and 140 mg/dl [6–8]. Control of brain tissue temperature at 34°C prevents catecholamine surge by about 50%; however, rapid induction of brain hypothermia to 32°C for neuroprotection causes an excessive reduction in serum catecholamines and unstable systemic circulation [3,7]. If it is difficult to control ICP at 34°C, two-step induction of brain hypothermia is required. This involves rapid early induction of brain hypothermia at 34°C initially, stabilization of vital signs, and then careful induction of brain hypothermia to 33°–32°C over about 3–6 h [5–7].

The management of hemoglobin function requires control of serum pH above 7.3, adequate oxygen delivery, and cerebral perfusion pressure (CPP) control above 80 mmHg with sufficient fluid resuscitation. If fluid resuscitation is not successful in maintaining the systolic blood pressure above 100 mmHg, temporal blockage of the abdominal aorta using an abdominal balloon catheter is available. Oxygen therapy focused on maintaining levels above 800 ml/min kg^{-1} with 22%–25% oxygen extraction ratio (O_2ER) is advised [5–7].

Prevention of Brain Damage by HPA Axis Neurohormonal Release

HPA axis activation following direct severe brain insult produces an excess release of HPA neuroendocrinological hormones such as catecholamines, vasopressin, and growth hormone. These neurohormonal reactions introduce a negative environment for the injured brain [2], for example, stimulation of the neuropeptide Y receptor in the hypothalamus promotes insulin-resistant hyperglycemia, vasopressin release activates blood–brain barrier (BBB) dysfunction, slow release of bound oxygen from hemoglobin associated with low 2,3-diphosphoglycerate (DPG) in hemoglobin, and rapid increases in brain tissue glucose and lactate levels [5–7]. These HPA axis neurohormonal changes occur within 5 min of injury. The early induction of brain hypothermia is only effective to prevent or minimize these stress-associated secondary brain damage mechanisms [6]. Hyperglycemia (>230 mg/dl) and hypo-albuminemia (<2.5 mg/dl) are serious conditions that require control of BBB dysfunction [7]. The management of hyperglycemia, replacement of albumin, control of AT-III above 100%, and administration of low molecular weight heparin (LWHP) are effective for management of BBB dysfunction in the acute stage [5–7].

Preclusion of Selective Neuronal Damage to Dopamine A10 Nervous System to Prevent Vegetation

Combination therapy of metoclopramide administration and control of brain tissue temperature to 32°–34°C

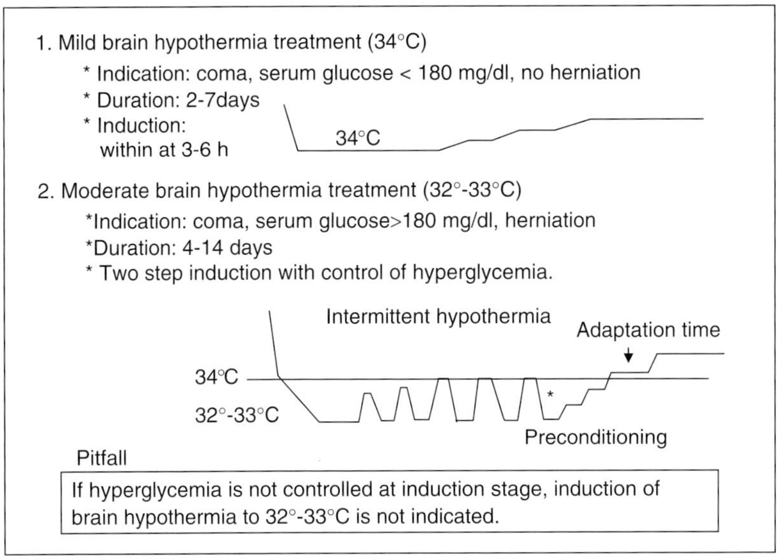

Fig. 39. The fundamental care plan for brain hypothermia treatment

is effective for the prevention of dopamine release [5,7]. The control of hemoglobin to above 11 g/dl, administration of vitamin C, and combination of brain hypothermia and pharmacological treatment with metoclopramide are useful to prevent selective radical damage to the dopamine A10 nervous system.

Selection of Mild or Moderate Brain Hypothermia Treatment

Mild Brain Hypothermia Treatment

Mild brain hypothermia (~34°C brain tissue temperature) is indicated in cases with Glasgow Coma Scale score (GCS) less than 8 with hyperglycemia (serum glucose levels less than 180 mg/dl) and no clinical signs of brain stem herniation. The early induction of brain hypothermia within 3 h is also an indication factor for mild brain hypothermia because the early induction allows much easier control of secondary brain damage after severe brain injury than does late induction. In special consideration of body tissue temperature, mild brain hypothermia is suitable after resuscitation following cardiac arrest. However, the tolerance of cardiac function to low serum catecholamines with moderate brain hypothermia is reduced. The duration is variable between 2 and 7 days (Fig. 39).

Moderate Brain Hypothermia

Moderate brain hypothermia (32°–33°C brain tissue temperature) is indicated in patients with GCS of 6 or less, and serum glucose levels above 180 mg/dl. The delayed (later than 3 h after insult) and late (later than 6 h after insult) induction of brain hypothermia are also possible even though effectiveness is limited. This is because many pathological changes are difficult to manage with a brain tissue temperature of 34°C over a short duration. The duration is variable at 4–14 days (Fig. 39) [5–7].

Management Plans for Brain Tissue Temperature

Two-step induction of brain hypothermia is a fundamental technique under anesthesia and analgesia. The brain tissue temperature is rapidly controlled to around 34°C and then the vital signs are stabilized. After control of hypopotassemia, arrhythmia, hyperglycemia, and elongation of the QT interval greater than 450 mm/s on the electrocardiogram (ECG), the second step requires careful induction of brain hypothermia to 32°–33°C depending on criteria. Rapid induction to 32°–33°C should be avoided to prevent the complications of unstable cardiac output, low blood pressure, immune dysfunction, and pituitary dysfunction. It takes about 4–6 h for two-step induction of 32°–33°C brain hypothermia [5–7].

Prolonged control of brain tissue temperature at 32°–33°C is necessary for the management of severely brain-injured patients. However, prolonged brain hypothermia below 33°C incurs unavoidable pituitary hormonal dysfunction and immune crisis. The pituitary dysfunction with immune crisis is one of the reasons for the high incidence of severe pneumonia during hypothermia treatment [3,8]. To avoid this complication, special consideration of brain tissue temperature management is required.

The intermittent elevation of brain tissue temperature from 32°–33°C to 34°C for short periods is a recognized technique of brain hypothermia. The physiological secretion of immune function-associated growth hormone occurs at around 18:00–22:00 hours in the evening to early night. The precise technique is described in Chaps. 34 and 44.

At the rewarming stage, the rewarming speed and time course are very important for the success of prolonged brain hypothermia treatment. The elevation of brain tissue temperature by 0.1°C requires 1 h. When the brain tissue is rewarmed to 34°–35°C, this temperature is maintained for 1–2 days to allow physiological adaptation. This technique is very successful in preventing rewarming stress. The adaptation times differ depending on the levels of hypothermia. Rapid elevation of blanket water temperature at the same time produces uncontrollable and marked brain swelling. The detailed technique is described in Chaps. 32 and 35.

Intensive Care Management During Brain Hypothermia Treatment

The control of brain tissue temperature at 32°–34°C for 1–2 weeks depends on the severity of brain injury. There are six major targets of ICU management during the cooling stage.

1. Stabilization of vital signs; sBP greater than 100 mmHg and PaO_2/FiO_2 ratio greater than 350.
2. Brain hypoxia; oxygen delivery (DO_2) greater than 800 ml/min, pH greater than 7.3, 6 l/min tidal volume with 6–12 cmH_2O PEEP, O_2ER: 23%–25%.
3. Management of cerebral blood flow (CBF) and metabolism; cerebral perfusion pressure greater than 80 mmHg, SjO_2 65%–70%, serum glucose 120–160 mg/dl.
4. Maintenance of systemic microcirculation; AT-III greater than 100%, gastric pHi greater than 7.3.
5. Prevention of cytokine encephalitis; AT-III greater than 100%, serum albumin greater than 3.0 mg/dl, CSF/serum albumin ratio less than 0.01.
6. Prevention of infections; washing of stomach, gastric juice pH less than 3.5, gastric pHi greater than 7.35, prevention of abdominal hypertension using long intestinal decompression catheter, nutritional considerations, digestive decontamination (intestinal administration of VCM + AMPH-B + albekasin), vitamin A greater than 50 μg/dl, AT-III + LWHP→serum albumin greater than 3.0 g/dl, cleaning of oral cavity and airway, intermittent culture study of air way secretions [5–7].

Rewarming Time

The timing of rewarming is one of the key points for successful brain hypothermia treatment. This is because the recovery of intracerebral pathophysiological changes is not obtained during the cooling stage. Stopped (or delayed) progression of pathophysiological changes caused by brain cooling and stopped or delayed secondary brain injury mechanisms, start again with rewarming. The reprogression of secondary brain injury mechanisms from the rewarming stage are made much worse by the metabolic shift from lipid to glucose, cytokine activation, and neurohormonal changes [1,6,7]. From the above reasons, the timing of rewarming requires a diagnosis that indicates at least some recovery. The recording of a θ-wave on the background of the δ-wave in trended EEG, no ICP elevation, SjO2 control between 60% and 75%, and no brain swelling on the computed tomography scan are indirect evaluation parameters to aid the decision to start rewarming [5–7].

Cerebral Dopamine Replacement Therapy

After brain hypothermia treatment, cases that show no recovery of consciousness should receive replacement therapy of cerebral dopamine [3–7]. Replacement of cerebral dopamine can occur by combination of pharmacological treatment and median nerve intermittent electrical stimulation (20 s on, 50 s off, 10–20 mA, 30 pulses/s, duration time 300 m/s) [5,7]. Reduced CSF dopamine after brain hypothermia is a good indicator for cerebral dopamine replacement therapy. In most cases of vegetative state after brain hypothermia treatment, more than 3 weeks of replacement therapy is appropriate. The response to cerebral dopamine replacement therapy is evaluated with increasing CSF dopamine/prolactin ratio.

References

1. Bioch M (1967) Cerebral effects of rewarming following prolonged hypothermia: significance for the management of severe cranio-cerebral injury and acute pyrexia. Brain 90:769–784
2. Corte FD, Mancini A, Valle D, Gallizzi F, Carducci P, Mignani V, De Marinis L (1998) Provocative hypothalamopituitary axis tests in severe head injury: correlation with severity and prognosis. Crit Care Med 26:1419–1426

3. Hayashi N (1995) Cerebral hypothermia treatment. In: Hayashi N (ed) Cerebral hypothermia treatment. Sogo Igaku Tokyo, pp 1–105
4. Hayashi N (1997) Combination therapy of cerebral hypothermia, pharmacological activation of the dopamine system, and hormonal replacement in severely brain damaged patients. J Jpn Intensive Care Med 4:191–197
5. Hayashi N (1997) Prevention of vegetation after severe head trauma and stroke by combination therapy of cerebral hypothermia and activation of immune-dopaminergic nervous system. Proceedings of the 6th annual meeting of Society for Treatment of Coma 6: 133–145
6. Hayashi N (2000) Enhanced neuronal damage in severely brain injured patients by hypothalamus, pituitary, and adrenal axis neuro-hormonal changes. In: Hayashi N (ed) Brain hypothermia. Springer Berlin Heidelberg New York Tokyo, pp 3–26
7. Hayashi N (2000) The clinical issue and effectiveness of brain hypothermia treatment for severe brain injured patients. In: Hayashi N (ed) Brain hypothermia. Springer, Berlin Heidelberg New York Tokyo, pp 121–151
8. Hayashi N, Hirayama T, Utagawa T, Ohata M (1994) Systemic management of cerebral edema based on a new concept in severe head injury patients. Acta Neurochir 60:541–543

33. Mistakes and Pitfalls of Brain Hypothermia Treatment

Improper Management of Brain Hypothermia

Early Administration of Manitol and Glycerol Create Cerebral Blood Flow Disturbances

To prevent brain edema, early administration of manitol and glycerol were recommended previously [21]. However, brain edema progresses not only as a secondary pathophysiological change [23] of directly injured brain tissue, but also by hypothalamus–pituitary–adrenal (HPA) axis neurohoromonal dysfunction [4,9] such as cardiopulmonary dysfunction caused by catecholamine surge [9], masking brain hypoxia [9], brain thermo-pooling [7,8,12], insulin-resistant hyperglycemia [7,9,12], and vasopressin-related blood–brain barrier (BBB) dysfunction [8,14]. Therefore, prevention of secondary brain damage caused by HPA axis neurohoromonal dysfunction should precede management of brain edema by administration of manitol and glycerol [9].

Brain hypothermia produces a 50%–60% reduction of serum catecholamine concentration at 34°C, and an 80% reduction at 32°C during moderate brain hypothermia [2,10,12]. The early administration of manitol and glycerol under hypothermia produces dehydration and can easily cause disturbances of microcirculation in the intestinal mucous membrane and brain tissue (Table 8). The basic concept of fluid resuscitation during brain hypothermia treatment contraindicates dehydration therapy. In brain hypothermia management, fluid resuscitation rather than dehydration can maintain sufficient administration of oxygen and metabolic substrates in injured brain tissue. The hyper-osmotic therapy obtained by administration of manitol and glycerol is a second-stage management strategy in brain hypothermia treatment.

However, the choice of manitol and glycerol during the management of brain hypothermia is still controversial. In the acute stage, insulin-resistant hyperglycemia associated with catecholamine surge is unavoidable [9]. A metabolic shift from glucose to lipid metabolism occurs following hypothermia [9,12]. Recent clinical studies using microdialysis suggested that administration of glycerol under the conditions of hyperglycemia activates lipid metabolism and converts glycogen to lactate. Hypothermia also activates these metabolic changes. Therefore, the combination of hypothermia, glycerol administration, lipid-dominant metabolism, and insulin-resistant hyperglycemia may be a bad combination, and can easily cause an increase in brain tissue lactate levels [19]. However, more detailed microdialysis studies of these clinical issues are required.

Brain edema is not an initial target of treatment in brain hypothermia treatment. The administration of manitol is indicated after stabilization of systemic circulation and during the second stage (cooling stage) for control of intracranial pressure (ICP) elevation. To prevent complications, dehydration therapy should be avoided and the normal systemic circulation maintained with more than 800 ml/min of oxygen because normal fluid resuscitation is important at the initial stage. To prevent the hazard of insulin-resistant hyperglycemia, progress of brain edema, and BBB dysfunction, about 1000 ml of 7% Acetic Ringer's solution should be infused with antithrombin-III (AT-III) and followed by 5% albumin.

Rapid Induction of Moderate Brain Hypothermia Increases Brain Tissue Lactate

The recent clinical studies of brain metabolism under the management of brain hypothermia using microdialysis suggest a negative effect from rapid induction of hypothermia [10]. Brain hypothermia with a lower body temperature produces diminished serum glucose expenditure. In some cases, we have recorded increased brain tissue glucose and serum glucose levels at 32°–33°C during moderate brain hypothermia when compared with 34°C during mild brain hypothermia (Fig. 28, Chap. 23). In these cases, brain tissue lactate levels also increased in proportion to increasing serum glucose levels [10]. Therefore, on metabolic considerations, man-

Table 8. The pitfalls of brain hypothermia treatment

Early manitol administration causes unstable microcirculation by combination with hypothermia-associated low serum catecholamines
Insulin-resistant hyperglycemia (>220 mg/dl) induces neuronal hypoxia with hemoglobin dysfunction and activates BBB dysfunction caused by vasopressin release
Normal CPP and PaO_2 are not sufficient for neuronal oxygenation
Short-duration hypothermia is not adequate to allow recovery and is limitted to halting the pathophysiology of brain damage
Complications of severe pneumonia and BBB dysfunction induce cytokine encephalitis with severe glutamate release
Early enteral and parenteral nutrition with BBB dysfunction results in an increase in brain tissue glutamate

BBB, Blood-brain barrier; CPP, cerebral perfusion pressure

agement of brain tissue temperature at 34°C is better than 32°–33°C. Without control of hyperglycemia, both forms of brain hypothermia are not effective for severe brain injury. Without due care, the rapid induction of brain hypothermia can easily be subject to this pitfall [10]. The brain tissue glucose and lactate levels begin to increase when serum glucose levels increase above 150–160 mg/dl. The critical level of serum glucose to produce dangerous levels of brain tissue lactate (>10–15 mmol/L) is more than 230 mg/dl.

Brain hypothermia at 32°–33°C is much more effective for the prevention of free radical attack and brain edema than brain hypothermia at 34°C; however, brain temperature at 32°–33°C is more likely to produce hyperglycemia than at 34°C. In intensive care unit (ICU) management of brain tissue temperature, careful management of serum glucose is important.

Delayed Control of Hyperglycemia Produces Anaerobic Brain Metabolism and BBB Dysfunction

The management of hyperglycemia in severely brain-injured patients is very important in the prevention of secondary brain damage; however, immediate control is very difficult. Before starting brain hypothermia, severe hyperglycemia is observed in all of severely brain-injured patients. Hyperglycemia is an unavoidable metabolic change associated with catecholamine surge caused by stimulation of the HPA axis in severely brain-injured patients [8]. In particular, excess release of epinephrine is more strongly correlated to the production of hyperglycemia than norepinephrine and dopamine.

Delayed control of hyperglycemia introduces, various negative factors for neuronal restoration during brain hypothermia treatment such as increased brain tissue glucose and lactate levels, increased lactate in systemic circulation, active anaerobic metabolism, low hemoglobin 2,3-diphosphoglycerate (DPG), and ineffective oxygen inhalation. In addition, recent clinical studies suggested hypothalamus neural control of macronutrient intake [15,16,20,24]. In acute hyperglycemia, vasopressin release occurs to prevent further intake of food. Our clinical studies in ICU using microdialysis suggested that prolonged hyperglycemia with serum glucose levels above 230 mg/dl produces excess release of vasopressin, BBB dysfunction, and increases proinflammatory cytokines [9]. The negative effects of hyperglycemia are not limited to the brain but also affect the major organs, liver, and heart. Associated with this hyperglycemia are increased levels of serum catecholamines and consumption of adenosine triphosphate (ATP) in the liver and heart. Therefore, ATP crisis in major organs, heart, and liver is hidden in stress-associated hyperglycemia after severe brain damage.

For management of hyperglycemia-associated stimulation of the HPA axis, early induction of brain hypothermia at 34°C is successful in the prevention of epinephrine release. Delayed control of hyperglycemia under the management of brain hypothermia negates the benefits of hypothermia toward brain damage. Delayed or rapid induction of moderate brain hypothermia (32°–33°C) may worsen hyperglycemia and make management more difficult. In a case of unavoidable late induction of brain hypothermia treatment, very careful management of hyperglycemia is necessary. The rapid induction of moderate brain hypothermia is dangerous without correcting hyperglycemia with serum glucose levels above 230 mg/dl.

Vasopressin release caused by the feedback mechanism of macronutrient neural control of hyperglycemia induces changes in BBB function, cerebral microcirculation, cerebrospinal fluid (CSF) cytokine, and pulmonary circulation [9,15–17,20,22]. The combination of hyperglycemia [6], vasopressin release [10], and inappropriate management of immune function during brain hypothermia [22] results in a condition that is susceptible to systemic infections and cytokine encephalitis [10].

The reduced effect of insulin caused by adrenocorticotropic hormone (ACTH) release, and reduced consumption of serum glucose in weakened skeletal muscle and the liver are made much worse by hyperglycemia. Special consideration of ICU management for insulin-resistant hyperglycemia is necessary.

Control of Normal PaO_2, Cerebral Perfusion Pressure, and ICP is not Enough Management

The maintenance of intracellular homeostasis is required in the initial management of severe brain injury. The control of normal values of PaO_2, cerebral blood blow (CBF), and ICP in such patients has long been an accepted approach. However, our recent clinical studies suggest that this approach is not appropriate, especially for severely brain-injured patients with Glasgow Coma Scale Score (GCS) less than 6. The masking brain hypoxia that includes the elevation of brain tissue temperature by brain thermo-pooling, slow release of bound oxygen from hemoglobin, insulin-resistant hyperglycemia associated with excess release of epinephrine, reduced oxygen delivery less than 800 ml/min caused by catecholamine surge, and blood shift into the intestinal side from excess release of dopamine, have been identified as causes of unsuitable management of normal PaO_2, CBF, and ICP for severely brain-injured patients [7–10,12]. This specific masking brain hypoxia in severely brain-injured patients also produces uncoupling of brain metabolism and CBF at the acute stage.

To avoid this masking brain hypoxia, maintenance of systemic circulation by fluid resuscitation, prevention of excess reaction to catecholamine surge by control of brain tissue temperature to 34°C, maintenance of systolic blood pressure higher than 100 mmHg to avoid brain thermo-pooling, management of serum phosphate, magnesium, and pH above 7.3 to prevent hemoglobin DPG reduction, management of oxygen delivery above 800 ml/min, and rapid control of hyperglycemia are important. Sometimes however, with normal CPP blood shift of systemic circulation to the intestinal side can easily introduce a pitfall of ICU CBF management [10]. Special dopamine-dominant circulation can be diagnosed by continuous monitoring of brain tissue temperature (or tympanic membrane temperature) and bladder temperature. Brain tissue temperature and tympanic membrane temperature are higher than bladder temperature; however, elevation of bladder temperature above brain tissue temperature occurs with blood shift to the intestinal site and localized inflammation of the bladder. Inversion of brain temperature and bladder temperature suggest an indirect parameter of CBF disturbance. The most common pitfall is lower cardiac output and a systolic blood pressure of 90–100 mmHg caused by reduced fluid resuscitation and early administration of manitol. The reduced cardiac output and lower systolic blood pressure make it difficult to wash out the elevated brain tissue temperature (brain thermo-pooling) without management of brain hypothermia [7].

Excessively rapid induction of moderate brain hypothermia (32°–33°C) introduces unstable cardiac function caused by oversuppressed catecholamine release and increased serum glucose level caused by reduced glucose expenditure. For correct management of brain hypothermia, the maintenance of sufficient cerebral oxygenation and adequate delivery of glucose with management of normal PaO_2, CBF, and ICP are very important [10,12].

Hypo-albuminemia Enteral-Intestinal Mucous Membrane Edema and Nonfunctioning Antibiotics

Acute phase responses, and increased interleukin-1 (IL-1) and interleukin-6 (IL-6) levels are common phenomenon following head injury [3]. IL-6 causes a dose- and time-dependent increase in the synthesis of serum α2-macroglobulin, fibrinogen, cysteine protease inhibitor, C-reactive protein, and α1-acid glycoprotein, and a decrease in albumin [3]. Therefore, hypo-albuminemia is mediated by cytokine elevation. Intravenous injection of recombinant tumor necrosis factor (TNF) into normal rabbits causes a dose-dependent depression of serum albumin levels [11]. In vitro exposure to murine IL-1 and TNF increases endothelial permeability to albumin and causes a time- and dose-dependent albumin leakage [18]. IL-1 and IL-6 decrease the mRNA synthesis of albumin. Thus, hypo albuminemia probably occurs because of increased vascular permeability and decreased synthesis. Causes of increased IL-1 and IL-6 levels after severe brain injury are known to include localized inflammatory reactions in directly injured brain tissue, stimulation of vascular endothelium by vasopressin release following the neural feedback mechanism of hyperglycemia, and activation of CD4 by release of HPA-axis growth hormone [3,4,9,13].

Without management of hypo-albuminemia in the acute stage, many complications can occur during brain hypothermia management. In conditions of serum albumin level less than 2.5 mg/dl, intestinal mucous edema, obstruction of the pancreatic duct, progression of brain edema, malfunction of hyperosmotic therapy to brain edema, unstable function of antibiotics, increases in free bacteria, and susceptibility to systemic infections are major clinical issues during brain hypothermia treatment [8].

The early management of hyperglycemia, prevention of excess release of growth hormone, and early replacement of serum albumin are important to prevent complications and ensure the success of brain hypothermia management [10]. The points of care management at each stage are summarized in Table 9.

Table 9. Management care point at each stage

Induction stage 1. Clean naso-oral cavity 2. Gastric leavage 3. Digestive decontamination 4. $\bar{D}O_2I > 600$ ml/min, $\bar{D}O_2 > 800$ ml/min	Precooling stage 1. Preconditioning: No severe infection, SG < 150 mg/dl, Vitamin A > 50 µg/dl, lymphocyte > 1500/mm^3, S. albumin > 3.5 mg/dl (prealbumin > 20 mg/dl), Hb > 12 mg/dl, DPG > 10 µmol/gHb, AT-III > 100%, platelet; 50 000–80 000, digastric decontamination, muscle massage, abdominal pressure < 10 mmHg 2. Antibiotics + γ-globulin 3. $\bar{D}O_2 > 800$ ml/min, O_2ER; 23%–25%
Cooling stage 1. Naso-oral cavity managment 2. Gastric juice pH < 3.5 3. prevent abdominal hypertension < 10 mmHg 4. Gastric decontamination antibiotics (GDC) 5. AT-III > 80%–100% & gastric pHi > 7.3 6. Gastric immune nutrition replacement > nutritional care 7. Ventilator care and urinary care 8. Breathing rehabilitation (alveoral dysfunction, atelectasis) 9. Intermittent elevation of BT from 32°C to 34°C at evening 10. Replacement of ZnCl, arginine with Hb > 11 mg/dl (if lympho-cytopenia occured, keep BT at 34°C + GH + γ-globulin add.) 11. Serum albumin > 3.5 mg/dl 12. Low dosage of antibiotics 13. O_2ER; 23%–25%, 2,3-DPG; 10–15 µmol/gHb	Rewarming stage 1. Very slow step up rewarming (0.1°C/h and stop at 34°–35°C) 2. Prevent rapid shift from lipid to glucose metabolism 3. Control of SG at 150–170 mg/dl 4. O_2ER; 23%–25% 5. Managment of neuromuscular junction 6. 34°–35°C BT keep for 2–3 days and BT > 36°C and then stop muscle relaxant > anesthesia 7. Nutritonal managment

DD: antibiotics associated colitis (diarrhea); treatment is stop the antibiotics, metronidazole 250 mg pr qi, (severe case IV) > oral vancomycine 125 mg qid

Pitfalls of Brain Hypothermia Treatment

Fall in Masking Neuronal Hypoxia

Brain hypoxia occurs in severe brain injury and is accompanied by brain swelling associated with neuronal energy crisis and neuronal hypoxia. This phenomenon is elicited by cardiac dysfunction with a 50 to 200-fold increase in catecholamine surge, and pulmonary dysfunction, reduced CPP, and elevation of ICP by space occupying lesions. The management of normal PaO_2, ICP, and CPP has long been considered as reasonable treatment for brain hypoxia and injured neuronal hypoxia. However, this management is not appropriate treatment, especially in severe cases (Fig. 19, Chap. 22).

Neuronal hypoxia occurs not only as a result of poor management of ICP, PaO_2, and CBF, but also because of slow release of bound oxygen from hemoglobin. Our recent clinical studies confirmed that the rapid progression of hemoglobin dysfunction is caused by reduced hemoglobin DPG levels (Fig. 20, Chap. 22). The time course of hemoglobin DPG decline is about 40–50 min in cases of cardiac-arrested whole brain ichemia (Fig. 12, Chap. 22). The elevation of brain tissue temperature by brain thermo-pooling (Fig. 12), the shift of systemic circulation into the intestinal organs by dopamine-dominant circulation, and oxygen delivery less than 500 ml/min are also causes of neuronal hypoxia in injured brain tissue. All of these new mechanisms of neuronal hypoxia are associated with stress to the HPA axis [10]. However, in experimental animal brain injury models, severe stress reaction of the HPA axis, 10- to 50-fold catecholamine surge, severe hyperglycemia, vasopressin release, and hemoglobin DPG reduction are not observed under anesthesia. In clinical ICU management of severely brain-injured patients, neuronal hypoxia in injured brain tissue occurs very commonly in the acute stage even with normal control of PaO_2, ICP, CPP, and CBF. Therefore, we refer to this neuronal hypoxia as "masking neuronal hypoxia." Without management of masking neuronal hypoxia, brain hypothermia treatment is unsuccessful in the ICU management of severe brain trauma, cerebral stroke, brain hypoxia, and brain resuscitation after cardiac arrest.

As previously described in this book, after reperfusion, body temperature elevated above 38°C combined with systolic blood pressure lower than 90–100 mmHg is a cause of brain thermo-pooling. Switching of the dopamine-dominant systemic circulation is a cause of the systemic circulation shift into the abdominal intestinal organs. Although dopamine increases cardiac output, it causes selective vasodilatation of intestinal vasculature and renal blood vessels. This specific dopamine-dominant catecholamine imbalance allows blood shift into the intestine rather than the brain despite normal CPP and oxygen delivery. Clinically, this phenomenon is recorded by elevated rectal temperature rather than brain tissue temperature or tympanic membrane temperature [12]. Under normal conditions, brain tissue temperature is always higher than rectal or bladder temperature. It is very difficult for brain-injured patients to survive when the brain tissue temperature/rectal temperature ratio (or tympanic membrane temperature/rectal temperature ratio) becomes less than 0.96 [12].

The management of masking neuronal hypoxia in injured brain tissue is important for the success of brain hypothermia treatment. The management of ICP, CBF, brain edema, oxygen delivery, hemoglobin dysfunction, prevention of catecholamine surge, and brain thermo-pooling can be achieved by a brain tissue temperature of 32°–34°C [11].

The critical level of oxygen delivery for the success of brain hypoxia ICU management is more than 600–700 ml/min [10]. This approach is applicable during brain hypothermia and also at normothermic brain tissue temperatures. There were no recorded differences in oxygen consumption between nonsurvival and survival groups; however, management of oxygen delivery above 700 ml/min showed better outcomes than for oxygen delivery less than 600 ml/min, as shown in Fig. 21, Chap. 22. The maintenance of oxygen delivery at the acute stage of severe brain injury is not easy because of reduced cardiac output and/or lower hemoglobin values in systemic circulation. Many factors are nominated as causes of reduced of cardiac output, such as the damage of cardiac muscles associated with coronary arterial spasm, contraction myocytolysis, difficult expansion of cardiac muscle contraction, and hyperglycemia caused by excess release of catecholamines. Excess release of catecholamines produces two metabolic disturbances: markedly increased cyclic adenosine monophosphate (AMP), and hyperglycemia with consumption of ATP and glycogen in the major organs, heart, and liver (Fig. 15, Chap. 22). Increased cyclic AMP levels immediately produce vascular contraction and cardiac ischemia due to coronary spasm and contraction myocytolysis. A similar pattern of ST elevation caused by cardiac infarction and prolongation of the QT interval to greater than 450 mm/sec is recorded on the electrocardiogram (ECG).

Hemoglobin dysfunction is an unexpected major issue for management of severely brain-injured patients. Slow release of bound oxygen from hemoglobin causes ineffective oxygen inhalation and respiratory management. In our recent clinical studies of cases with GCS less than 6, hemoglobin dysfunction was recorded in 41% of patients, shown as low arterial blood henoglobin-DPG (Hb-DPG) [10]. In these patients, severely reduced jugular venous Hb-DPG was recorded in 24% of cases (Fig. 20, Chap. 22).

Causes of reduced Hb-DPG were identified in our brain hypothermia studies as severe ketoacidosis, serum pH less than 7.2, hyperglycemia with serum glucose levels above 230 mg/dl, blood transfusion (>6000 ml), and continuous hemodiafiltration therapy. In most cases of reduced Hb-DPG, increased serum lactate levels were recorded [10]. This harmful stress-induced hyperglycemia and reduced Hb-DPG must be considered as important targets of initial management.

Normal control of ICP, CPP, and PaO_2 is not always suitable for the management of severely injured neurons. The control of brain tissue temperature at 32°–34°C can only prevent excess release of catecholamines and allow easy care of masking neuronal hypoxia. Prevention of apoptosis by suppression of caspase 3 and enhancing anti-apoptotic protein, prevention of gene damage in injured neurons, and suppression of free radical attack [7,10,13,24,29] are also neuroprotection effects of brain hypothermia management. Previously accepted methods of neuroprotection by the control of ICP, CBF, and prevention of brain edema are not adequate treatments for masking neuronal hypoxia.

Increased Brain Tissue Lactate Following Brain Hypothermia

For a long time, increased levels of brain tissue lactate have been considered to be produced by anaerobic metabolism in directly injured brain tissue. However, recent clinical study of brain hypothermia management found two further reasons of increased brain tissue lactate levels. In severely brain-injured patients, hyperglycemia associated with catecholamine surge is unavoidable [4,9,12,14]. Catecholamine surge could be reduced by early induction of brain hypothermia but cannot be prevented completely. The excess release of epinephrine during catecholamine surge is associated with stress reactions of the HPA axis and produces progressive glycogenesis. Epinephrine is a very strong promoter of these metabolic reactions by consuming ATP and glycogen in the liver (Fig. 15, Chap. 22). This HPA axis stress-associated hyperglycemia recorded at very high incidence in cases of brain trauma, hypertensive intracerebral hemorrhage, subarachnoid hemorrhage, acute onset of cerebral ischemia, and brain hypoxia with cardiac arrest (Figs. 16, 17, Chap. 22). Delayed induction of hypothermia, especially later than 3 h after severe brain injury, has difficulty controlling catetholamine surge-associated hyperglycemia and lactic acidosis in the injured brain tissue. This is because such hyperglycemia is resistant to insulin due to reduced insulin sensitivity, disturbed muscle protein synthesis, and suppression of insulin release (Fig. 14, Chap. 22). Therefore, to prevent these complications, early induction of brain hypothermia treatment is the most successful [13,14].

A second reason for hyperglycemia is the rapid induction of moderate brain hypothermia management (32°–33°C). This is the most common cause of increased brain tissue lactate level under brain hypothermia treatment. The rapid induction of hypothermia and excessive lower hypothermia produces hyperglycemia because of reduced consumption of serum glucose [13]. It has long been believed that hypothermia reduces the systemic metabolism; however, this concept is not correct. Following hypothermia, the metabolism shifts from glucose to lipid. The glucose metabolism reduction correlates to the hypothermia and lipid metabolism increases at lower body temperature. The brain tissue temperature at which the lipid metabolism becomes dominant is around 34°C [11,13,14]. Therefore, during the acute stage, two types of hyperglycemia must be controlled: that associated with the epinephrine surge caused by slow induction of hypothermia during the acute stage, and that caused by inadequate serum glucose consumption due to excessively low hypothermia in the cooling stage. Inadequate management of serum glucose during the cooling stage causes an increase in brain tissue lactate and pyruvate levels with increasing of brain tissue glucose as shown in Fig. 28, Chap. 23. In this case, brain tissue temperature should be controlled at 34°C rather than 33°C. The management of brain tissue temperature at 33°C produced increased brain tissue lactate level; however, no increase at 34°C was observed. Microdialysis studies suggested that the critical level of serum glucose to produce an increase in lactate is above 140 mg/dl at a brain tissue temperature of 33°C during the cooling stage.

Uncontrolled hyperglycemia during the acute stage produces many serious complications and unsuccessful hypothermia treatment. Increased brain tissue glucose level also produces the negative effect of increasing vasopressin release via the feedback mechanism of neural control of macronutrients [2,6,10,11,17,18,20,22].

Excess release of vasopressin changes the endothelial cell function and causes vascular contraction with CBF disturbances, as noted in previous animal studies. Our clinical studies using microdialysis suggested that, severe hyperglycemia produces increased brain tissue glucose level, vasopressin release, activates cytokines IL1 and IL6, and increases the permeability of the BBB [14]. This implies that brain edema and BBB dysfunction cannot be controlled successfully by hypothermia without good management of hyperglycemia [13]. Careful management of serum glucose to 120–140 mg/dl is recommended throughout brain hypothermia management. The management of this insulin-resistant hyperglycemia is very important for the success of hypothermia treatment. However, control of insulin-resistant hyperglycemia is not easy. The suggested management method during the induction and cooling stages are discussed in Chaps. 43 and 44.

Short Duration of Brain Hypothermia Worsens the Condition at Rewarming Stage

Brain hypothermia of short duration is not sufficient to induce significant recovery. The effect of brain hypothermia is limited to the prevention of secondary brain damage during the cooling stage, especially in severely brain-injured patients. The most serious clinical issue in these patients is that rewarming can worsen the overall condition (Fig. 40). Without recovery of injured brain tissue up until the rewarming stage, various pathophysiological changes that have been halted by hypothermia begin to occur again with elevation of brain tissue temperature. Rewarming from moderate brain hypothermia (32°–33°C) produces various negative events in the body [1]. The systemic metabolic shift from lipid to glucose occurs at a brain tissue temperature of about 34°C [8,10,12]. Activation of cytokine reactions caused by vasopressin release [10], brain hypoxia, and vascular engorgement are recorded during rewarming [12]. The overlap of these negative factors and re-progression of brain damage becomes worse with rewarming [1,9,25].

Before rewarming is commenced, care must be taken to determine whether the injured brain is on the way to recovery. Two days of brain hypothermia treatment that focuses on the prevention of brain edema is too short for the recovery of severely brain-injured patients. The necessary duration of brain hypothermia is theoretically variable.

In 400 cases with GCS less than 6, brain hypothermia management was carried out for 4–14 days in most cases and showed signs of recovery during this period. However, the longest hypothermia treatment was 40 days, from which the patient survived. This patient was a 27-year-old man who was involved in an automobile accident (Fig. 41). The diagnosis was diffuse brain injury with bilateral subdural hematomas and uncontrollable nasal bleeding (GCS was 4). Unfortunately, cardiac arrest occurred 15 min after removal of the bilateral subdural hematomas. Fifty-six days after surgery, the patient's eye opened with verbal stimulation. Three years later, he complained of lack of spontaneity, although personality and memory had been maintained.

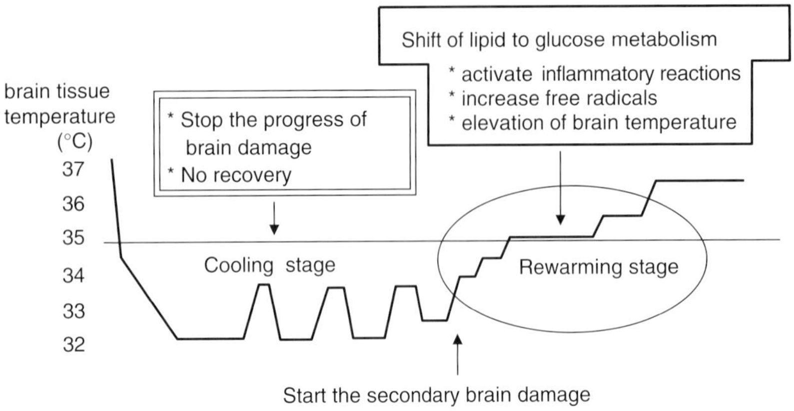

Fig. 40. The short duration of hypothermia without neuronal recovery causes secondary brain damage because of rewarming stress

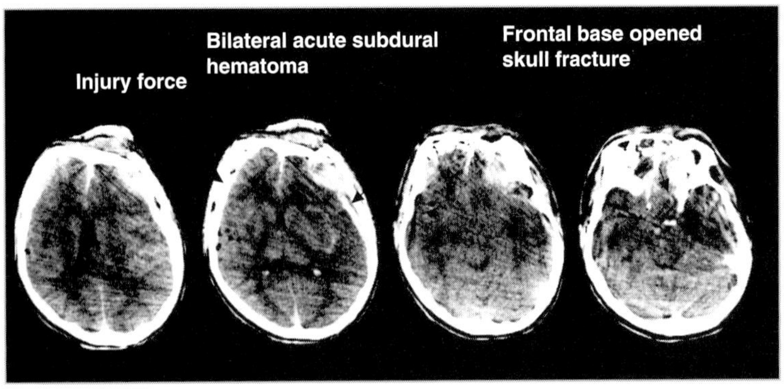

Fig. 41. Severe diffuse brain injury in a 28-year-old man with a bilateral thin subdural hematoma, bifrontal contusion, and hemorrhagic shock

It must be remembered that without skillful ICU management of systemic infection, immune crisis, neurohormomal abnormality, and hemoglobin dysfunction, brain hypothermia is difficult to continue for prolonged periods [5,6,8,10]. To provide an adequate duration of brain hypothermia, advanced care management to control of immune crisis, BBB dysfunction, cytokine encephalitis, intestinal mucous edema, pulmonary infection, and insulin-resistant hyperglycemia is required. The criteria to start rewarming is discussed in Chap. 45.

Reduced Immune Function Promotes Severe Pulmonary Infection and Cytokine Encephalitis

The complication of severe infection during brain hypothermia in severely brain-injured patients suggests unsuccessful management because of two possible reasons. One is the difficulty of continuing prolonged brain hypothermia. Brain hypothermia of short duration is not able to establish sufficient recovery for the indication of rewarming. Without recovery or at least partial recovery from brain damage, rewarming may worsen the outcome by overlapping rewarming stress and reprogression of initial brain damage (Fig. 40). Additional brain damage occurs because of cytokine encephalitis. In most cases, overlapping of cytokine encephalitis with severe brain damage produces uncontrollable increases in neurotoxic glutamate in the brain tissue and ICP elevation despite moderate brain hypothermia [10].

Severe damage to BBB function such as CSF/serum albumin ratio above 0.02 is a serious condition that accompanies increased cytokines in systemic circulation and pulmonary infection, and can lead to the additional complication of cytokines encephalitis (Fig. 27, Chap. 23). Our preliminary studies suggested that cytokine encephalitis produces a severe release of neuroteoxic glutamate in the brain tissue that is difficult to control using various ICU managements including moderate brain hypothermia.

Severe pulmonary infection is also a negative factor for brain injury because of brain hypoxia, vascular engorgement caused by hypercapnea, brain edema with progression of hypo-albuminemia, and cerebral venous congestion with increased mediastinal pressure.

The lower immune activity associated with reduced growth hormone (GH) levels is unavoidable during management of brain hypothermia (Fig. 42) [10]. This

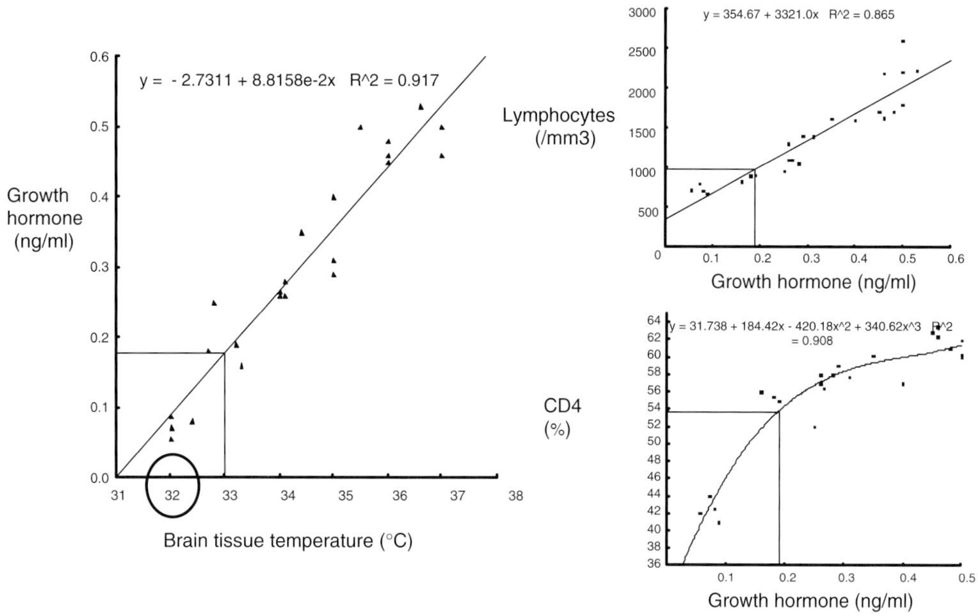

Fig. 42. Brain hypothermia management cannot avoid pituitary hypo-function and immune dysfunction. The critical brain tissue temperature for immune crisis is 32°C

phenomenon occurs when using brain hypothermia with any kind of brain cooling method, because successful brain hypothermia control is only obtained by precise control of circulating cerebral blood temperature. The low temperature of the pituitary gland is avoidable during brain hypothermia with the complication of low GH except at the induction stage. Before induction of brain hypothermia, GH level increases by stimulation of the HPA axis. Therefore, during brain hypothermia treatment, especially over prolonged periods, immune dysfunction is unavoidable [10,12].

Severe pulmonary infection is a serious complication during brain hypothermia treatment because of the disturbance of pulmonary function, worsening brain damage caused by cerebral vascular inflammation, increased vascular permeability, worsening brain edema, and increased neurotoxic glutamate levels caused by cytokine encephalitis. Put simply, the complications of systemic infection and pneumonia during brain hypothermia results in unsuccessful treatment.

The management of immune dysfunction, control of cytokine encephalitis, and prevention of infection during brain hypothermia treatment are not simple. The schedule for each particular treatment is the primary concern for ICU management during brain hypothermia treatment [5,6,12,15–18,20,22,24] and includes:

Control of brain tissue temperature
Replacement of neurohormones
Early management of catecholamine surge
Control of insulin-resistant hyperglycemia
Replacement of hypo-albuminemia
Management of BBB dysfunction
Management of gastric juice
Maintenance of microcirculation
Control of intestinal bacteria and bacterial translocation
Administration of effective antibiotics during hypothermia condition
Management of protein metabolism of skeletal muscle for increasing immune activity
Management of hemoglobin function
Maintenance of oxygen delivery
Detailed techniques for these treatments are discussed in Chaps. 44, 46, and 47.

Inadequate Nutrition Increases Brain Tissue Glutamate

In the ICU management of critically ill patients, early administration of parenteral and enteral nutrition is recommended, especially for the prevention of complications from infection. Enteral nutrition contains generous amounts of glucose, lipid, and amino acids to support immune functions and prevent energy crisis. However, hypothermia produce a metabolic shift from glucose to lipid. The brain tissue temperature of 34°C is the turning point between glucose and lipid metabolism [9,12]. Concerning the content of enteral nutrition, lipid is useful under the conditions of brain hypothermia,

Table 10. The changes in serum amino acids after parenteral nutrition of AMIZET and combination of AMIZET + glutamin

Serum amino acid (standard values: mmol/ml)	Nutrition	Brain tissue temperature (34°C)		Brain tissue temperature (36°C)	
Arginine	AMIZET + glutamin	86 ± 21.8	NS	126 ± 23.6	$P = 0.0105$
(54–130)	AMIZET XB	71 ± 10.1		62 ± 13.8	
Ornithine	AMIZET + glutamin	62 ± 14.6	NS	95 ± 25.0	$P = 0.0190$
(30–100)	AMIZET XB	72 ± 27.3		57 ± 12.2	
Citrulline	AMIZET + glutamin	18 ± 10.0	NS	25 ± 10.7	$P = 0.0105$
(17–43)	AMIZET XB	18 ± 6.4		12 ± 1.10	
Glutamine	AMIZET + glutamin	407 ± 50.0	NS	503 ± 91.7	NS
(430–700)	AMIZET XB	372 ± 48.1		421 ± 66.8	
Glutamate	AMIZET + glutamin	105 ± 23.7	NS	125 ± 23.6	NS
(12–63)	AMIZET XB	136 ± 65.3		137 ± 40.2	

AMIZET XB administration $n = 4$, AMIZET XB + glutamin administration $n = 6$
NS, Not significant

although the generous levels of glucose and glutamate may need to be reconsidered. The glucose metabolism is reduced by about 50% at a brain tissue temperature of 34°C. Administration of excess glucose causes an increase in serum glucose, brain tissue glucose, and an increase in brain tissue lactate [16,20,24]. Glutamate is the energy source of lymphocytes and is effective in maintaining immune function; however, increasing serum glutamate with BBB dysfunction is very dangerous for the injured brain tissue. Increasing levels of neurotoxic glutamate in injured brain tissue produces a neuroexcitation and delayed neuronal response. Our preliminary clinical studies suggest that about twice the neurotoxic level of glutamate is present in the serum after parenteral nutrition (Table 10). No increases in brain tissue glutamate levels were observed under the conditions of CSF/serum albumin ratio less than 0.01.

In cases of CSF/serum albumin ratio higher than 0.02, severe BBB dysfunction is likely and early nutrition produces an increase in neurotoxic glutamate in the injured brain tissue. The peak time of BBB dysfunction is about 2–4 days after trauma [12]. Therefore, other criteria for nutritional management during brain hypothermia treatment are preferred. In cases in which BBB dysfunction is not severe as shown by the CSF/serum albumin ratio less than 0.01, early nutrition that includes ZnCl, glutamine, and arginin for activation of immune function should start 2 days after trauma. However, in cases of CSF/serum albumin ratio higher than 0.01, initial enteral nutrition is limited to the administration of free glucose and saline with ZnCl. After 3–4 days, enteral administration of amino acid nutrition can begin, with monitoring of serum glutamate. We have observed uncontrollable increases in brain tissue glutamate even with moderate brain hypothermia (32°C) because of pulmonary infection under the conditions of CSF/serum albumin ratio more than 0.01. The misunderstanding of the timing of amino acid nutrition also produces unsuccessful brain hypothermia treatment.

References

1. Bioch M (1967) Cerebral effects of rewarming following prolonged hypothermia: significance for the management of severe cranio-cerebral injury and acute pyrexia. Brain 90:769–784
2. Boels PJ, Verbeuren TJ, Vanhoutte PM (1985) Moderate cooling depresses the accumulation and the release of newly synthesized catecholamines in isolated canine saphenous veins. Experientia 41:1374–1377
3. Castell JV, Andus T, Kunz D (1988) Interleukin-6. The major regulator of acute-phase protein synthesis in man and rat. Ann NY Acad Sci 557:87–101
4. Corte FD, Mancini A, Valle D, Gallizzi F, Carducci P, Mignani V, De Marinis L (1998) Provocative hypothalamopituitary axis tests in severe head injury: correlation with severity and prognosis. Crit Care Med 26:1419–1426
5. Davila DR, Breif S, Simon J, Hammer RE, Brinster RL, Kelley KW (1987) Role of growth hormone in regulating T-dependant immune events in aged, nude, and transgenic rodents. J Neurosci Res 18:108–116
6. Fedor EJ, Fisher ER, Lee SH, Weitzel WK, Fisher B (1956) Effect of hypothermia upon induced bacteremia. Proc Soc Exp Biol Med 93:510–512
7. Fukuda H, Tomimatsu T, Watanabe N, Mu JW, Kohzuki M, Endo M, Fujii E, Kanzaki T, Murata Y (2001) Post-ischemic hypothermia blocks caspase-3 activation in the newborn rat brain after hypoxia-ischemia. Brain Res 10: 187–191
8. Hayashi N (1995) Cerebral hypothermia treatment. In: Hayashi N (ed) Cerebral hypothermia treatment. Sogo Igaku Tokyo, pp 1–105
9. Hayashi N (1997) Prevention of vegetation after severe head trauma and stroke by combination therapy of cerebral hypothermia and activation of immune-dopaminergic nervous system. Proceedings of the 6th

annual meeting of Society for Treatment of Coma 6: 133–145
10. Hayashi N (2000) Enhanced neuronal damage in severely brain injured patients by hypothalamus, pituitary, and adrenal axis neuro-hormonal changes. In: Hayashi N (ed) Brain hypothermia. Springer, Berlin Heidelberg New York Tokyo, pp 3–26
11. Hayashi N (2000) The clinical issue and effectiveness of brain hypothermia treatment for severe brain injured patients. In: Hayashi N (ed) Brain hypothermia. Springer, Berlin Heidelberg New York Tokyo, pp 121–151
12. Hayashi N, Hirayama T, Utagawa A (1994) The cerebral thermo-pooling and hypothermia treatment of critical head injury patients. In: Nagai H (ed) Intracranial pressure IX. Springer, Berlin Heidelberg New York Tokyo, pp 589–599
13. Henning B, Honchel R, Goldblum SE, McClain CJ (1988) Tumor necrosis factor-mediated hypoalbuminemia in rabits. J Nur 118:1586–1590
14. Johnston MV, Trescher WH, Ishida A, Nakajima W (2000) Novel treatments after experimental brain injury. Semin Neonatol 5:75–86
15. Kagawa M, Nagao S, Bemana I (1996) Arginine vasopressin receptor antagonists for treatment of vasogenic brain edema: an experimental study. J Neurotrauma 13:273–279
16. Kossmann T, Hans V, Lenzlinger PM, Csuka E, Stsahel PF, Trentz O, Morgani-Kossmann MC (1996) Analysis of immune mediator production following traumatic brain injury. In: Schlag G, Redel H, Traber D (eds) Shock, sepsis and organ failure. Springer, Berlin Heidelberg New York Tokyo, pp 263–297
17. Kow LM, Pfaff DW (1986) Vasopressin excites ventromedial hypothalamus glucose-responsive neurons in vitro. Physiol Behav 37:153–158
18. Leibowitz SF (1999) Macronutrients and brain peptides: what they do and how they respond. In: Berthoud HR, Seeley RJ (eds) Neural and metabolic control of macronutrient intake. CRC, Boca Raton, pp 389–406
19. Lin TW, Kuo YS (1996) Acute pulmonary oedema following administration of vasopressin for control of massive GI tract haemorrhage in a major burn patient. Burns 22:73–75
20. MacIntosh TK (1994) Neurological sequele of traumatic brain injury: therapeutic implications. Cerebrovasc Brain Metab Rev 6:109–162
21. Maclain CJ, Henning B, Ott L, Goldblum S, Young AB (1988) Mechanisms and implications of hypoalbuminemia in head-injured patients. J Neurosurg 69:386–392
22. Montell E, Lerin C, Newgard CB, Gomez-Foix AM (2002) Effects of modulation of glycerol kinase expression on lipid and carbohydrate metabolism in human muscle cells. J Biol Chem 277: 2682–2686
23. Russwurm S, Stonans I, Schwerter K, Stonane E, Meissner W, Reinhart K (2002) Direct influence of mild hypothermia on cytokine expression and release in cultures of human peripheral blood mononuclear cells. J Interferon Cytokine Res 22:15–21
24. Slikker W, Desai VG, Duhart H, Feuers R, Imam SZ (2001) Hypothermia enhances bcl-2 expression and protects against oxidative stress-induced cell death in Chinese hamster ovary cells. Free Radic Biol Med 31:405–411
25. Stanley BG (1993) Neuropeptide Y in multiple hypothalamic sites controls eating behavior, endocrine, and autonomic system for body energy balance. In: Colmers WF, Wahlestedt C (eds) Biology of neuropeptide Y and related peptide. Humana Press, Totowa, NJ, pp 457–509
26. Suarez JI (2001) Treatment of acute brain edema. Rev Neurol 32:275–281
27. Temple DL (1994) The neuropeptide Y system (hypolhalamus) has a dense concentration of glucocorticoide (type II) receptors that mediate carbon hydrate intake. J Neuroendocrinol 6:479–501
28. Valeri CR, Cassidy G, Khuri S, Feingold H, Ragno G, Altschule MD (1978) Hypothermia-induced reversible platelet dysfunction. Ann Surg 205:175–181
29. Zhang Z, Sobel RA, Cheng D, Steinberg GK, Yenari MA (2001) Mild hypothermia increases Bcl-2 protein expression following global cerebral ischemia. Brain Res Mol Brain Res 95:75–85

34. Concepts in Brain Tissue Temperature Control

Mild or Moderate Brain Hypothermia?

The basic concept of brain hypothermia treatment is the management of adequate cerebral oxygenation, administration of sufficient metabolic substrates for injured neurons, control of neurohormonal function, and stabilization of cardiopulmonary function [4,6]. The previous concept of neuroprotection to tolerate brain ischemia by reduced brain metabolism makes it difficult for dying neurons in injured brain tissue to make a recovery. Therefore, stable systemic circulation and metabolism are important initially. In severely brain-injured patients, cardiopulmonary dysfunction occurs because of stress associated with the excess release of catecholamines [5]. This initial catecholamine surge [1,5] and neurohormonal response of the hypothalamus–pituitary–adrenal (HPA) axis [2] produces cardiac dysfunction not only by cardiac ischemia with coronary spasm but also by cardio-myocytolysis with prolonged contraction of cardiac muscles. To prevent this cardiopulmonary dysfunction, control of catecholamine surge by early induction of brain hypothermia is very useful [4,6]. However, brain hypothermia has biphasic effects to the systemic circulation. The early induction of brain hypothermia prevents the overreaction of catecholamine surge; however, severe brain hypothermia causes a drastic reduction in serum catecholamines and results in unstable systemic circulation [1,4,6]. The timing of brain tissue temperature control is one of the key points for successful brain hypothermia. Many types of hypothermia (not including brain hypothermia) have been administered and are as shown in Table 11.

Mild Brain Hypothermia Treatment (~34°C)

The strategy of brain tissue temperature control is decided by many factors such as the severity of brain damage, time to admission to the medical center after insult, cardiopulmonary dysfunction, severity of insulin-resistant hyperglycemia, presence of extracranial disease, and the level of medical care in hospital. Brain hypothermia at 34°–35°C known to have limited negative complications compared with treatment at 32°–33°C because reduction in serum catecholamines at 34°–35°C and metabolic shift from glucose to lipid are less than 50% [6]. The management of vital signs and homeometabolic changes is easier at 34°–35°C than at 32°–33°C brain temperature. Therefore, brain hypothermia treatment at 35°–34°C is preferred to early induction of brain hypothermia, which is the first step of moderate brain hypothermia (32°–33°C), in compromised patients, elderly patients with unstable systemic circulation, and patients with serious cardiopulmonary dysfunction including those resuscitated after cardiac arrest [6,12].

The early induction of brain hypothermia within 3h after insult is useful because it can prevent hemoglobin dysfunction and insulin-resistant hyperglycemia caused by excess release of catecholamines. However, if induction occurs later than 3h after insult, secondary brain damage caused by HPA axis abnormality progresses. In such cases, brain hypothermia treatment at 34°C is not enough. Late induction of brain hypothermia probably indicates brain hypothermia at 32°–33°C. Therefore, two-step induction of brain hypothermia is recommended in which brain hypothermia at 34°C is applied initially and, after stabilization of vital signs, the temperature is lowered to 32°–33°C. The duration is variable between 3–7 days, depending on the severity of brain damage.

The intensive care unit (ICU) management technique is also important because the difficulties encountered with brain hypothermia at 34°C and 32°–33°C are different. If the ICU care management technique and available personnel numbers are not adequate, brain hypothermia treatment at 34°C is recommended.

Moderate Brain Hypothermia Treatment (32°–33°C)

In severely brain-injured patients, the control of intracranial pressure (ICP) elevation is difficult with

Table 11. Recent clinical trials of mild to moderate hypothermia management

Author	Year	Body temperature	Cooling duration	Others
Clifton	1992	30°–32°C	1–8h	—
Gentilello	1992	35°C	3h	—
Marion	1997	32°C	48h	<10h
Signorini	2000	34°–35°C	~12h	—
Hickc	2000	33°C	24h	—
Reinert	2000	32°–35°C	48h	ICP ↑
Clifton	2000	32°–33°C	48h	<6h

management of the brain tissue temperature at 34°C. As a clinical issue for determining the brain tissue temperature at admission of severely brain-injured patients, the Glasgow Coma Scale (GCS) is not always practical for deciding the severity of brain damage and the prospects for effective brain hypothermia at 34°C. Insulin-resistant hyperglycemia is correlated to the severity of stress to the HPA axis in severe brain damage. Moderate brain hypothermia is indicated for patients with a GCS of 6 or less and a serum glucose level greater than 180mg/dl. However, without control of stress-related hyperglycemia at serum glucose levels lower than 180mg/dl, early induction of brain hypothermia at 32°–33°C is not indicated. The delayed and late induction of brain hypothermia treatment at 32°–33°C after control of serum glucose level to between 120 and 140mg/dl is probably appropriate [6]. The progress of pathophysiological changes of brain damage are difficult to control with mild hypothermia at 34°C. Pitfalls of brain hypothermia induction are the increasing levels of brain tissue glucose and lactate that are caused by brain hypothermia treatment. Our clinical studies using microdialysis suggest that rapid induction of moderate hypothermia (32°–33°C) produces an increase in serum glucose. The systemic metabolic shift from glucose to lipid metabolism also occurs following hypothermia. At a brain tissue temperature of 34°C, glucose metabolism and lipid metabolism become approximately equal, and below 34°C the expenditure of glucose rapidly decreases in the brain and extracranial major organs. Therefore, even though it may be possible to control serum glucose to near-normal levels around 34°C, the serum glucose level increases rapidly to more than 160mg/dl after induction of moderate brain hypothermia at 32°–33°C. In this case, brain tissue glucose increases two- to three-fold and brain tissue lactate increases about two-fold. The management of brain tissue temperature at 34°C is much better than 33°C in this case. This phenomenon occurs more readily in patients older than 75 years with reduced glucose consumption. During induction of brain hypothermia at 32°–33°C, if serum glucose levels of more than 180mg/dl are recorded, induction of brain hypothermia should stop until hyperglycemia is controlled. Under brain hypothermia at 34°C, careful management is necessary, especially that of hyperglycemia in patients with unstable cardiac function.

The duration of brain hypothermia at 32°–33°C is variable for between 4 and 14 days, depending on the severity of brain damage and the reversibility of neuronal damage [4,6]. A flat electroencephalogram (EEG) and auditory brainstem evoked potential (ABER), breathing arrest, and pupil dilatation are not signs of contraindication in the acute stage. However, after 3–6h, these critical clinical signs do suggest contraindication of brain hypothermia treatment.

The Time Schedule for Management of Brain Tissue Temperature

The purpose of brain cooling at each stage of treatment is different depending on the time after insult. Within 3–6h after severe brain injury, prevention of catecholamine surge, management of hemoglobin dysfunction, maintenance of neuronal oxygenation in injured brain tissue, management of harmful stress-associated hyperglycemia, prevention of brain thermo-pooling, and prevention of blood–brain barrier (BBB) dysfunction caused by excess release of vasopressin are major targets of treatment [5,8–11,13]. After 6h, in the cooling stage, neuroprotection facilitated by administration of adequate oxygen and metabolic substrates is the most important management strategy to prevent secondary brain damage caused by brain edema, brain ischemia, and ICP elevation. At this stage, ICU management must also focus on the negative factors of brain hypothermia such as immune crisis and ease of infection [3,5], unstable cardiopulmonary function [1,5], hyperglycemia, hypokalemia, and thrombocytopenia [5].

Before starting rewarming, it is important to affirm that brain damage is on the way to recovery, systemic infections are absent, immune activity has increased, and hyperglycemia is under control in order to reduce the worsening of brain damage caused by rewarming stress [4,6].

The early and rapid induction of brain hypothermia to 34°C within 3h after insult is fundamental care management. However, management of temperatures below 34°C requires care and slow induction of brain hypothermia, because rapid induction of moderate brain hypothermia produces biphasic effects on the injured brain tissue. Moderate brain hypothermia is

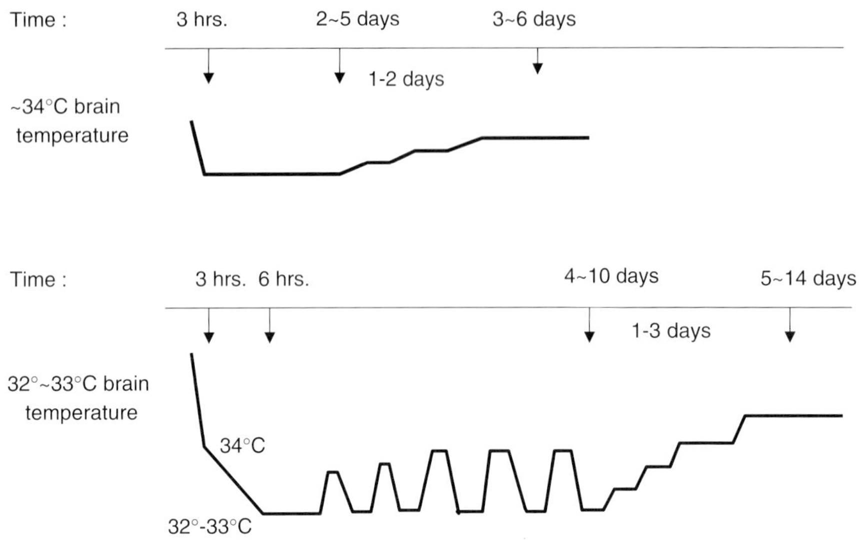

Fig. 43. The time schedule of brain hypothermia treatment

more effective than mild brain hypothermia for the prevention of free radical reactions and the prevention of brain edema; however, imbalance in brain metabolism can easily occur. The acute increase in serum glucose level associated with reduced glucose consumption contributes to increasing levels of brain tissue glucose and lactate. The rapid induction of mild brain hypothermia to 34°C showed no serious complications with management of fluid resuscitation and well-organized anesthesia. However, below 34°C, moderate brain hypothermia produced dramatic changes in systemic circulation caused by reduced serum catecholamines and increased brain tissue glucose related to hyperglycemia associated with the metabolic shift from glucose to lipid [6]. Therefore, hyperglycemia occurs during the acute stage of brain hypothermia because of two reasons: one is no control of catecholamine surge, and the other is reduced glucose consumption arising from metabolic shift from glucose to lipid at temperatures lower than 34°C. As a strategy for brain hypothermia treatment, two different time schedules of brain hypothermia treatment should be considered as shown in Fig. 43.

Mild Brain Hypothermia Treatment (~34°C)

The timing of induction of brain hypothermia to 34°–35°C is very simple. GCS less than 8, stabilized vital signs, and no arrhythmia are criteria for early induction of brain hypothermia treatment. If the level of available medical care is not ideal, mild brain hypothermia at 34°–35°C is also recommended. Before the induction of brain hypothermia, the water temperature of the cooling device should be set between 15° and 17°C and the brain tissue temperature reduced to 34°C rapidly. If the patient requires surgery to remove intracranial hematoma, the surgical operation can be carried out under the control of brain tissue temperature at around 34°C. Surgical operations at brain tissue temperatures below 34°C are not recommended except in cases in which systemic circulation can be maintained using a special circulating device. This is because the serum catecholamine level becomes too low and it is difficult to maintain stabilized systemic circulation during surgery.

After obtaining stabilized systemic circulation, oxygen delivery, and cardiopulmonary function, brain tissue temperature is maintained at about 34°C for 3–7 days until evidence of recovery of the brain injury is observed. The most important ICU management issues are the prevention of pulmonary infection and cytokine encephalitis with management of neuroprotection for brain edema, cerebral blood flow (CBF) disturbances, brain hypoxia, metabolic imbalance, and ICP elevation [3–5,7,11,13]. The management technique for the prevention of infection at a brain tissue temperature around 34°C is not difficult. Desirable management goals during the cooling stage and before the rewarming preconditioning stage are:

Serum albumin higher than 3.5 mg/dl
CSF/serum albumin ratio lower than 0.01
Serum glucose level between 120 and 140 mg/dl
Vitamin A higher than 50 mg/dl
Hemoglobin (Hb) higher than 12 mg/dl 2,3-Diphosphoglycerate higher than 10 mmol/g Hb
Antithrombin-III higher than 100%
Platelet count 50 000–80 000/cu mm
Digastrics decontamination
Muscle massage
Abdominal pressure less than 10 mmHg.

The detailed ICU management techniques are discussed in Chaps. 44 and 46. These preconditioning ICU management strategies are very useful to prevent worsening of rewarming-stage infections. If ICP is not controlled to below 20 mmHg within 12 h or to less than 15 mmHg within 24 h when using brain hypothermia at 34°C, moderate brain hypothermia is indicated.

The time course and speed of rewarming are very important for the success of prolonged brain hypothermia treatment. Fundamentally, rewarming of brain tissue temperature by 0.1°C requires 1 h. This technique is especially important for brain hypothermia treatment that is prolonged for more than 3 days. It is important to allow time for adaptation to neurohormonal changes, cardiovascular changes, rapid increases in brain metabolism, and various enzymatic changes. However, in cases of short-duration brain hypothermia (such as 2 days), a rewarming speed of 0.5°C per hour is acceptable (Fig. 43).

To prevent rewarming stress and various complications, rewarming should be halted at 35°C and this temperature maintained for 1–2 days. This period is known as "physiological adaptation time." In our ICU, the rewarming speed is 1 day to raise the brain tissue temperature by 1°C. After rewarming, the control of brain tissue temperature at around 36°–36.5°C is also important. As a technique, the localized cooling of the head and neck for 3–5 days, even after rewarming is finished, is useful.

Moderate Brain Hypothermia Treatment (32°–34°C)

Moderate brain hypothermia treatment is indicated as a second stage treatment in cases that show no response to brain hypothermia treatment at 34°C. The induction in two steps at different speeds is very safe and is a successful restoration therapy for neuronal recovery in injured brain tissue. Rapid induction of brain hypothermia to 34°C is performed initially. ICU management then focuses on the stabilization of systemic circulation, control of serum glucose at 120–150 mg/dl (at least lower than 180 mg/dl), management of cardiopulmonary dysfunction such as arrhythmia and elongation of the QT interval greater than 450 mm/sec, and replacement of hypokalemia. After stabilizing these clinical issues, brain tissue temperature is reduced to 32°–33°C, step by step, and spending 5–6 h at this temperature as shown in Fig. 43.

The management of brain tissue temperature is very successful for the prevention of free radical reactions, neurotoxic neurotransmitter release, vascular engorgement, and progressing brain edema; however, it is very stressful to the systemic circulation and immune function by reducing the HPA axis neurohormonal functions. Prolonged continuous control of brain tissue temperature at 32°C is not recommended because diminished pituitary hormonal function may result. In turn, this results in a reduction in growth hormone (GH) level, diminished CD4 activity, lymphocytopenia, and immune crisis [5,6].

The question of how to manage such complications for the success of prolonged brain hypothermia treatment is important. The intermittent control of moderate brain hypothermia is a basic technique for prolonged brain hypothermia without complications of immune crisis and infection. To prevent pituitary dysfunction and increases of hormonal release from the pituitary gland, temporary elevation of brain tissue temperature from 32°–33°C to 34°C is recommended. The timing of brain tissue temperature elevation during moderate brain hypothermia is also important. Because 18:00–22:00 hours is the time during which serum levels of GH increase naturally in humans, temporal elevation of brain tissue temperature should be conducted during this time to prevent immune crisis (Fig. 8, Chap. 23). Intermittent control of brain tissue temperature during moderate brain hypothermia produces a low rate of GH replacement, GH-associated hyperglycemia, immune crisis, and a high incidence of complications due to pulmonary infection.

Moderate brain hypothermia is indicated in severely brain-injured patients and in cases of delayed induction of brain hypothermia treatment. Without some recovery from brain damage, the brain injury mechanism reprogresses with rewarming of the brain tissue. For the recovery of severely brain-injured patients, prolonged brain hypothermia is necessary.

Another clinical issue of prolonged brain hypothermia is the metabolic shift from glucose-dominant metabolism to lipid-dominant metabolism. This issue is discussed in Chap. 43. The reduction of all metabolic paths during hypothermia is not a correct concept. Therefore, during the rewarming stage, a patient undergoing prolonged hypothermia treatment requires an adaptation time for the shift in metabolism from lipid to glucose. Careful, step-by-step rewarming with 1–2 days adaptation times at a brain tissue temperature of 35°C is important, as shown in Fig. 43.

The Rewarming Time

The use of brain hypothermia for 2–3 days to prevent brain edema and free radical reactions is reported in recent papers. Such treatment is very dangerous for severely brain-injured patients. The short duration of brain hypothermia does not provide sufficient time to allow recovery from severe brain injury. Although short-duration brain hypothermia stops pathophysiological changes or delays the progress of them, without recovery from brain injury during the cooling stage, rewarming promotes the progression of pathophysiological changes again and worsens the condition due to rewarming stress [6]. Therefore, before rewarming is commenced, injured tissue must be on the way to recovery. Overlapping of rewarming stress and reprogression of brain-injury pathophysiology are made much worse by rewarming. Forms of rewarming stress include the metabolic shift from lipid to glucose, increasing levels of serum catecholamines, imbalance between hyperglycemia and delayed glucose expenditure, cerebral vascular engorgement, activation of HPA axis neurohormones, activation of cytokines, and activation of infectious bacteria. Certainly, 2-day brain hypothermia treatment is too short for recovery of severely brain-injured patients. The adequate duration of brain hypothermia is theoretically variable because of the aforementioned reasons.

However, prolonged brain hypothermia treatment that provides enough time to allow recovery from severe brain damage may be easily complicated by immune crisis with reduced GH and severe systemic infections. To retain an adequate duration of brain hypothermia for recovery from various levels of brain damage, skillful care techniques for the control of immune crisis and infections are required. Criteria for the rewarming procedure for severely brain-injured patients are also needed.

From the aforementioned reasons, the decision to start rewarming must be made with precise evidence of recovery of injured tissue or a diagnosis that indicates recovery has begun. The appearance of a θ-wave on the background of the δ-wave on the trended EEG, no ICP elevation, SjO_2 control at 60%–75%, and no brain swelling observed on the computed tomography-scan are indirect evaluation parameters for the decision to start rewarming. The absence of severe BBB dysfunction (CSF/serum albumin < 0.01), hypo-albuminemia (<3.0 mg/dl), and hyperglycemia (>180 mg/dl) are also further indications to prevent worsening of brain damage. Very strong replacement therapy of serum albumin and control of the serum glucose level to between 120 and 140 mg/dl are recommended before the start of rewarming. The complication of pneumonia at the rewarming stage is a strong contributor to unsuccessful brain hypothermia treatment.

References

1. Boels PJ, Verbeuren TJ, Vanhoutte PM (1985) Moderate cooling depresses the accumulation and the release of newly synthesized catecholamines in isolated canine saphenous veins. Experientia 41:1374–1377
2. Corte FD, Mancini A, Valle D, Gallizzi F, Carducci P, Mignani V, De Marinis L (1998) Provocative hypothalamopituitary axis tests in severe head injury: correlation with severity and prognosis. Crit Care Med 26:1419–1426
3. Fedor EJ, Fisher ER, Lee SH, Weitzel WK, Fisher B (1956) Effect of hypothermia upon induced bacteremia. Proc Soc Exp Biol Med 93:510–512
4. Hayashi N (1997) Prevention of vegetation after severe head trauma and stroke by combination therapy of cerebral hypothermia and activation of immune-dopaminergic nervous system. Proceedings of the 6th annual meeting of Society for Treatment of Coma 6: 133–145
5. Hayashi N (2000) Enhanced neuronal damage in severely brain injured patients by hypothalamus, pituitary, and adrenal axis neuro-hormonal changes. In: Hayashi (ed) Brain hypothermia. Springer, Berlin Heidelberg New York Tokyo, pp 3–26
6. Hayashi N (2000) The clinical issue and effectiveness of brain hypothermia treatment for severe brain injured patients. In: Hayashi (ed) Brain hypothermia. Springer, Berlin Heidelberg New York Tokyo, pp 121–151
7. Hayashi N, Hirayama T, Utagawa A (1994) The cerebral thermo-pooling and hypothermia treatment of critical head injury patients. In: Nagai H (ed) Intracranial pressure IX. Springer, Berlin Heidelberg New York Tokyo, pp 589–599
8. Kagawa M, Nagao S, Bemana I (1996) Arginine vasopressin receptor antagonists for treatment of vasogenic brain edema: an experimental study. J Neurotrauma 13: 273–279
9. Leibowitz SF (1999) Macronutrients and brain peptides: what they do and how they respond. In: Berthoud HR, Seeley RJ (eds) Neural and metabolic control of macronutrient intake. CRC, Boca Raton, pp 389–406
10. Lin TW, Kuo YS (1996) Acute pulmonary oedema following administration of vasopressin for control of massive GI tract haemorrhage in a major burn patient. Burns 22:73–75
11. MacIntosh TK (1994) Neurological sequele of traumatic brain injury: therapeutic implications. Cerebrovasc Brain Metab Rev 6:109–162
12. Nagao K, Hayashi N, Kanmatsuse K, Arima K, Ohtsuki J, Kikushima K, Watanabe I (2000) Cardiopulmonary cerebral resuscitation using emergency cardiopulmonary bypass, coronary reperfusion therapy and mild hypothermia in patients with cardiac arrest outside the hospital. J Am Coll Cardiol 36:776–783
13. Suarez JI (2001) Treatment of acute brain edema. Rev Neurol 32:275–281

35. Management of Brain Tissue Temperature

Fundamental Technique of Brain Tissue Temperature Control

The management of brain tissue temperature with precise control of cerebral blood flow (CBF) blood temperature is a fundamental technique for the management of brain hypothermia [4]. The precise control of brain hypothermia can be obtained by control of the systemic circulatory blood temperature using the blanket technique [2–4]. Cooling of systemic circulatory blood causes homogeneous whole-brain hypothermia, because blood circulates through all of the brain tissue. The cerebrospinal fluid (CSF) cooling approach for brain hypothermia directly reduces the surface temperature of the brain to a depth of a few millimeters; however, deep brain tissue is not cooled suffiently without cooling of the brain circulatory blood. Localized cooling of the skull and nasal cavity reduces CSF temperature, but not that of all of the brain tissue.

An isolated and selective brain-cooling technique by infusion of cooled saline into the carotid artery provides precise control of the systemic circulatory blood temperature. However, precise control of brain tissue temperature using this technique is very difficult at the rewarming stage. This is because the cessation of cooled saline infusion into the brain produces an immediate and rapid elevation of brain tissue temperature caused by recirculation of warm blood. Also, excess infusion of saline for brain cooling is a negative factor for the prevention of brain edema. The combination of isolated, selective brain cooling and mild hypothermia using the blanket technique will reduce the negative effects of excess saline infusion. Direct cooling of the systemic circulation is a very effective cooling method for the management of brain tissue hypothermia. As direct blood-cooling methods, two techniques have been developed. One technique is blood cooling by using an external systemic circulation system, with a combination of balloon pumping and insertion of a pacemaker [5]. This technique is useful for resuscitated cardiac arrest patients. The other is direct blood cooling by insertion of a cooling device into the blood vessels, carotid artery, and abdominal vein. The Innercool method by Celsius Control has been reported [1]. The direct method is the most convenient for the control of brain tissue temperature. However, these techniques are all limited to short-duration brain hypothermia and require direct insertion of a cooling catheter in the vena cava via the femoral vein or in the aortic arch via the abdominal aorta. Prolonged catheterization is very difficult in terms of safety because of a high incidence of infection and vascular thrombosis.

The indirect method of brain hypothermia using the cold water blanket technique to reduce the systemic blood temperature is the most popular technique [2–4]. Figures 44 and 45 show the blanket technique for brain cooling (Modified Blanketrol II, Nihon MDM, Tokyo, Japan). Figure 46 shows the same cooling system Medi Therm II by Gaymer Industries Orchard Park, NY, USA). The patient is placed on a dry towel that has been placed on the cooling blanket. The patient is then covered with a dry towel and a second cooling blanket before the patient and cooling blankets are completely wrapped in a large dry towel. Exposure of the body to room temperature should be avoided to stabilize the brain tissue temperature. If the patient weighs more than 80 kg, the cooling system should be separated into ventral and dorsal systems by using two machines.

The time course for the management of blanket water temperature is important. The recommended control of blanket water temperature for brain hypothermia at 32°–34°C is shown in Fig. 47. The detailed technique is described in Chap. 35. If it is difficult to control brain hypothermia or difficult to induce brain hypothermia for short time, repeat and repeat the management cycle of blanket water temperature with more dynamic large friction is successful as shown in Fig. 48.

Prolonged brain hypothermia cannot avoid pituitary hormonal dysfunction, regardless of the brain hypothermia method because cooling of the brain tissue results in cooling of the pituitary gland. Reduced growth hormone levels lower the cellular immune activity, reduce the lipid metabolism, and can easily introduce

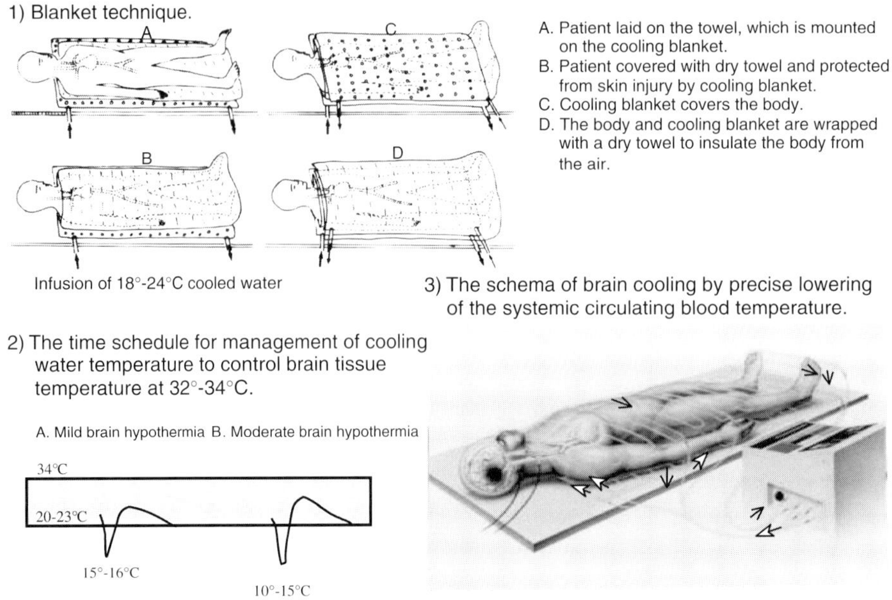

Fig. 44. Brain cooling technique using the cooling water blanket and modified Blanketrol II

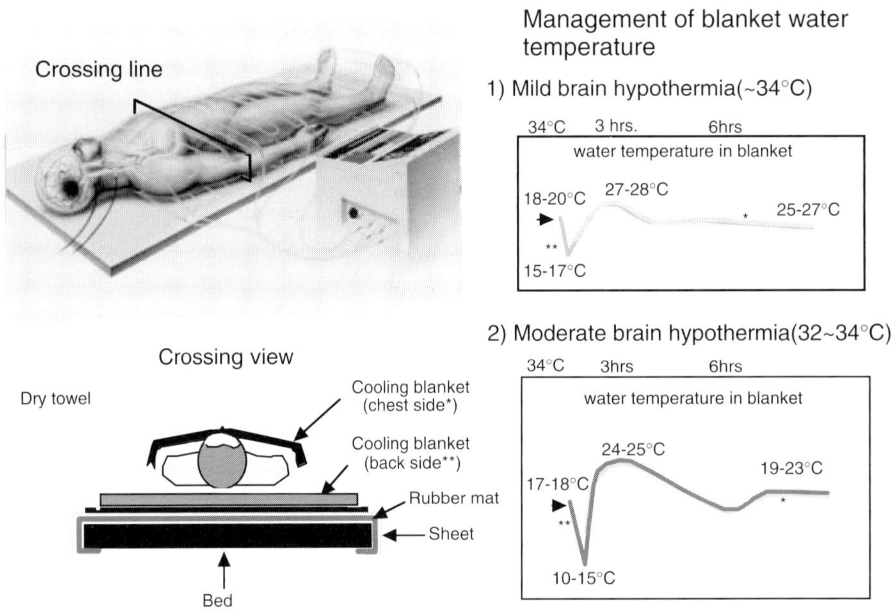

Fig. 45. Brain cooling technique using chilled water blanket and cooling device

the complication of severe pneumonia. Therefore, prolonged brain hypothermia requires special consideration for management of immune dysfunction and mild replacement of growth hormones. Excess administration of growth hormone produces hyperglycemia as a complication [2–4].

Rapid Induction of Mild Brain Hypothermia

For rapid induction of mild brain hypothermia, the water temperature of the cooling device should be initially set between 10° and 15°C. The water temperature should then be very slowly elevated to 24°–25°C, with

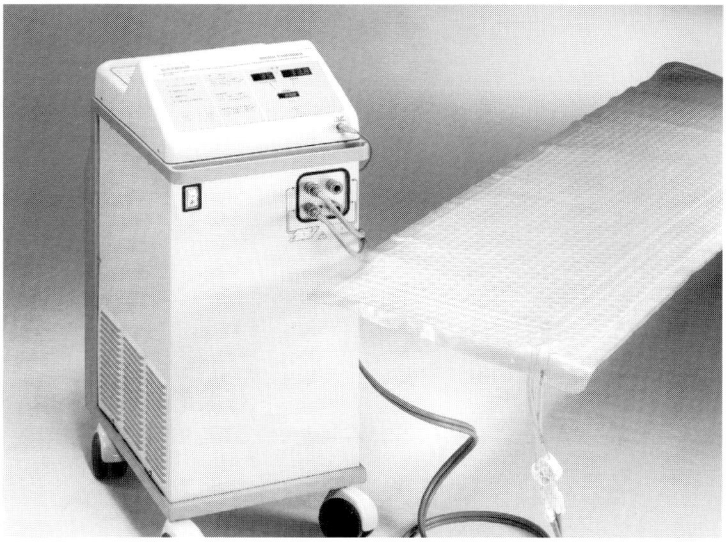

Fig. 46. Blanket cooling system for brain hypothermia treatment

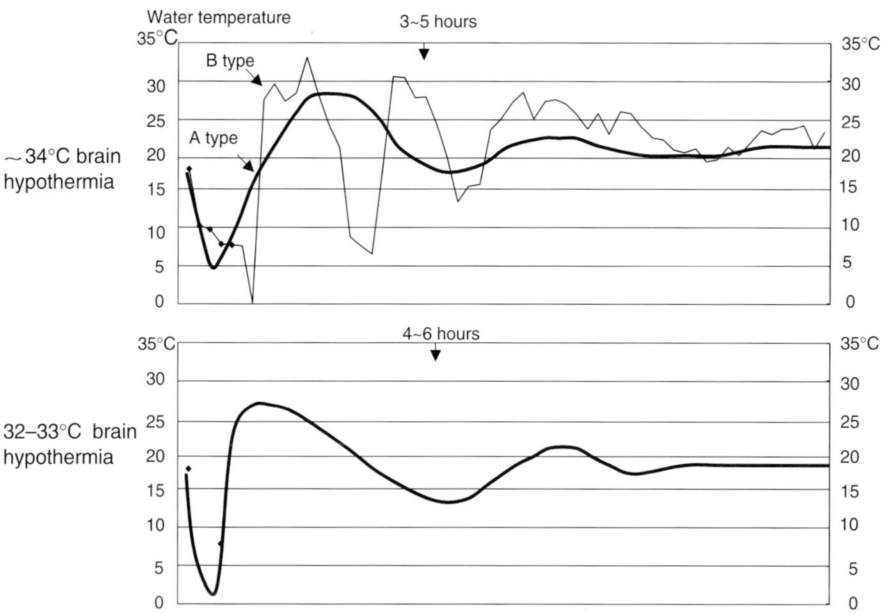

Fig. 47. The management of blanket water temperature for induction of ~34°C and 32°–33°C brain hypothermia

monitoring of brain tissue temperature. Complete wrapping of the patient's body, removed of heat-producting medical devices from around the bed, control of room temperature at 18°–20°C, and maintaining air flow around the bed are all helpful techniques for maintaining stable brain hypothermia.

Safe Induction of Moderate Brain Hypothermia

After induction of mild brain hypothermia to give a stable brain tissue temperature of 33.5°–34°C, the systemic circulation and cardiopulmonary functions should be stabilized. The brain tissue temperature should then be reduced to 32°–33°C for periods of 5–6h (Fig. 43, Chap. 34). Intermittent elevation of the brain tissue temperature from 32°–33°C to 34°C is desirable for prolonged brain hypothermia to prevent pituitary hormonal crisis, immune dysfunction, and the accumulation of brain tissue glucose and lactate because of reduced glucose consumption [2–4]. To achieve intermittent elevation of the brain tissue temperature, careful removal of the cooling blanket from the body without changes of the blanket water temperature is recommended. Elevation of the brain tissue temperature to 34°C is best performed when physiological growth hormone levels increase naturally between 1800 and 2200 hours.

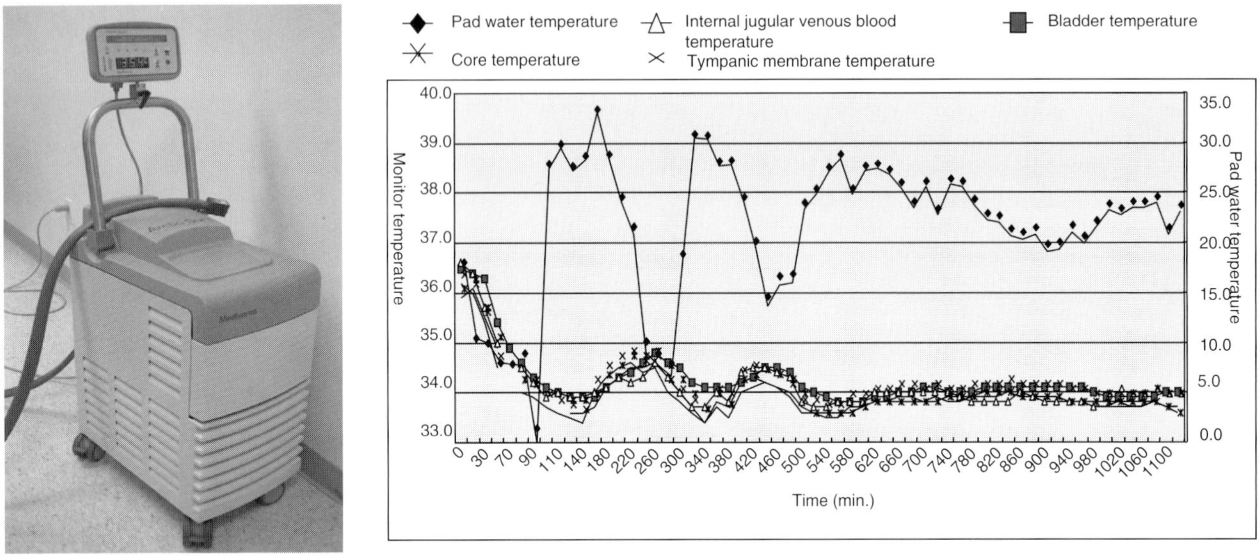

Fig. 48. Automatic control device for mild brain hypothermia manufactured by Medivance. The plot shows the relationships between the blanket water temperature and internal jugular venous blood temperature, bladder temperature, core temperature, and tympanic membrane temperature

One of the most important techniques in brain hypothermia treatment is rewarming without complications. Rapid elevation of blanket water temperature produces an uncontrollable and marked elevation of brain tissue temperature. To avoid rapid elevation of brain tissue temperature at the rewarming stage, blanket water temperature should be elevated from 22° to 26° or 27°C very slowly (0.1°C/h) and the brain tissue temperature controlled with step-by-step elevation as shown in Fig. 43 (Chap. 34). When the brain tissue temperature is elevated to 34°–35°C, this temperature is maintained for 1–2 days to allow physiological adaptation to changes of the systemic metabolism from lipid to glucose, increased serum glucose levels caused by serum catecholamine surge, imbalance between glucose consumption and production, vascular engorgement, and activation of CD4. This adaptation time is maintained by recooling the blanket water from 27°–28°C to 26°–25°C. This management of blanket water temperature prevents spontaneous elevation of brain tissue temperature from 34°–35°C.

After adaptation time, the brain tissue temperature should be very carefully elevated to 36°–37°C. Reduced contact area between the cooling blanket and the patient allows safe control of brain tissue rewarming. This technique is much simpler when rewarming above 34°–35°C. The slow and steady rate of rewarming is less inclined to cause complications. In cases of prolonged brain hypothermia of more than 4 days, adaptation times are necessary to stabilize metabolic changes.

Compartment Cooling Blanket Technique

To control the blood temperature of the systemic circulation, the small-blanket cooling method is not capable of reducing the systemic circulating blood temperature to 32°–33°C. The two-compartment blanket cooling technique allows easier control of brain tissue temperature. The thorough wrapping of the patient in the blanket, a stable, heat-conductive blanket sheet, and strong circulation of cooled water in the blanket are important to maintain stable brain tissue hypothermia. The compartment cooling blanket technique using two cooling machines is very successful in obtaining stable brain tissue hypothermia.

Cooling Suit Technique

In recent clinical studies, a new cooling pad developed by Medivance (www. medivance.com Louisville, CO, USA) was described. The Arctic Sun Energy Transfer Pads allow much easier management of brain hypothermia patients in the intensive care unit (ICU) than blankets (Fig. 49). The cooling pad consists of five small separated pads that cover the chest, abdomen, back, and bilateral thigh. The exterior of the pad is made of soft nonheat-conducting material, and the inside surface that contacts with the body is sealed with a translucent

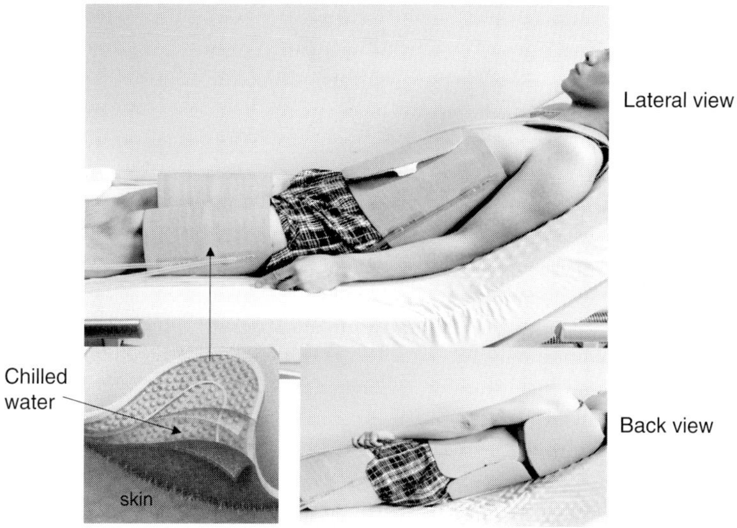

Fig. 49. Cooling suit for brain hypothermia treatment

thin film. This film is covered with adhesive gelatinous material (Fig. 49). Therefore, the cooling effect on body temperature is very powerful with a small cooling pad. Figure 49 shows the general view of how the five cooling pads are worn. This system allows easy care of catheterization, fluid resuscitation, and peripheral massage for the prevention of venous thrombosis. No skin allergic responses to the adhesive cooling pad were experienced in cases of prolonged brain hypothermia treatment. The Arctic Sun system has an automatic induction program for mild brain hypothermia treatment. The automatic management of prolonged moderate brain hypothermia remains in the design stage with clinical studies.

Many types of cooling suits have been developed in NASA projects. The Allon 2000 device was released by Advanced Technologies (Israel) for brain hypothermia treatment of children. However, we have no experience with this system.

Direct Blood-Cooling Techniques

Monan and Kanem Method [5]. The systemic circulatory blood is cooled in an external shunt system with coil cooling and continuous hemodiafiltration (CHDF) that was developed in our ICU. French size 12 heparin zed catheter is inserted into the femoral artery and blood is diverted into the external direct blood cooling system. The cooled blood is returned to the systemic circulation via the inferior vena cava (Fig. 50). The direct blood-cooling method is effective for control of brain tissue temperature for patients resuscitated after cardiac arrest. This method is suitable for maintaining brain circulation in cases of poor peripheral circulation, cardiac dysfunction, muscle weakness, immune dysfunction, and respiratory weakness. As a clinical issue of this method, anticoagulation management is necessary to maintain external circulation. Therefore, hemorrhagic disease such as hypertensive intracerebral hemorrhage, subarachnoid hemorrhage, and severe head trauma with epidural, subdural hematoma, and diffuse brain injury are contraindicated. The whole brain ischemia–hypoxia after cardiac arrest with cardiac disease, obstructive air way disease, and hanging.

Inner Cool by Celsius Control System [1]. The Celsius Control Catheter has its own cooling system that, when inserted into the vena cava through the femoral vein, cools the venous blood directly (Fig. 51). The cooled abdominal venous blood circulates into the brain and begins to cool the brain tissue directly. The direct control technology of the Celsius system has a limited rate of brain tissue cooling and is limited to short-duration therapy because of the catheterization technique. Although it is still undergoing clinical studies, this technique is convenient for the control of brain tissue temperature, with intermittent temperature changes controlled by computer. This system was released by Coolest (San Diego, CA, USA).

CSF Cooling Technique

A continuous CSF cooling technique by perfusion of cooled artificial CSF from ventricles to the lumbar subarachnoid space using a shunting system has been developed (Medivance Arctic Sun Units). This technique is not sufficient for cooling the whole brain, and is limited to cooling the surface of the brain tissue to a depth of about 1 cm because warmed blood (about 37°C) circu-

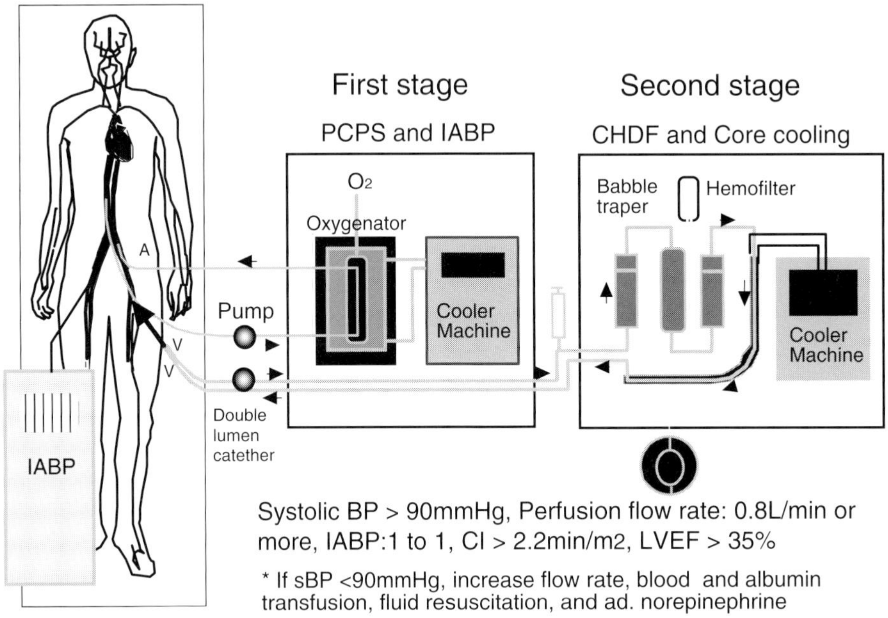

Fig. 50. The direct blood cooling system for cardiac arrest patients. PCPS, percutaneous cardiopulmonary support; IABP, intra-aortic balloon pumping; CHDF, continuos hemodia filtration

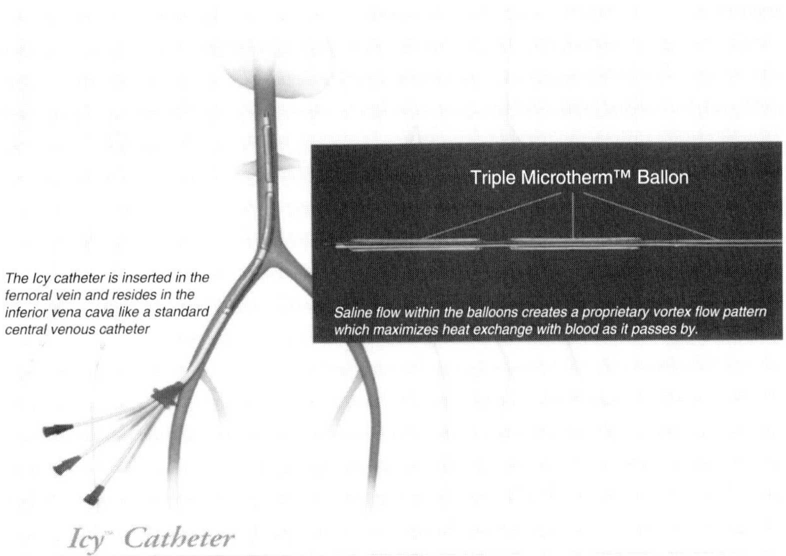

Fig. 51. Direct blood cooling abdominal catheter

lates in the brain parenchyma. However, this technique has potential for the development of a new brain hypothermia treatment approach by combination with another blood-cooling method. One of the management difficulties is maintenance of neural oxygenation because of slow release of bound oxygen from hemoglobin as a result of rapid reduction in hemoglobin 2,3-diphosphoglycerate (DPG) in severely brain-injured patients. Administration of fluorocarbon oxygen carrier with cooled artificial CSF into the ventricles could be a breakthrough for treatment of neural hypoxia that occurs by hemoglobin dysfunction. This approach is still under research in our ICU.

Additional Supporting Cooling Methods

Gastrolavage Cooling Method. After cranial surgery, we prefer the gastrolavage method with cooled saline to prevent Mendelson's pneumonia. Washing the stomach with iced saline is very successful in the prevention of severe chemical pneumonia and maintains stable low blood temperature. However, with this additional cooling method, excess rapid cooling and volumes of saline above 200 ml should be avoided. Too rapid a cooling rate and deep hypothermia can easily introduce cardiac dysfunction by arrhythmia or atrial–ventricular block. Washing the stomach with more than 200 ml of saline may disrupt gastric juice production and also may cause abdominal hypertension.

Alcohol Cooling. This cooling method is very useful over short periods, but is not suitable without prior maintenance of stable systemic circulation and vital signs. This technique is very easy to administer and shows good success in young children and babies. However, this cooling method rapidly reduces the systemic circulation and therefore must be used with care.

Pharmacological Cooling. As an initial fluid resuscitation to prevent insulin-resistant hyperglycemia, maintain adequate fluid resuscitation, and avoid brain thermo-pooling, 7% Acetic Ringer's solution should be infused with the antipyretic acetaminophen (650 mg).

References

1. Georgiadis D, Schwarz S, Kollmar R, Schwab S (2001) Endovascular cooling for moderate hypothermia in patients with acute stroke: first results of a novel approach. Stroke 32:2550–2553
2. Hayashi N (1995) Cerebral hypothermia treatment. In: Hayashi N (ed) Cerebral hypothermia treatment. Sogo Igaku, Tokyo, pp 1–105
3. Hayashi N (1997) Prevention of vegetation after severe head trauma and stroke by combination therapy of cerebral hypothermia and activation of immune-dopaminergic nervous system. Proceedings of the 6th annual meeting of Society for Treatment of Coma 6: 133–145
4. Hayashi N (2000) The clinical issue and effectiveness of brain hypothermia treatment for severe brain injured patients. In: Hayashi N (ed) Brain hypothermia. Springer, Berlin Heidelberg New York Tokyo, pp 121–151
5. Okamoto K, Nagao K, Miki T, Nitobe E, Arima K, Hayashi N (2000) New hypothermia method using blood cooling system: Monan and Kanem method. In: Hayashi N (ed) Brain Hypothermia Springer, Berlin Heidelberg New York Tokyo, pp 203–212

36. Intensive Care Unit Bed Design for Brain Hypothermia

Stable body temperature is required for the success of brain hypothermia treatment. As part of brain hypothermia treatment, cooling methods have been discussed previously. However, there are many factors that can affect attempts to stabilize brain tissue hypothermia. Bed configuration is also an important consideration for the success of stable hypothermia management.

Brain hypothermia treatment requires a bed configuration with low heat conduction from the patients body and suitable softness to prevent pressure sores, and allows easy management of pulmonary rehabilitation, easy vibration tapping of the back, and easy rehabilitation of kinetic function [1] on the bed. Some types of Roto bed can provide these functions; however, a bed that is ideal for brain hypothermia treatment is still not available. Prolonged bed rest can easily induce various complications such as pulmonary dysfunction, peripheral venous thrombosis, pulmonary atelectasis, reduced bowel function, muscle weakness, immune dysfunction, leakage of Ca^{++} from bone marrow, high incidence of renal calcification, and decubitus. The Roto bed is very effective in preventing these complications.

We use an ordinary hospital bed for brain hypothermia treatment. A rubber sheet is laid on the mat, upon which an aluminum sheet is placed to prevent heat conduction between the patient and the mat. The mat and sheets are then covered by a cotton sheet. The patient is placed on a dry towel and is positioned on the cooling blanket. The patient is then covered with a dry towel and cooling blanket, after which the patient and cooler blanket are completely wrapped with a large dry towel (Fig. 45, Chap. 35) [2,3].

The compartmental cooling suit technique developed using Arctic Sun energy transfer pads (Medivance, 500 South Arthur Aveneu Suite 100 Lauisville, Colorado 80027, www.medivance.com) (Fig. 49, Chap. 35) is also useful for management of brain tissue hypothermia.

References

1. Green BA, Green KL, Klose KJ (1980) Kinetic nursing for acute spinal cord injury patients. Paraplegia 18:181–186
2. Hayashi N (1995) Cerebral hypothermia treatment. In: Hayashi N (ed) Cerebral hypothermia treatment. Sogo Igaku, Tokyo, pp 1–105
3. Hayashi N (2000) The clinical issue and effectiveness of brain hypothermia treatment for severe brain injured patients. In: Hayashi N (ed) Brain hypothermia. Springer, Berlin Heidelberg New York Tokyo, pp 121–151

37. Design of the Intensive Care Unit for Brain Hypothermia Treatment

Careful management of temperature around the bedside assists in maintaining stable brain hypothermia. Air conditioning, heat-generating medical devices and monitors around the bed, air convection, room size, and weather are all factors that may affect the management of brain tissue temperature (Fig. 52).

We have designed a separate system of atmospheric convection for three compartments in the large room of the intensive care unit (ICU). The airflow and retention of heated air around the bed in each compartment is controlled by two different air conditioners. One is the air conditioner that services the entire ICU and the other is a localized air conditioner that services a few beds. All of the air around each bed is removed via a vent in the ceiling over the bed. Such control of airflow and temperature in the ICU are very effective for minimizing the effects of heat-generating medical devices around the bed, and also are very effective for preventing the spread of infections in the ICU.

The room temperature in the ICU is controlled at about 20°–23°C. However, in an open style ICU as shown in Fig. 52, a corner bed is not recommended because a higher room temperature and poor atmospheric convection results in unstable management of brain tissue hypothermia.

Each bed in our ICU has air compressors to drive medical devices such as the bed and ventilator, with no electric power motors. No heat production and limited noise in the ICU is more comfortable for the patient. If air compressors are not used in the ICU, more space is required to set up medical devices further from the bed. Very close positioning of heat-generating medical devices to the patient's bed results in poor management of brain hypothermia. Atmospheric convection, room temperature, the air-outlet system, and heat-generating devices around the bed are negative factors for management of stable, mild to moderate brain hypothermia in ICU.

Reference

1. Hayashi N (1995) Cerebral hypothermia treatment. In: Hayashi N (ed) Cerebral hypothermia treatment. Sogo Igaku, Tokyo, pp 1–105

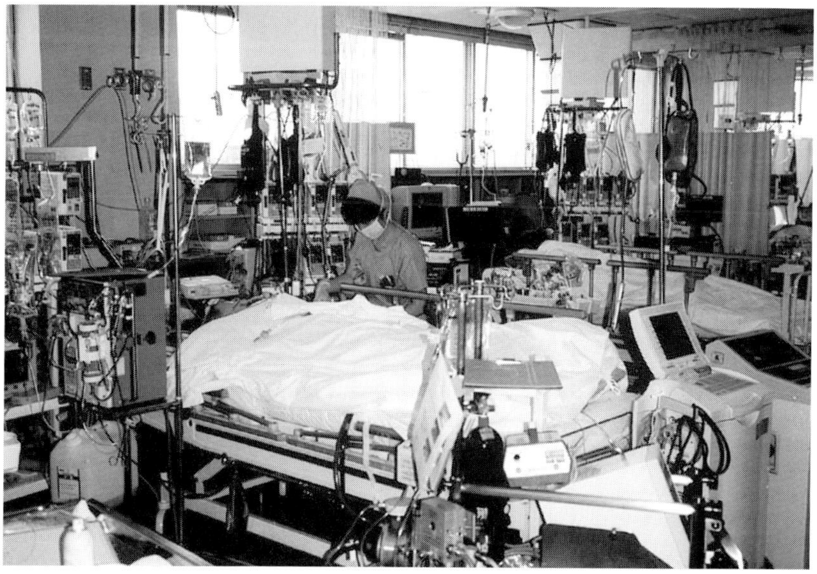

Fig. 52. Brain hypothermia treatment for cardiac-arrest patient in the intensive care unit

38. Preparation for Management of Brain Hypothermia

Preconditioning for Brain Hypothermia in Patients

Stabilized systemic circulation and cardiac function is important from the beginning of treatment because serum catecholamines progressively decrease in proportion to the severity of brain tissue hypothermia [1]. Early dehydration management to prevent brain edema introduces difficult conditions for the induction of brain hypothermia treatment because of reduced systemic circulation volume and unstable cardiac output. An arrhythmia-prolonged QT-interval of more than 450 mm/s, hyperglycemia, and hypopotassemia must be controlled before the induction of hypothermia. The complication of severe pneumonia produces unsuccessful brain hypothermia because of uncontrollable increases in brain tissue glutamate associated with cytokine encephalitis. To prevent pneumonia (Mendelson's syndrome), food and gastric juice in the stomach should be washed out by gastric lavage with 1000 ml of cooled saline, immune function should be managed by maintaining microcirculation of the intestinal organs by replacement of antithrombin III (AT-III) to above the 100% level, intestinal mucous membrane edema can be prevented by management of serum albumin levels above 3.0 g/dl, and serum glucose levels should be carefully maintained between 120 and 140 mg/dl [1–3]. The nurse prepares the gastric lavage during surgery.

The equipment list for gastric lavage is:

1. Nasagastric tube (1 tube)
2. Cooled saline at about 10°C (2000 ml, 4 bottles)
3. 20-ml syringe (1 syringe)
4. Stethoscope
5. Bucket
6. Xerokaine jelly
7. G gauze
8. Plaster tape

Preparation of Medical Devices and Instruments for Brain Hypothermia

The list of medical instruments and devices is:

1. Cooling device (1–2)
2. Plasty pad blanket (2–3)
3. Sterilized, cooled saline (about 10°–15°C, 7 l)
4. Dry towel (2–3)
5. Towel sheet (1–2)

Preparation and Management of the Cooling Machine

The cooling device and system should be set up for use at any time. The cooling device is filled with about 7 l of sterilized, cooled saline, and connected to the plasty pad cooling blanket. The device temperature is set at 10°–15°C in preparation for brain hypothermia treatment (Fig. 46, Chap. 35).

The Time Schedule for Cooling Blanket Water Temperature

The time schedule for cooling blanket water temperature is different for mild brain hypothermia (~34°C) and moderate brain hypothermia (32°–33°C). For the success of early and rapid induction to moderate brain hypothermia and prevention of catecholamine surge, two-step control of plasty pad blanket water temperature is recommended, as shown in Fig. 33 (Chap. 26). If possible, two cooling devices to separately cool the chest and back side plasty pad blanket should be used to obtain stable hypothermia [1,3].

Mild Brain Hypothermia

The time schedule for cooling the brain tissue is described in Chap 32. To attain a brain tissue temperature of about 34°C, the water temperature of the back side plasty pad blanket is set at 15°C before the start of brain hypothermia. The patient is initally placed on their back on the cooling plasty pad. The patient is then covered with a dry towel and the chest-abdominal cooling blanket is laid over, after which the patient and the cooler blanket are completely wrapped with large dry towel. Communication of body temperature and room temperature should be avoided to attain stable brain tissue temperature.

The water temperature of the back-side plasty pad blanket should be elevated very slowly to 22°–23°C with monitoring of brain tissue temperature. The chest-side blanket water temperature should be set between 27°–28°C and then be allowed to drop to 20°–26°C. When brain tissue temperature is stabilized at around 34°C, the water temperature of both cooling blankets should be set at 20°–26°C [1,3]. The time window for the control of brain hypothermia is shown in Fig. 47 (Chap. 35).

In cases in which induction of brain hypothermia for a short time is difficult, repetition of the management cycle of blanket water temperature with more dynamic large friction is successful as shown in Fig. 48 (Chap. 35).

Moderate Brain Hypothermia

Water temperature in the back-side plasty pad blanket is initially set at 10°C and the cooled water is circulated for 10 min. When the patient is placed on the plasty pad blanket, the water temperature of the chest-side blanket is set between 24° and 25°C. Body cooling then begins with monitoring of brain tissue temperature. The change of blanket water temperature is then only focused on the back-side plasty pad blanket. The back-side plasty pad blanket water temperature is carefully elevated to 26°–28°C with monitoring of brain tissue temperature. When the brain tissue temperature reaches 34°C, brain cooling is stopped temporarily, and the vital signs are checked: cardiopulmonary function, presence of hypopotassemia (<3.0 mEq/dl), hyperglycemia, arrhythmia, and elongation of QT interval (QT interval > 450 mm/s) on the electrocardiogram (ECG) [1,3]. After management of these parameters, brain hypothermia is recommenced and moderate brain hypothermia is attained by lowering the blanket water temperature from 27°–28°C to about 19°–25°C. The time schedule after restarting brain hypothermia is important. The reduction in serum catecholamines and rapid progression of serum hyperglycemia are major negative issues for management of brain hypothermia below 34°C. To avoid the complication of unstable systemic circulation, careful, slow induction of moderate brain hypothermia is recommended. We take about 5–6 h for the induction of moderate brain hypothermia. Moderate brain hypothermia is obtained by control of blanket water temperature at around 19°–23°C in most cases. If moderate brain hypothermia is not obtained by this technique, other factors in the ICU management technique are not being satisfactorily addressed.

Preparation for Fluid Resuscitation

The replacement of circulation volume, control of hyperglycemia associated with catecholamine surge, prevention of progression of blood–brain barrier (BBB) dysfunction, normalization of acidosis, replacement of hyponatremia, and maintenance of cardiac output are the major purposes of fluid resuscitation. Early hyperosmotic dehydration therapy for the prevention of brain edema is contraindicated because reduced circulation volume combined with low serum catecholamines, caused by hypothermia, can easily produce disturbances of cardiac function and systemic circulation. The administration of 7% Acetic Ringer's solution (500–1000 ml) with suppository and 650 mg acetaminophen, as an initial fluid resuscitation, followed by 4% saline and 5% albumin and/or 0.9% Acetic Ringer's solution, are recommended.

To prevent hemoglobin and platelet dysfunction, administration of potassium phosphate (7 mg/kg i.v. for a 1-mg/dl elevation of serum phosphate) is successful. As a maintenance fluid, Actit solution that includes 10 mEq/dl potassium phosphate, 5 mEq/dl Mg^{++}, and 5.0 g/dl glucose is recommended. Activation of the lipid metabolism by vitamin A during hypothermia and prevention of seizures by the administration of vitamin B are additional considerations.

Preparation of the Monitors

Four main monitors are necessary for management of brain hypothermia treatment. Monitoring of cardiopulmonary function, brain thermal regulation, neural function, immune function and digestive organ function, interaction between changes in systemic circulation and metabolism to cerebral blood flow (CBF) and brain metabolism, and intracranial pathophysiological changes such as CBF, brain metabolism, and intracranial pressure (ICP) are major topics.

1. Analysis of cardiopulmonary dysfunction
   ECG
   Arterial blood pressure
   SaO_2

Blood gas analysis
FiO_2 and PaO_2/FiO_2
CVP
$ETCO_2$
Swan Ganz catheter (CO, CI, DO_2, VO_2, O_2ER, SVR, PWP, PVR)
Alveolar capillary CO_2 permeability index (ACCPI) = ETCO2/CO·$PvCO_2$;0,1-0,2

2. Brain thermo-regulation
Core temperature
Tympanic membrane temperature (TmT)
Jugular venous blood temperature (JvT)
Bladder temperature
Brain tissue temperature (BTT)

3. CBF and brain metabolism
Serum glucose
BBB function (CSF/serum albumin ratio < 0.01)
Serum albumin > 3.5 mg/dl
JvT/TmT or BTT/TmT (cerebral thermal index; 1.01–1.03)
SjO_2 (65%–75%)
Brain thermo-pooling: $(JvT - TmT) \geq 1$
Blood shift to intestine: bladder temperature > TmT
BSO_2
ICP < 15 mmHg
Microdialysis

4. Neuronal function
Trend EEG
Auditory brainstem evoked response (ABER)
Dopamine A10 nervous function: CSF dopamine/CSF prolactin > 0.5

5. Digestive organs and immune function
Intestinal pressure throughout the gastric tube
Gastric pHi by tonometer method (pHi < 7.3)
Abdominal hypertension: bladder pressure or ileum pressure (<15 mmHg)
Lymphocytes $> 1500\,mm^{-3}$

References

1. Hayashi N (1995) Cerebral hypothermia treatment. In: Hayashi N (ed) Cerebral hypothermia treatment. Sogo Igaku, Tokyo, pp 1–105
2. Hayashi N (2000) Enhanced neuronal damage in severely brain injured patients by hypothalamus, pituitary, and adrenal axis neuro-hormonal changes. In: Hayashi N (ed) Brain hypothermia. Springer, Berlin Heidelberg New York Tokyo, pp 3–26
3. Hayashi N (2000) The clinical issue and effectiveness of brain hypothermia treatment for severe brain injured patients. In: Hayashi N (ed) Brain hypothermia. Springer, Berlin Heidelberg New York Tokyo, pp 121–151

39. Noninvasive Monitoring of Brain Damage

The monitoring of brain tissue temperature, intracranial pressure (ICP), SjO_2, oxygen delivery, and cerebral perfusion pressure (CPP) is necessary in intensive care unit (ICU) brain hypothermia management as fundamentals of the technique [1,8]. However, these monitors require considerable skill, are invasive to critically ill patients, and are difficult to perform in the early part of the acute stage. In addition, information about the severity of the catecholamine surge, blood–brain barrier (BBB) dysfunction, cerebral blood flow (CBF) disturbances, microcirculatory disturbances, brain metabolism and release of neurotoxic amino acids are useful to ICU brain hypothermia management [1,8]. However, these monitors cannot always be used because of practical limitations that include small medical teams at night, no monitoring system for the microdialysis technique, no high-speed liquid chromatography, limited insurance cover for brain hypothermia management, and limited economic support of these advanced monitors [8]. In addition, we have no times to monitors by abruptly rapid fall to critical conditions. Therefore, the noninvasive diagnosis of patient pathophysiology without high technology and expensive monitoring systems (Table 12) is important.

The alternate and indirect evaluation methods of monitoring changes in brain tissue temperature, brain thermo-pooling, ICP elevation, low CPP, BBB dysfunction, sufficient oxygen delivery, reduced 2,3-diphosphoglycerate (DPG) hemoglobin (Hb) dysfunction, disturbance of microcirculation, catecholamine surge, and reduced ·NO radical scavenging must be understood. Our methods are described in Fig. 53 [1,4].

Figure 15 (Chap. 22) shows the main points of ICU management of brain hypothermia without invasive monitors and without expensive medical equipment. The systolic blood pressure higher than 100 mmHg, QT interval shorter than 450 mm/s on the electrocardiogram (ECG), no arrhythmia, and hypopotassemia are indirect parameters of stabilized vital signs and brain tissue temperature [1–3].

Neuronal oxygenation and administration of adequate metabolic substrates are most important for restoration of injured neurons in initial treatment. For this treatment to succeed, enough arterial oxygenation, normal oxygen delivery with sufficient CPP, easy release of oxygen from Hb in the brain, and adequate serum glucose [1–3] and phosphate for production of adenosine triphosphate (ATP) [6] in the injured brain tissue are necessary. The ratio of $PaO_2/FiO_2 > 300$ is an indirect parameter of arterial oxygenation. Management of Hb > 11 mg/dl, $ETCO_2$ 34–38 mmHg, and $PaCO_2$ 32–38 mmHg simultaneously indicates more than 800 ml of oxygen delivery [1,2,7,8]. Hemoglobin dysfunction caused by reduced DPG levels produces slow release of bound oxygen from Hb [2]. That means the progression of neuronal hypoxia or brain tissue hypoxia despite normal control of PaO_2, CPP, and oxygen delivery. To maintain Hb function, normalization of serum pH, serum micronutrients, and macronutrients such as serum pH > 7.3, serum glucose (120–140 mg/dl), serum phosphate (3–4 mg/dl), and serum magnesium (1.4–1.8 mEq/l), are fundamental care strategies.

The brain tissue temperature is evaluated by monitoring the jugular venous blood temperature [1,2]. However, this is not the case at the terminal stage because of shunting of the external carotid blood flow into the jugular venous blood with nonfilling or poor feeding caused by severely elevated intracranial pressure of more than 60–70 mmHg. At the normal physiological condition, the metabolic component of brain temperature is about 0.4°–0.7°C [3]. Therefore, under normal conditions, the brain tissue temperature is 0.4°–0.7°C higher than core temperature.

The tympanic membrane temperature is mainly determined by the microcirculation around the tympanic membrane. Therefore, external carotid blood flow and carotid blood flow strongly influence the tympanic membrane temperature [2]. The tympanic membrane temperature is useful as an indirect parameter of the external carotid blood flow, carotid blood flow, and shunting of internal to external carotid blood flow. If the brain tissue temperature is higher than tympanic membrane temperature, combined with elevation of brain tissue temperature or elevated jugular venous blood temperature indicates there is brain thermo-pooling due to reduced CBF. The monitoring of CBF distur-

Table 12. Basic monitors for ICU care management

1. Stability of vital signs
sBP > 100 mmHg
QT < 450 mm/s
K^+ > 3.0 mEq/dl, no arrhythmia
2. Oxygenation
PaO_2/FiO_2 > 300
Hb > 12 mg/dl
$ETCO_2$ 34–38 mmHg
$PaCO_2$ 32–38 mmHg
pH ≥ 7.3, serum phosphate 3–4 mg/dl
Serum glucose 120~140 mg/dl
3. Control of brain temperature
Brain tissue temperature (BTT) (32°–34°C)
TmT > bladder temperature
Jugular venous blood temperature = BTT
4. Maintenance of microcirculation
ICP < 15 mmHg
AT-III > 100%
BTT/TmT 1.01–1.03
5. Prevention of infection
Serum glucose 120–140 mg/dl
Serum albumin > 3.0–3.5 mg/dl
Gastric juice pH < 3.5
Care of immune function
Lymphonode > 1000 m^3
L-alginine 30 g/30 min per day (drip)
early immune enteral nutrition
GluminS, 10 g × 3/day, L-dopa, 500 mg/day, bromocriptine 2.5 g
Enteral nutrition start from 3–4 days
Muscle massage
Care of respiratory muscle weakness
K_2HPO_2, Mg, vitamin A > 50 mg/dl
Cleaning of oral cavity
VCM · AMPH-B · LVFX enteral nutrition
PEEP ≤ 5 cmH_2O
6. Prevention of cytokine encephalitis
Albumin > 3.5 mg/dl
AT-III > 100%, low molecular weight heparine
Antibiotics
CSF/serm albumin < 0.01

bance at the bedside is important for the management of severely brain-injured patients. The accurate, continuous monitoring of CBF at the bedside is technically very difficult. However, indirect and continuous monitoring of CBF disturbance at the bedside is not so difficult using a computed monitoring method. The brain thermo-pooling associated with CBF disturbances produces an increasing difference between brain tissue temperature and tympanic membrane temperature. Conversely, when the tympanic membrane temperature is higher than the brain tissue temperature and the jugular venous blood temperature, this suggests poor filling of brain circulation. Therefore, computed monitoring of the difference between brain tissue temperature and tympanic membrane temperature or the cerebral thermal index (CTI) (brain tissue temperature/tympanic membrane temperature) is useful as a monitor of CBF disturbance. The normal value of the CTI is 1.01–1.03. The critical values of the CTI for the diagnosis of CBF disturbance is higher than 1.05 and non- or poor-filling CBF disturbances are indicated at less than 1.0 [1,2].

The continuous computed monitoring of CTI and the pattern of CTI changes are very useful to diagnose CBF disturbances at the bedside. These CBF disturbances are also detected when the brain tissue temperature is lower than the bladder temperature. As an alternative indicator to diagnose CBF disturbances, tympanic membrane temperature lower than bladder or rectal temperature is also useful. The progressive reduction of CBF by elevation of ICP produces the shift of systemic blood circulation from the brain to the intestinal site. The dopamine-dominant systemic circulation also produces a shift of the systemic circulation from the cranial site to the intestinal site even with normal CPP. This is because vascular dilatation of the intestinal organs and renal blood vessels occur specifically by dopamine-

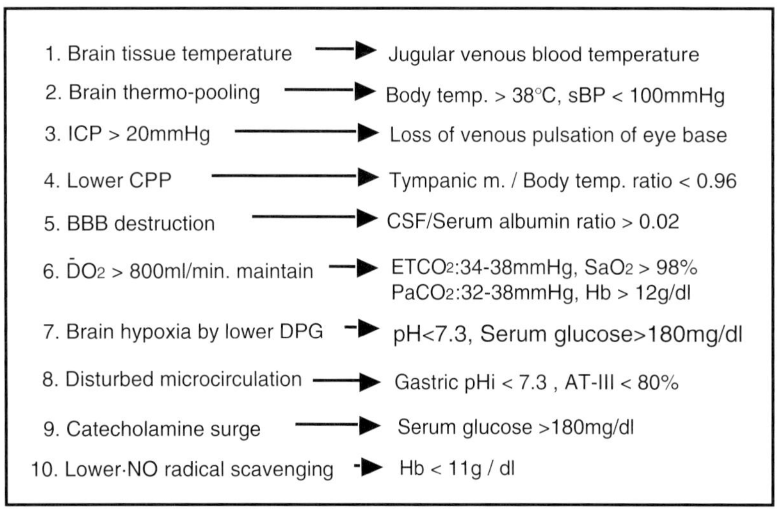

Fig. 53. Noninvasive monitoring for brain hypothermia treatment

dominate circulation. During brain hypothermia treatment, monitoring of the jugular venous blood temperature is also useful except in eases of poor filling of CBF with ICP more than 60–70 mmHg. The monitoring of tympanic membrane temperature is also useful as an alternative method for the evaluation of brain tissue temperature; however, tympanic membrane temperature is difficult to use as an indirect parameter of brain tissue temperature under conditions of CBF disturbance. The monitoring of jugular venous blood temperature is useful at the ICU bedside because there is no need for the surgical procedure of craniotomy [1,2].

Causes of CBF disturbances include reduced CPP, ICP elevation, and disturbance of microcirculation. The brain is a prothrombin-rich organ. Prothrombin can easily induce a metabolic shift for thrombin and increase of thrombin in the bloodstream can lead to formation of a microthrombus in injured brain tissue. Antithrombin-III (AT-III) is a stabilizer of increased thrombin caused by hemolytic function. Changes in AT-III levels can be evaluated as an indirect parameter of microcirculation. The intestinal mucous membrane is very sensitive to microcirculation disturbance from a microthrombus. This phenomenon is diagnosed by monitoring reducing gastric pHi < 7.3 using the tonometor method [2]. The critical value of AT-III for induction of gastric pHi lower than 7.3 is less than 100%. Therefore, detection of AT-III levels lower than 100% and gastric pHi less than 7.3 suggest the disturbance of microcirculation in the brain and in intestinal digestive organs. To prevent microcirculation disturbance in the brain tissue, control of ICP below 15 mmHg and management of AT-III above 100% by replacement therapy is recommended.

On the management of brain hypothermia treatment, the complication of severe pulmonary infection with severe damage to the BBB is a very dangerous condition. This is because increased cytokines in the bloodstream are allowed into the injured brain tissue [2,3] and introduce the complication of cytokine chemical encephalitis. We have recorded uncontrollable release of neurotoxic brain glutamate in injured brain tissue despite management of brain tissue temperature at 32°C (Fig. 54). In such cases, the question of how to diagnose the severity of BBB dysfunction at the bedside is important. Albumin is a large molecule and permeates the BBB with difficulty under normal conditions. The indirect parameter of BBB dysfunction, CSF/serum albumin ratio, was initially reported in experimental studies by Kossman et al. [5]. In clinical studies with normal BBB function, CSF/serum albumin ratio was less than 0.007 [2,3]. However, neurotoxic glutamate began to increase at CSF/serum albumin ratio above 0.01 with the complication of pneumonia. Severe brain edema is observed with elevation of CSF/serum albumin ratio above 0.02. Therefore, we could diagnose BBB dysfunction at the ICU bedside by monitoring of the CSF/serum albumin ratio. A CSF/serum albumin ratio above 0.02 suggests severe damage of BBB function, 0.01–0.02 suggests moderate damage of BBB function, and 0.01–0.007 suggests mild BBB dysfunction. These diagnostic criteria for the severity of BBB dysfunction were ascertained from microdialysis studies in our ICU (Fig. 55). During brain hypothermia treatment, complication of severe pulmonary infections and CSF/serum albumin ratio above 0.02 suggest the unsuccessful management of brain hypothermia treatment. Effective management methods of BBB dysfunction are the prevention of microthrombus by replacement of AT-III, administration of low molecular weight heparin to prevent vascular inflammatory reactions, and serum albumin maintained above 3.0 mg/dl. The goal of BBB

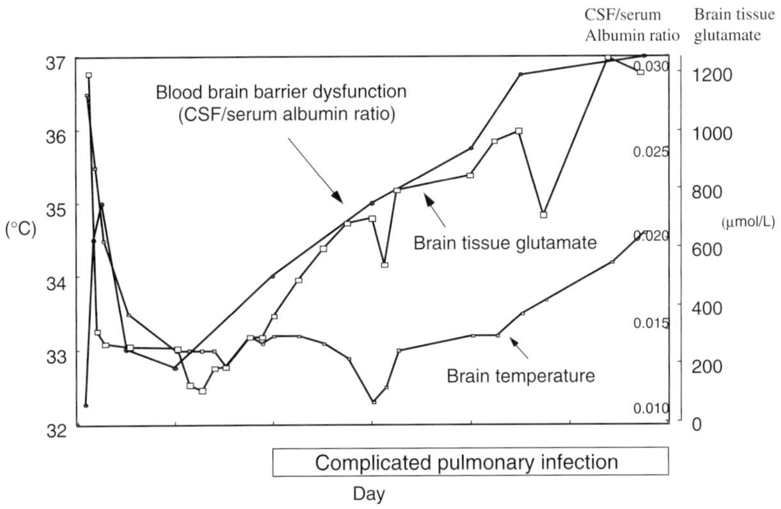

Fig. 54. Uncontrollable increase of neurotoxic brain tissue glutamate by complication of pneumonia with severe blood–brain barrier dysfunction

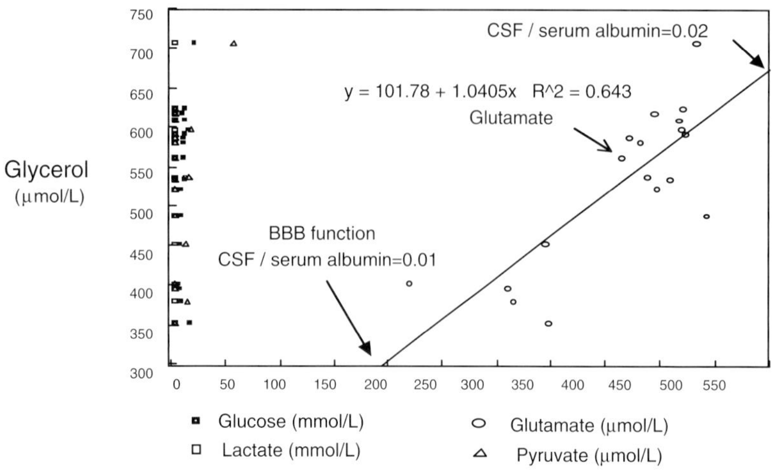

Fig. 55. The interrelationships between changes of the neuronal cell membrane damage agent glycerol, and various metabolic substrates in the bloodstream under the changes of BBB dysfunction. The increasing of CSF/serum ratio more than 0.01 produces the neurotoxic effects of serum glutamate for neuronal cell membrane function

dysfunction management is a CSF/serum albumin ratio less than 0.01.

References

1. Hayashi N (1995) Cerebral hypothermia treatment. In: Hayashi N (ed) Cerebral hypothermia treatment. Sogo Igaku, Tokyo, pp 1–105
2. Hayashi N, (2000) Enhanced neuronal damage in severely brain injured patients by hypothalamus, pituitary, and adrenal axis neuro-hormonal changes. In: Hayashi N (ed) Brain hypothermia. Springer, Berlin Heidelberg New York Tokyo, pp 3–26
3. Hayashi N (2000) The clinical issue and effectiveness of brain hypothermia treatment for severe brain injured patients. In: Hayashi N (ed) Brain hypothermia. Springer, Berlin Heidelberg New York Tokyo, pp 121–151
4. Hayashi N, Utagawa A, Kinosita K, Izumi T (1999) Application of a novel technique for clinical evaluation of nitric oxide-induced free radical reactions in ICU patients. Cell Mol Neurobiol 19:3–17
5. Kossmann T, Hans V, Lenzlinger PM, Csuka E, Stsahel PF, Trentz O, Morgani-Kossmann MC (1996) Analysis of immune mediator production following traumatic brain injury. In: Schlag G, Redel H, Traber D (eds) Shock, sepsis and organ failure. Springer, Berlin Heidelberg New York, pp 263–297
6. Pasko SA, Volosheniuk TG (1990) Disordered phosphorus metabolism and its correction in the acute period of severe craniocerebral trauma. Zh Vopr Neirokhir Im NN Burdenko 3:14–16
7. Shoemaker WC, Apple PL, Kram HB, Waxman K, Lee T (1988) Prospective trial of supernormal values of survivors as therapeutic goals in high-risk surgical patients. Chest 94:1176–1186
8. Swan HJC, Ganz W (1983) Hemodynamic measurements in clinical practice: a decade in review. J Am Coll Cardiol 1:103–113

40. Neuron Protection in Injured Brain Tissue During Surgery

Acute brain swelling or the explosion of injured brain from the opened skull during surgery provides no indication for brain hypothermia treatment because multiple mechanical brain tissue lacerations occur in the deep brain. To prevent these complications or the worsening of brain injury, strategies are required that concern anesthesia, surgical position, lowering of brain and core temperature, surgical considerations, and equipment for monitoring the patient in the intensive care unit (ICU).

Anesthesia for Surgery

Early anesthesia is important to prevent excess neurohormonal reactions of the hypothalamus–pituitary–adrenal (HPA) axis that produce neuronal hypoxia and secondary brain damage despite control of intracranial pressure (ICP), cerebral perfusion pressure (CPP), cerebral blood flow (CBF), and PaO_2 within normal limits [4,5]. These specific brain injury mechanisms of nonanesthetized patients have been described previously. After fluid resuscitation, patients were placed on ventilation while under anesthesia.

The combined management of anesthesia, analgesia, and cerebral dopamine antirelease medication is introduced to prevent more damage to injured neuron and dopamine A10 nerve cells [5]. The induction of anesthesia occurs with the initial drip of propofol (1–2 mg/kg, i.v.), followed by administration of lidocaine (1–2 mg/kg) anesthesia [5–8], fentanyl (0.1 mg, i.v.) analgesia, and muscle relaxation with vecronium (0.02 mg/kg, i.v.) [2]. This anesthesia allows easy tracheal intimation and is also effective in removing the stress to the HPA neuronal axis. After administration of complete muscle relaxation with succinylcholine (1.5 mg/kg, i.v.), cranial surgery is carried out under the persistent combined anesthesia of isoflurane and fentanyl. Administration of metoclopramide [10] is also performed to prevent excess release of cerebral dopamine. The combined management of brain hypothermia and pharmacological treatment of cerebral antidopamine release is very powerful for the prevention of selective radical damage to the dopamine A10 nervous system and prevention of vegetation.

Surgical Position

The main aims of neurological surgery are the removal of acute subdural hematoma, halting hemorrhage of contused brain tissue, evacuation of necrosed brain tissue, removal of pressure to the upper brain stem, and external decompression for accidental brain swelling at the rewarming stage. The injured brain is cooled directly by applying cooling saline throughout surgery. The body temperature is controlled between 34° and 36°C.

On the operation table and after stabilization of anesthesia and vital signs, patients' hair is trimmed away, the scalp is cleaned, and an elastic bandage is applied to prevent shock when the dura is opened. If it is difficult to maintain the systemic circulation after multiple trauma, insertion of a balloon catheter into the abdominal aorta is suitable for maintaining the circulation of CBF and the coronary cardiac feeding artery. The preliminary procedure of applying an elastic bandage to the extremities and insertion of a balloon catheter is very useful for maintaining circulation to the brain, heart, and lungs in the case of unexpected shock during surgery such as opening of the dura, delayed masking bleeding, and allergic shock [5]. The craniotomy is carried out in the 20° head-up position to prevent venous stasis and further ICP elevation. ICP elevated above the capillary pressure of 34–40 mmHg by brain swelling produces brain explosion from the surgically opened dura (Fig. 56). This rapid acute brain swelling and protrusion of brain tissue from the surgical field produces multiple tissue lacerations in the deep brain. Prevention of acute brain swelling requires modification of the surgical position, brain tissue cooling, and careful consideration of anesthesia.

In cases of severe brain injury that are expected to show acute brain swelling upon dura opening, patients should be operated on in the supine head-up position initially. Before opening the dura, the head position should be switched to about 35°–40° from 15°–20° to

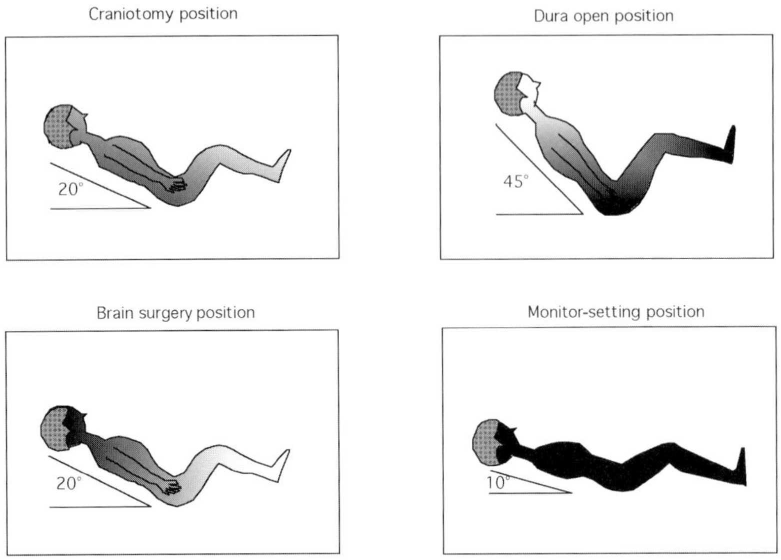

Fig. 56. Surgical positions for surgery on herniated, severely brain-injured patients

prevent brain explosion from the surgical field of dura incisions (Fig. 56). Although this technique is very successful, the complication of brain ischemia is unavoidable with this technique. Fluid resuscitation using 7% ascorbic Ringer's solution, application of elastic bandages to the extremities, control of hypercapnea, use of the legs-up position, mild brain hypothermia (34°C), and control of neuronal oxygenation are important before switching to a head-up position of 35°–40°. Whole brain ischemia caused by the head-up position provides a better chance of survival than acute brain swelling and cerebral explosion from the surgical field. If it is difficult to control hypotension, it may be necessary to shift to the head-down position or control the CPP with an abdominal balloon catheter. After stabilization of brain swelling and after removal of hematoma, the surgical position can be returned to the 20° head-up position with sufficient neuronal oxygenation and adequate control of serum glucose.

Lowering Brain Tissue and Core Temperatures

The cooling of injured brain tissue with sufficient cerebral oxygenation during surgery is important if patients are to survive. Irrigation of the surgical field with chilled artificial cerebrospinal fluid (CSF) that includes amino acids, electrolytes, oncotic agent, and fluorocarbon oxygen carrier (F44E emulsion) is effective for the restoration of injured neurons [3,9]. However, this technique is not capable of cooling the whole brain and cooling is limited to a depth of 1 cm from the brain surface and ventricular wall. Clinical results in cases in which cooling of deep brain tissue was attempted using CSF cooled below 28°C were not satisfactory because cellular homeostasis is difficult to maintain below 28°C. Therefore, for maintenance of satisfactory whole-brain hypothermia during surgery, irrigation of brain tissue with chilled artificial CSF can be combined with management of core temperature to 34°C. The major advantage of this technique is that sufficient oxygen for injured brain tissue is administered directly, despite the presence of hemoglobin dysfunction and slow release of bound oxygen from hemoglobin by reduced 2,3-diphosphoglycerate [4].

Surgical Considerations

The removal of acute subdural hematoma, stopping hemorrhage from contusion in the brain tissue, evacuation of necrosed brain tissue, removal of the compression pressure from the upper brain stem, and external decompression to allow adaptation to accidental brain swelling at the rewarming stage are the major purposes of neurological surgery. Cooling of the injured brain tissue below 33°C and simultaneous direct administration of oxygen by applying artificial CSF that includes fluorocarbon oxygen carrier, is a new approach to minimize neuronal damage. Body temperature is controlled between 33° and 34°C.

Large-scale craniotomy and external decompression that include the lower portions of temporal bones are basic approaches for herniated patients. Removal of the lower portion of the temporal bone is effective in minimizing the mechanical pressure to the upper brain stem. Without consideration of this surgical approach, it is difficult for herniated, severely brain-injured patients to survive. One of the difficulties of management in ICU during brain hypothermia treatment is the complication of cytokine encephalitis associated with severe pulmonary infection combined with severe blood–brain barrier dysfunction [5]. Severe brain swelling and ICP elevation are unavoidable after surgery even with management of brain tissue temperature at 32°–33°C. Large patching of dura on the surgically decompressed area and loose suturing of the dura closure can be used to prevent hydrocephalus caused by CSF leakage in the subcutaneous space. Draining of subcutaneous CSF is helpful in controlling acute ICP elevation with hydrocephalus. ICP elevation may also be controlled with early implementation of VP shunting and is important for management of severely brain-injured patients. Large-scale external decompression surgery also increases the tolerance toward brain swelling during the rewarming stage.

Debridement of necrotic contused brain tissue allows easy ICP management during brain hypothermia treatment. Because necrotic brain tissue promotes the production of · OH^- radicals and stimulates the release of glutamate and cytokines, the identification of necrotic brain tissue during surgery is important. However, there are no easy means of doing this. We manage contused brain tissue by repeated irrigation with saline, and then the floated brain tissue is removed via a 1-mm diameter suction tube. Normal brain tissue is difficult to remove with such a small-diameter suction tube.

A potential pitfall of brain surgery is the rapid progression of other acute subdural hematomas on the other side, after removal of the primary hematoma. If unsuccessful internal decompression is observed, even with evacuation of the subdural hematoma, progression of other hematomas must be considered. In such cases, immediate surgical operation on the other side of the brain must be carried out. Computed tomography is not recommended at this stage for the correct diagnosis of other hematoma because it wastes valuable time in attempts to save severely brain-injured patients.

Monitors for ICU Management

Before closing the craniotomy site, various sensor devices and a microdialysis catheter (M60 catheter, internal/external diameter 0.15/1.0mm, Fig. 57) are set near the injured brain tissue to monitor ICP (Fig. 58), brain tissue oxygen level and metabolism, release of neurotoxic glutamate [1,4], and brain tissue temperature. The combination of these monitors is a very effective component of successful ICU management of brain hypothermia treatment.

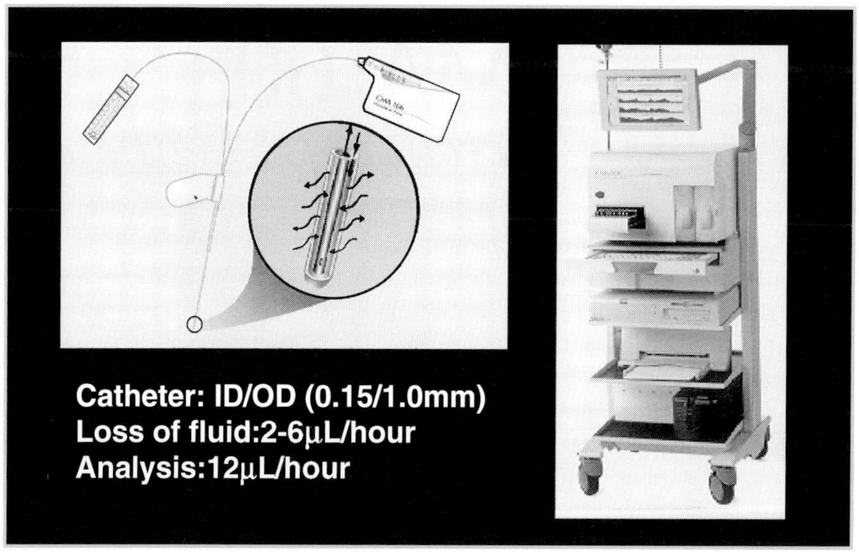

Fig. 57. The microdialysis monitor (CMA60/106) for brain metabolism and neuronal functions

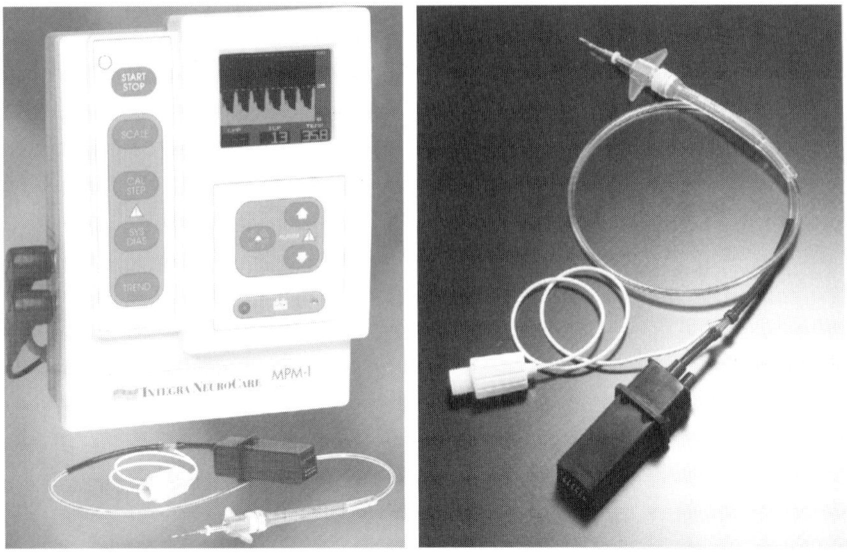

Fig. 58. Monitoring system for intracranial pressure and brain tissue temperature (Integra Neuroscience, San Diego, CA 92121-4309, USA)

References

1. Binnert C, Tappy L (2002) Microdialysis in the intensive care unit: a novel tool for clinical investigation or monitoring? Curr Opin Clin Nutr Metab Care 5:185–188
2. Caldwell JE, Heier T, Wright PM, Lin S, McCarthy G, Szenohradszky J, Sharma ML, Hing JP, Schroeder M, Sessler DI (2000) Temperature-dependent pharmacokinetics and pharmacodynamics of vecuronium. Anesthesiology 92:84–93
3. Clark LC Jr, Spokane RB, Hoffmann RE, Sudan R, Homan MM, Maloney AC, Jacobs SJ, Stroup TL, Winston PE (1988) Polarographic cerebral oxygen availability, fluorocarbon blood levels and efficacy of oxygen transport by emulsions. Biomater Artif Cells Artif Organs. 16:375–393
4. Hayashi N (2000) Enhanced neuronal damage in severely brain injured patients by hypothalamus, pituitary, and adrenal axis neuro-hormonal changes. In: Hayashi N (ed) Brain hypothermia. Springer, Berlin Heidelberg New York Tokyo, pp 3–26
5. Hayashi N (2000) The clinical issue and effectiveness of brain hypothermia treatment for severe brain injured patients. In: Hayashi N (ed) Brain hypothermia. Springer, Berlin Heidelberg New York Tokyo, pp 121–151
6. Leslie K, Bjorksten AR, Ugoni A, Mitchell P (2002) Mild core hypothermia and anesthetic requirement for loss of responsiveness during propofol anesthesia for craniotomy. Anesth Analg 94:1298–1303
7. Sahin A, Aypar U (2002) Effect of amino acid solutions on intraoperative hypothermia and postoperative shivering. Comparison of two anesthetic regimens. Acta Anaesthesiol Scand 46:64–67
8. Spitzfaden AC, Jimenez DF, Tobias JD (1999) Propofol for sedation and control of intracranial pressure in children. Pediatr Neurosurg 31:194–200
9. Triolo AJ, Osterholm JL, Alexander GM, Bell RD, Frazer GD (1990) Local cerebral glucose metabolism after global ischemia: treatment by ventriculocisternal perfusion with a fluorocarbon emulsion. Neurosurgery 26:487–488
10. Zis AP, McGarvey KA, Clark CM, Lam RW, Adams SA (1992) The role of dopamine in seizure-induced prolactin release in humans. Convuls Ther 8:126–130

41. Prolonged Anesthesia for Brain Hypothermia Treatment in ICU

The effects of analgesic agents and mucle relaxants on intracranial pressure (ICP), cerebral blood flow (CBF), and blood pressure are listed in Table 13. Short duration of brain hypothermia, such as 48 h, is ineffective in preventing brain edema and can make the overall condition much worse [3]. In treatment of severe brain injury, short duration of moderate brain hypothermia (34°C) does not allow recovery and only halts the progression of neuronal damage and pathophysiology. In this case, rewarming can worsen the outcome because of re-progression of secondary brain damage and overlapping rewarming stress. This means that recovery of injured brain tissue or at least part-recovery are criteria to commence rewarming. Therefore, in severely brain-injured patients, prolonged brain hypothermia is required.

In the intensive care unit (ICU), initial anesthesia for induction of brain hypothermia or continuous anesthesia after surgery is administered using a drip of propofol (1–2 mg/kg) [3,4,6]. After stabilization of cardiopulmonary function and systemic circulation, patients are administered a continuous drip of midazolam (0.15–0.25 mg/kg h^{-1}) anesthesia, combined with pancuronium (0.05 mg/kg h^{-1}) muscle relaxation, and buprenorphine (1.0–2.0 mg/kg h^{-1}) analgesia [1,3–6]. Brain hypothermia treatment is carried out under this anesthesia until the middle of the adaptation time at the end of the rewarming stage. Propofol allows much easier management of cardiopulmonary function and adaptation for rapid progression of hypermetabolism than midazolam. Although the mechanism of anesthesia, the low incidence of cardiopulmonary dysfunction, and the small complication of renal dysfunction are similar, propofol is a short acting anesthesia when compared with midazolam. Midazolam is suited to use for prolonged anesthesia during the cooling stage without cardiopulmonary and renal dysfunction. However, propofol is useful as a short-acting anesthesia at the beginning of the induction stage and late in the rewarming stage. Propofol allows much easier management for response to unstable cardiopulmonary function than does midazolam. At the end of the rewarming stage, we change the anesthesia from midazolam to propopfol.

Brain hypothermia treatment is administered while patients are monitored for ICP, SjO_2, SvO_2, SaO_2, cerebral perfusion pressure, cardiac output, oxygen delivery ($\bar{D}O_2$), oxygen extraction ratio, brain tissue temperature and/or jugular venous blood temperature, tympanic membrane temperature, bladder temperature,

Table 13. The effects of analgesic agents and muscle relaxants on blood pressure, ICP, and CBF

Analgesic agents	Initial i.v. dosage	Maintenace	Blood pressure	ICP	CBF
Benzodiazepines					
Midazolam	0.03–0.3 mg/kg	0.05–0.5 μg/kg min^{-1}	— or ↓	— or ↓	↓
Lorazepam	0.04 mg/kg		↓	—	↓
Diazepam	0.1–0.2 mg/kg		↓	—	↓
Others					
Propofol	1–2 mg/kg	5–50 μg/kg min^{-1}	↓↓	↓	↓
Etomidate	0.3–0.4 mg/kg		↓	↓	↓
Narcotics					
Morphine	2–5 mg	2–5 mg/h	↓	↑	—
Fentanyl	25–50 mg	50–100 μg/h	↓	↑	—
Alfentanyl	10–15 μg/kg	0.5–3 μg/kg min^{-1}	↓	↑	—
Sufentanyl	0.2–0.6 μg/kg	0.01–0.05 μg/kg min^{-1}	↓	↑	—
Depolarizing					
Succinylcholine	1 mg/kg		—	↑	—
Nondepolarizing					
Pancuronium	0.1 mg/kg	4–8 g/h	↑	—	—

ICP, intracranial pressure; CBF, cerebral blood flow; —, 110 change pulmonary arterial pressure, and end-tidal CO_2 [2]. Brain hypoxia is evaluated by changes in PaO_2, SaO_2, 2,3-diphosphoglycerate, brain tissue temperature, and $\bar{D}O_2$. The CBF-metabolic imbalance is evaluated from interacted changes in SjO_2 and the cerebral thermal index (brain tissue temperature/tympanic membrane temperature) [2]. All patients are cared for in ICU with direct participation of educational doctors using computerized management systems.

References

1. Caldwell JE, Heier T, Wright PM, Lin S, McCarthy G, Szenohradszky J, Sharma ML, Hing JP, Schroeder M, Sessler DI (2000) Temperature-dependent pharmacokinetics and pharmacodynamics of vecuronium. Anesthesiology 92:84–93
2. Hayashi N (2000) Enhanced neuronal damage in severely brain injured patients by hypothalamus, pituitary, and adrenal axis neuro-hormonal changes. In: Hayashi N (ed) Brain hypothermia. Springer, Berlin Heidelberg New York Tokyo, pp 3–26
3. Hayashi N (2000) The clinical issue and effectiveness of brain hypothermia treatment for severe brain injured patients. In: Hayashi N (ed) Brain hypothermia. Springer, Berlin Heidelberg New York Tokyo, pp 121–151
4. Leslie K, Bjorksten AR, Ugoni A, Mitchell P (2002) Mild core hypothermia and anesthetic requirement for loss of responsiveness during propofol anesthesia for craniotomy. Anesth Analg 94:1298–1303
5. Sahin A, Aypar U (2002) Effect of amino acid solutions on intraoperative hypothermia and postoperative shivering. Comparison of two anesthetic regimens. Acta Anaesthesiol Scand 46:64–67
6. Spitzfaden AC, Jimenez DF, Tobias JD (1999) Propofol for sedation and control of intracranial pressure in children. Pediatr Neurosurg 31:194–200

42. Imaging and Monitoring for Brain Hypothermia Management

Computed Tomography Imaging After Surgery

The presence of residual hematoma, rebleeding of subdural hematomas on the other side of the brain, complication of acute hydrocephalus, diffuse brain swelling, and brain stem compression are all dangerous conditions. Computed tomography (CT) imaging is recommended as soon as possible after surgery. Further surgery should not be delayed if indications for surgical intervention have been observed. One of the difficulties of surgery is the misdiagnosis of progression of any subdural hematoma on the other side of the brain that was not observed on the preoperative CT scan. Brain swelling after removal of a subdural hematoma suggests the possibility of progression of other thin subdural hematomas, presence of residual subdural hematoma in the nonsurgical field, or rebleeding of a silent hematoma that was not observed on the CT scan because of mechanical compression of the initial subdural hematoma. If residual hematoma is suspected, further surgical craniotomy should be done immediately. To make a correct diagnosis of other subdural hematomas, examination of the CT scan after surgery followed by scheduling for re-operation is, theoretically, a reasonable approach. However, this surgical approach is too late for the survival of the patient without vegetation in most severely brain-injured patients. The strategy of surgical treatment and examination of the CT scan is important.

In intensive case unit (ICU) management, the severity of brain swelling, narrowing of lateral ventricles, inconsistency between gray and white matter, the severity of contusion in injured tissue, and development of intracerebral hematoma in contusion are check points. In multiple trauma patients, additional studies of abdominal CT scan, chest CT scan, and pelvic CT scan are required for diagnosis of masking intra-abdominal hemorrhage, silent dissection aneurysm of the aortic arch, complication of hemopneumothorax, and vascular injury of the femoral artery.

ICU Management Before Brain Hypothermia Treatment

Before Induction of Brain Hypothermia

Monitoring of Vital Signs

The initial requirement of ICU management is stabilization of vital signs. Maintenance of systolic blood pressure above 100 mmHg, clear breathing sounds, and no arrhythmia are important for maintaining uniform brain hypothermia. Unstable blood pressure is unfavorable for the induction of brain hypothermia treatment because cardiac insufficiency can easily occur with reduced serum catecholamine caused by hypothermia [9,10]. Difficult control of brain tissue hypothermia caused by slow washout of thermo-pooled blood in the brain tissue [12] and insufficient administration of oxygen and metabolic substrates are basic clinical issues of unstable systemic circulation [1,16]. To avoid this complication, fluid resuscitation with 7% ascorbic Ringer's solution without manitol for the prevention of brain edema are recommended initially. Then, the application of elastic bandages to the extremities for mechanical elevation of peripheral vascular resistance is successful in preventing disturbances of the microcirculation of major organs under brain hypothermia treatment. Intermittent elastic bandaging of the extremities not only prevents an over hydration by fluid resuscitation, but also, indirectly, reduces the chances of progression of brain edema. Another benefit of bandaging the extremities is the prevention of pulmonary micro-embolus formation and disturbance of pulmonary circulation by preventing venous stasis and venous thrombosis in peripheral extremities (Fig. 59) [9]. The critical level of dehydration for the disturbance of microcirculation is observed with the presence of dry skin, and is higher than 40% of Ht, with a shock index (pulse number/systolic blood pressure) higher than 0.5–0.7.

Hypertensive medicines are not recommended for maintaining systolic blood pressure above 100 mmHg. This is because harmful stress-induced catecholamine surge, the hazard of cardiopulmonary dysfunction

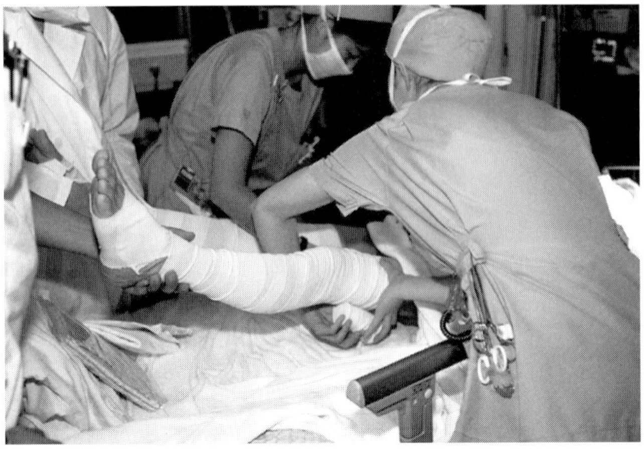

Fig. 59. Elastic bandage technique for stabilizing systemic circulation during brain hypothermia treatment

caused by coronary spasm, and cardiac muscle contraction will be promoted by administration of hypertensive medications. Cardiac ischemia can be monitored by a shift of ST junction on the Fig. 64 (EEG), the J-wave, and increasing levels of serum troponin I [11,16,18,22].

Head Position

After surgery, the head-up position for the prevention of intracranial pressure (ICP) elevation is not recommended. The initial target of ICU management is preventing neuronal hypoxia and dysoxia and ensuring an adequate supply of metabolic substrates and glucose [9,10].

The maintenance of cerebral blood flow (CBF) is an initial care management requirement after surgery. For the success of this management, the head-up position is less preferred to the flat position. Without special complications of acute brain swelling, the flat position is recommended for the prevention of brain ischemia during the 12h period after brain damage. The purpose of the head-up position is to accelerate the venous outflow and prevent brain swelling and brain edema [6,21]. However, these complications occur as a result of unsuccessful management of brain ischemia, brain hypoxia, and inadequate supply of metabolic substrates. In most cases of severely brain-injured patients, the autoregulation mechanism of CBF is damaged and therefore, the head-up position after surgery produces added severe brain ischemia and can trigger development of brain edema. The time window of care management of the head position is important. Use of the flat position for 6h–12h after successful surgical management, followed by a head-up position of 5°–7° to prevent ICP elevation is recommended.

Analysis of Blood Gases and Neuronal Hypoxia

The analysis of blood gases is important for the design of strategies for brain hypothermia treatment. PaO_2 less than 60mmHg means respiratory insufficiency, and less than 38mmHg is the critical level of hypoxia for neuronal recovery. The PaO_2/FiO_2 ratio is useful a marker to evaluate the oxygen uptake by pulmonary function. The control of PaO_2/FiO_2 to above 350mmHg is a basic respiratory care requirement during brain hypothermia treatment. PaO_2/FiO_2 less than 250 suggests lung injury that includes the damage of alveolar epithelium, and PaO_2/FiO_2 less than 200 suggests the complication of acute respiratory distress syndrome (ARDS). During brain hypothermia, this condition requires pressure-controlled inverse ratio ventilation, lower PEEP pressure, administration of a radical scavenger, management of antithrombin-III (AT-III) above 100%, serum albumin greater than 3.5g/dl, control of PaO_2/FiO_2 greater than 300, activation of respiratory muscle protein metabolism, maintenance of immune function with control of growth hormone, prevention of infection, and care of the hemoglobin function [9,11]. The management of oxygen delivery at more than 700–800ml/min and maintenance of PaO_2/FiO_2 greater than 350 are not enough to ensure neuronal oxygenation. The management of hemoglobin function to allow efficient binding of inhalated oxygen and fast release of bound oxygen from hemoglobin in the brain tissue is also important. The 2,3-diphosphoglycerate (DPG) in hemoglobin is a regulator of hemoglobin function. The management of serum pH greater than 7.3, serum phosphate at 3–5mg/dl, serum magnesium at 1.2–1.8mEq/l, and serum glucose at 120–140mg/dl are the minimum requirements for maintaining hemoglobin functions. In the condition of serum pH lower than 7.2, hemoglobin DPG progressively reduces to critical levels at which conditions difficult are for the release of bound oxygen from hemoglobin in injured brain tissue [9–11]. This means unsuccessful neuronal oxygenation despite normal PaO_2 and oxygen administration. In our clinical studies of changes in hemoglobin DPG levels in severely brain-injured patients [Glasgow Coma Scale score (GCS) less than 6], results suggested that hemoglobin DPG was severely reduced in about 42% of patients, and in 25% of patients was reduced to critical levels with ineffective oxygen inhalation despite a normal level of PaO_2.

The control of $PaCO_2$ between 34 and 38mmHg during brain hypothermia treatment is recommended [12]. The actual $PaCO_2$ is 2–5mmHg lower than the data for $PaCO_2$ monitored under brain hypothermia conditions. Therefore under brain hypothermia conditions of 33°–34°C, a recorded $PaCO_2$ value of 34–38mmHg implies an actual value of 28–31 mmHg. The critical level of $PaCO_2$ to produce cerebral vascular contraction and CBF disturbance is below 24 mmHg. Hyperventilation therapy to reduce the ICP during brain hypothermia treatment is not recommended. This is because increasing CBF by control of low ICP is temporary and prolonged $PaCO_2$ control below 28 mmHg can easily produce CBF disturbances [9,11] On the contrary, increased $PaCO_2$ above 45 mmHg causes relaxation of vascular smooth muscle. Acute brain swelling caused by vascular engorgement is a major complication of hypercapnea. The $PaCO_2$ threshold for the occurrence of vascular engorgement is more than 50 mmHg. The contraction power of cardiac muscle also reduces because of flaccid cardiac muscle tonus at this level.

Hyperglycemia

In severely brain-injured patients with trauma, hemorrhagic cerebral stroke, and ischemic cerebral stroke, stress-associated hyperglycemia caused by epinephrine surge is unavoidable. Severe hyperglycemia, with serum glucose levels of more than 230 mg/dl, produces increased levels of brain tissue glucose and lactate. Without management of hyperglycemia, induction of moderate brain hypothermia (32°–33°C) is complicated by the rapid progression of anaerobic brain metabolism and increasing levels of brain tissue lactate. The complication of severe hyperglycemia is caused by reduced glucose consumption in the whole body associated with the metabolic shift from glucose to lipid at a brain tissue temperature of 34°C [9–11]. Therefore, before induction of hypothermia, stress-associated hyperglycemia must be controlled to serum glucose levels of 120–140 mg/dl. The negative effects of hyperglycemia are not simple. Slow release of bound oxygen from hemoglobin caused by reduced DPG is another issue [9–11]. This complication is a serious clinical issue for the management of severely brain-injured patients at the acute stage, with ineffective oxygen inhalation and unsuccessful neuronal oxygenation, despite management of normal PaO_2, oxygen delivery, ICP, and CBF. Our clinical studies recorded severe hemoglobin DPG reduction in about 44% of severe brain trauma patients. If serum glucose increased above 180–230 mg/dl, we believe that the feedback mechanism of macronutrient neural control requests no further nutrition. This feedback mechanism is controlled by the release of vasopressin and insulin [9–11]. The excess release of vasopressin promotes proinflammatory cytokines and blood–brain barrier (BBB) dysfunction as shown in Fig. 36.

Therefore, stress-associated hyperglycemia with serum glucose levels above 180–230 mg/dl makes induction of brain hypothermia difficult and is a contraindication for moderate brain hypothermia (32°–33°C), because of ineffective oxygen inhalation, progress of anaerobic metabolism, increased brain tissue lactate levels, progress of brain edema, and high incidence of complications in major organs [9,11]. To control hyperglycemia, insulin is the first-choice medication. However, in severely brain-injured patients, ordinal administration of insulin is not so effective, because the serum level of insulin is reduced by harmful stress-associated catecholamine surge, insulin sensitivity is reduced by stress-related glucocorticoid release, and consumption of glucose is reduced because of muscle weakness and the release of glucagon. The release of alanine and glutamate from skeletal muscles following severe brain damage produces weakness of skeletal and respiratory muscles [9,10]. These pathophysiological changes are the background to the difficult control of stress-associated hyperglycemia. Therefore, the initial method to prevent insulin-resistant hyperglycemia is to minimize epinephrine release and reduce stimulation of the hypothalamus–pituitary–adrenal (HPA) axis. The early induction of brain hypothermia (within 3 h of brain damage), control of brain temperature at 33°–34°C, replacement of insulin, no administration of steroid, activation of protein synthesis by administration of salbutamol and glutamine, inhibition of protein catabolism by administration of amurinone, and kinetic therapy are recommended.

Hypo-albuminemia

Hypo-albuminemia is a common complication in severely brain-injured patients [14] and is classified into grades of severe, moderate, and mild hypo-albuminemia. For the management of severely brain-injured patients, severe hypo-albuminemia (serum albumin <2.5 mg/dl) includes many negative factors such as limited effects of hyper-osmotic therapy to prevent brain edema, intestinal mucous membrane edema and difficult enteral nutrition, reduced lymphocyte count caused by intestinal edema, susceptibility to pulmonary edema, increased free bacteria and the complication of infection, and unstable pharmacological effectiveness (Fig. 60) [11]. About 70% of medical drugs are stabilized by binding to albumin in the bloodstream (Table 14). Our preliminary study under hypothermia conditions of 32°–33° suggested that the activities of albumin-binding antibiotics such as vancomycine were reduced. On the other hand, the activity of non-albumin-binding antibiotics such as albekasin were not affected (Fig. 61). Albekasin is one of the most useful antibiotics for methicillin resistant staphylococcus aureus (MRSA) during hypo-albuminemia and hypothermia conditions. The increase of free bacteria under the conditions of severe hypo-

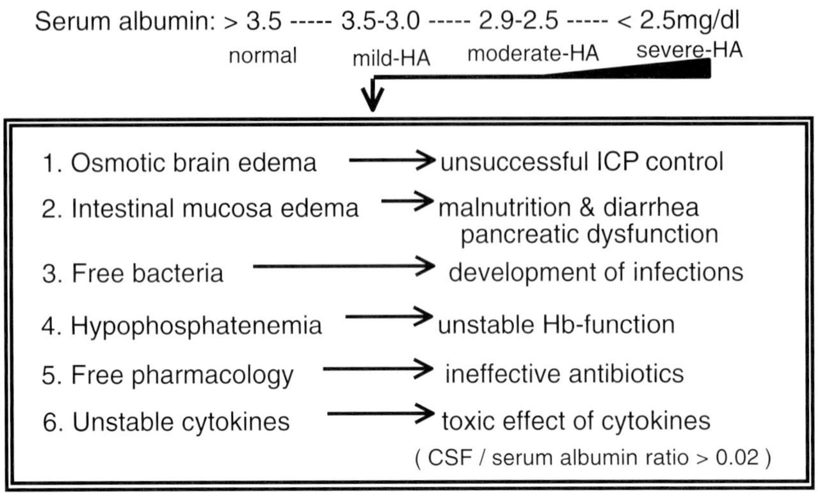

Fig. 60. Negative effects of hypo-albuminemia (*HA*) during brain hypothermia treatment. *ICP*, intracranial pressure; *Hb*, hemoglobin; *CSF*, cerebrospinal fluid

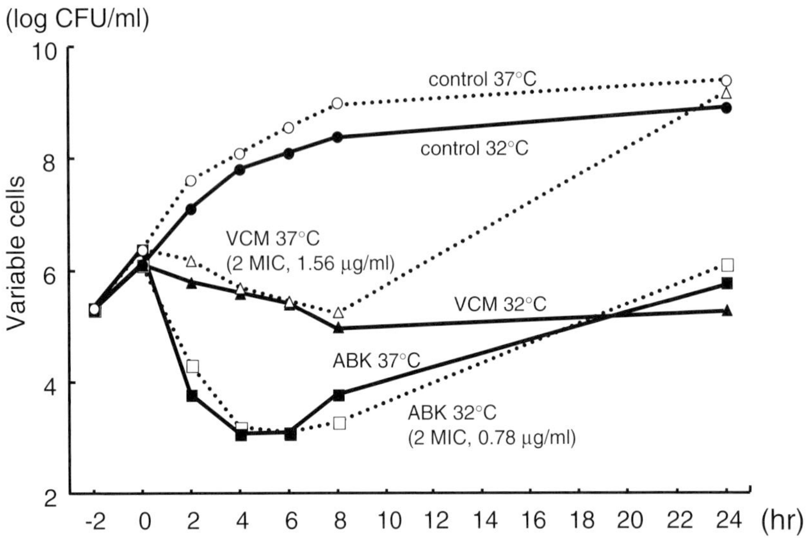

Fig. 61. Time-kill curve for arbekacin (*ABK*) and vancomycin (*VCM*) for MRSA NI-2 at 37°C and 32°C

albuminemia is also a big issue for the management of systemic infections. This is because with spreading of infection, the BBB function will decrease with hypo-albuminemia, cytokines can easily permeate the BBB, and brain tissue glutamate levels increase with the complication of cytokine encephalitis, resulting in unsuccessful brain hypothermia treatment. The preliminary management of hypo-albuminemia before the induction of brain hypothermia treatment is very important for the success of treatment. The management of serum albumin above 3.0–3.5 mg/dl is recommended.

Antithrombin III

The brain is a very rich organ of prothrombin. Severe brain damage causes release of prothrombin and activates thrombin function (Fig. 62). Therefore, antithrombin-III (AT-III) is very rapidly consumed to prevent micro-embolus formation following severe brain injury. The change in AT-III level is a good indirect parameter of possible microcirculation disturbance. This concept also probably applies to the conditions of microcirculation in other major organs. The intestinal mucous membrane is very sensitive to disturbances of microcirculation. The severity of intestinal mucous membrane damage caused by ischemia is indirectly diagnosed by changes in the pH of the gastric wall tissue (gastric pHi). The use of the tonometor technique allows the monitoring of gastric pHi changes. Our clinical studies suggest that gastric pHi is very sensitive to changes in the AT-III level. This means that AT-III reduction not only promotes the disturbance of cerebral microcirculation, but also produces intestinal organ ischemia [9,11]. The critical level of AT-III to cause aci-

Table 14. Protein binding type antibiotics

Antibiotics	Abbreviation	Protein binding (%)	Renal out	Metabolize
Cefdinir	CFDN	73.1	○	
Cefuroxime	CXM-AX	35	○	
Cefixime	CFIX	63	○	
Cefteram pivoxil	CFTM-PI	74.6	○	
Cefcapene pivoxil	CFPN-PI	45	40	
Cefalotin	CET	70	52	
Cefazolin	CEZ	72	93	
Cefmetazole	CMZ	84	○	
Cefoxitin	CFX	73	78	
Cefamandole	CMD	75	96	
Cefotetan	CTT	90.9	○	
Cefbuperazone	CBPZ	54.9	○	
Cefsulodin	CFS	90	54	
Cefoperazone	CPZ	90		○
Cefotaxime	CTX	38	○	
Ceftizoxime	CZX	30–50	○	
Cefmenoxime	CMX	80	○	
Cefpiramide	CPM	96.3		○
Ceftriaxone	CTRX	88	55	45
Cefodizime	CDZM	86	○	
Cefminox	CMNX	69	○	
Latamoxef	LMOX	60	○	
Flomoxef	FMOX	35	○	
Aztreonam	AZT	52.6–55.7	○	
Faropenem	FRPM	82.6–92.1		
Panipenem/Betamipron	PAPM/BP	PAPM 7.0 BP 73.1		
Sulbactam/Cefoperazone	SBT/CPZ	CPZ 90.4	○ SBT	
Vancomycin	VCM	34.3	85	
Chloramphenicol	CP	60		○
Ticarcillin	TIPC	45	○	
Benzylpenicillin	PCG	40–60	○	
Gentamicin	GM	35	○	
Strepomycin	SM	30	○	
Doxycycline	DOXY	87	40	○
Minocycline	MINO	75		○
	ST	50	9	○
Nalidixic	NA	88–91	○	
Enoxacin	ENX	31.9	○	
Ciprofloxacin	CPFX	30	○	
Lomefloxacin	LFLX	24.4	○	
Tosufloxacin	TFLX	37.4	○	
Fleroxacin	FLRX	32	77.3	
Sparfloxacin	SPFX	42.2	10	○
Levofloxacin	LVFX	47–52	88.5	3.9
Clarithromycin	CAM	42–70	○	○
Erythromycin	EM	70–75	10	○
Roxithromycin	RXM	98.3		○
Lincomycin	LCM	70–80	10	○
Clindamycin	CLDM	60–95	5	○

dosis of the gastric wall (pHi 7.3) is about 90%–100% (see Fig. 63). Therefore, replacement of AT-III is recommended to increase the serum AT-III level to above 100%. This management of AT-III is useful for the prevention of CBF disturbance and the complication of bacterial translocation from intestinal organs during brain hypothermia treatment.

Electrocardiogram

There are many types of cardiac dysfunction that are recorded during brain hypothermia treatment of severely brain-injured patients. Before induction of brain hypothermia, cardiac ischema is recorded with an excess release of catecholamines. In our series of clinical

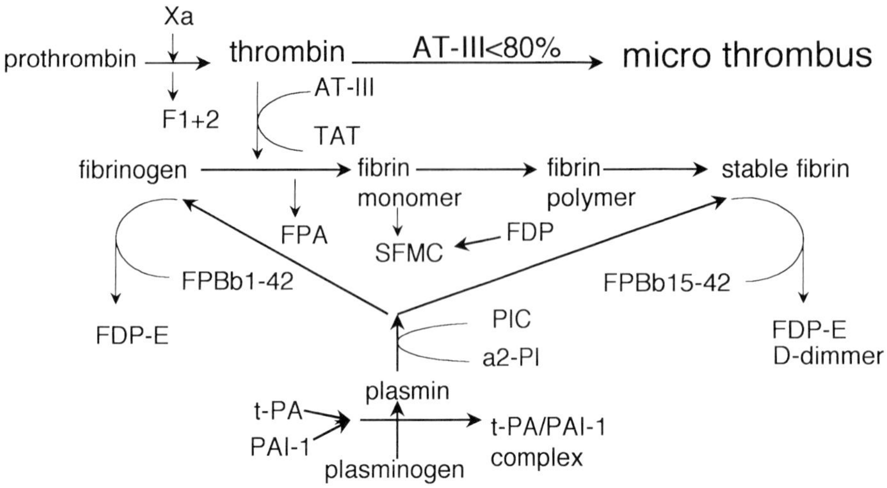

Fig. 62. The schema for the mechanism of changes that occur in coagulation and fibrinolysis after severe brain damage

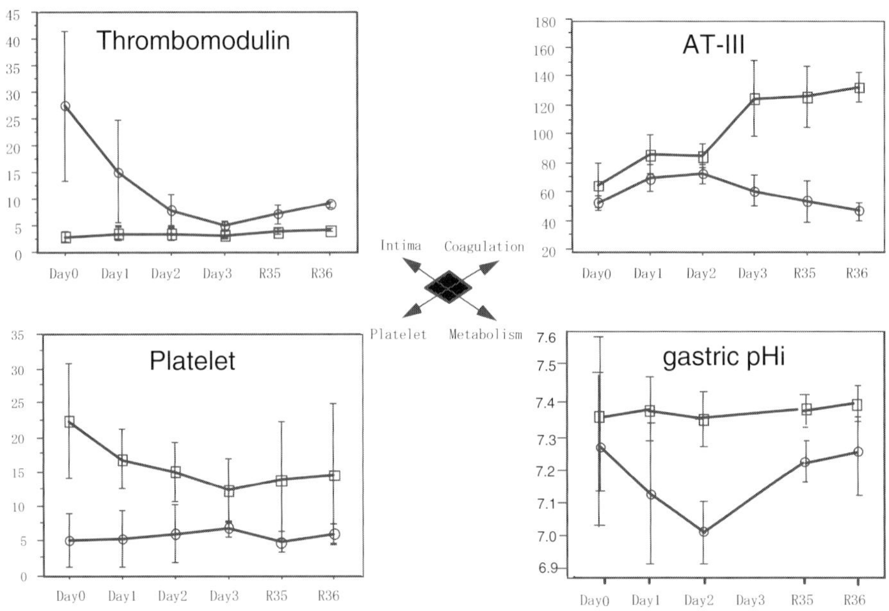

Fig. 63. The changes of thrombomodulin, antithrombin III (*AT-III*), platelet, and gastric pHi during the acute stage, under the management of brain hypothermia treatment ($n = 14$). *Circles*, disseminated intravascular coagulopathy (DIC) group; *squares*, nonDIC group

studies, catecholamine surge of 20–200 times normal levels were recorded about 3h after severe brain injury. Coronary spasm and contraction myocytolysis are major causes of cardiac damage after severe brain damage. This cardiac ischemia is monitored by ST changes on the electrocardiogram (ECG) and increased serum troponin I.

Another clinical issue concerns the fact that hypothermia itself produces changes in cardiac function. The major clinical issue of cardiac function following brain hypothermia is mainly produced by reduced serum catecholamine levels. Lower cardiac output occurs following brain hypothermia with temperatures lower than 33°–33.5°C (Fig. 8, Chap. 28). Changes in the circulating blood volume caused by dehydration therapy for the prevention of brain edema can easily disturb cerebral microcirculation and that of other major organs during moderate brain hypothermia. On the ECG, the ST changes of more than 1mm J-wave and QT interval of more than 450mm/s have been considered as warning signs. The management of cardiac ischemia and hypoxia is required before induction of brain hypothermia management. Cardiac arrhythmia associated with hypocalemia is another cardiac complication during brain hypothermia treatment. The precise mechanism of hypopocalemia following hypothermia has not been clarified.

The intracellular ion changes in the cardiac muscle are recorded as the J-wave (Osborn wave) on the ECG following hypothermia [8,22]. The appearance of the J-wave on the ECG depends on the core temperature (Fig. 64). After more than 2 days of prolonged brain hypothermia, the recorded J-wave intensities were 15%,

30%, and 50% at 34°C, 33°C, and 32°C brain tissue temperature, respectively. However, no cardiopulmonary hemodynamic changes were recorded by the J-wave in our ICU clinical study (Fig. 65). The recording of AF on the ECG suggests the possibility of brain infarction. Observation of low AT-III, Ht greater than 40%, high serum osmolarity, difference in bilateral tympanic membrane temperatures of more than 0.8°C, and difference in bilateral neurological reactions provide an early diagnosis of brain infarction.

Urinary Drainage

Urinary drainage provides information concerning renal function, dehydration, systemic metabolic conditions, renal elimination of metabolic substrates for ·NO radicals, and abdominal hypertension. Urinary drainage is also a basic technique for the prevention of ICP elevation caused by abdominal hypertension. Therefore, continuous urinary drainage not only prevents ICP elevation, but also bowel ischemia, venous stasis of the liver, and pulmonary interstitial tissue pressure rises. We have no reliable monitors of abdominal hypertension, and as an alternate method, the urinary bladder pressure is monitored as an indirect parameter. With abdominal pressure lower than 10 mmHg, there are no effects on ICP and systemic circulation; however, about at 15 mmHg, venous stasis occurs in intestinal digestive organs and liver circulation. Abdominal hypertension above 17 mmHg produces ischemia in the intestinal digestive organs, venous stasis of the liver and lungs, complication of pulmonary edema, and immune dys-

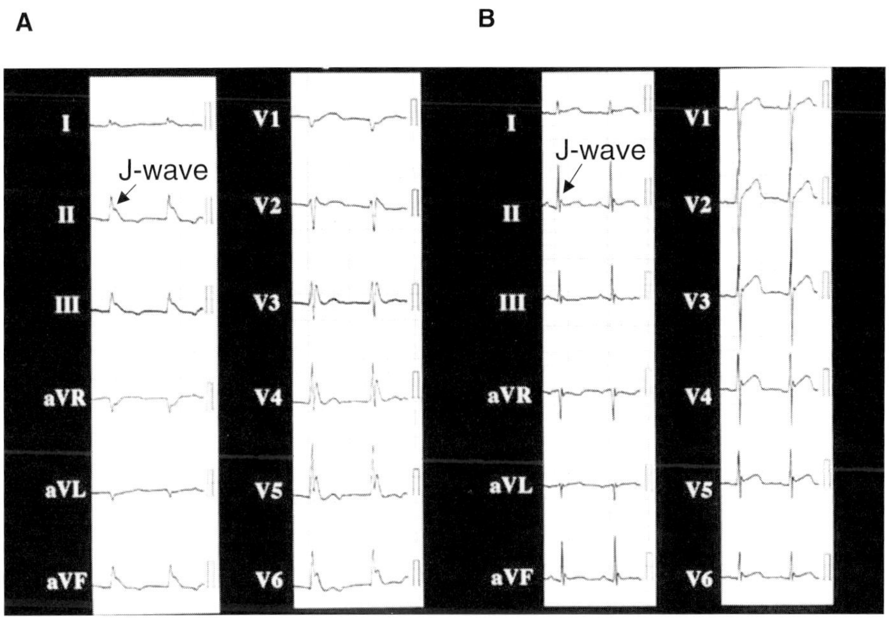

Fig. 64. J-wave on electrocardiogram from 28°C accidental hypothermia (**A**) and 32°C controlled hypothermia (**B**)

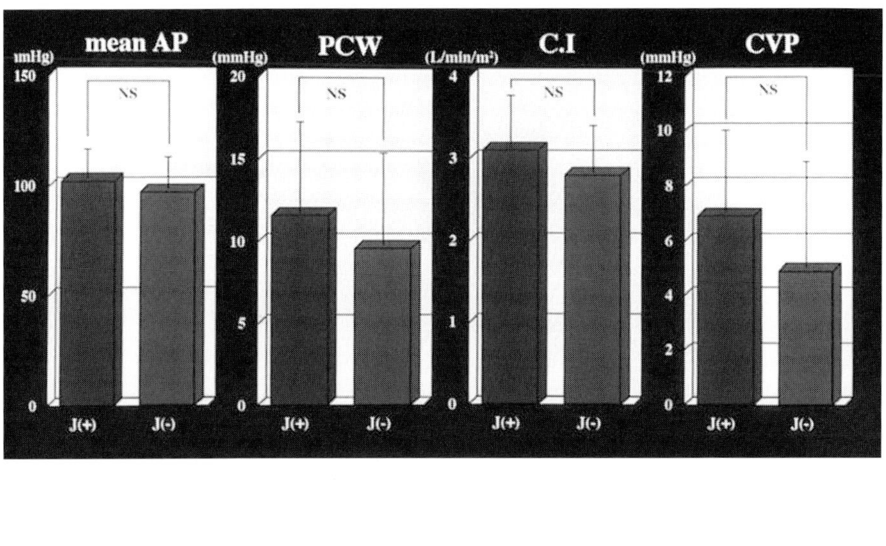

Fig. 65. Cardiopulmonary hemodynamic changes. *J*(*t*), during presence of J-wave; *J*(−), no presence of J-wave. *AP*, arterial pressure; *PCW*, pulmonary capillary wedge pressure; *CI*, cardiac index; *CVP*, central venous pressure; *NS*, not significant

function. The critical abdominal pressure for the production of cardiac congestion and ICP elevation is about 25 mmHg.

Gastric Lavage

Gastric lavage is necessary to prevent abdominal hypertension, ischemia of the digestive organs, oral bacterial translocation, and aspiration pneumonia. Aspiration pneumonia, in particular, is a very serious complication because of progression of alveolar infections caused by enteral bacteria and chemical damage of alveolar epithelium caused by acid gastric juice [9–11].

Immune dysfunction is unavoidable during brain hypothermia, especially at temperatures lower than 34°C used in moderate brain hypothermia treatment. This is because of reduced levels of growth hormone, ploractin, and adrenocorticotropic-hormone (ACTH) that are recorded with poor pituitary function correlated to brain tissue hypothermia [4,5,10]. Aspiration pneumonia is very difficult to manage under the condition of immune dysfunction. To prevent the serious complication of pneumonia, gastric lavage is a very important part of initial care management. In preparation for gastric lavage, the air in the stomach should be removed and the contents of the full stomach aspirated. To prevent a gastric air trap in the stomach during gastric lavage, the right-side position and positional drainage are recommended. After that, gastric lavage should be started with cooled saline. The recommended temperature of the saline is about 34°C. The use of too much cooled saline may trigger cardiac arrhythmia because the heart is located very close to the esophagus and stomach. The infusion volume of cooled saline should never be more than 250 ml. Rapid infusion of more than 250 ml of saline into the stomach could trigger vomiting and increase abdominal hypertension.

Monitoring of Tympanic Membrane Temperature

Changes in tympanic membrane temperature can be used as an indirect monitor of carotid blood flow. The tympanic membrane temperature is determined by balance of the core temperature, localized ear tissue metabolism, blood flow around the tympanic membrane, and the temperature of the surrounding air. The heat production from the localized ear tissue metabolism around the tympanic membrane is very low and may be lower than 0.01°C [9,10]. The temperature of the surrounding air is stable and is lower than body temperature. Therefore, the influences of localized ear tissue metabolism and temperature of the surrounding air on the tympanic membrane temperature are negligible. The tympanic membrane temperature is elevated by carrying of the core temperature by the external carotid blood flow and washout these temperature throughout venous outflow in the ears. In most cases, excepting ear blood flow disturbances, changes in tympanic membrane temperature depend on changes of core temperature, carotid blood flow, and external carotid blood flow. Therefore, the basic temperature of tympanic membrane is mainly determined by core temperature, although the dynamic changes of tympanic membrane temperature provides are produced by changes in carotid blood flow. The tympanic membrane temperature can be used as an indirect clinical parameter for the conditions of external carotid blood flow and is also very close to being an indirect parameter for conditions of carotid blood flow [9,10].

Clinical utilization of tympanic membrane temperature provides differentiation between the right and left side. It is lower than the bladder temperature and reveals the difference between brain tissue temperature and jugular venous blood temperature. An unusually low tympanic membrane temperature combined with high bladder temperature is a sign of CBF disturbance. The cerebral oxygen metabolism and CBF disturbances can be diagnosed more precisely by monitoring the cerebral thermal index (CTI, defined as the brain tissue temperature/tympanic membrane temperature ratio and jugular venous oxygen saturation) [9,10]. The diagnostic methods for the detection of CBF disturbance and cerebral oxygen metabolism are summarized in Table 15. The early diagnosis of CBF disturbances during brain thermo-pooling and cerebral vasospasm at the bedside is straightforward as shown in Figs. 9 (in Chap. 25) and 66, respectively. As an alternative parameter of brain tissue temperature/tympanic membrane temperature, the ratio of jugular venous blood temperature/tympanic membrane temperature is also available, except under non-feeling conditions.

Table 15. The diagnostic parameters for distrubances of cerebral blood flow and metabolism at the bedside

	CTI	$SjvO_2$
Hypermetabolism	→	↘
Hypometabolism	→	↗
Ischemia	↗	↘
Ischemic hypometabolism	↑	→↗
Ischemic hypermetabolism	↗	→↘
Nonfilling	<1	↗↘
Luxury perfusion	↘	↗
Recovery	↘	↘

CTI, cerebral thermal index (brain tissue temperature/tympanic membrane temperature ratio); $SjvO_2$, jugular venous blood oxygen saturation

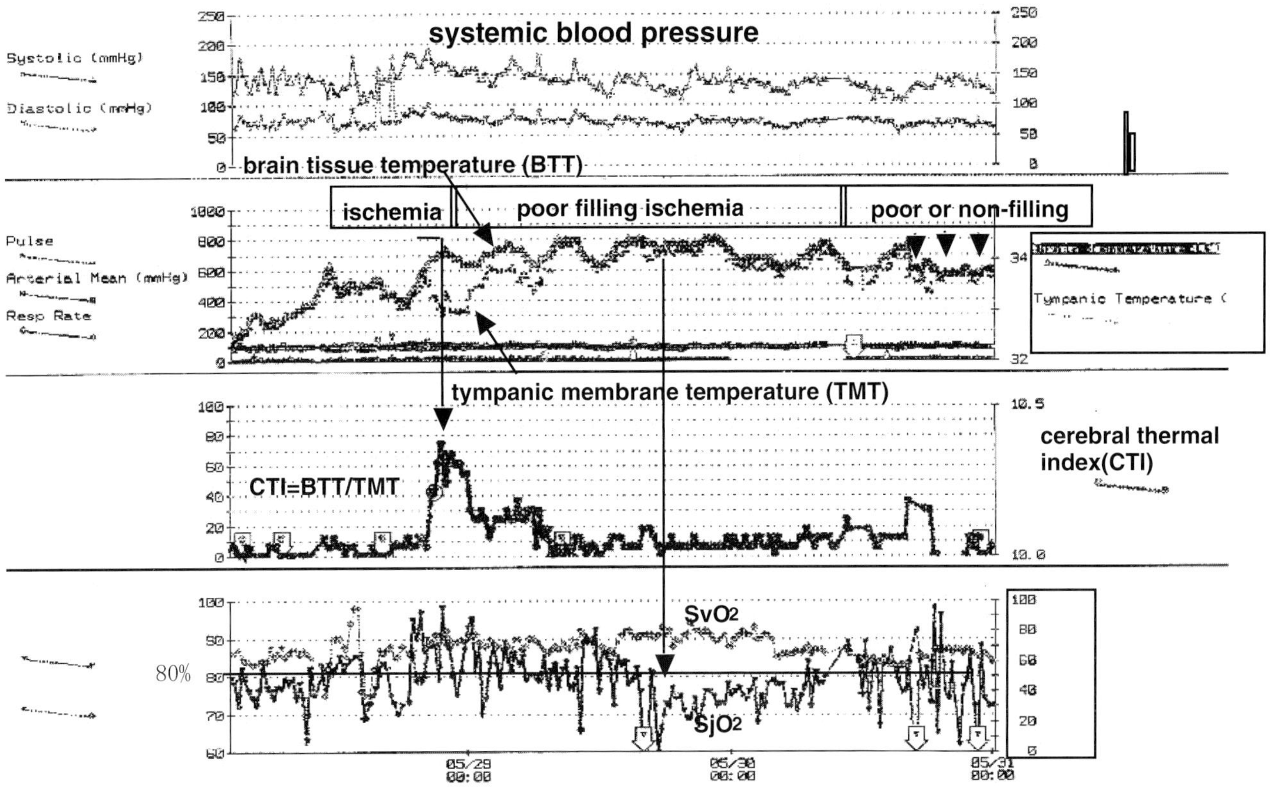

Fig. 66. Cerebral hemodynamic changes at the rewarming stage. Cerebral vasospasm was detected by divergence of brain tissue temperature (*BTT*) and tympanic membrane temperature (*TMT*), that follows the progressive fluctuating elevation of BTT and TMT. The BTT becomes equal to TMT when cerebral thermo-pooling reaches the teminal stage of brain metabolism

In ICU management, continuous monitoring of the tympanic membrane temperature by the heat clearance method is more useful than an infrared monitor of the inner ear. Because changes of the tympanic membrane temperature are very delicate computed continuous recording is useful (Fig. 67). To monitor the tympanic membrane temperature, the external ears must be clean, earwax should be removed, and the ears disinfected.

Monitoring of Cardiac Output and Cardiac Index

The Swan Ganz catheter is very useful for management of cardiopulmonary function during brain hypothermia treatment (Figs. 68, 69). The reduction of serum catecholamines and low cardiac output are unavoidable physiological reactions during brain hypothermia treatment [9,11]. To maintain stable neuronal oxygenation and metabolic substrates administration for injured tissue, the management of reduced cardiac output, maintenance of CPP, and adequate oxygen delivery are important. Dehydration therapy for the prevention of brain edema is contraindicated before the induction of brain hypothermia treatment. The information concerning oxygen delivery and oxygen consumption is obtained through the Swan Ganz catheter (Fig. 70). The desired oxygen delivery ($\bar{D}O_2$) is higher than 800 ml/dl, and the oxygen extraction ratio (O_2ER) is controlled between 20% and 25%. Fluid resuscitation, maintenance of the cardiac index above 3 l/kg, hemoglobin >11 g/dl, and SaO_2 >98% are required in initial ICU management.

Preparation for Monitoring Cardiac Output and Oxygen Extraction Ratio

Swan Ganz catheter kit
Sterilization kit
Surgical cover sheets
Local anesthesia
Five-milliter syringe and 20 ml of saline
Five percent heparinized saline (500 ml)
Automatic oxygen delivery monitoring device

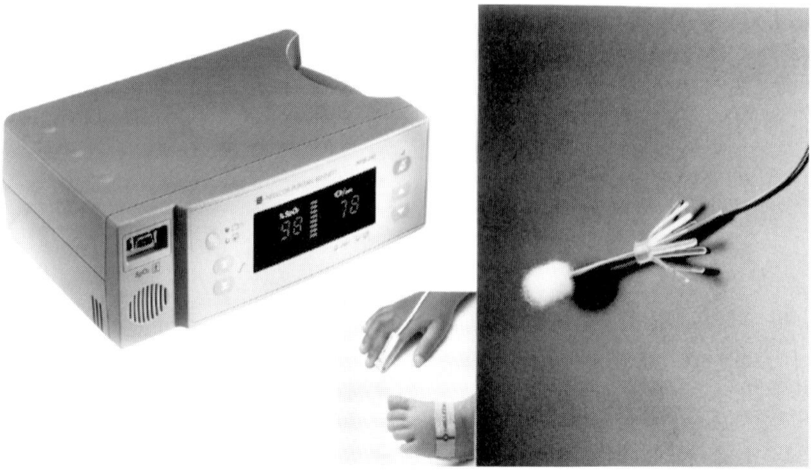

Fig. 67. The continuous monitoring system for tympanic membrane temperature

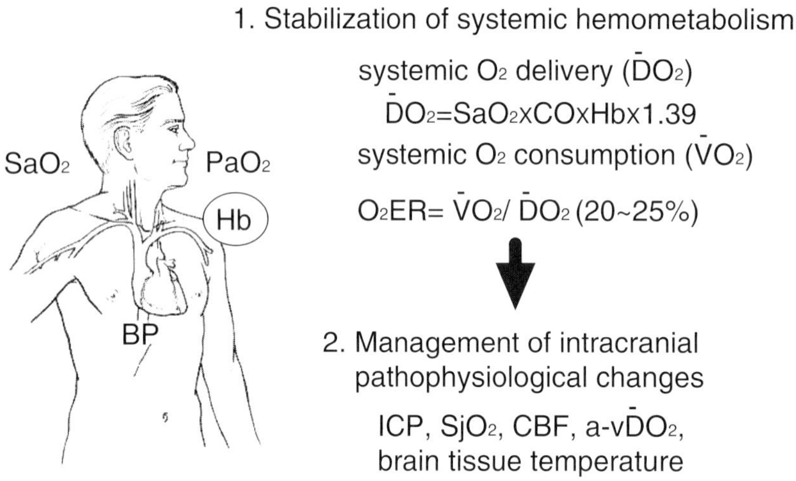

Fig. 68. The management of systemic circulation and metabolism using Swan Ganz monitor technique

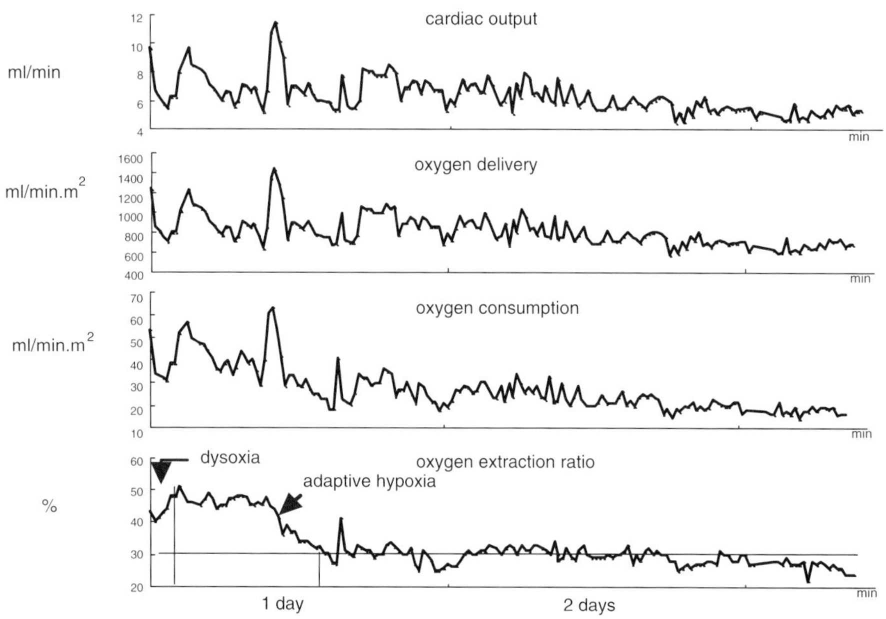

Fig. 69. The alteration of systemic hemo-metabolism after surgery on acute subdural hematoma (Glasgom Coma Scale score 6)

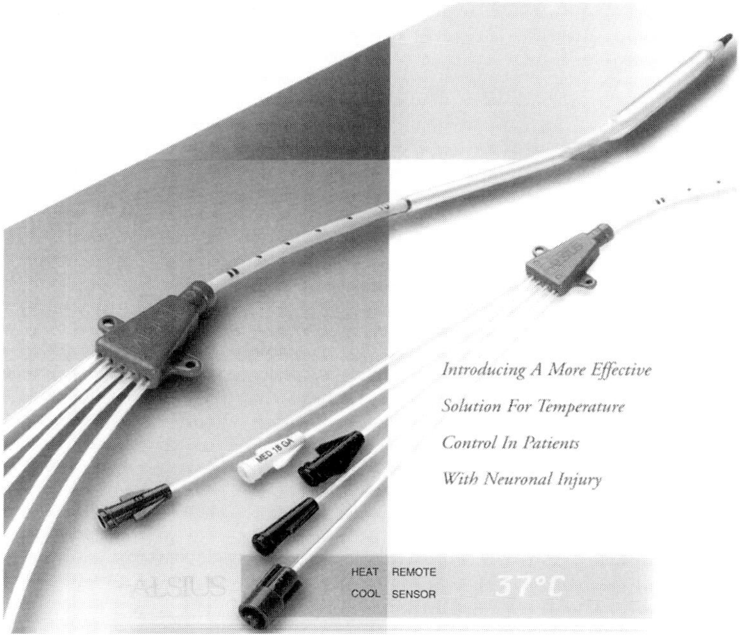

Fig. 70. Swan Ganz catheter for monitoring cardiac output

Insertion of Catheter

The Swan Ganz catheter is inserted into the pulmonary artery through the right ventricle with puncture of the subclavian vein from the lateral side at the middle of the clavicle line. If the puncture is from the inner side of the middle of the clavicle line, the catheter will easily go up into the jugular vein. The location of the catheter tip can be easily determined by monitoring the pressure wave as shown in Fig. 71.

Management of Swan Ganz Catheter

Care should be taken with the use of the Swan Ganz catheter in a closed system. Prolonged insertion of the Swan Ganz catheter of more than 6 days in the pulmonary artery is not recommended. A high incidence of fibrin formation on the tip of the Swan Ganz catheter has been observed. Because antibiotics cannot be delivered to infected parts of the catheter, management of catheter infection with prolonged insertion into the pulmonary artery is very difficult to control.

After Induction of Brain Hypothermia

Intracranial Pressure Monitor

The monitoring of ICP is useful for ICU brain hypothermia management after surgery (Fig. 58, Chap. 40). However, the interpreted meaning of ICP and its effect on the brain tissue are different depending on the condition of the closed or semi-closed skull after surgical external decompression. ICP elevation caused by mass lesion or brain edema, in the closed skull, produces whole brain ischemia caused by reduced perfusion pressure. However, intercompartmental pressure differences, such as those between the supra- and infratentorial pressure and/or right and left supratentorial pressure are limited to very small values by Pascal's theory. The CBF and ICP are maintained at relatively constant levels even with changes in blood pressure, cerebral perfusion pressure (CPP), and head position. However, in a case of disturbance of CBF autoregulation, ICP will be increased according to increasing blood pressure and the complication of acute brain swelling. The ICP sensor is already inserted in the brain tissue at the end of surgery. The calibration of the zero point of ICP is adjusted to the midpoint between the bragma and the external auditory canal.

In cases of a semi-closed skull after external decompression, the zero point must be set at heart level. The ventricular cerebrospinal fluid (CSF) pressure is the most accurate method of monitoring ICP in such patients. This is because the brain tissue pressure is not an accurate parameter for evaluation of ICP under the environment of an open skull. The electrical distortion sensor is used to monitor brain tissue pressure, and therefore, in the open skull, brain tissue pressure is influenced by the compression force of tissue weight and atmospheric pressure. Monitoring of brain tissue pressure shows high pressure in the lower portion of the

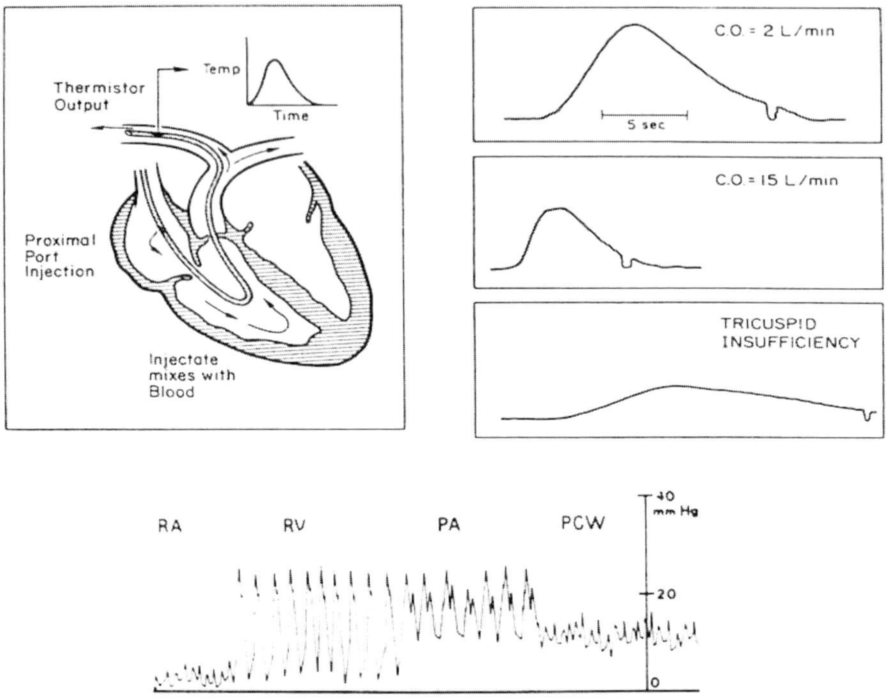

Fig. 71. Monitoring of cardiac output (*CO*) by heat clearance curve determined from Swan Ganz catheter. The catheter tip position is determined by monitoring of pressure wave as shown in the *lower* part

brain than other side at rotation of head position. The weight of brain tissue causes high pressure in the under side electrical distortion sensor brain than upper side brain electrical distortion sensor in the open skull.

Above 1010hPa, the atmospheric pressure acts as a positive compression pressure on the brain tissue. However, below 1010hPa, atmospheric pressure acts as a negative pressure toward the brain tissue. In the ICU management of ICP, bad weather with atmospheric pressure lower than 1010hPa can cause the brain to swell out through the surgical cavity. Therefore, the management of brain edema, vascular engorgement, cerebral venous circulation, high mediastinal pressure, hypercapnea, and head position are important during bad weather with atmospheric pressure lower than 1010hPa.

Monitoring of epidural pressure using the Spiel Berg ICP sensor is an alternative method of monitoring the ventricular CSF pressure in externally decompressed patients (Fig. 72) [9]. The CPP is calculated from the difference between the mean arterial blood pressure and ICP. Elevated ICP produces a CBF reduction with reduced CPP. However, critical levels of ICP to produce CBF disturbance are not consistent and vary between patients. Because, in the consistent volume of cranial cavity, buffer effect by CSF, soft brain tissue, and blood volume occur to the mass effect. This effect changes not only with the size of the mass lesion and buffer capacity, but also with the speed of ICP elevation.

For the management of ICP, understanding the relationships between changes of ICP and vascular pressure in the brain tissue is very useful. This is especially so for changes between capillary pressure caused by ICP elevation and reduction in water filtration rate from elevation of cerebral venous pressure and brain tissue pressure (Fig. 2, Chap. 20).

Monitoring Jugular Venous Blood Temperature and Oxygen Saturation

The H-catheter was designed by the author for the simultaneous measurement of internal jugular venous blood temperature and oxygen saturation (Fig. 73). The internal jugular venous blood temperature of the dominant venous outflow vessels can be used as an indirect indicator of the brain tissue temperature (Fig. 11, Chap. 22) [9,10]. This concept is supported by clinical data and evidence of brain tissue temperature washout by cerebral venous circulation (Figs. 10, 11, Chap. 22). In most patients, the jugular venous outflow is not the same on the right and left. The jugular venous blood temperature of the dominant venous outflow side reflects the

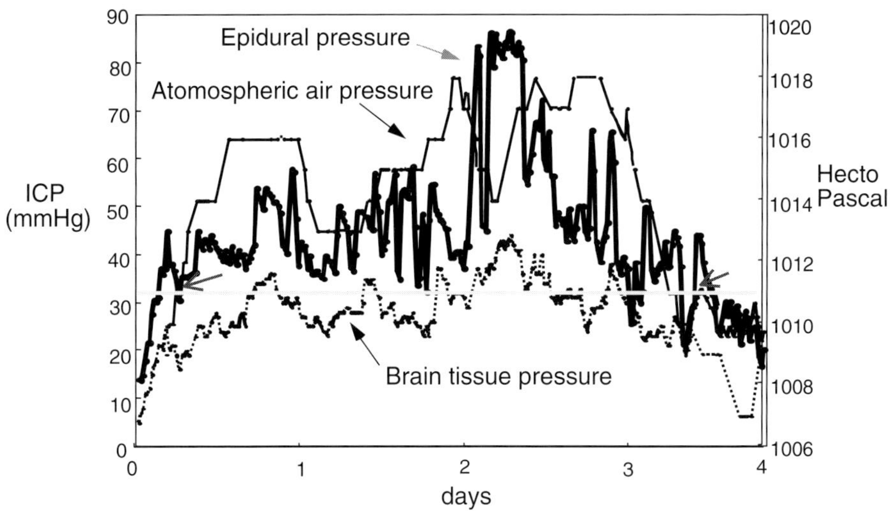

Fig. 72. Trends in atmospheric air pressure, brain tissue pressure, and epidural pressure for an externally decompressed semi-closed skull

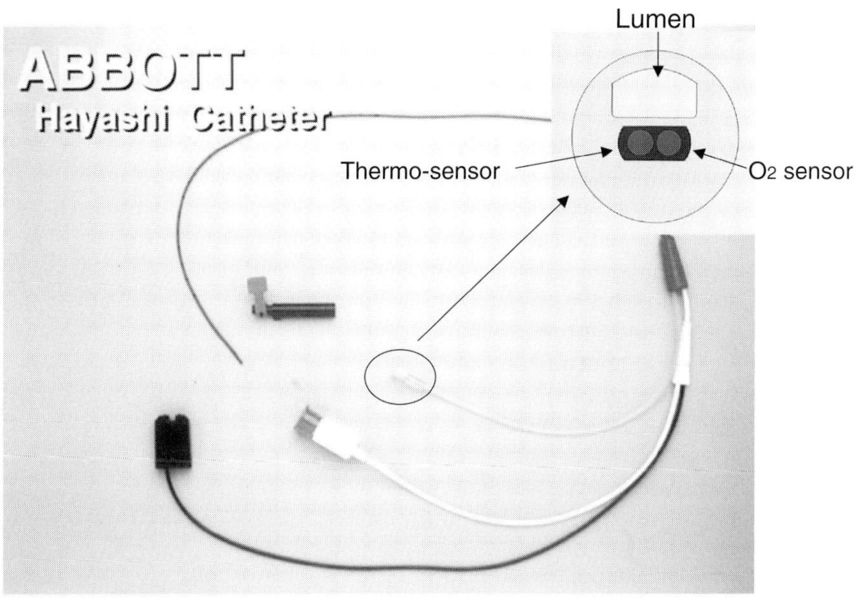

Fig. 73. Hayashi catheter (H-catheter) for monitoring jugular venous blood temperature and oxygen saturation

more correct brain tissue temperature. The dominant venous outflow side of the jugular vein is diagnosed from the higher ICP elevation after unilateral neck compression. Catheter tip position is another potential pitfall of monitoring the jugular venous blood temperature as an indicator of brain tissue temperature because the extracranial venous circulation flows into the internal jugular vain at high neck position.

The jugular venous blood oxygen saturation ($SjvO_2$) provides two points of information [20]. One concerns oxygen expenditure in the brain tissue and the other, the degree difficulty in the release of oxygen from binding hemoglobin. The measurement of low hemoglobin DPG suggests slow release of oxygen from binding hemoglobin and neuronal hypoxia despite normal PaO_2 and normal oxygen delivery. This phenomenon is known as masking neuronal hypoxia. Figure 74 shows the hemodynamic changes at the terminal stage of herniation caused by diffuse brain injury and bilateral subdural hematoma.

Requirements for Measurement of Jugular Venous Blood Temperature and Oxygen Saturation

H-catheter kit
Sterilization kit
Surgical cover sheets
Local anesthesia
Five-milliliter syringe and saline (20 ml)

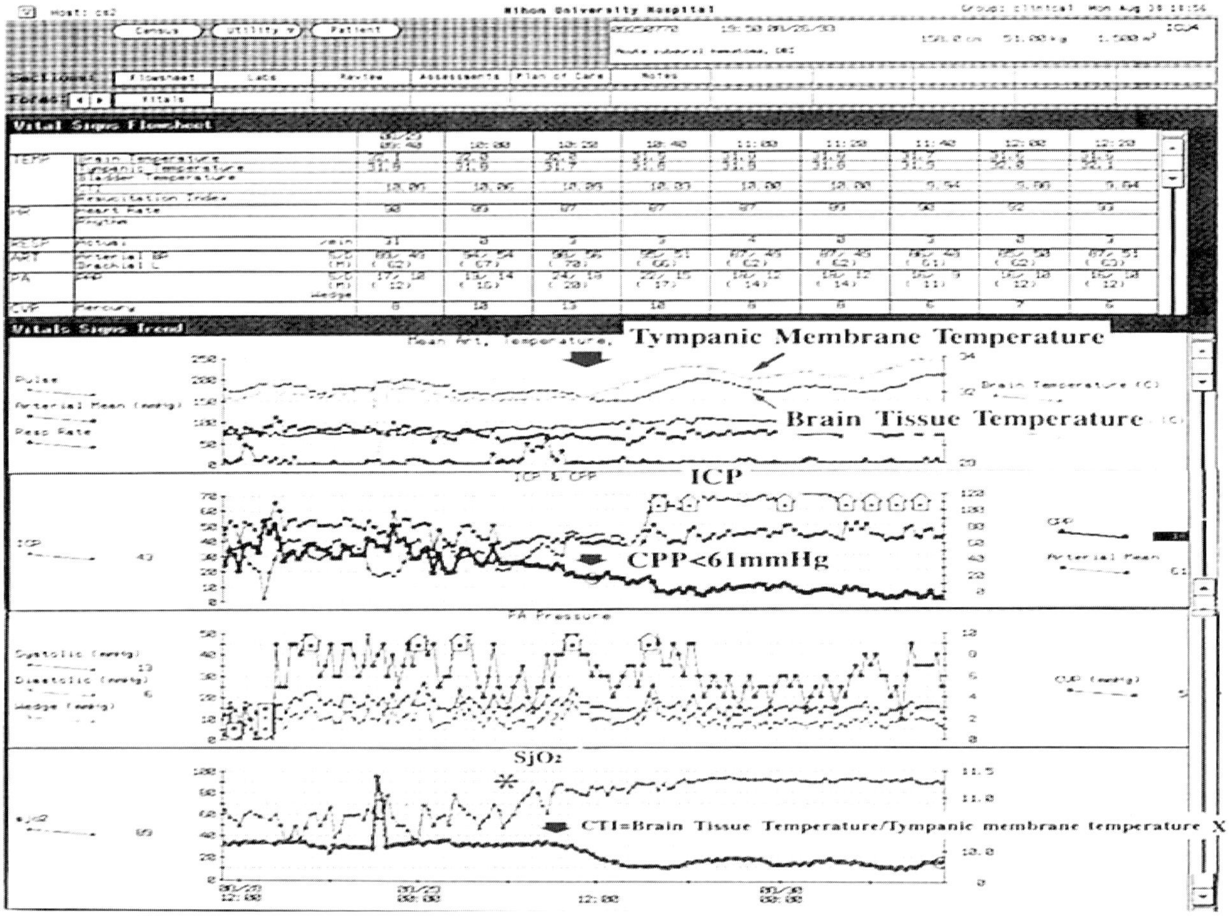

Fig. 74. The changes of jugular venous oxygen saturation (SjO_2) and jugular venous blood temperature (*brain tissue temperature*) at terminal stage of herniation in severe head injury

Five percent heparinized saline (500 ml)
Monitoring device

Technique of H-Catheter Insertion

Positioning of the neck is important for successful canulations. The patient's neck should be slightly extended and then the head turned about 45° away from the site of insertion. The entire neck, right and left supraclavicle areas, and the precodial region are disinfected with povidone iodine skin sterilization. The recommended insertion site is in the apex of the triangle formed by the sterna and clavicle heads of the sterno-cleido-mastoid muscle. Cannulation from this site is safer than from other sites because the line between the insertion site and the jugular bulb is straight and sufficiently long. A local anesthetic agent is administered to anesthetize the skin. A trial insertion is then performed. After insertion of the needle into the skin, carefully advance the needle with continuous aspiration force on the syringe. This trial insertion is performed using a 5-ml syringe with 23-gauge needle. A catheter needle is not required because the jugular vein can be reached by advancing the needle about 3 cm from the puncture site.

When back flushing of blood into the syringe is noticed, the direction and depth of the needle, and the color of the blood in the syringe should be confirmed to rule out erroneous penetration of an artery. After confirming successful penetration, the needle is removed with fingers and placed at the skin level to mark the depth of penetration. The main penetration is then performed using the introducer. The needle is advanced with aspiration of the syringe and a slight resistance will be felt when the needle tip meets the vein. After noticing back flushing of venous blood into the syringe, the needle should be advanced about 2 mm.

Correct positioning of the needle can be confirmed by pushing and pulling the plunger several times to obtain smooth flushing and withdrawal of venous blood. The inner needle is removed while keeping the outer needle steady with the remaining hand. After the guide wire of the H-catheter is inserted into the jugular vein through the sheath, the outer needle is removed to leave the guide wire in the jugular vein. A 2- to 3-mm skin incision is made surrounding the puncture site. An introducer with a 5 French sheath attached is advanced over the guide wire, and is inserted into the jugular vein by pushing and rotating the introducer. When the needle is pushed deep enough to attach it to the skin with the wing of the introducer, only the introducer is then removed to secure the sheath in the correct position.

The optical corner of the H-catheter is attached to the optical module, and pre-insertion calibration can be performed. After advancing the H-catheter into the jugular vein by about 17 cm, resistance against further advancement will be felt in many cases. When such resistance is felt, the H-catheter should be withdrawn about 5 mm. At this time, radiography should be performed to confirm the position of the catheter tip.

When the catheter tip has been successfully positioned into the jugular bulb, the tip will be between the external acoustic canal and the tip of the mamillary process in the lateral position. The catheter tip will be in the center of the eye socket on the frontal view. After confirming successful placement of the catheter tip, the light intensity of the catheter should be adjusted to within the normal range, and then the intensity calibration performed.

Brain Tissue Oxygen

Oxygenation of the injured brain has been evaluated by monitoring PaO_2, oxygen delivery, jugular venous oxygen saturation (SjO_2), and brain tissue oxygen. However, brain tissue oxygen tension was monitored as hemoglobin binding type tissue oxygen. The monitoring of pure free brain tissue oxygen tension has been technically difficult. However, recent technical development has produced the pure oxygen monitor for brain tissue from Licox (Integra NeuroSciences Plainsboro, NJ). In clinical studies with the Licox brain tissue oxygen monitor, brain tissue oxygen did not correlate to the changes in CPP [18] and SjO_2 [7,19]. Therefore, the reliability of devices for monitoring neuronal oxygenation in injured brain tissue is open to question. However, there is a simple explanation for why pure brain tissue oxygen tension does not correlate to changes in CPP and SjO_2. Hemoglobin dysfunction, observed as slow release of oxygen from binding hemoglobin caused by reduced DPG levels, occurs in severely brain-injured patients with HPA axis stress reactions [10]. Our clinical studies of changes in DPG levels during trauma (GCS < 6) and whole brain ischemia caused by cardiac arrest recorded high incidence of DPG reduction of 44% [10] and 70%, respectively, at 30–40 min after insult. These very important clinical issues are discussed in Chap. 33. The high values of SjO_2 means not only reduced neuronal oxygen consumption in the injured brain tissue, but also slow release of oxygen from binding hemoglobin. Therefore, direct monitoring of pure oxygen tension in injured brain tissue using the Licox system could be evaluated as a more reliable monitor than previous oxygen monitoring systems.

Microdialysis Monitor and Biochemical Cerebrospinal Fluid Monitor

The microdialysis monitor directly records changes in brain tissue metabolism and neurotoxic glutamate release in injured brain tissue [2,10,15,17]. The complications observed by CT and clinical worsening were not recorded by monitoring of microdialysis (Fig. 75). The changes in brain tissue glucose related to changes in serum glucose, brain tissue pyruvic acid, brain tissue lactate, and neuro-toxic glutamate analyses are shown in Fig. 76. This monitor is very powerful for confirmation of correct management.

However, the quality of the medical device is very important for monitoring microdialysis [10]. This is because during sampling, extracellular fluid in the brain

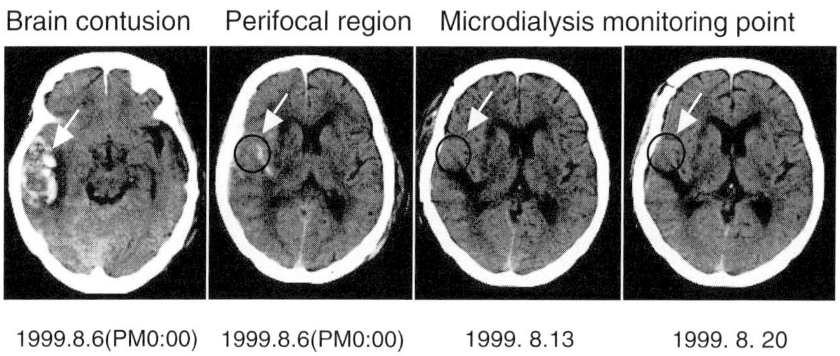

Fig. 75. Changes in computed tomography scans during monitoring of microdialysis in the intensive care unit. No brain tissue damage was recorded. Diameter of catheter: 0.15/1 mm, flow: 0.3 μl/min

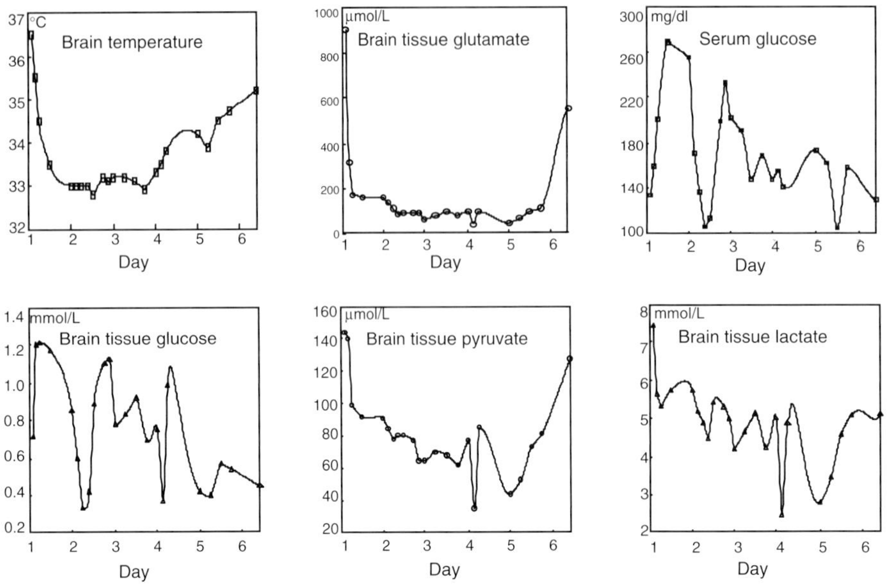

Fig. 76. The changes in brain tissue metabolites, including glutamate, following 33°C brain hypothermia. The level of neurotoxic glutamate is reduced by induction of brain hypothermia at 33°C

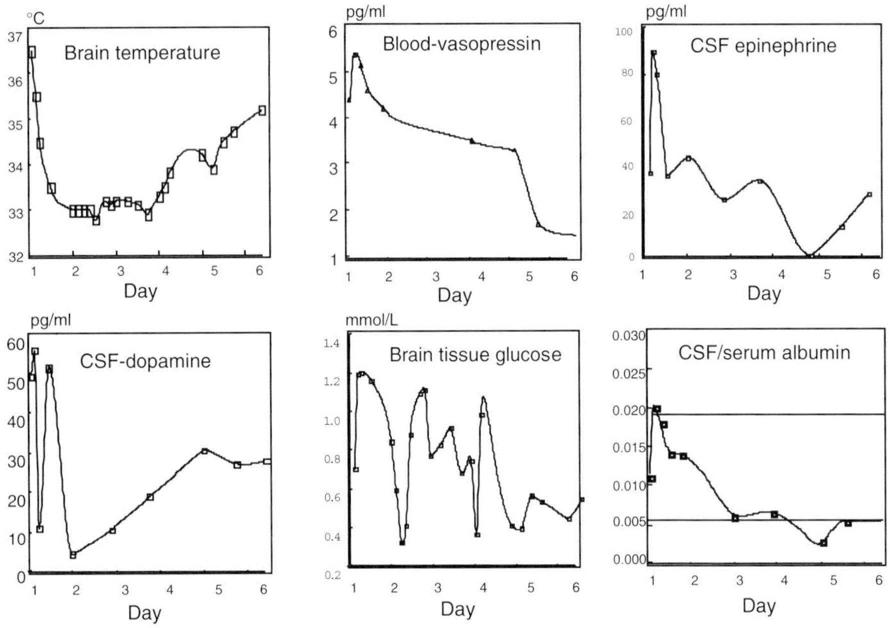

Fig. 77. Sequential changes of vasoactive neurohormones, metabolic substrates and blood–brain barrier function [evaluated with changes of cerebrospinal fluid (*CSF*)/serum albumin] following brain hypothermia treatment for traumatic brain injury

tissue is obtained by exchange with artificial CSF in the microdialysis catheter. The exchange speed of both fluids is decided by the permeability of the semi-permeable catheter tip membrane. The complication of brain edema occurs when monitoring microdialysis with a microdialysis catheter that does not use very limited fluid exchange. To prevent this complication, the permeable volume of the catheter tip membrane should be less than 10 μl/h. Therefore, without a high-quality micro-analyzer and small sampling, this study is difficult. At present, the CMA60/106 Microdialysis AB (Roslagsvagen, Stockholm, Sweden) is the only acceptable instrument (Fig. 57, Chap. 40).

The technique of setting the catheter is similar to that used in ICP monitoring. In this discussion, typical case studies of microdialysis monitoring, are useful.

A 62-year-old man suffering coma was admitted following a traffic accident. The diagnosis was bilateral diffuse brain injury, GCS 4 with brain stem herniation. At 2 h after brain injury, brain hypothermia treatment was induced (Fig. 77). The brain tissue temperature was controlled at 33°C for 4 days with oxygen delivery higher than 800 ml/min. The excess release of glutamate was completely blocked by brain hypothermia for 6 days. No increase in brain tissue lactate was recorded during this management [11].

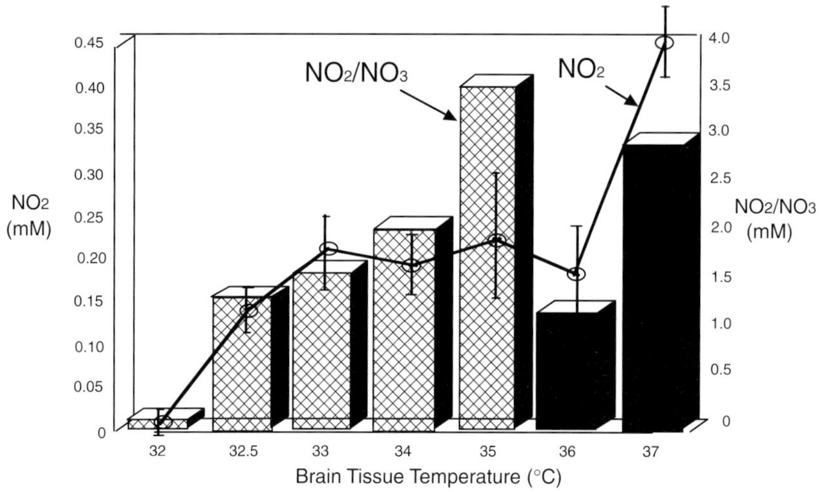

Fig. 78. Brain hypothermia is effective in reducing ·NO radicals. Brain hypothermia at 32°–33°C is more effective in controlling radical reactions that 34°C. $n = 8$

Biochemical monitoring of CSF/serum albumin ratio, CSF dopamine/prolactin ratio, and serum glucose are very effective to indirectly analyze the BBB function, the possibility of vegetation, and the severity of stress reactions [9–11]. Albumin is a high molecular weight protein such that it is difficult for it to permeate the normal BBB. The CSF/serum albumin ratio is less than 0.007 in normal patients; however, CSF/serum albumin ratio higher than 0.007 suggests BBB dysfunction. Our clinical studies suggest that a ratio higher than 0.01 causes increases in brain tissue glutamate and systemic infection. Severe BBB dysfunction, with a CSF/serum albumin ratio of more than 0.02, produced uncontrollable increases of neurotoxic glutamate even with 33°C brain hypothermia management. In this patient, CSF/serum albumin ratio of 0.01–0.02 (moderate BBB dysfunction) continued for 2 days and was recovered at 3 days by replacement of albumin, AT-III, and immune activation as shown in Fig. 77.

The release of intracerebral dopamine following severe brain damage produces·OH^- radicals and suppresses the production of prolactin during the acute stage. From experimental studies, the mechanism of ·NO radical production is understood to be the reaction of brain tissue oxygen with dopamine (Fig. 33, Chap. 26). These radical formations caused by dopamine release suggest that selective dopamine nervous system by radical attack. The early induction brain hypothermia to temperatures lower than 34°C is successful in preventing the release of cerebral dopamine. This is the main reason why early induction of brain hypothermia treatment is recommended.

The precise management of hyperglycemia at the induction stage and the early cooling stages of brain hypothermia is especially important. Because of not only increase brain tissue lactate, hemoglobin dysfunction which caused by reduction of hemoglobin DPG, increasing vasopressin release, and also difficult to induce the 32–33°C moderate brain hypothermia for prevent of NO radical production. The systemic·NO radical reaction is also evaluated by monitoring the NO_2/NO_3 ratio and $NO_2 + NO_3$ (Fig. 78) [13].

References

1. Almeida A, Delgado-Esteban M, Bolanos JP, Medina JM (2002) Oxygen and glucose deprivation induces mitochondrial dysfunction and oxidative stress in neurones but not in astrocytes in primary culture. Neurochem 81:207–217
2. Binnert C, Tappy L (2002) Microdialysis in the intensive care unit: a novel tool for clinical investigation or monitoring? Curr Opin Clin Nutr Metab Care 5:185–188
3. Birman H, Haq A, Hew E, Aberman A (1984) Continuous monitoring of mixed venous oxygen saturation in hemodynamically unstable patients. Chest 86:753–756
4. Chiolero R, Lemarchand TH, Schutz Y, de Tribolet N, Felber JP, Freeman J, Jequier E (1988) Plasma pituitary hormone levels in severe trauma with or without head injury. J Trauma 28:1368–1374
5. Corte FD, Mancini A, Valle D, Gallizzi F, Carducci P, Mignani V, De Marinis L (1998) Provocative hypotha-lamopituitary axis tests in severe head injury: correlation with severity and prognosis. Crit Care Med 26:1419–1426
6. Feng H, Huang G, Gao L, Tan H, Liao X (2000) Effect of intracranial pressure and cerebral perfusion pressure on outcome prediction of severe traumatic brain injury. Chin J Traumatol 3:226–230
7. Filippi R, Reisch R, Mauer D, Perneczky A (2000) Brain tissue pO_2 related to $SjvO_2$, ICP, and CPP in severe brain injury. Neurosurg Rev 23:94–97

8. Gussak I, Chaitman BR, Kopecky SL, Nerbonne JM (2000) Rapid ventricular repolarization in rodents: electrocardiographic manifestations, molecular mechanisms, and clinical insights. J Electrocardiol 33:159–170
9. Hayashi N (1995) Cerebral hypothermia treatment. In: Hayashi N (ed) Cerebral hypothermia treatment. Sogo Igaku, Tokyo, pp 1–105
10. Hayashi N (2000) Enhanced neuronal damage in severely brain injured patients by hypothalamus, pituitary, and adrenal axis neuro-hormonal changes. In: Hayashi N (ed) Brain hypothermia. Springer, Berlin Heidelberg New York Tokyo, pp 3–26
11. Hayashi N (2000) The clinical issue and effectiveness of brain hypothermia treatment for severe brain injured patients. In: Hayashi N (ed) Brain hypothermia. Springer, Berlin Heidelberg New York Tokyo, pp 121–151
12. Hayashi N, Hirayama T, Utagawa T, Ohata M (1994) Systemic management of cerebral edema based on a new concept in severe head injury patients. Acta Neurochir [Suppl] 60:541–543
13. Hayashi N, Utagawa A, Kinosita K, Izumi T (1999) Application of a novel technique for clinical evaluation of nitric oxide-induced free radiacal reactions in ICU patients. Cell Molec Neurobiol 19:3–17
14. MaClain CJ, Henning B, Ott L, Goldblum S, Young AB (1988) Mechanisms and implications of hypoalbuminemia in head-injured patients. J Neurosurg 69:386–392
15. Nilsson OG, Saveland H, Boris-Moller F, Brandt L, Wieloch T (1996) Increased levels of glutamate in patients with subarachnoid haemorrhage as measured by intracerebral microdialysis. Acta Neurochir [Suppl] 67:45–47
16. Pool JL, Kessler L (1958) Mechanism and control of centrally induced cardiac irregularities during hypothermia. J Neurosurg 15:52–63
17. Rothman SM (1984) Synaptic release of excitatory amino acid neurotransmitter mediates anoxic neuronal death. J Neurosci 4:1884–1891
18. Sahuquillo J, Amoros S, Santos A (2000) Does an increase in cerebral perfusion pressure always mean a better oxygenated brain? A study in head-injured patients. Acta Neurochir [Suppl] 76:457–462
19. Sarrafzadeh AS, Kiening KL, Bardt TF, Schneider GH, Unterberg AW, Lanksch WR (1998) Cerebral oxygenation in contusioned vs. nonlesioned brain tissue: monitoring of PtiO2 with Licox and Paratrend. Acta Neurochir [Suppl] 71:186–189
20. Sheinberg M, Kanter MJ, Robertson CS, Contant CF, Narayan RK, Grossman RGI (1992) Continuous monitoring of jugular venous oxygen saturation in head-injury patients. J Neurosurg 76:212–217
21. Suarez JI (2001) Treatment of acute brain edema. Rev Neurol 32:275–281
22. Vassallo SU, Delaney KA, Hoffman RS, Slater W, Goldfrank LR (1999) A prospective evaluation of the electrocardiographic manifestations of hypothermia. Acad Emerg Med 6:1121–1126

43. Induction of Brain Hypothermia Treatment

Mild brain hypothermia treatment (34°C) is indicated in patients with a Glasgow Coma Scalescore (GCS) of 8 or less, serum glucose concentration less than 230 mg/dl, and no clinical signs of herniation. The duration is variable at 3–7 days, and brain hypothermia should be started within 3 h after insult (Fig. 28, Chap. 23). Moderate brain hypothermia (32°–33°C) is indicated in patients with a GCS of 6 or less, and serum glucose concentration less than 180 mg/dl. The duration is variable at 4–14 days. Early brain hypothermia treatment is indicated for the prevention of vegetation. A flat electroencephalogram (EEG) and no response of the auditory brain stem evoked potential (ABER), breathing arrest, and pupil dilatation are not signs of contraindication at admission (Fig. 79). This is because, despite the disappearance of cell membrane potentials shortly after brain damage, many neuronal cells remain alive. However, these critical signs suggest the contraindication of brain hypothermia treatment 3–6 h after brain trauma and stroke.

Control of brain tissue temperature using the cold water blanket technique to reduce the systemic blood temperature is a fundamental technique [2–5]. Selective cooling of the head and neck produce insufficient lowering of brain tissue temperature and cause uncontrollable brain tissue temperature elevation at the rewarming stage. This is because warmed systemic blood passes through the entire brain after selective cooling of the head and neck is stopped. The rapid cerebral circulation with warmed blood produces a rebounding elevation of brain tissue temperature. This unsuitable management of brain tissue temperature also produces vascular engorgement and acute brain swelling. Figure 45 (Chap. 35) shows the concept of brain cooling using the blanket technique [2,3,5] (modified Blanketrol II, Cincinnati Sub-Zero and Medivance, Louisville, CO, USA).

Preliminary Refrigeration and Use of the Cooling Blanket

The preliminary cooling of blanket water before induction of brain hypothermia saves time during brain hypothermia treatment. Disinfected, chilled saline (15°–20°C) perfuses and cools the blanket. The patient is rested on the cooled blanket covered by a dry towel, and the management of vital signs is commenced and the required monitoring instrumentation is set up as described in Chap. 35. The cooling blanket technique is summarized in the following discussion.

The patient is positioned on the precooled blanket and is covered with a dry towel and a second cooling blanket. The patient and the cooling blankets are then wrapped completely with a large dry towel. It is essential that the body be insulated from room temperature to stabilize brain tissue temperature. If the patient weighs more than 80 kg, the cooling system should be separated into ventral and dorsal circulation by using two cooling machines [2].

After stabilization of vital signs and addressing the basic parameters for maintaining brain function, the cooling device should be set at 10°–15°C for brain hypothermia treatment. Two techniques for management of the chilled water temperature are useful. The water temperature can be set at 26°–27°C after bed rest with monitoring of brain temperature (or tympanic membrane temperature). When the brain tissue temperature reaches 34.5°C, the blanket water temperature is reduced to 20°–23°C. Brain hypothermia can be stabilized at around 34°C within at 2–3 h. This cooling technique is described in Fig. 44 (Chap. 35) [2,5]. As an alternative, the blanket water temperature can be cycled dynamically between 0° and 30°C, and the cooling cycle repeated three to four times as shown in Fig. 47 (Chap. 35). Careful control of the device used to monitor brain tissue temperature or jugular venous blood temperature is important.

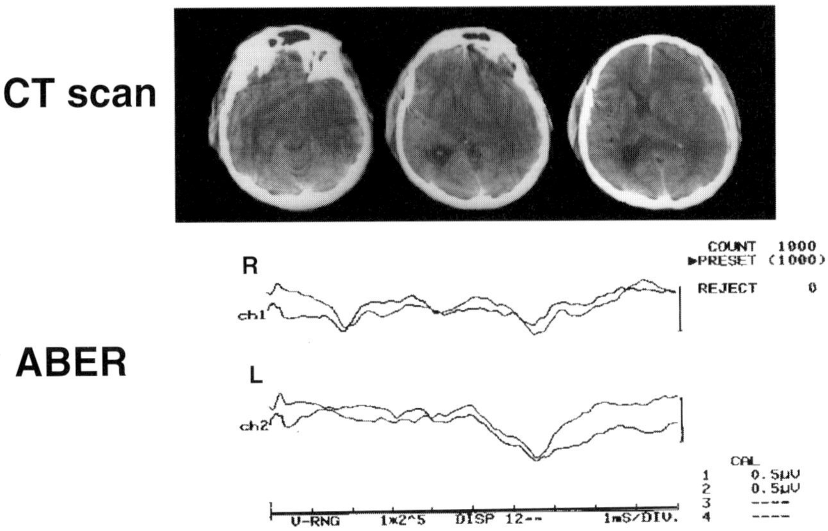

Fig. 79. Alteration of computed tomography (CT) scan and ABER (Glasgow Coma Scale score 4)

The Time Schedule for Management of Brain Tissue Temperature

Mild Brain Hypothermia Management (~34°C)

Brain tissue temperature can be rapidly brought to 34°C while under the control of anesthesia, analgesia, and muscle relaxants. The cooling duration is about 3–7 days depending on the reversibility of the brain injury. Forty-eight hours of brain hypothermia is not sufficient for the prevention of brain edema in severely brain-injured patients. With such short-duration treatment, it is difficult for recovery from severe brain damage to occur and is limited to preventing worsening of secondary brain injury mechanisms. Such short-duration brain hypothermia results in reprogression of brain injury mechanism during the rewarming stage. As a result, reprogression of the brain injury mechanism during the rewarming stage is worsened by rapidly increasing glucose and oxygen consumption, vascular engorgement, and activation of inflammatory cytokines. The criteria for rewarming are discussed in Chap. 45.

Moderate Brain Hypothermia Management (32°–33°C)

Brain tissue temperature is rapidly reduced to 34°C while under the control of anesthesia, analgesia, and muscle relaxants. At 34°C, further brain cooling is halted to allow stabilization of vital signs, control of hyperglycemia, management of abnormal electrocardiogram (ECG), and replacement of serum albumin and antithrombin-III (AT-III). Brain hypothermia is then carefully resumed to achieve moderate brain hypothermia (32°–33°C) over a period of about 5–6h. This is because progressive reduction of hypothalamus-pituitary-adrenal (HPA) neuronal hormones and systemic metabolic shift from glucose to lipid occur at brain tissue temperatures below 34°C. To allow adaptation to these stressful body changes, time is important. As a technique of brain hypothermia induction, the two-step induction with rapid cooling to 34°C and slow induction to 33°–32°C is recommended [2,3,5]. The time schedule for the control of saline temperature in the cooling device is described earlier and is shown in Figs. 46, 47 (Chap. 35).

Serious complications may arise during the second stage of cooling to moderate brain hypothermia, including cardiac arrhythmia, hypokalemia, elongation of the QT interval to greater than 450mm/s on the ECG, and hyperglycemia with serum glucose levels above 180mg/dl [2]. In such cases, further cooling should be stopped and warning signs immediately addressed.

By reducing the body temperature, consumption of tissue glucose is dramatically reduced, and especially so at brain tissue temperature lower than 34°C. In that time, the serum glucose level increases abruptly, as do levels of brain tissue glucose and lactate. Microdialysis studies suggest that management of mild brain hypothermia is preferable to moderate brain hypothermia with hyperglycemia. Therefore, careful management of serum hyperglycemia is very important at the induction stage. The rapid induction of brain hypothermia without management of hyperglycemia is a major pitfall of brain hypothermia treatment.

Fundamental Care Management of Systemic Circulation and Oxygen Metabolism

The most important care management consideration during the induction stage is neuronal oxygenation and adequate administration of metabolic substrates in the injured brain tissue. To ensure that these requirements are met, stable systemic circulation, good brain circulation, and sufficient pulmonary oxygen uptake are necessary. To maintain stable systemic circulation and pulmonary oxygen uptake, dehydration management for the prevention of brain edema at the induction stage is not recommended [2,5–7]. This is because serum catecholamine levels decrease with lower brain tissue temperature, and of the difficulty maintaining stable systemic circulation with hypothermia and dehydration management. The early administration of high osmotic solution such as manitol and glycerol to prevent brain edema destabilizes systemic circulation, cerebral microcirculation, and oxygen metabolism. Therefore, normovolemic fluid therapy is the preferred care management therapy during induction time.

About 3h after brain injury, dopamine-dominant systemic circulation occurs [4]. The negative effect of dopamine-dominant systemic circulation is accumulation of blood in the intestinal organs and a reduction in cerebral perfusion pressure (CPP). The administration of dopamine to maintain blood pressure 3h after brain injury accelerates these negative events. Dopamine administration after 3h is not recommended.

Normovolemic fluid resuscitation, maintenance of cardiac function by administration of doputorex, potassium phosphate, and magnesium, elastic bandaging of extremities to retain perfusion pressure to major organs (Fig. 59, Chap. 42), and adequate selection of hypertensive are important care management considerations. Within 1 hour of brain injury, for a short duration, epinephrine or vasopressin is recommended in cases without severe hyperglycemia. At 1–3h after brain injury, epinephrine and norepinephreine combined with doptorex are recommended for the maintenance of blood pressure. However, prolonged administration of this treatment induces adenosine triphosphate (ATP) crisis in major organs and insulin-resistant hyperglycemia. Prolonged administration of vasopressin also causes blood–brain barrier (BBB) dysfunction, increases brain tissue glucose levels, and promotes pulmonary edema. From 6h after trauma and ischemic insults, however, fluid resuscitation with small hypertensive medication is fundamental. To support these clinical issues, early insertion of a balloon catheter into the abdominal aorta is useful for maintaining the carotid and coronal artery circulation. Temporary and partial occlusion of the abdominal blood flow by balloon catheter (Fig. 31, Chap. 26) may be very successful for maintaining stable cardiopulmonary function and neuronal restoration of dying neurons during the acute stage. Management of serum hypophosphate at 3–4mg/dl, serum pH above 7.3, serum glucose at 120–140mg/dl, AT-III above 100%, and albumin above 3.0g/dl are also important for maintaining the stable systemic circulation and oxygen metabolism.

Management of Cardiopulmonary Function Without Swan Ganz Catheter

The management of cardiopulmonary function with monitoring of cardiac output (CO), cardiac index, and oxygen extraction ratio is very successful in severely brain-injured patients undergoing brain hypothermia treatment. The Swan Ganz Catheter technique is routinely introduced in intensive care unit (ICU) management. However, this invasive technique is not always available because of many reasons, such as insufficient time for rapidly worsening patients, unavailability of trained staff, and lack of monitoring systems at the bedside to analyze the CO. Similarly, in these severely brain-injured patients, normal management of blood pressure, PaO_2, intracranial pressure (ICP), and CPP is not always effective without maintenance of oxygen delivery higher than 700–800ml/min, control of stress-associated hyperglycemia, and management of hemoglobin dysfunction. The precise management of oxygen delivery and administration of suitable metabolic substrates are especially important at the initial stage.

Our method for the management of CO of more than 700–800ml/min without the Swan Ganz catheter technique is described.

The end tidal CO_2 ($ETCO_2$) increases in proportion with increasing CO and $PvCO_2$. The oxygen delivery ($\bar{D}O_2$) also increases in proportion with CO, Hb, and SaO_2. $PvCO_2$ is very similar to $PaCO_2$ and the relationship between of $ETCO_2$ and $PaCO_2$ for maintaining oxygen delivery higher than 700ml/min is presented in Fig. 21 (Chap 22). The relationship between $ETCO_2$ and $PaCO_2$ changes depending on the alveolar permeability (K). Therefore, simultaneous monitoring of $ETCO_2$ and $PaCO_2$ can allow diagnosis of the correct ICU management technique, means to deliver sufficient oxygen and CO.

During brain hypothermia treatment, control of $PaCO_2$ slightly higher than normal $PaCO_2$ at about 34–38 mmHg is recommended for the control of ICP. This is because under the condition of hypothermia, real $PaCO_2$ is calibrated at a lower level. Therefore, to maintain oxygen delivery at more than 800 ml/min, $ETCO_2$ must be controlled between 32 and 38 mmHg. In cases of pulmonary dysfunction with increased alveolar permeability, $K = 0.19$, and high values of $PaCO_2$, $ETCO_2$ must also be controlled at high levels at around 38 mmHg. The actual management of $ETCO_2$ at 32–38 mmHg, $PaCO_2$ between 34 and 38 mmHg, hemoglobin higher than 11–12 g/dl, and SaO_2 higher than 98% are management goals to ensure oxygen delivery higher than 800 ml/min without the Swan Ganz catheter technique [2].

Management of Neuronal Oxygenation

The management of neuronal oxygenation is the most important ICU issue at the induction stage of brain hypothermia treatment. Neuronal restoration therapy is more important than the previous concept that neuroprotection therapy should be an initial treatment of brain hypothermia treatment. Administration of sufficient oxygen and adequate metabolic substrates to the dying neurons in injured brain tissue in conjunction with neurohormonal control at 32°–34°C brain tissue temperature is a basic management concept. Neuroprotection achieved by reducing oxygen demand, hypometabolism, and prevention of brain edema cannot restore dying neurons in injured brain tissue. The control of ICP, cerebral blood flow (CBF), and PaO_2 to normal levels with normal oxygen delivery is not sufficient initial treatment for severely brain-injured patients. Slow release of bound oxygen from hemoglobin and ineffective oxygen inhalation is caused by reduced hemoglobin 2,3-diphosphoglycerate (DPG) levels associated with severe acidosis, pH lower than 7.2, hyperglycemia with serum glucose level above 230 mg/dl, and preserved blood transfusion. Furthermore, elevated brain tissue temperature activates the demand for oxygen and glucose in injured neurons. Therefore, as an initial treatment of neuronal oxygenation, detailed and novel ICU management techniques are required.

A checklist for management of neuronal oxygenation in injured brain tissue is summarized as follows: PaO_2/FiO_2 ratio >350, serum glucose 120–140 mg/dl, $\bar{D}O_2 > 700$–800 ml/min, serum pH > 7.3, hemoglobin-DPG 12–15 μg/dl, CPP > 80 mmHg, systolic blood pressure (SBP) > 100 mmHg, and tympanic membrane temperature should be greater than bladder temperature [5].

Management of Metabolic Substrates and Hyperglycemia for Injured Brain Tissue

Adequate administration of glucose is one of the most difficult aspects of initial management of brain hypothermia treatment. In severely brain-injured patients, insulin-resistant hyperglycemia is unavoidable because of neurohormonal stress reactions such as catecholamine surge and adranocorticotropic hormore (ACTH) release. Stress-associated hyperglycemia that is difficult to control at the acute stage includes extensive pathophysiological background [4]. Epinephrine reduces the serum insulin level and simultaneously metabolizes ATP and glycogen into glucose. Harmful stress-associated vasopressin and ACTH release also occur and reduce the sensitivity of insulin [1,2,4,9,10,13,14]. The liver and skeletal muscle are sites of significant consumption of serum glucose and help to normalize the hyperglycemia. The activation of the hypothalamus–pituitary–adrenal (HPA) axis promotes the release of alanine and glutamine from skeletal muscles. These metabolic changes in the skeletal muscles make control of hyperglycemia difficult and can easily introduce the complication of immune dysfunction. All severely brain-injured patients with HPA-axis neurohormonal dysfunction exhibit insulin-resistant hyperglycemia that is very difficult to control [9,10,13,14]. Severe hyperglycemia with serum glucose levels above 230 mg/dl produces the complication of marked increases of brain tissue glucose and lactate [4]. The vasoconstrictive hormone, vasopressin, is also released by the feedback mechanism of neural control of macronutrient hyperglycemia [2]. Vasopressin is a very strong vasoconstrictor of arterioles. This reaction can easily result in the complications of pulmonary edema, systemic microcirculatory disturbance, and brain edema. Therefore, hyperglycemia during the acute stage is a very dangerous condition.

In brain hypothermia treatment, there is a time limit for the management of hyperglycemia. This is because at brain tissue temperatures lower than 34°C, the decreased consumption of serum glucose caused by the metabolic shift from glucose to lipid metabolism results in increased serum glucose (Fig. 80). Therefore, the control of serum hyperglycemia must be achieved before the induction of moderate brain hypothermia

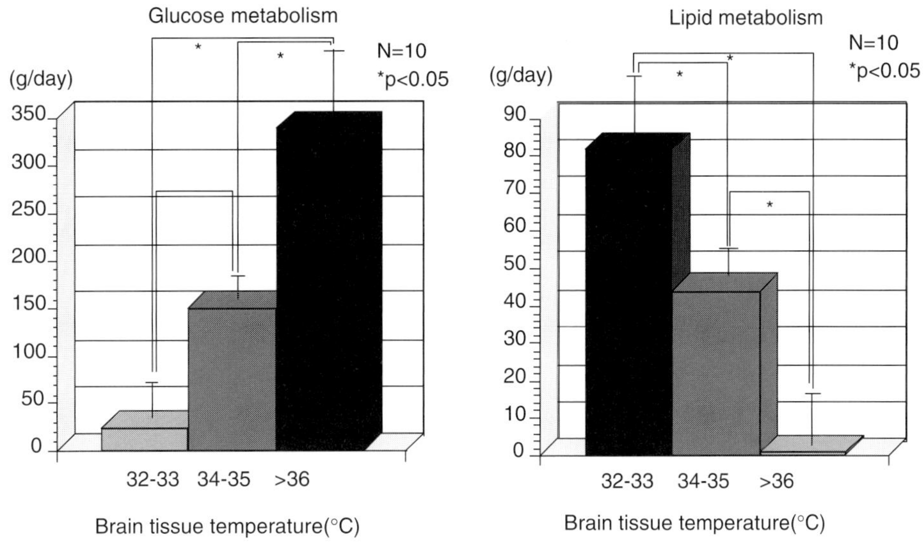

Fig. 80. The metabolic shift from glucose to lipid following induction of brain hypothermia

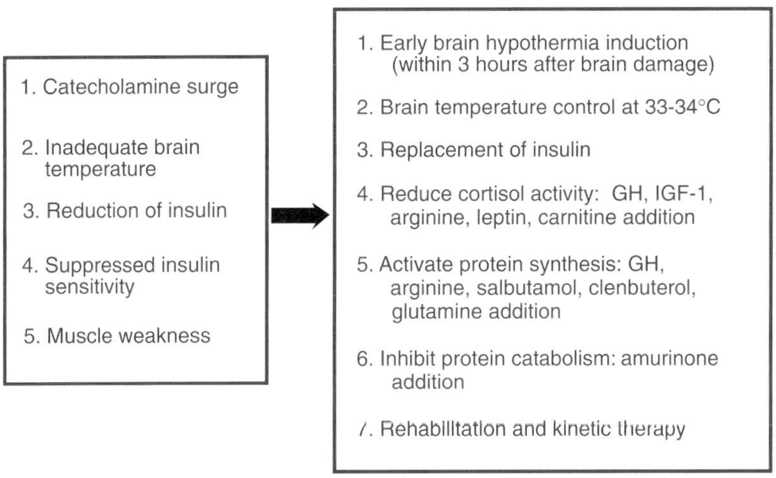

Fig. 81. The management of hyperglycemia associated with severe brain injury. *GH*, growth hormone; *IGF-1*, insulin like growth factor-1

(32°–33°C). Our clinical studies of brain hypothermia treatment suggested that without control of serum glucose to between 120 and 140 mg/dl, brain tissue glucose increases significantly due to reduced serum glucose consumption and the metabolic shift from glucose to lipid metabolism at brain tissue temperature less than 34°C.

The circumstances of hyperglycemia are different for mild and moderate brain hypothermia. In mild brain hypothermia, hyperglycemia is produced by catecholamine surge; however, hyperglycemia in moderate brain hypothermia is produced by combination of catecholamine surge and a reduction of glucose expenditure.

As a management strategy, early induction of brain hypothermia within 3 h after brain injury is the most successful for preventing catecholamine surge; Brain hypothermia at about 33°–34°C is effective in reducing serum catecholamines by about 70%; however, rapid induction of moderate brain hypothermia produces unstable systemic circulation because of an excess reduction of serum catecholamines [2,4]. Catecholamine surge lowers the release of serum insulin, and therefore, in most cases of severe brain injury, the serum insulin level is very low. For management of stress-associated hyperglycemia, more insulin administration is necessary than for ordinary diabetic patients.

As a pharmacological treatment, recommended steps include administration of insulin to activate the uptake of serum glucose into the skeletal muscles, administration of growth hormone and arginine to increase insulin sensitivity and increase uptake of serum glucose into the muscles, and administration of amurinone to stabilize the muscle function by inhibiting protein catabolism. Muscle massage and kinetic therapy are also effective for the control of catecholamine surge-associated hyperglycemia (Fig. 81).

Table 16. Fluid resuscitation for severe brain damage

5% Albumin, 7% acetic Ringer + 650 mg acetaminophen	
prevention of BBB dysfunction, hyperglycemia, and hyperthermia	
Triple H therapy	
Hemodilusion	$\bar{D}O_2 > 700$ ml/min, CI > 4 ml/min m^{-2}
Hypervolemia	No brain edema or pulmonary edema
Hypertension	Mean ABP > 80 mmHg
Prevention of brain edema	
Manitol	
Serum albumin > 3.5 mg/dl	
Glycerol ←	serum glucose > 140 mg/dl
no indication	brain temperature < 33°C

BBB, blood–brain barrier; DO_2, oxygen delivery; CI, cardiac index; ABP, arterial blood pressure

Fluid Resuscitation at Induction Stage

Fluid resuscitation during brain hypothermia treatment is very important. This is because dehydration produces unstable systemic circulation caused by reduced serum catecholamines with hypothermia. Normovolemic fluid resuscitation is fundamental care management.

Concerning the content of fluid resuscitation, low-glucose content fluid is necessary. This is because stress-associated hyperglycemia is unavoidable and produces hemoglobin dysfunction, promotes BBB dysfunction by vasopressin release, activates brain tissue acidosis by increasing the brain tissue lactate level, and activates proinflammatory cytokines by a macronutrient feedback mechanism. Therefore, glucose-free fluid resuscitation such as 7% acetic Ringer solution, Veen F, or Salin Hess solution are preferred at the induction stage, except in cases of hypoglycemia.

The replacement of potassium phosphate, vitamin A, vitamin B, Mg^{++}, 5% albumin, and AT-III are recommended as part of of fluid resuscitation at the induction stage. Potassium phosphate is a source of ATP production in oxygen carrier hemoglobin and neurons in injured brain tissue. Most phosphate is stabilized by inorganic type combined with lipid; therefore, vitamin A is also required to stabilize lipid metabolism at brain tissue temperature below 34°C [5,12]. Magnesium chloride combined with potassium phosphate is also important to prevent respiratory muscle weakness. Respiratory muscle weakness is a very dangerous complication because of reduced adaptation to prolonged hypoxia, induction of pulmonary atelectasis, and ease of severe pulmonary infection. Vitamin B is necessary to prevent epileptic seizure after severe brain injury. The replacement of serum albumin is very successful for the prevention of brain edema, the maintenance of immune function by prevention of intestinal mucosa edema, the stabilization of antibiotic function, and the suppression of proinflammatory cytokines. Anti-thrombin-III prevents micro-embolus and disturbances of microcirculation in the brain, lungs, heart, and intestinal organs. We prefer the control of serum glucose at 120–140 mg/dl, serum phosphate at 3–4 mg/dl, serum magnesium at 1.4–2.0 mEq/l, vitamin A at 50–100 µg/dl, AT-III greater than 100%, and serum pH greater than 7.3 for prevention of these complications.

Pharmacological Management for Neuroprotection

Management of Microcirculation and Vascular Inflammation

The brain is a prothrombin-rich organ, and therefore, in injured brain tissue, thrombin is easily released and protects against more bleeding in the lesions. However, thrombin is one of the sources of micro-embolus formation. AT-III neutralizes these excess reactions in the injured brain and protects against disturbances of microcirculation. The reduction of AT-III level suggests not only the severity of brain tissue damage but also the consumption of AT-III in preventing micro-embolus formation and disturbances of microcirculation [4]. The dangerous condition of systemic disturbance of microcirculation is diagnosed by reduced level of AT-III. The intestinal mucous membrane is very sensitive to ischemia and disturbance of microcirculation. These secondary patho-physiological changes and intestinal organ ischemia can be diagnosed by monitoring the gastric mucous membrane pH (gastric pHi) using the tonometer method. Less than 80% of AT-III and gastric pHi lower than 7.3 suggests the complication of systemic disturbance of microcirculation in severely brain-injured patients.

The management of AT-III above 100% by replacement of AT-III is recommended during brain hypothermia treatment to prevent disturbances of microcirculation in the brain and the nutritional supporting intestinal organs. Another pharmacological intervention of AT-III has been reported as an anti-inflammatory for vascular endothelium. Recent basic research suggested that the combination of AT-III and low molecular weight heparin is very effective in preventing vascular inflammation and the development of disseminated intravascular coagulations (DIC). Triple H-therapy is widely used for preventing disturbances of cerebral microcirculation (Table 17).

Anti-Ca^{++} and Management of Serum Magnesium

Changes in calcium ion level plays a major role in neuronal degeneration following damage to the central nervous system. Other studies have suggested that changes in calcium ion homeostasis underlie delayed neuronal cell death, brain engorgement, and vasospasm following experimentally induced intraparenchymal and subarachnoid hemorrhage, and plays a role in neuronal death associated with cerebral ischemia.

As pharmacological interventions, two types of anti-Ca^{++} have been reported. One is the use of calcium channel inhibitors (Nimodipine, Celestat, and Selfotel) and the other is the use of calcium channel modulators (ACEA-1021, and ZD9379) as shown in Table 18. Anti-calcium medicines are regulators of Ca^{++} channels in cell membranes and intracellular homoeostasis. To stabilize Ca^{++} channels, Mg^{++} ion channels must be stabilized with sufficient ATP. Therefore, for clinical management, combination of anti-calcium medicines, administration of magnesium, a source of ATP production, and sufficient oxygenation are important during brain hypothermia treatment.

Magnesium is considered to be a regulator of calcium channels in cell membranes in the brain and heart. Recent animal studies suggested that maintenance of magnesium ion homeostasis is extremely important for bio-energetic and metabolic function. Magnesium in the brain is involved in a number of critical cellular processes including glycolysis and oxidative phosphorylation, cellular respiration, and synthesis of DNA, RNA, and protein. Magnesium is mandatory for all enzyme reactions that involve ATP. The presence of magnesium is also essential for mitochondrial and plasma membrane integrity. Recent experimental studies suggested that the total tissue magnesium concentration increases acutely in the injury site at 10 min postinjury and then falls precipitously to remain significantly depressed for up to 24 h after injury. These changes in magnesium levels were directly correlated with the severity of the injury and the outcome. Magnesium is not only essential in the brain, but also for the maintenance of protein metabolism in the respiratory and skeletal muscles. The muscle is very important for stabilization of harmful stress-associated hyperglycemia and for the prevention of immune dysfunction by acting as an energy source for immune cells during brain hypothermia treatment.

In the management of these complications during neuronal restoration, adequate muscle function to prevent infection and maintain hemoglobin function for neuronal oxygenation, and combined administration of magnesium chloride and potassium phosphate are important. The management of serum magnesium at 1.6 ± 0.20 mEq/l and serum phosphate at 3–4 mg/dl is the initial target at the acute stage. A low magnesium level is easily diagnosed when urine magnesium is reduced by 2 mEq/day. The serum phosphate level increases at the acute stage after severe brain damage, however, rapid reduction of serum phosphate level occurs during the cooling stage in most cases.

Table 17. Indication of triple H therapy

Triple H therapy	Indication
Hemodilusion	$\bar{D}O_2 > 700$ ml/min
Hypervolemia	No brain edema or pulmonary edema
Hypertonic saline	No hypernatoremia and pH > 7.3

Table 18. Current status of various neuroprotective agents

Class	Mechanism	Medications	Status
Ca channel inhibitors	Voltage sensitive Ca channel antagonists	Nimodipine	Phase III
	Noncompetitive NMDA antagonist	CNS1102 (Cerestst)	Phase III
	Competitive NMDA antagonist	CGS-19755 (Selfotel)	Phase III
Ca channel modulators	Glycine site antagonists	ACEA-1021	Phase II
		ZD9379	Phase II
Presynaptic glutamate inhibition	Presynaptic voltage sensitive	BW19C89	Phase II
	Sodium channel antagonists	Fos-phenytoin	Phase III
	Unclear mechanism	Lubeluzole	Phase III
Other ion channels	AMPA receptor antagonists	NBQX	Phase II
	Plasma membrane abuse-dependent antagonism	Monogangliosides	Phase III
Agents directed against delayed effects of ischemia	Lipid peroxidation inhibitor	Tirilizad	Phase III
	Anti-adhesive molecules	CD11b/18	Phase II
		ICAM-1 (enlimolab)	Phase III
	Synthesis of phsophatidylcholine	Citicoline	Phase III

NMDA, N-methyl-D-asparaginic acid; AMPA, α-amino-3-hyroxy-5-methyl-4-isoxazole propionic acid

Prevention of Vasopressin Release and BBB Dysfunction

BBB dysfunction in the severely injured brain produces not only increased interstitial fluid, but also an increase in neurotoxic cytokines. The disturbance of cerebrovascular autoregulation, severe brain tissue acidosis, hypercapnea, and radical attack to cerebral blood vessels have been considered as causes of BBB dysfunction. The management of blood gases and pH are basic care strategies to prevent the progression of BBB dysfunction.

Our recent clinical studies using microdialysis suggested that vasopressin also correlated to the changes in BBB dysfunction, as shown in Fig. 23 (Chap. 22) [5]. The release of vasopressin is produced by HPA axis stress-associated hyperglycemia. Therefore, early management of excess vasopressin release is also important to prevent BBB dysfunction [9]. The vasopressin-induced BBB dysfunction was not recorded in experimental animal studies because stress to the HPA axis is very limited in experimental animal models under anesthesia. The management of excess release of vasopressin is not easy without early induction of mild brain hypothermia. This is because the excess release of vasopressin is triggered by direct damage of the hypothalmus and the feedback mechanism of neural control of stress-associated hyperglycemia [1,4,13,14]. The control of stress-associated hyperglycemia is also not simple without stopping excess release of epinephrine from catecholamine surge with early induction of mild brain hypothermia management. The stress to the HPA axis with severe brain damage produces excess release of vasopressin and epinephrine. The serum epinephrine level increases by about 20–200 times because of HPA axis stress, and then this epinephrine stimulates glucose production to give a serum glucose level of more than 230 mg/dl [4]. These metabolic changes are made more severe by other neurohormonal reactions such as glucagon release and reduced insulin sensitivity because of release of ACTH. The reduced glucose consumption by skeletal muscles is also a reason for the difficult control of stress-associated hyperglycemia at the acute stage. For the management of vasopressin-related BBB dysfunction, early induction of brain hypothermia and care management of stress-associated hyperglycemia are important.

The use of steroids is another pharmacological treatment for the prevention of BBB dysfunction. However, in the management of brain hypothermia treatment, the use of steroids is not recommended without control of stress-associated hyperglycemia in the acute stage. The hyperglycemia sensitive hypothalamus neuropeptide Y receptors respond to vasopressin release and the presence of glucocorticoid simultaneously [1,13,14]. Without control of hyperglycemia, steroid administration may stimulate vasopressin release more severely, and then induce BBB dysfunction. Our preliminary clinical studies suggest that activation of interleukin 1 (IL1) and IL6 cytokines involve these reactions, as shown in Fig. 23 (Chap. 22).

Albumin is a large molecule and therefore permeates the BBB with difficulty. In cases of no damage to the BBB, the cerebrospinal fluid (CSF)/serum albumin ratio (BBB index) is less than 0.007. A BBB index of 0.007–0.01 suggests mild BBB dysfunction, and an index of 0.01–0.02 suggests moderate BBB dysfunction. Severe BBB dysfunctiom is indicated by a BBB index of more than 0.02.

The critical level of BBB dysfunction to produce cytokine encephalitis associated with systemic infection is with a BBB index greater than 0.02 (Fig. 55, Chap. 39). A BBB index of more than 0.01 indicates the replacement of serum albumin. However, the effect of anti-vasopressin on the prevention of BBB dysfunction remains unstudied.

Prevention of Nitrous Oxide Radical Formation and Lipid Peroxidation

Highly reactive free radicals cause the peroxidation of membrane phospholipids, the oxidation of cellular proteins, and intracellular Ca^{++} attack in neurons and cerebral blood vessels. For the scavenging of free radicals, many pharmacological interventions have been attempted in experimental studies. However, in clinical studies, manitol, vitamins E and C, and the pharmacological medicine Radicut have been administered as pharmacological treatment. The timing of the administration of these radical scavengers is very important. At the induction stage of brain hypothermia treatment, Radicut is recommended, however, prolonged administration of Radicut to the end of the cooling stage is not recommended. Although Radicut is removed via liver metabolism, liver function is reduced during brain hypothermia management and liver dysfunction can arise from prolonged administration.

Hemoglobin is a known scavenger of ·NO radicals. Brain hypothermia treatment with management of hemoglobin levels higher than 11 g/dl is very successful in removing ·NO radicals [8]. Hypothermia also reduces the production of ·NO radicals. Our clinical studies of brain tissue temperature (very close to core temperature) suggest that a brain tissue temperature of 34°C is not sufficient for the prevention of ·NO radical production. Mild brain hypothermia (34°C) reduces ·NO radical production by about 50% and moderate brain hypothermia reduces if further, by about 80% at 33°C and by more than 90% at 32°C [2].

Effective brain tissue hypothermia for prevention of ·NO radical formation requires brain tissue temperature lower than 32°–33°C. To succeed in the induction of moderate brain hypothermia, early control of stress-associated hyperglycemia and stabilization of vital signs are important.

Prevention of Brain Edema

There are many misunderstandings concerning the management of brain edema. Brain edema is caused or worsened by brain ischemia, brain hypoxia, energy crisis, imbalance of input and output of cerebral circulation, and neurotoxic neurotransmitter release. Therefore, these conditions should be managed by prior hyperosmotic dehydration therapies to prevent brain edema. The early administration of hyperosmotic solution such as manitol produces a volume deficit for maintaining cerebral microcirculation and lower CPP under the conditions of reduced serum catecholamines by induction of brain hypothermia.

The prevention of brain edema needs special consideration at the induction stage of brain hypothermia treatment. The use of hyperosmotic solution, such as manitol or glycerol, and pharmacological reduction of CSF formation are not recommended as initial treatment for brain edema.

The recommended management of brain edema at the induction stage of brain hypothermia treatment is the replacement of albumin to maintain the serum albumin level above 3.5 g/dl, normovolemic circulation, flat position, CPP greater than 70–80 mmHg, DO_2 greater than 700–800 ml/min, PaO_2/FiO_2 greater than 350, serum pH greater than 7.3, serum phosphate greater than 3.0 mg/dl, control of serum glucose at 120–140 mg/dl, prevention of abdominal hypertension, serum hemoglobin greater than 11 mg/dl, pharmacological management to prevent selective ·NO radical damage to the dopamine A10 nervous system, and early induction of mild brain hypothermia. In most cases, early administration of hyperosmotic solution such as manitol or glycerol was not necessary in our clinical series.

If external carotid venous dilatation is observed, this suggests elevation of mediastinal pressure, acute pulmonary edema, airway obstruction, or cardiac insufficiency. Therefore, the management of cardio-pulmonary dysfunction and 5°–10° head-up position are recommended. Hyperosmotic dehydration therapy is recommended after stabilizing cardiopulmonary function, dehydration, and control of hypo-albuminemia. The hyperosmotic solution cannot reduce brain edema under the condition of hypo-albuminemia, such as that with serum albumin lower than 2.5 mg/dl. This mechanism is described in detail in Chap. 42 on the management and monitoring of ICP.

Control of Aspiration Pneumonia

The complication of aspiration pneumonia is a negative factor for the success of brain hypothermia treatment. Limited cerebral oxygenation, worsening of brain edema by infiltration of cytokines through the damaged BBB, and difficult management of pulmonary infection are clinical issues. Enteral bacterial translocation, acid chemical alveolar damage, disturbed microcirculation because of prolonged bed rest, and reduced immune function caused by hypothermia are reasons for difficult management. Gastric lavage of the stomach and one-shot enteral administration of nonabsorbable antibiotics: levofloxacin (Cravit, 200 mg) + amphotericin B (100–300 mg), and combination of antibiotic therapy with panipenem beta amipron (Carbenin 500 mg × 2/day), or second choice: ceftazidinme (Modasin 1 g × 2/day) for prevent of pseudomonas aspiration pneumonia and enteral bacterial translocation are useful.

Criteria for Induction or Halting of Brain Hypothermia

The indications and contraindications for brain hypothermia treatment are listed in Chap. 28 and 29. Brain hypothermia treatment can be started after management of various contraindicated factors, such as shock, arrhythmia, severe hyperglycemia, and cardiac insufficiency.

The management of mild brain hypothermia is easy; however, moderate brain hypothermia requires special consideration and careful management. Two-step induction is successful in avoiding the complications of brain hypothermia treatment. The rapid induction of brain hypothermia to a brain tissue temperature of 34°C is possible; however, rapid induction of brain hypothermia to lower than 34°C is not recommended. This is because the metabolic shift from glucose to lipid occurs following hypothermia. During mild brain hypothermia, the metabolic balance between glucose and lipid, becomes equal. However, at brain tissue temperature lower than 34°C, lipid metabolism becomes dominant in all major organs and rapidly reduces the consumption of serum glucose in the brain, liver, heart, lungs, and skeletal muscles. Without careful management of serum glucose, hyperglycemia rapidly develops at brain tissue temperatures below 34°C. Unsuccessful management of hyperglycemia at temperatures below 34°C produces many negative complications for the management of injured brain tissue. Neuronal hypoxia occurs despite normal care management of PaO_2 and oxygen delivery. Rapidly increasing brain tissue glucose can stimulate increased levels of brain tissue lactate and excess release of vasopressin, and can easily worsen brain injury despite control of brain hypothermia. In such cases, further induction of mild brain hypothermia should be avoided until the serum glucose level is controlled to 120–140 mg/dl.

Criteria for induction of moderate brain hypothermia are stabilization of vital signs, DO_2 more than 700–800 ml/min, serum glucose less than 150 mg/dl, correct any hypopotassemia and maintain above 3 mEq/dl, no arrhythmia and QT interval less than 450 mm/s on the ECG after induction of mild brain hypothermia. After management of these pathophysiological changes, brain hypothermia treatment can be extended to temperature below 34°C. Physiological reactions of brain hypothermia treatment include hypopotassemia, J wave on ECG, elongation of the QT interval, reduced cardiac output below 33°C, ventricular fibrillation, hypocalcemia, hyperglycemia, consumption of vitamin A with unstable membrane phosphate metabolism, prolonged muscle relaxation, shivering, and prolonged coagulation time.

References

1. Corte FD, Mancini A, Valle D, Gallizzi F, Carducci P, Mignani V, De Marinis L (1998) Provocative hypothalamopituitary axis tests in severe head injury: correlation with severity and prognosis. Crit Care Med 26:1419–1426
2. Hayashi N (1995) Cerebral hypothermia treatment. In: Hayashi N (ed) Cerebral hypothermia treatment. Sogo Igaku, Tokyo, pp 1–105
3. Hayashi N (1997) Prevention of vegetation after severe head trauma and stroke by combination therapy of cerebral hypothermia and activation of immune-dopaminergic nervous system. Proceedings of the 6th annual meeting of Society for Treatment of Coma 6:133–145
4. Hayashi N (2000) Enhanced neuronal damage in severely brain injured patients by hypothalamus, pituitary, and adrenal axis neuro-hormonal changes. In: Hayashi N (ed) Brain hypothermia. Springer, Berlin Heidelberg New York Tokyo, pp 3–26
5. Hayashi N (2000) The clinical issue and effectiveness of brain hypothermia treatment for severe brain injured patients. In Hayashi N (ed) Brain hypothermia. Springer, Berlin Heidelberg New York Tokyo, pp 121–151
6. Hayashi N, Hirayama T, Utagawa A (1994) The cerebral thermo-pooling and hypothermia treatment of critical head injury patients. In: Nagai H (ed) Intracranial pressure IX. Springer, Tokyo, pp 589–599
7. Hayashi N, Hirayama T, Utagawa T, Ohata M (1994) Systemic management of cerebral edema based on a new concept in severe head injury patients. Acta Neurochir [Suppl] 60:541–543
8. Hayashi N, Utagawa A, Kinosita K, Izumi T (1999) Application of a novel technique for clinical evaluation of nitric oxide-induced free radical reactions in ICU patients. Cellular and Molecular Neurobiology 19:3–17
9. Kagawa M, Nagao S, Bemana I (1996) Arginine vasopressin receptor antagonists for treatment of vasogenic brain edema: an experimental study. J Neurotrauma 13:273–279
10. Kow LM, Pfaff DW (1986) Vasopressin excites ventromedial hypothalamus glucose-responsive neurons in vitro. Physiol Behav 37:153–158
11. Lin TW, Kuo YS (1996) Acute pulmonary oedema following administration of vasopressin for control of massive GI tract haemorrhage in a major burn patient. Burns 22:73–75
12. Pasko SA, Volosheniuk TG (1990) Disordered phosphorus metabolism and its correction in the acute period of severe craniocerebral trauma. Zh Vopr Neirokhir Im NN Burdenko 3:14–16
13. Stanley BG (1993) Neuropeptide Y in multiple hypothalamic sites controls eating behavior, endocrine, and autonomic system for body energy balance. In: Colmers WF, Wahlestedt C (eds) Biology of neuropeptide Y and related peptide. Humana Press, Totowa, NJ, p 457–509
14. Temple DL, Leibowitz SF (1994) The neuropeptide Y system (hypothalamus) has a dense concentration of glucocorticoide (type II) receptors that mediate carbon hydrate intake. J Neuroendocrinol 6:479–501
15. Swan HJC, Ganz W (1983) Hemodynamic measurements in clinical practice: a decade in review. J Am Coll Cardiol 1:103–113

44. Management During the Cooling Stage

The Target of Management During the Cooling Stage

The restoration of dying neurons and neuroprotection against secondary brain damage are the main goals of intensive care unit (ICU) management during the cooling stage of brain hypothermia treatment [22,24]. Management of neuroprotection against the progression of brain edema, ischemia, intracranial pressure (ICP) elevation, free radical attack, and neuroexcitation is not sufficient for severely brain-injured patients. Prior to neuroprotection management, restoration therapy should be considered for severely brain-injured patients affected by trauma, stroke, hypoxia, or cardiac arrest.

The administration of sufficient oxygen and suitable metabolic substrates such as glucose and phosphate are fundamental for neuronal restoration in injured brain tissue [1,12,33,36,41]. For the success of this treatment, stable systemic circulation, control of hemoglobin dysfunction [13,21,22,24], management of insulin-resistant hyperglycemia [23,24,27], control of blood–brain barrier (BBB) function [11], prevention of neurotoxic glutamate release [3,5], and care management of hypothalamus–pituitary–adrenal (HPA) axis neurohormonal abnormality [4,10,17,24,29] under brain hypothermia are all required at the start of treatment.

The next step of neuroprotection, such as management of ICP elevation [37], brain edema [41], BBB dysfunction [35], disturbance of microcirculation [33], free radical reactions [18,20,23], and elevation of brain tissue temperature by brain thermo-pooling [23,25,26] must be achieved with the prevention of hypothermia-associated complications [2,14,35,43]. In the management of severely brain-injured patients, special consideration of memory disturbance, emotional dysfunction, and vegetation is required, even at the acute stage [20–22,24].

The management targets at the initial cooling stage are:

Systolic blood pressure >100 mmHg
$PaO_2/FiO_2 > 300$
Serum glucose 120–140 mg/dl
Oxygen delivery >700–800 ml/min (Other monitor markers $ETCO_2$ 32–38 mmHg, $PaCO_2$ 34–38 mmHg, Hb > 11 g/dl, SaO_2 > 98%)
O_2ER 22%–25%
Serum pH 7.3–7.4
Serum phosphate 3–5 mg/dl
Serum potassium 4–5 mg/dl
Serum magnesium 1.5–2.0 mEq/l
Serum albumin >3.0–3.5 mg/dl
Antithrombin-III (AT-III) >100%
Ht < 35%
ICP < 15 mmHg
SjO2 60%–80%
Brain tissue temperature 32°–34°C intermittent control
Vitamin A >50 μg/dl
Abdominal pressure <15 mmHg
Gastric juice pH < 3.5
QT interval <450 mm/s and no arrhythmia

Time Schedule for Management of Brain Tissue Temperature

The time schedules for mild (34°C) and moderate (32°–33°C) brain hypothermia are different during the cooling stage (Fig. 43, Chap. 34). This is because at brain temperature of 34°–37°C, pituitary hormonal release is not severely suppressed and a low incidence of immune dysfunction is associated with a reduction in growth hormone level [9]. Also, glucose metabolism is dominant over lipid metabolism until the brain tissue temperature reaches 34°C [20,24]. However, below 34°C, there are dramatic changes in systemic circulation, metabolism, and immune function that are caused by reduced serum catecholamines, increased brain tissue glucose caused by hyperglycemia associated with a metabolic shift from glucose to lipid, and a reduced growth hormone level, respectively [22,24]. Therefore, in the management of moderate brain hypothermia, special consideration must be given to prevent these complications.

Mild Brain Hypothermia

Mild brain hypothermia treatment is indicated for cases in which Glasgow Coma Scale score (GCS) is less than 8, and there are no signs of herniation or cardiopulmonary dysfunction, as described in Chaps 28 and 29. If a full medical team is not available, induction of mild brain hypothermia treatment is also recommended.

Brain tissue temperature should be controlled at about 34°C for 3–7 days until evidence of recovery or partial recovery of the brain injury is observed (Figs. 39, Chap. 32; 43, Chap. 34). Therefore, the cooling duration depends on the severity of brain injury or stroke. The most important ICU requirements are the prevention of pulmonary infection and cytokine encephalitis, with neuro-protection against brain edema, cerebral blood flow (CBF) disturbances, brain hypoxia, metabolic imbalance, and ICP elevation [24]. The technique for the prevention of infection during mild brain hypothermia is not difficult. The required management criteria are the control of serum albumin level above 3.5 g/dl, cerebrospiral fluid (CSF)/serum albumin ratio to less than 0.01, serum glucose level to 120–140 mg/dl, replacement of vitamin A to greater than 50 mg/dl, hemoglobin (Hb) greater than 12 g/dl, 2,3-diphosphoglycerate (DPG) greater than 10 mmol/gHb, AT-III greater than 100%, platelet count 50 000–80 000/cu mm, digastrics decontamination, muscle massage, abdominal pressure less than 10 mmHg during the cooling stage and before the rewarming preconditioning stage [22,24]. The detailed ICU management technique is discussed later in this section. Such ICU management is very useful for preventing worsening of rewarming stage infections.

Moderate Brain Hypothermia

Moderate brain hypothermia is indicated as a second stage treatment in cases that show no effects from mild brain hypothermia treatment. Two-step variable speed induction is very safe and effective as restoration therapy for neuronal recovery in injured brain tissue [22,24]. Rapid induction of brain hypothermia to 34°C is scheduled initially. ICU management then focuses on stabilization of systemic circulation, control of serum glucose at 120–140 mg/dl (at least lower than 180 mg/dl), management of cardiopulmonary dysfunction such as arrhythmia and elongation of the QT interval to greater than 450 mm/s on the electrocardiogram (ECG), and treatment of hypopotassemia. After stabilizing these clinical issues, the brain tissue temperature is then reduced to 32°–33°C for periods of 5–6 h, as shown in Fig. 39 (Chap. 32).

Prolonged moderate brain hypothermia is very successful for the prevention of free radical reactions (Fig. 77, Chap. 42), neurotoxic neurotransmitter release (Fig. 76, Chap. 42) [5,21,24,27], vascular engorgement, and the progression of brain edema; however, it is very stressful to the systemic circulation and immune function because of reduced HPA axis neurohormone function [22,24]. Prolonged continuous control of brain tissue temperature at 32°C is not recommended because of diminished pituitary hormonal release. The reduction of growth hormone (GH) produces diminished CD4 activity, lymphocytopenia, reduces lypolytic action, and results in immune crisis (Fig. 42, Chap. 33) [20,24].

To prevent these complications, the use of intermittent moderate brain hypothermia is useful [24]. Temporary brain tissue temperature elevation from 32°–33°C to 34°C for a short duration prevents the excessive reduction in pituitary hormones. In this management, the timing of temporary brain tissue temperature elevation is also important. Because the physiological release of GH occurs in the early evening and into the night, the temporary elevation of brain tissue temperature should be scheduled at 18:00–22:00 hours to prevent immune crisis and pituitary dysfunction (Fig. 39, Chap. 32).

This intermittent control of brain tissue temperature during moderate brain hypothermia produces lower incidence of GH replacement, GH-associated hyperglycemia, immune crisis, and complications of pulmonary infection. The time schedule for the management of cooling at 32°–33°C is provided in Fig. 43 (Chap. 34).

Restoration Therapy for Injured Neurons

For a long time, neuroprotection therapy has been considered to be the main goal of management in brain-injured patients because it is difficult for injured neurons to make a recovery. Prevention of further secondary damage was the main purpose in ICU management. However, recent clinical studies in ICU management demonstrated the presence of new brain injury mechanisms that were not observed in anesthetized experimental animal models [23,25,26]. Slow release of bound oxygen from hemoglobin in the brain, systemic bloodstream shifts to the intestinal organs, increasing brain tissue glucose and lactate levels caused by insulin-resistant hyperglycemia, and reduced neuronal activity occur due to stress to the HPA axis neurohormonal immune system following

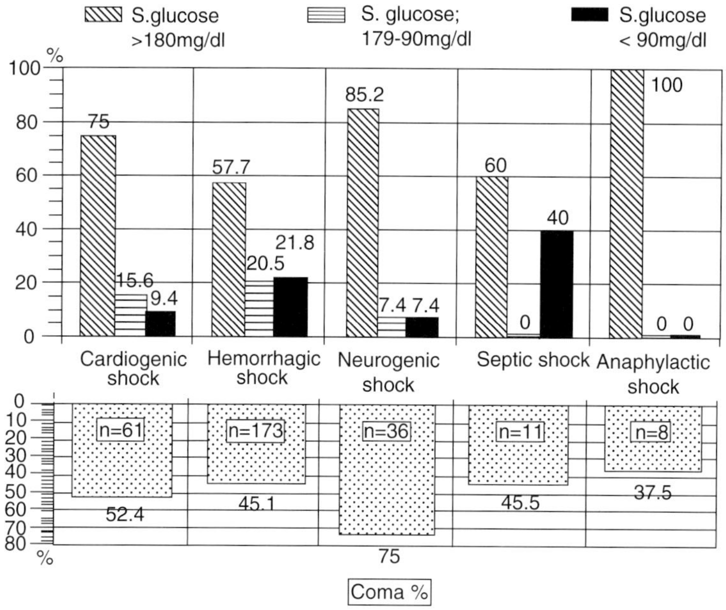

Fig. 82. The incidence of stress-associated hyperglycemia and coma in various shock patients

severe brain injury [23]. Changes in management to accommodate these new findings of brain injury mechanisms have produced unexpectedly excellent clinical results in cases of injury that were considered to be difficult to survive or would provide little neuronal recovery. Put simply, correct management for severely brain-injured patients has not been performed using previously accepted hypothermia treatment. The neuron is in fact stronger than was previously thought.

Management of Systemic Circulation and Metabolism

In the cooling stage of brain hypothermia treatment, unstable systemic circulation is produced by two main reasons. One is cardiac dysfunction produced by cardiac ischemia and hypoxia by the excess release of catecholamines and hemoglobin dysfunction [5,24]. The other is poor management of the hypothermia technique, in particular rapid induction of hypothermia without management of dehydration [7].

Harmful stress stimulates the HPA axis and produces an excess release of catecholamines, epinephrine, norepinephrine, and dopamine in the bloodstream [23]. The severity of these catecholamine surges is correlated to changes in rapid stress, severity, and the type of disease [8]. In our clinical studies, anaphylactic shock, cardiac arrest caused by heart infarction, diffuse brain injury and acute subdural hematoma, subarachnoid hemorrhage, and neurogenic shock produced the most severe excess releases of catecholamines and produced hyperglycemia (Fig. 82).

Delayed induction of hypothermia produces catecholamine surge-associated cardiac dysfunction because of coronary vasoconstriction and contraction myocytolisis of cardiac muscles. This means persistent cardiac contraction, difficult cardiac muscle relaxation, and cardiac ischemia [23]. To escape these cardiac hazards, early induction of hypothermia is successful; however, overly rapid induction of hypothermia and cooling below 34°C produces an excessive reduction in serum catecholamines. Therefore, the management of brain temperature must be conducted carefully with step-by-step monitoring of the ECG, vital signs, PaO_2, and serum glucose level.

Another cause of unstable systemic circulation during brain hypothermia treatment is early administration of hyperosmotic solution. At a brain tissue temperature of 34°C, serum dopamine is reduced to very low levels and epinephrine and norepinephrine are reduced by about 50%. Early administration of manitol during the cooling stage causes a volume deficit for the maintenance of microcirculation combined with reduced cardiac output. The intestinal organs and renal flow are very sensitive to ischemia caused by severe hypothermia. The complication of AT-III lower than 80% and dehydration by manitol administration produces a high risk of intestinal ischemia and renal ischemia. These complications can easily cause systemic infections, liver dysfunction, malnutrition, immune dysfunction, and severe pulmonary infection [14,24].

Basic management of systemic circulation and metabolism at the initial cooling stage of brain hypothermia requires normovolemic fluid resuscitation, maintenance of cardiac function by sufficient administration of oxygen, and adequate control of potassium phosphate, magnesium, and serum glucose (Fig. 30, Chap. 26) [20,22,24]. The application of elastic bandages to the extremities to prevent excess fluid resuscitation, and the use of the abdominal balloon catheter technique are also successful for maintaining stable cardiopulmonary–brain circulation (Figs. 31, Chap. 26; 59, Chap. 42).

As a pharmacological treatment, administration of phosphodiesterase inhibitors with adrenergic agents doputamine (selective β1-adrenergic effects; Doptorex) is recommended to maintain cardiac output. However, early administration of dopamine is not recommended for two reasons. One is the activation of the blood shift to the intestinal organs and promotion of masking brain hypoxia even with normal cerebral perfusion pressure (CPP), the other is the possibility of hydroperoxide radical formation in injured brain tissue [3,40] by chemical reaction of dopamine with oxygen under the conditions of severe damage to the BBB. This is because serum dopamine may be permeable to the damaged BBB and diffuse into the injured brain tissue. As another pharmacological treatment for maintaining systemic circulation, the administration of AT-III is useful for maintaining microcirculation in the brain and intestinal organs [24,33].

Hypertonic crystalloid solutions of 7% ascorbic Ringer solution (limit of 1000 ml) combined with colloids and 5% albumin is our initial choice for fluid resuscitation to prevent the various complications of catecholamine surge-associated hyperglycemia. After stabilizing the systemic circulation, normovolemic and isotonic fluid is used with balanced Na^+, K^+, Cl^-, magnesium chloride, and potassium phosphate.

The severe brain trauma patient often suffers other hemorrhagic trauma at the same time. It is very difficult to maintain cerebral circulation and coronary circulation in such cases. The insertion of a balloon catheter into the abdominal aorta produces some chance of survival. Temporary and incomplete occlusion of abdominal blood flow by the balloon catheter (Fig. 31, Chap. 26) is sometimes very successful in maintaining stable cardiopulmonary function and aiding neuronal restoration of dying neurons in cases of multiple trauma. Control of serum hypophosphatemia to 3–4 mg/dl, serum pH higher than 7.3, PaO_2/FiO_2 greater than 300, serum glucose at 120–140 mg/dl, management of AT-III higher than 100%, and replacement of serum albumin to greater than 3.0 mg/dl are also very successful measures for the maintenance of systemic circulation and oxygen metabolism.

Management of Hemoglobin Dysfunction

Hemoglobin is a very strong carrier of oxygen into the brain. However, without the hemoglobin enzyme 2,3-diphosphoglycerate (DPG), bound oxygen cannot be released from hemoglobin in the brain. This complication has already been reported in the replacement of preserved blood and hemofiltration therapy [13]. This means that oxygen inhalation with normal PaO_2 is not adequate care management. Normal oxygen delivery into the brain with no administration of oxygen for dying neurons is a serious situation in attempts to restore injured brain tissue. Recent chemical research initiated the technique of direct measurement of serum DPG and hemoglobin-binding DPG. The simultaneous measurement of hemoglobin-binding DPG in arterial blood and in internal jugular venous blood gives very useful information about neuronal hypoxia. In severe brain trauma patients (GCS less than 6), hemoglobin-binding DPG in jugular venous blood was reduced in 47% of patients and was at seriously low levels in 24% of patients [23]. Severe hyperglycemia, severe acidosis ($pH < 7.2$), reduced potassium phosphate, and loss of magnesium are known causes of DPG reduction [23,27].

The management of hemoglobin dysfunction requires the replacement of potassium phosphate and control of serum phosphate at 3–5 mg/dl, replacement of magnesium chloride and control of serum magnesium to about 1.6 ± 0.20 mEq/l, maintenance of serum pH above 7.3, control of serum glucose at 120–140 mg/dl, and prevention of red blood cell aggregation by maintaining serum AT-III higher than 100% [24].

An alternate management strategy for neuronal hypoxia that is produced by hemoglobin dysfunction is the perfusion of a fluorocarbon oxygen carrier (F44E emulsion-Revoxyn) as part of the CSF technique, and has been developed in experimental studies by Triolo et al. [42]. This management strategy is still undergoing clinical research; however, this method may become a new ICU method for critical brain-injured patients affected by trauma, cardiac arrest, or stroke.

Control of Insulin-Resistant Hyperglycemia

The considerations and care management methods for hyperglycemia are presented in the description of induction care management (Fig. 81, Chap. 43). At the cooling stage, management of hyperglycemia is important. Serum glucose is maintained at 120–140 mg/dl by

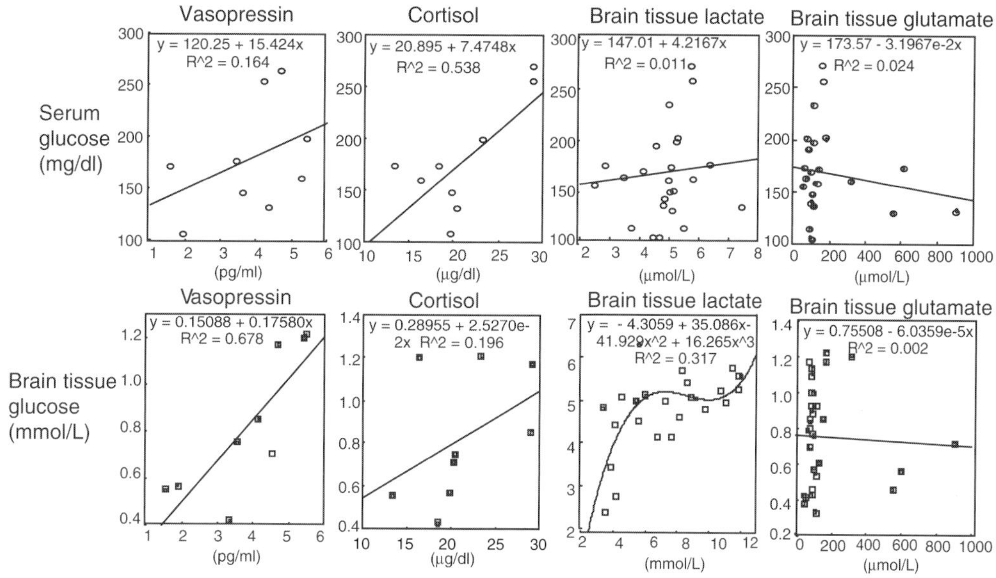

Fig. 83. The effects of hyperglycemia increasing brain tissue glucose on changes of brain tissue lactate and neuronal hormones

Table 19. The effect of neuronal hormones on the metabolism of macronutrients

Neuronal hormones	Insulin release	Muscle glucose uptake	Hepatic glucogenesis	Proteolysis	Lipolysis	Ketogenesis
Catecholamines	↓	↓	↑	↑	↑	↑
Glucagon			↑			↑
Growth hormone	↓	↓		↓	↑	↑
Glucocorticoids		↓	↑	↑	↑	↑
Thyroid hormones			↑	↑	↑	↑

↓, Decrease; ↑, increase

a continuous drip of insulin included with saline (Humarin-R 50U + saline 100ml). There are many causes of unsuccessful management of hyperglycemia. Excessive lowering of the body temperature produces a shift from glucose to lipid metabolism and reduces the glucose expenditure. The control of hyperglycemia then becomes very difficult by ordinary administration of insulin. Further administration of insulin or elevation of body temperature by about 0.5°–1.0°C is advised. At the same time, prolonged hypothermia reduces liver and skeletal muscle metabolism and glucose consumption, reduces dramatically and produces insulin-resistant hyperglycemia [23,24]. The ability of the body to metabolize many pharmacological medicines such as antibiotics and radical scavengers also decreases during prolonged brain hypothermia treatment. Therefore, overdoses of pharmacological medicines can occur very easily and can also reduce the liver function. This poor iatrogenic management also promotes insulin-resistant hyperglycemia during brain hypothermia treatment. Stabilized albumin-binding antibiotics complicate liver dysfunction because serum hypo-albuminemia may easily occur with reduced liver function during prolonged hypothermia. Selection of non-albumin-binding antibiotics, low dosages of antibiotics, replacement of serum albumin, and liver protection are required. The effects of hyperglycemia and increased brain tissue glucose on brain tissue lactate levels and neurohormonal changes are presented in Fig. 83. The critical concentration of serum glucose to produce increases in brain tissue lactate is 180–200mg/dl.

Management of HPA Axis Neurohormone Dysfunction

After severe brain injury, HPA axis neurohormonal function is stimulated and releases vasopressin, GH, adrenocorticotropic hormone (ACTH), and catecholamines into the bloodstream (Table 19) [6,17,30,31]. All of these reactions are defense mechanisms against brain stress and brain damage. However, excess release of these neurohormones produces further hazard to the injured brain by the occurrence of hemoglobin dysfunction, insulin-resistant hyperglycemia, promotion of BBB dysfunction, and neuronal hypoxia [23]. No management of these defense responses is also a dangerous condition in the injured brain [8,9,17]. How to suitably manage and control these defense reactions is very important for the preservation of injured neurons at the cooling stage. The neurohormone reactions is nonanesthetized patients could be prevented by early induction of brain hypothermia to less than 34°C. However, prolonged treatment at lower than 34°C produces an excessive reduction in neurohomone release and causes immune dysfunction and loss of animation activity [10,21–23]. In the management of critical brain-injured patients, prolonged moderate brain hypothermia management must be used to prevent brain edema, free radical neuronal damage, and ICP elevation [20,24,27]. To prevent the loss of animate activity associated with prolonged hypothermia, intermittent control of brain tissue temperature between 32° and 34°C with neurohormone replacement therapy is successful [24].

Hypothalamus Dysfunction

The direct damage of the hypothalamus produces a reduction in vasopressin release. As complications, hypoosmotic urinalysis, dehydration, reduction of systemic circulation, hyponatremia, and diabetes mellitus can occur. The excessive administration of manitol during hypothalamus dysfunction produces severe dehydration and worsens the microcirculation of major organs, the brain, heart, lungs, and intestinal organs [7,24].

The management of serum vasopressin is not simple during the cooling stage of brain hypothermia. The release of vasopressin is accelerated by serum hyperosmotic pressure and the feedback mechanism of neural control of macronutrient intake such as hyperglycemia [23,30,31]. The management of vasopressin release is very important to determine the prognosis. Overly rapid induction of moderate brain hypothermia reduces vasopressin release and complicates diabetes mellitus. Dehydration under brain hypothermia is very dangerous, and promotes ischemia in the intestinal organs with immune crisis and CBF disturbances by reason of reduced serum catecholamines and circulation blood volume [24,27]. Therefore, before the administration of manitol, stabilization of the systemic circulation by normovolemic fluid resuscitation is important. Excessive reduction of serum catecholamines during the cooling stage is prevented by intermittent control between moderate (32°–33°C) and mild (34°–35°C) brain hypothermia, as shown in Fig. 43 (Chap. 35). The pharmacological administration of phosphodiesterase inhibitors combined with adrenergic agents such as doputamine is an additional care method. On the other hand, excessive release of vasopressin occurs because of unsuitable management of hyperglycemia during brain hypothermia at 33°–34°C [24]. The activation of BBB dysfunction, induction of proinflammatory cytokines, and induction of cytokine encephalitis with combination of systemic or severe pulmonary infection were recorded in our clinical studies using microdialysis [23,24]. Hyperglycemia with glucose serum levels higher than 230 mg/dl, with severe BBB dysfunction (evaluated by CSF/serum albumin >0.02), serum albumin less than 2.5 g/dl, and pulmonary infection is a very dangerous situation at the cooling stage [24]. The excessive reduction or release of vasopressin during cooling stage of brain hypothermia are also clinical issues.

Hypopituitarism

Pituitary gland hypothermia is unavoidable during brain hypothermia treatment. ACTH is the most sensitive of the pituitary hormones to hypothermia (Fig. 24, Chap. 23). ACTH is a regulator of neutrophil; therefore, the control of brain hypothermia below 34°C is an interesting technique to prevent neutrophil-associated inflammatory reactions [10]. Brain hypothermia at temperatures below 32°–33°C reduces levels of thyroid stimulating hormone (TSH) and GH. Recent clinical studies demonstrated that GH not only activates human growth, but also regulates the immune functions. Our preliminary studies suggested that GH stimulates the CD4 immune system and suppresses the CD8 immune system [20,23,24]. In addition, the number of lymphocytes is strictly correlated to changes of GH under brain hypothermia [9]. From these clinical studies, GH appears to activate the cellular immune functions such as interleukin I (IL1) and IL6; however, anti-inflammatory immune function such as IL8 and IL10 may be suppressed [20]. An indirect indicator of reduced GH level is lymphocytopenia, lower than $1000/mm^3$. The replacement of GH is very useful to provide recovery from immune dysfunction during brain hypothermia treatment. However, replacement of GH produces clinical issues; one is the high cost and the other is hyperglycemia [24]. To prevent immune dysfunction associated with reduced GH, there are two choices. One is to temporarily elevate the brain tissue temperature from 32°–33°C to around 34°C from 18:00 to 22:00 hours. The other is pharmacological stimulation for the production of GH. Administration of L-arginine and IGF-1 is successful in providing recovery of immune function during brain hypothermia treatment [24]. However, before this pharmacological treatment, careful management of hyperglycemia is recommended because GH reduces the glucose uptake from skeletal muscles.

Neuroprotection Therapy

Neuroprotection therapy is not directly effective in providing neuronal recovery. However, without such management, neuronal restoration in injured brain tissue is difficult.

Prevention of Brain Thermo-pooling and Vascular Engorgement

The elevation of brain tissue temperature by brain thermo-pooling occurs when the body temperature is greater than 38°C, systolic blood pressure is lower than 90–100 mmHg, and during reperfusion of CBF [23,25,26]. Figure 84 shows a typical case of brain thermo-pooling after ischemic reperfusion. These specific conditions occur during the acute stage and the induction stage of brain hypothermia treatment. Unsuccessful management of brain thermo-pooling suggests poor prognosis even with normal control of ICP. The brain thermo-pooling phenomenon is not recorded under the management of brain hypothermia. However, rapid elevation of brain tissue temperature of 1°–2°C produces acute brain swelling by vascular engorgement at the early cooling stage. This is because the pathophysiology of the brain thermo-pooling phenomenon includes elevation of brain tissue temperature, increased metabolic demand, and disturbance of autoregulation of CBF.

To prevent pituitary hormonal dysfunction, immune dysfunction, and liver dysfunction, control of brain tissue temperature between mild and moderate brain hypothermia must be carried out very carefully (Figs. 39, Chap. 32, 43, Chap. 34) [20,22,24]. As a technique for intermittent elevation of brain tissue temperature from 32°–33°C to 34°C, the removal of the cooling blanket

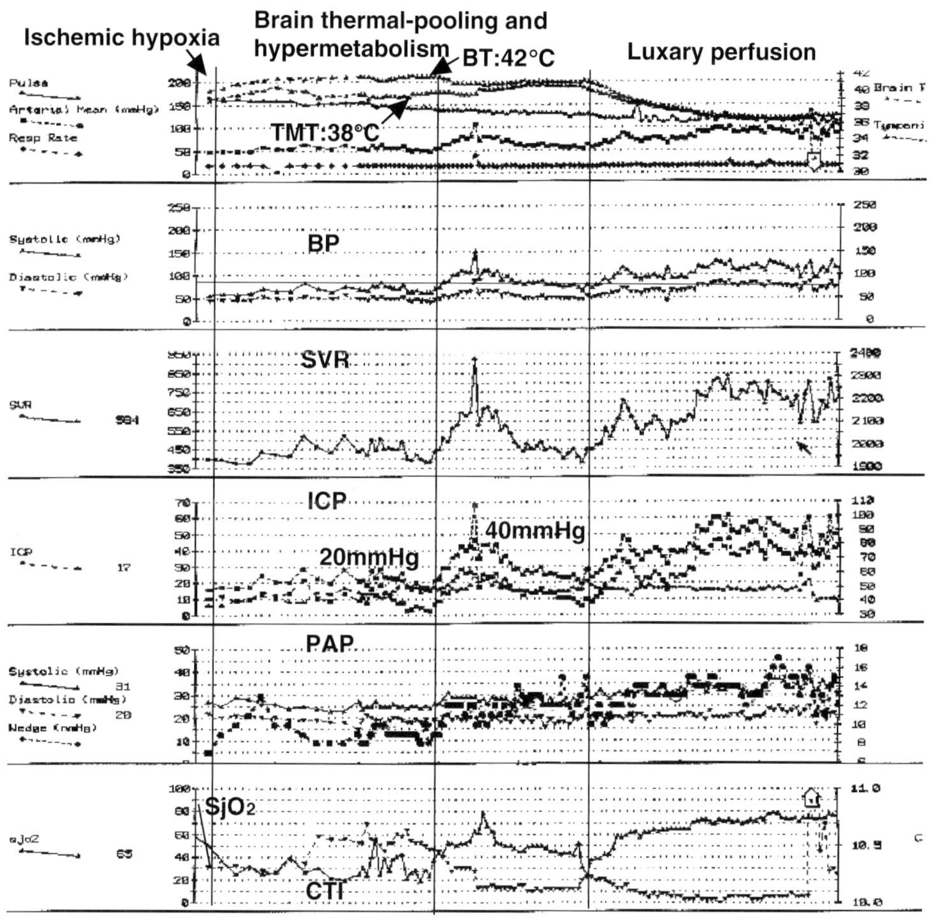

Fig. 84. Typical cases of brain thermo-pooling and ischemic hypermetabolism after reperfusion of severe brain ischemia. *TMT*, Tympanic membrane temperature; *BT*, brain tissue temperature; *BP*, blood pressure; *SVR*, systemic vascular resistance; *ICP*, intracranial pressure; *PAP*, pulmonary arterial pressure; *CTI*, cerebral theramal index; *SjO2*; jugular venous oxygen

from the patient's body, little by little, is recommended. The careful elevation of cooling blanket water temperature is not recommended because it is very difficult to reduce the brain tissue temperature rapidly if the brain tissue temperature is elevated by more than 1°C. The technique of reducing the cooling area without changing the cooling blanket temperature is safe and is much easier for the control of intermittent elevation of brain tissue temperature.

Prevention of Excess Release of Cerebral Dopamine and Free Radical Reactions

A number of compounds with free radical scavenging properties have been studied with the hope that they will reduce the toxic effects of free radicals. Many effective radical scavengers have been reported; however, in clinical studies, successful pharmacological scavengers have not yet been identified. Recent phase II clinical studies of the effectiveness of tirilazad (U-74006F), a 21-aminosteroid, suggested no clinical improvement in overall functional outcome of stroke patients [12,33].

As metabolic substrates of ·NO radicals, the NO_2/NO_3 ratio is a good indicator of ·NO radical reactions (Fig. 78, Chap. 42) [27]. Our clinical studies suggested that low NO_2/NO_3 in serum was very sensitive to the hemoglobin content. The critical level of hemoglobin for increasing NO_2/NO_3 was less than 10–11 mg/dl. Hemoglobin is a very useful physiological radical scavenger in systemic circulation. To prevent various complications that are associated with free radicals, such as pneumonia, liver dysfunction, intestinal dysfunction, and many other organic disturbances, the management of hemoglobin above 11 mg/dl is favored by reasons of maintaining oxygen delivery and also for radical scavenging. Hemoglobin is a powerful physiological scavenger in severely brain-injured patients. The management of hemoglobin above 11 mg/dl is effective in maintaining of sufficient oxygen delivery and prevents free radical reactions in the brain, lungs, and intestinal digestive organs.

In the management of severe brain damage caused by trauma, stroke, or cardiac arrest, the prevention of vegetation and memory disturbances are very important. In our recent clinical studies, selective radical attack of the dopamine A10 nervous system has been pointed out as a mechanism of emotion–memory disturbances in severely brain-injured patients. The dopamine A10 nervous system is the center of neuronal function for memory, emotion, volition, love, and anxiety (Fig. 34, Chap. 26). Therefore, damage to the A10 nervous system can easily result in vegetation. The precise damage mechanism of the dopamine nerve system has been clarified by experimental animal studies [3]. The brain ischemic stroke produces the release of dopamine. In the brain, this released dopamine reacts with oxygen and produces quinine and hydrogen peroxide. Hydrogen peroxide is then easily converted to the neurotoxic $\cdot OH^-$ radical [40]. These chemical reactions in severely injured brain tissue are thought to produce the selective radical damage to the dopamine nervous system (Fig. 33, Chap. 26).

For the management of selective radical damage to the dopamine A10 nervous system, the administration of a radical scavenger and prevention of dopamine release from the dopamine A10 nervous system may be considered. The administration of a pharmacological radical scavenger such as Radicut, vitamins E and C, and control of hemoglobin above 11 g/dl are basic techniques to prevent selective radical attack to the dopamine A10 nervous system. The prevention of dopamine release in the injured brain by early induction of brain hypothermia to below 34°C, and pharmacological treatment with metoclopramide at the acute stage are another treatment (Fig. 30, Chap. 26).

Prevention of Excess Release of Cerebral Glutamate

The management of brain tissue hypothermia is very successful for the prevention of neurotoxic glutamate release [16] in injured brain tissue [24]. This neuroprotection effect is correlated to lowering of brain tissue temperature. Our clinical studies using microdialysis suggest that the release of brain tissue glutamate can be reduced to 5%–15% of normal levels under moderate brain hypothermia and about 40% under mild brain hypothermia, as shown in Fig. 78 (Chap. 42).

The effect of hypothermia to prevent glutamate release is not simple. The toxicity of brain tissue glutamate increases in the presence of lactate as shown by increased neuronal cell membrane damage indicated by the marker glycerol (Fig. 85). The severity of BBB dysfunction combined with systemic infection also affect the responsiveness of glutamate release during the cooling stage of brain hypothermia. Severe systemic infection produces increases of proinflammatory cytokines in the bloodstream. These cytokines may go into the injured brain tissue via the damaged BBB. The increased CSF IL6 correlated with the severity of BBB damage in some patients (Fig. 23, Chap. 22). The critical level of BBB dysfunction to produce cytokine encephalitis is a CSF/serum albumin ratio higher than 0.01 (Fig. 55, Chap. 39). In this patient, management of brain tissue hypothermia was not effective in reducing

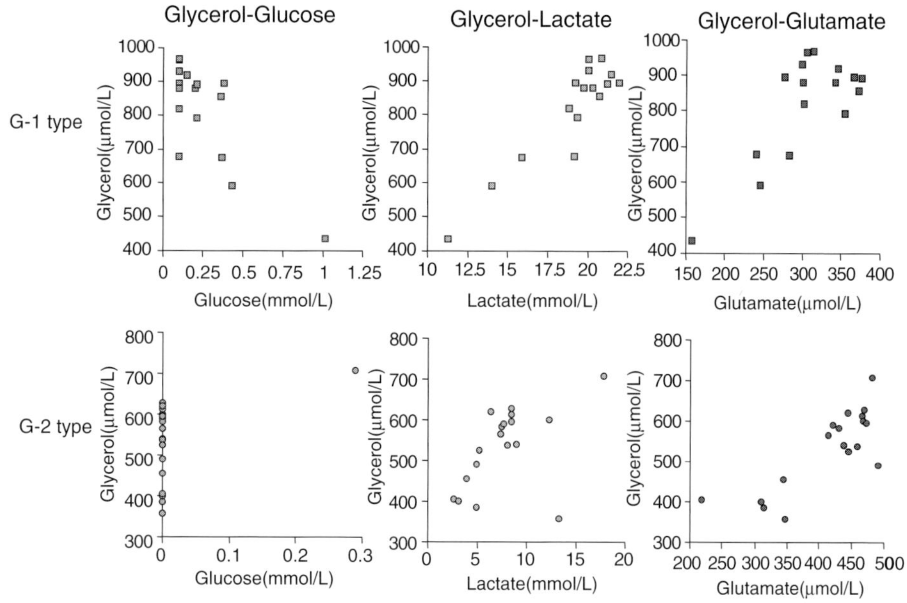

Fig. 85. The neuronal toxicity of brain tissue glutamate correlated to increasing brain tissue lactate

the glutamate release even with management of brain hypothermia at 32°C. The serum proinflammatory cytokines are produced, not only by severe brain tissue damage, but also, by damage of the lungs and intestinal organs. From these results, management of extracerebral organs and prevention of severe infection must be taken with the same level of care as the management of brain injury. Therefore, in the ICU management of the cooling stage, careful management of the injured brain and extracerebral major organs, and prevention of pneumonia are required. The complications of severe or prolonged pulmonary infection and inappropriate management of the BBB during brain hypothermia treatment suggest unsuccessful treatment. These concepts must be considered for the success of brain hypothermia treatment.

Management of BBB Dysfunction

Damage to the BBB has, for a long time, been considered to be a result of brain ischemia and direct brain tissue destruction. Recent basic studies demonstrated that induction of serum cytokines associated with disturbances of microcirculation also cause damage of the vascular intimae, and, possibly, the changes in the BBB. These proinflammatory cytokines in injured tissue may be produced by a number of factors, including injured vascular endothelium, proliferation of macrophages, and infiltration of microglias. The proinflammatory cytokines, such as IL1, IL6, and tumor necrosis factor (TNF), activate the coagulation factor thrombin, reduce tissue plasminogen activator, stimulate micro-embolus formation, and change the vascular permeability. However, recent clinical studies suggested that stress-associated neurohormone vascular reactive hormones and vasopressin also stimulate IL1 and IL6 production and change the BBB function. The precise mechanism of the central neurohormone influence on BBB function is not yet clarified.

In the management of BBB dysfunction, steroids have long been used. The effectiveness of anti-edema is still controversial. In experimental animal studies with anti-edema, the effect of the steroid is positive; however, in clinical studies, negative results have been reported in the acute stage of severe brain injury. However, steroid is very effective for brain edema produced by metastatic brain edema.

The recent clinical studies provided similar answers about this discrepancy of the anti-effect of brain edema. The harmful stress-associated hyperglycemia following severe brain damage is not serious in anesthetized experimental animals; however, stress-associated hyperglycemia is a very serious condition in nonanesthetized clinical brain-injured patients. This severe hyperglycemia stimulates neuropeptide Y receptors in the hypothalamus appetite center and produces vasopressin release as a mechanism of neural control of the macronutrient feedback mechanism [30,31]. Steroid also stimulates the neuropeptide Y receptor, because these receptors include the glucocorticoid type II receptors. The administration of steroid under the conditions of hyperglycemia produces further stimulation of vasopressin release. Vasopressin is not only a vasoconstrictor, but also stimulates the induction of proinflammatory cytokines IL1 and IL6. Steroid is not recommended in cases of stress-associated hyperglycemia to prevent brain edema in the acute stage.

Animal studies suggested that vasopressin release could be prevented by moderate hypothermia [9]. However, in clinical studies, vasopressin release could not be prevented by moderate brain hypothermia (32°–33°C) under the conditions of hyperglycemia with serum glucose level above 230 mg/dl.

For management of BBB dysfunction during the cooling stage of brain hypothermia, the control of serum glucose at 120–140 mg/dl is fundamental. Early control of brain tissue temperature at 34°C prevents catecholamine surge and the release of vasopressin. For pharmacological management of BBB dysfunction, administration of AT-III is effective in preventing endothelial vascular reaction and micro-embolus formation. During brain hypothermia treatment, AT-III level higher than 100% is recommended. Combination therapy of AT-III with low molecular weight heparin is recommended for severely damaged BBB function, such as in cases with CSF/serum albumin ratio greater than 0.01. After management of endovascular inflammatory reactions, replacement of serum albumin to a level higher than 3.0 g/dl is useful [24]. The high osmotic pressure reduces the permeability of the BBB and stabilizing of anti-inflammatory cytokines justifies replacement of serum albumin. The management of serum albumin is also very important to prevent intestinal mucous edema.

The management of serum glucose, serum albumin, and AT-III are important for management of BBB dysfunction and brain edema at the cooling stage of brain hypothermia treatment. These combined treatments for BBB dysfunction strongly affect the prognosis of children.

Prevention of Brain Edema

Brain edema can have multiple causes; cellular edema is caused by dysfunction of cell membrane functions and intracellular homeostasis in glia and neuron cells; vasogenic edema results from impairment of the BBB; hydrostatic edema occurs after disruption of autoregulation, most often after rapid decompression of acute subdural hematoma; and osmotic edema results from serum hypo-osmolarity associated with hypoalbuminemia and hyponatremia [41]. In the ICU management of severely brain-injured patients, these multiple causes of brain edema can be observed simultaneously. Combination of various types of brain edema will change with each cases and over time. The early selection and implementation of the management procedure for the various types of brain edema are important for the success of the cooling stage of brain hypothermia treatment.

The initial target of brain edema treatment is the prevention of cellular swelling of glia and neurons. The management of brain hypoxia and adequate administration of metabolic substrates without disturbances of microcirculation are important for management of cellular swelling. To prevent cytotoxic brain edema, essential management criteria include systolic blood pressure greater than 100 mmHg, PaO_2/FiO_2 greater than 300, serum glucose 120–140 mg/dl, oxygen delivery greater than 700–800 ml/min, Hb greater than 11 mg/dl, SaO_2 greater than 98%, serum pH 7.3–7.4, serum phosphate 3–5 mg/dl, serum magnesium 1.2–2.0 mEq/l, serum albumin greater than 3.0 mg/dl, AT-III greater than 100%, and ICP less than 15 mmHg. The head position should be kept flat to maintain sufficient CBF [39]. Early administration of hyperosmotic agents, manitol and glycerol, is not recommended during brain hypothermia treatment. This is because unstable systemic circulation will be activated very easily because of reduced circulation volume under the conditions of reduced serum catecholamines and hypothermia. In addition, glycerol could produce more brain tissue lactate with hyperglycemia. Therefore, glycerol is not the first choice for hyperosmotic therapy in the cooling stage in cases of stress-associated hyperglycemia.

After 6–12 h from brain damage, vasogenic edema becomes a major target of ICU management. The management of BBB dysfunction by control of serum glucose at 120–140 mg/dl, serum albumin greater than 3.0 g/dl, and AT-III greater than 100% are useful to stabilize vasogenic edema. Hyperosmotic agents, manitol and glycerol, are very successful in removing the interstitial edema at the stabilized condition of systemic circulation. After normovolemic fluid resuscitation, the combination therapy of manitol 500–1000 ml/day with frusemide (20–100 mg/day) is successful for the temporary recovery from severe brain edema and pulmonary edema. The administration of manitol under the condition of hypo-albuminemia (albumin lower than 2.5 g/dl) cannot expect an osmotic anti-edema effect. After 6–12 h of brain damage and with controlled stable systemic circulation, the head-up position (5°–10°) is recommended to maintain an easy venous outflow circulation. The head-up position helps reduce brain edema and prevent venous stasis.

Control of ICP

The development of intracranial hypertension is accompanied by rebleeding from injured brain tissue, neurological deterioration caused by brain edema and hydrocephalus, venous stasis with elevation of mediastinal pressure, and intestinal organ dysfunction with abdominal hypertension during the cooling stage of brain hypothermia treatment. As results of these complications, elevation of ICP can produce a reduction of CPP, brain ischemia, neuronal hypoxia, acceleration of brain swelling, and herniation at the final stage. The relationships between ICP elevation and pathophysiological changes in the brain tissue are described earlier in Chap. 20. Therefore, this discussion will describe the management of ICP elevation during brain hypothermia treatment.

To control ICP during brain hypothermia treatment, the sources of accompanying complications such as rebleeding, hydrocephalus, development of brain edema, pulmonary obstructions, and abdominal hypertension should be dealt with initially. The management of normovolemic fluid resuscitation, sufficient oxygen delivery (>700–800 ml/min), and adequate serum glucose (120–140 mg/dl) are fundamental before the control of ICP.

Head Position

Slight head-up position of 5°–8° helps to keep cerebral venous outflow. Therefore, the head-up position is recommended for control of ICP elevation. However, in severely brain-injured patients, most cases suffer unstable systemic circulation. The reduced cardiac output caused by cardiac ischemia and changed peripheral vascular resistance due to excess release of catecholamines are causes of unstable systemic circulation. Furthermore, injured neurons need sufficient oxygen and adequate metabolic substrates for neuronal restoration through the stabilized systemic circulation. Brain edema and ICP elevation progress as results of insufficient care. To avoid these consequences, head position should be kept flat until stabilized systemic circulation is obtained at the initial time of the cooling stage [24]. These management techniques are especially important for the induction of the cooling stage of brain hypothermia treatment.

Pharmacological Sedation and Muscle Relaxation

The negative effects of excess neurohormone reactions that cause harmful stress to the HPA axis have been described previously. However, induced hypothermia as management of severe brain injury is also stressful to the human body. Pharmacological sedation, muscle relaxation, and neuroleptanalgesia are necessary to avoid hypothermia stress even with coma patients. However, the sedative pharmacology and analgesia must be chosen carefully because these drugs also effect changes of CBF, brain metabolism, and ICP elevation. Table 13 (Chap. 41) summarizes the physiological characteristics of sedative and analgesic agents. For the pharmacological management to maintain sedation during brain hypothermia treatment, the combination of midazolam, fentanyl, and pancuronium is recommended. Midazolam is the first choice for prolonged anesthesia without major complications of cardiovascular and renal dysfunction. Midazolam is not only effective for sedation, but is also effective in preventing traumatic convulsions and ischemia seizures. Propofol can be used with hypertensive patients at the acute stage with normovolemic fluid resuscitation.

Osmotic Management

Increasing the serum osmotic pressure is a simple mechanical method to remove interstitial brain edema. As a pharmacological drug, manitol is the first choice. Glycerol is not indicated in cases of harmful stress-associated hyperglycemia because of increasing brain tissue lactate. However, in hypo-albuminemia, the hyperosmotic effects for reducing brain edema will expire. Therefore, hyperosmotic management must be scheduled in the absence of hypo-albuminemia. The early administration of manitol is not indicated at the induction of brain hypothermia treatment where there is unstable systemic circulation with reduced circulation volume. At the cooling stage, osmotic management must occur with stabilized systemic circulation.

CSF Drainage

The retention of CSF in severe brain injury increases ICP and reduces the absorption of interstitial edema and neurotoxic substrates throughout the ventricular CSF circulation. In the acute stage, the release of neurotoxic neurotransmitters, such as glutamate and dopamine, are major targets of treatment. Brain hypothermia treatment is very successful in preventing the release of these neuronal transmitters; however, brain hypothermia management is not useful for removing previously released neurotoxic glutamate and dopamine. CSF drainage in the acute stage is the only effective means of removing these neurotoxic neurotransmitters. Prolonged retention of these neurotransmitters may produce synaptic dysfunction. CSF drainage can be expected to reduce the prolonged retention of these neurotoxic neurotransmitters with or without ICP elevated hydrocephalus. The three major purposes of CSF drainage are reduction of ICP elevation, the recovery of interstitial edema, and removal of neurotoxic neurotransmitters. For these reasons, we prefer CSF drainage, if possible, in the acute stage even with normal ICP.

Prevention of Pulmonary Obstruction and High Mediastinal Pressure

Airway obstruction during the management of severe brain injury with brain hypothermia treatment is a serious complication. Brain hypoxia and cerebral venous stasis are clinical issues of airway obstruction. When the cerebral venous pressure is about 15 mmHg and the saggital sinus pressure is 5 mmHg, a mediastinal pressure higher than 15–20 mmHg will produce ICP elevation. We control the ventilator with an airway pressure at 17–20 mmHg, and keep PEEP pressure lower than about 10 mmHg during brain hypothermia treatment.

An airway pressure higher than 25 mmHg, can produce increased cerebral venous pressure, portal venous stasis, and congestion of intestinal organs. However, with the complication of severe pulmonary infection with pulmonary congestion, the airway pressure should be controlled at 20–25 mmHg for short durations with PaO_2/FiO_2 higher than 300.

Control of Abdominal Hypertension

Abdominal pressure is lower than 5 mmHg under normal physiological conditions. Abdominal hypertension produces dysfunction in various intestinal organs. Urinary obstruction, paralytic ileuses, and the complication of abdominal bleeding are causes of abdominal hypertension. Mild abdominal hypertension, 10–15 mmHg, reduces the disturbance of microcirculation in digestive intestinal organs. Venous congestion of the liver and lungs develop at abdominal pressures higher than 17–20 mmHg. ICP elevation with venous stasis and cardiac congestion develop at abdominal pressures higher than 25 mmHg. To prevent abdominal hypertension, urinary drainage and insertion of an ileum catheter is fundamental. Gastric lavage on the first day, followed by insertion of an ileum catheter into the ileum beyond the Trize ligament on the second day is an ideal schedule for control of abdominal hypertension, ischemia of digestive organs, and early enteral nutrition [24].

Other Treatment

The basic pathophysiology of cytotoxic and vasogenic brain edema is the destruction of cell membrane function complicated with disturbances of intracellular homeostasis in neurons, glia, and vascular intimae. The stabilization of ion channels and morphological reconstitution of cell membranes in these neuronal and vascular cells are fundamental management strategies. Sufficient oxygenation, adequate administration of glucose, replacement of phosphate with vitamin A, replacement of magnesium, and inhibition of lipid peroxidation are required to stabilize cell membrane functions and prevent brain edema. The management criteria required to prevent cellular swelling are oxygen delivery greater than 700–800 ml/min, Hb greater than 11 mg/dl, SaO_2 greater than 98%, serum pH 7.3–7.4, serum phosphate 3–5 mg/dl, serum magnesium 1.6 ± 0.2 mEq/l, serum albumin greater than 3.0 g/dl, and AT-III greater than 100%.

To inhibit lipid peroxidation, lipid soluble seleno–organic compound (Ebselen) and glutathione peroxides are introduced in clinical treatment. Recent clinical studies in which 300 patients were randomized within 48 h of ischemic stroke to either Ebselen or placebo showed that Ebselen-treated patients had a significantly better outcome, especially if treated within 24 h of onset.

Sodium channel antagonists, anticonvulsants, phenytoin and its water-soluble derivative fosphenytoin, and lamotrigine and related compounds BW-1003C87 and sipatrigine (BW-619C89) are all sodium channel antagonists with cytoprotective properties are being developed. Phenytoin and fosphenytoin have demonstrated neuroprotective ability in animal studies of cerebral ischemia. A multicentre placebo-controlled clinical study of fosphenytoin, lamotrigine, BW-1003C87, sipatrigine (BW-619C89), lubeluzole which acts as a sodium channel blocker and inhibits glutamate release and nitrite oxide-medicated toxicity, and lifarizine which possesses both sodium and calcium channel modulating properties, is in progress.

Pitfalls of ICP Management During Brain Hypothermia

Early administration of manitol and dopamine at the acute stage is dangerous in a condition of unstable systemic circulation with BBB dysfunction. To prevent the progression of brain edema, rapid administration of manitol and glycerol in the acute stage produces dehydration, circulating volume reduction, and intravascular slugging in microcirculation. Furthermore, during brain hypothermia treatment at 32°–34°C, serum catecholamines will be reduced to less than 50% of normal levels [20,24,27]. Therefore, early administration of manitol without suitable fluid resuscitation causes unstable systemic circulation and disturbance of cerebral microcirculation. Before starting anti-edema therapy, maintenance of cerebral circulation with administration of sufficient oxygen and adequate glucose is important. Brain edema develops with unsatisfactory management of cerebral circulation, neuronal oxygenation, and brain metabolism. The early administration of dopamine to maintain systolic blood pressure above 100 mmHg is not recommended for two reasons. The administration of dopamine in cases of severely damaged BBB function with a CSF/serum albumin ratio of more than 0.01 causes an increase of serum dopamine penetration into the injured brain tissue [24]. Increased cerebral dopamine in the injured brain tissue produces neurotoxic radical formation. The other argument against dopamine administration is the shift of the systemic circulation into the intestinal organs caused by pharmacological vasodilatation of the kidneys and intestinal digestive organs. Normovolemic fluid resuscitation with good cerebral oxygenation and careful management of harmful stress-associated hyperglycemia are very important at the cooling stage.

Prevention of Convulsion

The exact incidence of posttraumatic epilepsy after severe brain injury is difficult to evaluate because of prophylactic administration of phenytoin and inconsistency in injury severity and treatment. However, posttraumatic epilepsy during brain hypothermia treatment is a serious complication. Hyperemia, release of excitatory neurotransmitters, consumption of residual brain energy, and brain ischemia after convulsions all worsen brain damage. The critical persistent time of epilepsy for the development of neuronal necrosis is about 20–30 min. Therefore, prophylactic treatment against epileptic seizure is very important during the cooling stage.

The key points for management of posttraumatic epilepsy are:

1. Type is divided into early epilepsy (≤7 days) and late epilepsy (>7 days) after head trauma.
2. Prophylactic anticonvulsant does not reduce the frequency of late seizures.
3. Anticonvulsants should be used to prevent early seizures in high risk patients such as those with GCS ≤ 8 on admission.
4. Cases with acute subdural, epidural, or intracerebral hematoma, open depressed skull fracture with parenchyma injury, cortical injury, or penetrating injury, and history of significant alcoholic abuse are recorded in high incidence.
5. Discontinue anticonvulsants after 1 week in most uncomplicated cases.

To understand indications and select anticonvulsant medicines, modes of action, metabolism, dosage, and side effects are summarized in Table 20.

Table 20. The pharmacological characteristics of various anti-epieptic medicines

	Benzodiazepines	Midazolam	Phenytoin	Valproate	Phenobarbital
Mode of action	Postsynaptic Bz1 (anti-convulsant, anxiolytic effects) Presynaptic Bz2 (sedation, and hypnotic) receptor mediated	Activate GABA neurons with binding of post synaptic Bz1 receptors	Membrane stabilizer Prevent Na^+ influx	Inhibitor of GABA transaminase and glutamate decarboxylase	Depressant effect on neuronal membranes
Metabolism	Receptor binding. The highest density of receptors in cerebral cortex, with low density in cerebellum, basal ganglia, limbic system, and brain stem	Liver and intestine	Liver Can saturate enzyme systems Long half life	Liver Protein bound Short variable half life	Liver or excreted in urine unchanged Long half life
Dosage	5–10 mg i.v. Peak effects are seen in 5–10 min	0.15–0.3 mg/kg (i.v.) Maintenance: half or same dosase of 0.15–0.3 mg/kg	Can be given as single dosage e.g., 150–400 mg at night	2–3 × daily 600 mg to 3 g total daily dosage	Can be given as single dosage, e.g., 90 mg at night
Side effects	Allergic reaction Memory impairment	Low incidence of arrythmia and hypotension	Gum hypertrophy Cerebellar dysfunction at toxic levels	Gastrointestinal upset Thrombocytoprnia Drug-induced hepatitis Hair loss Tremor/chorea	Sedation Depression Behavioural disturbances in children Skin rashes Withdrawal seisures

The initiation of antiepileptic medicine such as benzodiazepines for cortical damage, midazolam for damage of the basal ganglia, and followed by phenytoin for neuroprotection of cerebellum are recommend within 3–6 h after severe brain damage. Phenytoin is also effective for the prevention of cytotoxic brain edema by acting as a membrane stabilizer, and prevents Na^+ influx in severely brain-injured patients. Vitamin B is nesessary to prevent epileptic seizure after severe brain injury.

Phenobarbital has been utilized to control seizures and ICP elevation for a long time; however, phenobarbital blocks the hydrogen transport system in mitochondria and causes severe reduction of adenosine triphosphate (ATP) production. This negative effect is a serious condition for neuronal restoration in severely brain-injured patients, especially under the conditions of brain hypothermia. For the success of neuronal restoration, dying neurons require ATP production even under the conditions of brain hypothermia. The administration of phenobarbital is not recommended for the restoration of dying neurons except under special conditions such as prolonged epilepsy and uncontrolled ICP elevation despite the use of various treatments.

The combination of phenobarbital and brain hypothermia is very powerful for reducing ICP elevation; however, reduction of brain tissue ATP is a very dangerous condition for dying neurons in injured brain tissue. Our preliminary clinical studies of the combination of brain hypothermia and phenobarbital administration suggested poor prognosis even with normalization of ICP elevation.

Other ICU Management Issues

Control of $PaCO_2$

Animal studies have suggested the use of a closed circulation system to measure oxygen consumption and carbon dioxide production. During brain hypothermia with low blood temperature, the production of carbon dioxide will be low. For moderate brain hypothermia, $PaCO_2$ will be 2–4 mmHg lower than that at 37°C. Therefore, $PaCO_2$ greater than 40 mmHg during brain hypothermia treatment suggests the possibility of trouble within the respiratory system. On the other hand, hyperventilation during brain hypothermia treatment can cause a large reduction in $PaCO_2$ with disturbance of the systemic microcirculation. The control of $PaCO_2$ at 32–36 mmHg during brain hypothermia treatment is recommended.

Fluid Selection

The basic choice for fluid selection requires normal osmotic pressure, low glucose content, adequate phosphate and magnesium, and the normal valance electrolytes sodium, potassium, and chloride. Prevention of harmful stress-associated hyperglycemia is important to avoid hemoglobin dysfunction, excess release of vasopressin, increased brain tissue lactate, and activation of proinflamatory cytokines [23,24].

The early management of BBB dysfunction is also as important as early fluid resuscitation. The replacement of AT-III to prevent endovascular inflammatory reactions, followed by 5% albumin is useful for the management of BBB dysfunction. The management of AT-III at higher than 100% under brain hypothermia (32°–34°C) is successful for the prevention of endovascular damage and micro-embolus formation in the systemic circulation [20,22,24]. Hypo-albuminemia after severe brain injury is a common complication [34]. The replacement of albumin and maintenance of serum albumin higher than 3.0 g/dl is very successful for the prevention of brain edema with normalization of BBB dysfunction, and also prevents infection during the cooling stage of brain hypothermia [20,22,24]. The effect of albumin in preventing infection is discussed later in this section.

The use of magnesium chloride with potassium phosphate is also important to prevent respiratory muscle weakness. Respiratory muscle weakness is a very dangerous complication because of activated immune crisis, reduced adaptation to prolonged hypoxia, induction of pulmonary atelectasis, and susceptibility to severe pulmonary infection. The management of protein synthesis of respiratory muscle is helpful in avoiding these complications.

Management of Digestive Organs

The major targets for the management of the digestive organs during the cooling stage are:

Prevention of abdominal hypertension
Control of intestinal mucous edema
Maintenance of microcirculation to intestinal organs
Prevention of pulmonary hypertension
Removal of the contents of a full stomach
Control of gastric juice pH
Control of intra-ileum lumina pressure
Control of macronutrient intake feedback reaction
Prevention of bacterial translocation
Management of digastrics decontamination
Enteral nutrition
Maintenance of energy source to intestinal immune cells

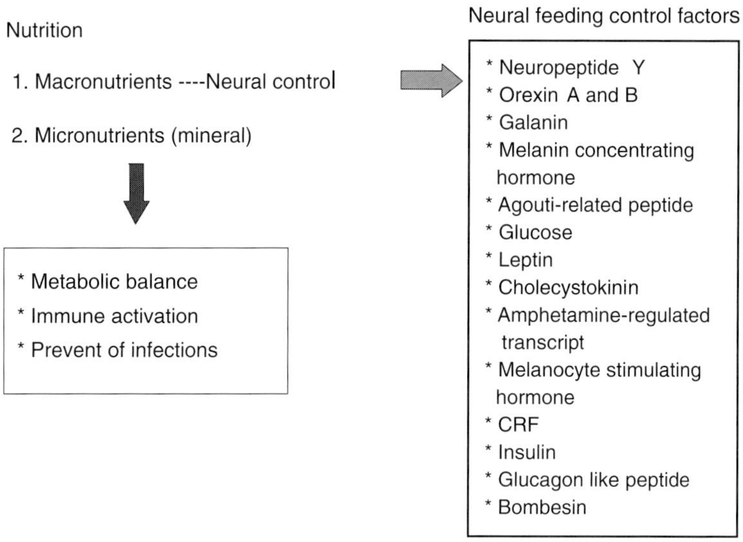

Fig. 86. Basic nutritional consideration in severely brain-injured patients. CRF, corticotropin releasing factor

The abdominal pressure can be controlled to less than 10 mmHg to prevent ischemia of the intestinal organs, portal venous stasis, and ICP elevation, by insertion of an ileum tube. The management of hypo-albuminemia (higher than 3.0 mg/dl of serum albumin), replacement of AT-III (higher than 100%,) and prevention of abdominal hypertension are important to prevent intestinal mucous edema and for the management of the digestive organs. Unsuccessful management of intestinal mucous edema produces various complications such as diarrhea during enteral nutritional administration, pancreatic dysfunction because of pancreatic duct obstruction, immune dysfunction, and activation of bacterial translocation [24].

Pulmonary hypertension can also produce congestion of the portal vein, venous stasis of the digestive organs, and intestinal mucous edema. We prefer the use of a ventilator with low tidal volume and PEEP pressure lower than 15 mmHg. The critical airway pressure to produce intestinal dysfunction is 35 mmHg. Gastric lavage after cranial surgery is important to prevent abdominal hypertension and pneumonia (Mendelson's syndrome). Washing of the stomach with normothermic saline and control of gastric juice pH lower than 3.5 are very useful for the prevention of intestinal bacterial translocation thoughout the mouth and trachea. Gastric juice pH greater than 4.0 sees the breakdown of the chemical acid barrier to intestinal bacteria. The insertion of an ileum tube distal to the Traiz ligament is useful for the control of intestinal ischemia by reducing intra-luminal pressure. The management of digastrics decontamination with nonabsorbable and hypothermia-active antibiotics (combination of levofloxacin (Cravit, 200 mg) + amphotericin B 100–300 mg) and early administration of enteral nutrition are useful to prevent systemic infections. The energy source of intestinal immune cells is glutamine that is produced in the lungs and skeletal muscles. Therefore, management of pulmonary infection and muscle weakness is also important to prevent immune crisis during brain hypothermia treatment.

Nutritional Management

Nutritional considerations are divided between the use of macronutrients and micronutrients (Fig. 86). The metabolic nutritional phase is divided into the metabolic ebb phase and metabolic flow phase (Fig. 87). In the ICU management of critically ill patients, early administration of parenteral and enteral nutrition is recommended. However, enteral and parenteral nutrition that is too early can increase neurotoxic glutamate in injured brain tissue because serum glutamate is approximately doubled by enteral and parenteral nutrition (Table 10, Chap. 33). Neurotoxic serum glutamate can be permeable to the damaged BBB and worsen the condition. Before deciding upon enteral nutrition, the severity of BBB dysfunction (determined by CSF/serum albumin ratio) and the level of hypo-albuminemia must be determined. During brain hypothermia treatment, serum glucose rapidly increases because of reduced glucose expenditure after the brain temperature falls below 33°C. Hyperglycemia with serum glucose greater than 230 mg/dl activates vasopressin release and changes BBB function (Fig. 88). Hypo-albuminemia also produces increased permeability of the BBB by an osmotic mechanism. Early enteral nutrition is very effective for the prevention of infection by maintaining glutamine and providing energy to immune cells.

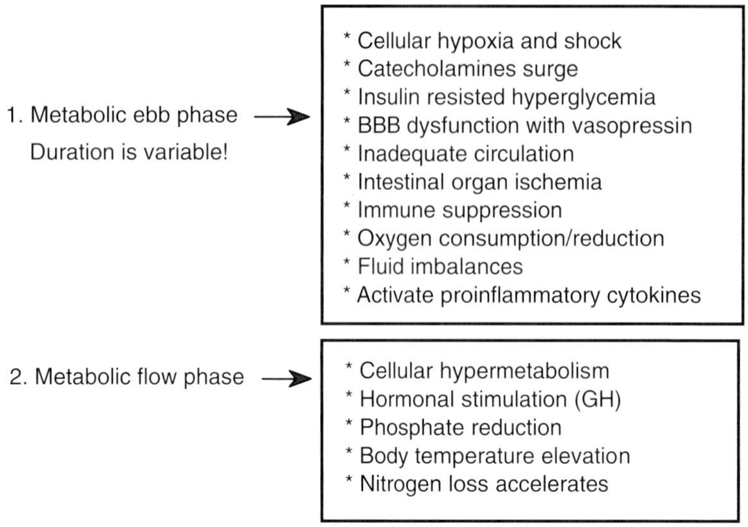

Fig. 87. Two metabolic nutritional phases and related pathophysiology

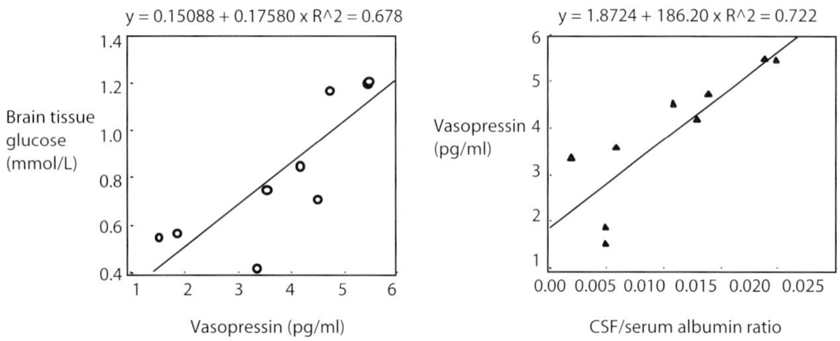

Fig. 88. The relationships between changes of brain tissue glucose, cerebrospinal fluid (CSF) vasopressin and CSF/serum albumin ratio [blood–brain barrier (BBB) dysfunction marker]. Increasing brain tissue glucose promotes excess release of vasopressin by macronutrient neural feed back mechanism and changes of BBB dysfunction

However, glutamine is a very neurotoxic substrate. The serum glutamine concentration increases twofold after enteral and parenteral nutrition. Therefore, early enteral nutrition under the conditions of severe BBB dysfunction (CSF/serum albumin ratio ≥0.01) can promote the progression of delayed neuronal death by increasing the brain tissue glutamate level. Because the peak time of BBB dysfunction will be about 3–4 days after brain injury, glutamine-free enteral nutrition is recommended for this period. However, there is no correct answer regarding enteral nutrition during brain hypothermia treatment. Increasing brain tissue glutamate was not recorded with the following strategy of nutritional management during brain hypothermia.

For cases in which BBB dysfunction is not severe (CSF/serum albumin ratio <0.01), early enteral nutrition, that includes 1% $ZnCl_2$, glutamine (Glumin-S, Kyowa Hakko, Tokyo, Japan), arginine (arginine hydrochloride, Ajinomoto-pharuma, Tokyo, Japan), and amino acid for activation of immune function, should start from 2 days after trauma. However, in cases in which the CSF/serum albumin ratio is higher than 0.02, initial enteral nutrition is limited to saline with $ZnCl_2$ initially and is then followed by ω-3 unsaturated fatty acid enteral nutrition (Fibren-HY, Meiji, Tokyo, Japan) (Fig. 89). During brain hypothermia treatment, glucose metabolism shifts to lipid metabolism. At 34°C during mild brain hypothermia, the division between glucose and lipid metabolism is about equal. However, at 32°C lipid metabolism becomes dominant (about 82%) over glucose metabolism (about 18%). The ω-3 unsaturated fatty acid enteral nutrition is reasonable as nutrition during brain hypothermia treatment. The enteral nutrition of Fibren-HY is very successful for the prevention of activation of harmful stress-associated hyperglycemia even at the early stage. After stabilizing BBB function amino acid nutrition with glutamine can begin about 3–4 days after brain damage with monitoring of serum glutamate. Enteral nutrition is very useful for preventing severe systemic infections and for the management of immune crisis during brain hypothermia treatment.

Prevention of Immune Crisis

The mechanism of immune dysfunction under hypothermia has not been elucidated previously. Our recent clinical study suggested that GH is a regulator of

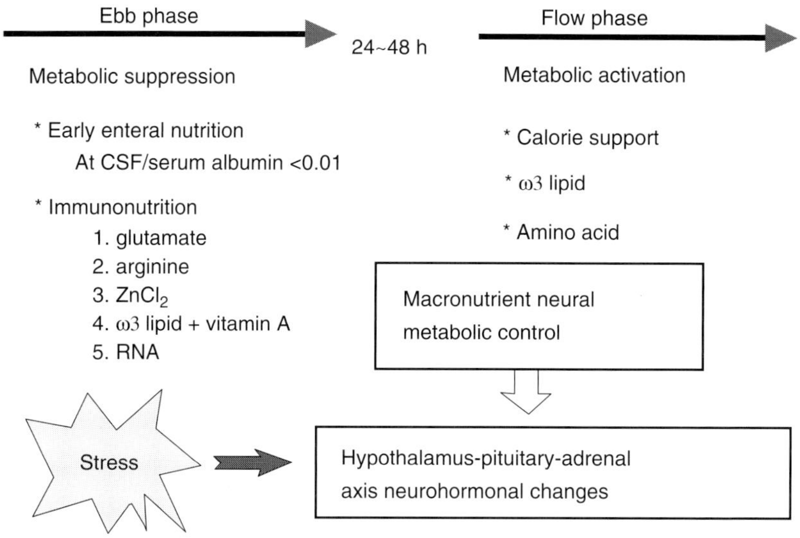

Fig. 89. Nutritional considerations for severely brain-injured patients

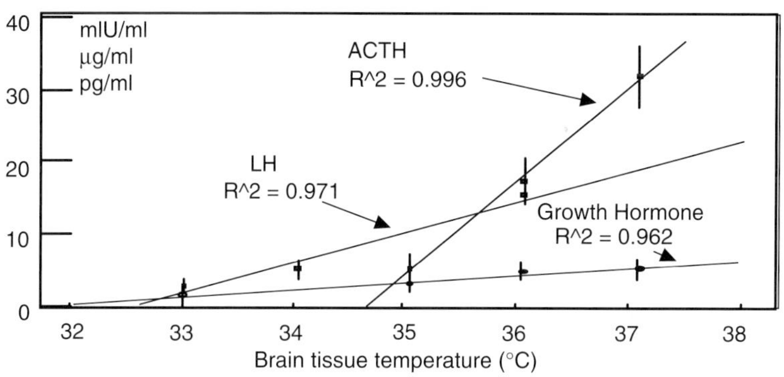

Hormone	Immunologic Function
ACTH	Stimulates NK-cell activity, Stimulates B-cell proliferation Suppression of IFN-γ synthesis Suppress MHC class II expression by macrophage
GH	Enhances the generation of cytotoxic T cells (IL2,IL5,IL6) Suppress the antiinflamatory cytokines Stimulates the production of O_2 by macrophages

Fig. 90. Brain hypothermia produces pituitary hypo-function and immune dysfunction. *ACTH*, adrenocorticotropic hormone; *GH*, growth hormore; *LH*, luteinizing hormone

the immune response (Fig. 90) [24]. The use of brain hypothermia cannot avoid subjecting the pituitary gland to low temperature and results in a reduction of serum GH level. GH activates CD4 and cellular immune function and produces increased levels of proinflammatory cytokines IL1 and IL6 [9,20]. However, CD8 associated with anti-inflammatory cytokine IL10 and fluid immune function will be suppressed (Fig. 37, Chap. 27). Therefore, we believe that excessive release of GH causes the activation of proinflammatory cytokines and worsening of systemic infections. On the other hand, excessive reduction of GH caused by brain hypothermia causes cellular immune suppression and susceptibility to infection. The number of lymphocytes strongly correlates to the release of serum GH during brain hypothermia treatment as shown in Fig. 42 (Chap. 33). Lymphocytopenia lower than $1000\,mm^3$ is an indirect critical measure of immune dysfunction during brain hypothermia treatment. Glutamic acid is an energy source for lymphocytes and is produced in the lungs and skeletal organs. Therefore, prevention of pulmonary infection and administration of glutamine, alanine, potassium phosphate, and magnesium chloride are also important to prevent immune crisis during brain hypothermia treatment. Administration of growth hormone and arginine is a direct treatment to prevent immune crisis. However, it is difficult to prevent immune crisis by these replacement therapies alone. The use of intermittent brain hypothermia and prevention of pituitary hormonal crisis is a novel technique for the prevention of infection during prolonged brain hypothermia treatment [20,22,24].

In the use of intermittent brain hypothermia, the brain tissue temperature is elevated slightly from 32°–33°C to 34°C during the evening period of 1800–2000 hours which is the time of physiological GH increase without the complication of hyperglycemia. In cases of severe infection with reduced immune function, we controlled brain tissue temperature at 34°C using various treatments as described previously.

The management of immune crisis during brain hypothermia treatment requires:

Prevention of pulmonary infection
Management of respiratory muscle metabolism
Management of skeletal muscle (massage and prevention of venous stasis)
Replacement of phosphate, magnesium, alanine, and glutamine
Administration of arginine with normal levels of hemoglobin (>11 g/dl)
Intermittent brain hypothermia control
Early enteral nutrition that includes glutamine

Special Consideration for Prevention of Infection During Hypothermia

During the management of brain hypothermia treatment, control of infection is very important and directly affects the prognosis [14]. Increasing serum cytokines under the condition of severe BBB damage results in cytokine encephalitis. The complication of cytokine encephalitis in severe brain injury produces brain edema and release of neurotoxic glutamate that is difficult to control even with 32°–34°C brain hypothermia. Therefore, the complication of pneumonia and systemic infection during brain hypothermia means unsuccessful treatment. The major causes of infection during brain hypothermia treatment are HPA axis neurohormone dysfunction, suppression of immune function, energy crisis in immune cells, hypo-albuminemia, metabolic suppression of skeletal muscles, enteral bacterial translocation, and inadequate parenteral and enteral nutrition (Table 21) [24].

Fundamental Management for Prevention of Infection During Brain Hypothermia

All severely brain-damaged patients affected by trauma, stroke, hypoxia, or cardiac arrest produce stress neurohormonal reactions and release excess HPA axis hormones [8,23]. These stress reactions are not severe in anesthetized animal models. However, specific HPA axis neurohormonal reactions of clinical patients produces insulin-resistant hyperglycemia, activation of cytokines, hypo-albuminemia, pulmonary edema, and immune dysfunction [23].

Table 21. The causes of severe infection during brain hypothermia treatment

Unsuitable management of hypothalamus-pituitary-adrenal axis neuroendocrinological dysfunction
Hyperglycemia caused by catecholamine surge
Excess stimulation of neuropeptide Y receptors
Respiratory muscle weakness caused by reduced insulin
Immunological dysfunction caused by muscle weakness
Hypo-albuminemia
Reduced release of growth hormone caused by hypothermia
Cellular immune dysfunction
Lymphocytopenia
Poor enteral care management
Gastric mucous edema caused by hypo-albuminemia
Abdominal hypertension
Unsuitable nutritional care management
Increase of serum glutamate and brain tissue glutamate caused by early nutrition: if CSF/serum albumin > 0.02

CSF, cerebrospinal fluid

Delayed induction of brain hypothermia produces an excess release of catecholamines and severe hyperglycemia [23]. Severe hyperglycemia (serum glucose >230 mg/dl) stimulates the release of vasopressin [30,31], and activates proinflammatory cytokines, BBB dysfunction, hemoglobin dysfunction, and disturbances of microcirculation in the brain, lungs, and heart [23,24]. Excessive stimulation of cytokines results in damage during DNA synthesis of albumin. Of these factors, hypo-albuminemia (serum albumin <2.5 mg/dl) is a big issue for the management of infections because of intestinal mucous edema, pancreatic duct obstruction, inaction of albumin-binding antibiotics, and BBB dysfunction. The intestinal mucous edema can easily reduce digestive immune function and hinders early enteral nutrition because of diarrhea. Therefore, hyperglycemia and hypo-albuminemia combined is a very dangerous condition for worsening systemic infections.

On the other hand, overly prolonged suppression of the HPA axis neurohormonal reaction also results in susceptibility to infection. Brain tissue temperature lower than 34°C reduces the levels of GH and ACTH. GH is a very important regulator of immune function of CD4 and lymphocytes. The critical brain tissue temperature for maintaining immune function and lymphocytes activity is about 32°C as shown in Fig. 4 (Chap. 20). Therefore, in moderate brain hypothermia below 34°C, immune dysfunction can easily complicate systemic infection. The early induction of brain

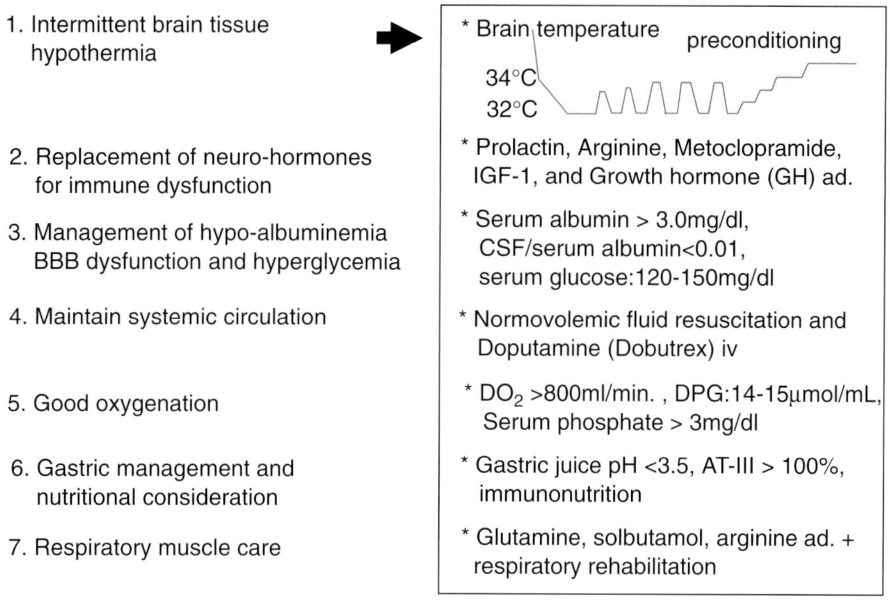

Fig. 91. Basic infectious control management during brain hypothermia treatment. BBB, blood–brain barrier; IGF-1, insulin like growth factor; CSF, cerebrospinal fluid; DPG, 2,3-diphosphoglycerate

hypothermia and intermittent brain hypothermia management with well-organized hyperglycemia and hypoalbuminemia is most important to prevent easy infection. The fundamentals of infectious care management during brain hypothermia are summarized in Fig. 91 and are different to previous antibacterial infection management criteria.

Early Management of Pulmonary Infection

Gastric lavage using normothermic saline is fundamental for the prevention of Mendelson's syndrome pneumonia. This management is also effective in preventing abdominal hypertension and bacterial translocation when combined with control of gastric juice pH at about 3.0–3.5. Iced saline is useful for early induction of hypothermia; however, at the cooling stage, gastric lavage with too much cooled saline can easily cause arrhythmia and AV block, especially in cases showing dehydration, hypokalemia, or cardiac disease.

The high incidence of infection during brain hypothermia treatment is mainly produced by bacterial translocation of intestinal bacteria and immune suppression (Table 22). The early management of intestinal bacterial translocation and immune dysfunction is very successful for the prevention of infection during brain hypothermia treatment. Pseudomonas and gram-negative enteral bacteria are most common bacteria that cause pneumonia. Immipenem cilastain sodium (Tienam 1–2 g/day ×3) or meropenem trihydrate (Meropn, 1–2 g/day ×4) are recommended as first choice antibiotics for gram-negative bacteria and Pseudomonas at the cooling stage.

Early nutrition is very successful in preventing infection, as previously described. However, before starting

Table 22. Bacterial infection and the immunocompromised host

Microorganisms	Immunocompromised host
Pseudomonas	Insufficiency of macrophages
Staphylococcus	
Enterobacter	
Candida	
Aspergillus	
Herpes	Abnormal T-cells
Cytomegalo virus	
Toxoplasma	
Legionella	
Mycobacteria	
Histoplasma	
Pseudomonas	Abnormal B-cells
Pneumocytis carini	
Streptococcus pneumoniae	
Streptococcus pneumoniae	Insufficiency of compliments
Nisseria	

enteral nutrition, intestinal organ ischemia must be controlled. Intestinal ischemia is produced by microembolus formation associated with reduced AT-III (≤80%), abdominal hypertension (≥15 mmHg), and mucous membrane edema caused by severe hypoalbuminemia (≤2.5 mg/dl). The presence of severe BBB damage with a CSF/serum albumin ratio of more than 0.01 is also a negative factor for early enteral nutrition. For early nutrition, the CSF/serum albumin ratio must be higher than 0.01.

To prevent complications, two-step enteral nutrition is preferred. Initially, no glutamine should be included in enteral nutrition (such as Ensure) that combines with replacement of AT-III and serum albumin for 3–4 days after brain injury. Glutamine can then be included in enteral nutrition as shown in Fig. 89.

Control of hyperglycemia prevents the excess release of vasopressin, induction of IL1 and IL6, and BBB dysfunction through the reduction of macronutrient responses. These increased serum cytokines, such as IL1 and IL6, can easily permeate the damaged BBB and cause severe brain edema. Additional cytokine encephalitis with infection during brain hypothermia is a very dangerous complication.

ICU Care for Prevention of Systemic Infection

The basic steps of ICU care to prevent infection are:

1. Intermittent elevation of brain tissue temperature from 32°C to 34°C during the evening
2. Naso–oral cavity cleaning
3. Gastric juice pH < 3.5
4. Prevent abdominal hypertension <10 mmHg
5. Digestive decontamination antibiotics
6. AT-III > 80% to 100% and gastric pHi > 7.3
7. Serum albumin >3.5 mg/dl
8. Replacement of $ZnCl_2$, arginine, and Hb > 11 g/dl
9. Gastric immune nutrition replacement followed by nutritional care
10. Ventilator care and urinary care
11. Breathing rehabilitation
12. Management of lymphocytopenia (34°C brain hypothermia, GH, γ-globulin)
13. Low dosage of antibiotics and nonprotein-binding antibiotics
14. O_2ER 23%–25%; DPG 12–15 mmol/gHb
15. Muscle rehabilitation

Management of Severe Pulmonary Infection

If severe infection occurs during brain hypothermia treatment, steps must be taken to:

Isolate the infectious source
Prevent systemic inflammatory reactions
Administer hypothermia-effective antibiotics
Recover immune function
Manage intestinal ischemia
Prevent intestinal bacterial translocation
Replace albumin
Control hyperglycemia

To minimize the effect of infection on brain damage, the management of BBB dysfunction is also important.

Removal of Infectious Source. In most cases, enteral bacteria from the patient are the infectious source. The enteral administration of amphotericin B, vancomycin, or albekacin in combination with intravenous injection of hypothermia-effective antibiotics such as cefmetazole, flomoxef, or arbekacin or bacteria-sensitive antibiotics is basic treatment. The management of gastric juice pH to less than 3.5 provides a barrier to the enteral bacteria translocation through the mouth and trachea.

Direct Management and Anti-inflammatory Treatment for Infected Organs. The administration of hypothermia-effective antibiotics, delivery of sufficient oxygen (≥700–800 ml/min), and stabilization of vital signs are effective in the management of infected organs. The sensitivity of antibiotics under the conditions of brain hypothermia has not been studied. Our recent clinical studies suggested that cefmetazole, flomoxef, and arbekacin were effective even under the conditions of hypothermia. However, further studies of the effects of hypothermia on the action of antibiotics are required.

Prevention of Systemic Inflammatory Reactions. Anti-inflammatory medicine such as aspirin, AT-III, or AT-III combined with low molecular weight heparin are treatments of choice. AT-III is very sensitive for the prevention of vascular inflammation. Steroid pulse therapy for the prevention of inflammatory reactions is not recommended during brain hypothermia treatment. Under the condition of hyperglycemia the steroid may overstimulate the neuropeptide Y receptor in the vascular wall of the lungs, brain, and heart. The stimulation of the hypothalamus neuropeptide Y receptor by steroid and hyperglycemia also produces the release of vasopressin. These pathophysiological reactions produce increased vascular permeability and disturbances of microcirculation. During brain hypothermia treatment, serum glucose increases because of reduced glucose expenditure. Therefore, steroid is not recommended for the prevention of systemic inflammatory reactions during brain hypothermia treatment. The management of hyperglycemia is also effective in preventing cytokine reactions, indirectly associated with preventing the excess release of vasopressin.

Recovery of Immune Function. The intravenous administration of GH and/or L-arginine is very powerful in boosting immune functions (Fig. 92). Although GH is very useful for increasing the immune activity and lymphocyte action, GH is very expensive and is difficult to use for a prolonged period. As an alternate medication, L-arginine is much easier to use in ICU management.

Control of Intestinal Bacteria and Prevention of Bacterial Translocation. Digastrics decontamination with enteral administration of nonabsorbable antibiotics, early enteral nutrition for immune cells, control of abdominal hypertension, prevention of intestinal mucous edema, and management of AT-III to prevent disturbances of intestinal microcirculation are effective management steps for the control of bacterial translocation.

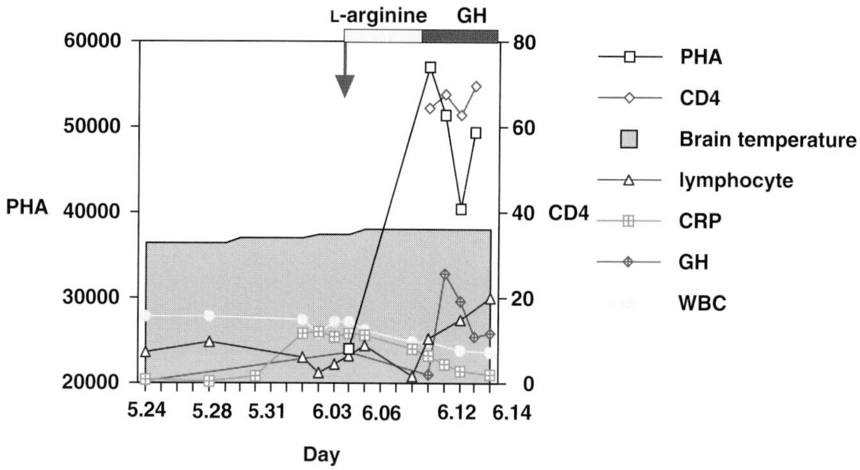

Fig. 92. The successful recovery of immune function by administration of L-arginine and growth hormone (*GH*) in severe pneumonia. PHA, phytohemagglutinin; CD4, CD4-T cell; CRP, C-reactive protein; GH, growth hormone; WBC, white blood cell

Protection of BBB. It is difficult to prevent cytokine chemical encephalitis without management of BBB. Proinflammatory cytokines in the bloodstream may easily permeate the damaged BBB in cases of systemic infection. Cytokine encephalitis produces an uncontrollable increase of neurotoxic glutamate in injured brain tissue even with moderate brain hypothermia. The critical level of BBB dysfunction is evaluated with a CSF/serum albumin ratio higher than 0.01. For treatment of BBB dysfunction, administration of AT-III combined with low molecular weight heparin to prevent vascular inflammation and micro-embolus formation is used initially. After that, replacement of serum albumin to more than 3.0–3.5 mg/dl is basic management for injured BBB. The use of steroid is not recommended under the presence of stress-associated hyperglycemia.

Antimicrobial Therapy. The choice of antibiotics is determined by a culture study of antimicrobial sensitivity. In our clinical studies of pneumonia bacteria, 46.8% were gram-negative, 35.9% were gram-positive, and fungal infection accounted for 14.5%. In these bacteria, methicillin resistant *staphylococcus aureus* (MRSA) was most common at 15.8%, and followed *Pseudomonas aeruginosa* 9.7%, *Klebsiella pneumoniae* 7.6%, *Eenterococcus faecalis* 6.9%, *Escherichia coli* 4.1%, and *Streptococcus pneumoniae* 2.1%. The antimicrobial effects of antibiotics are influenced by body temperature, serum albumin level, and liver and renal function. Before starting antimicrobial therapy, diagnosis of the antibiotic sensitivity, the presence of hypo-albuminemia, and the hepatic–renal functions are important. However, information concerning the antimicrobial effects toward bacteria under hypothermia is limited. Our clinical studies suggested that the antimicrobial effects of cefoperazone, which is metabolized in the liver, was much more effective than the renally eliminated antibiotics cefmetazole, flomoxef, and arbekacin under hypothermia. The antimicrobial effects of arbekacin, vancomycin, amino glycosides, and β-lactams, which are almost totally eliminated by the kidneys, are not effective with the conditions of mild brain hypothermia without renal dysfunction. If hepatic–renal function is reduced by about 50%, the required dose of these antibiotics is about 50% of a normal dose. Multi bacteria infections occur in many cases during brain hypothermia, and therefore, double-drug therapy is recommended. In brain hypothermia treatment, compromised host patients with immune dysfunction and enteral ischemia with unsuitable neurohormone management are commonly infected. Intravenous administration of antipseudomonal penicillin with amino glycoside and/or vancomycin is the medication of first choice for severe pulmonary infections. Prophylactic enteral administration of amphotericin B, vancomycin, or albekasin is very successful to prevent the occurrence of severe pulmonary infections. Antibiotic therapy should not be continued for more than 2 weeks.

Outcomes. The clinical results of management of systemic infection during brain hypothermia treatment are summarized in Table 23. We experienced a high incidence (64.2%) of severe infection at the initial stage in the period 1991–1993. However, complication of severe infection during brain hypothermia treatment is currently limited to about 5.2% by using the abovementioned infectious control management strategies.

Management of Disseminated Intravascular Coagulopathy and Sepsis

The activation of intravascular coagulation during the cooling stage and activation of fibrinolysis at the rewarming stage is the major target of management

Table 23. The advances in management of pulmonary infection during brain hypothermia treatment

Period	Treatment	Cases	Percentage
1991–1993	Antibiotics γ-Globulin Physiological rehabilitation Prevention of hypoproteinemia	9/14	64.2%
1994–1995	GL-washing O_2ER control at 23%–25% Kinetic therapy Early intestinal nutrition Electrical muscle stimulation	16/50	32.0%
1996–1998	Replacement of growth hormone L-Arginine, glutamine, Zn immune Hemoglobin > 12 mg/dl Vitamin A and lipid nutrition at rewarming stage	21/16	12.5%
1999–2001	Intermittent hypothermia Serum glucose 120–140 mg/dl Serum albumin > 3.5 mg/dl Two-step enteral nutrition Digestive decontamination Immune care management	1/19	5.2%

GL, gastric lavage

Table 24. The changes of coagulation and fibrinolysis markers between disseminated intravascular coagulation (DIC) and non-DIC during cooling stage and at rewarming stage

	Day 0		Day 1		Day 2	
	DIC	non-DIC	DIC	non-DIC	DIC	non-DIC
Cooling phase						
PLT (/mm³)	7.6 ± 4.2**	23.3 ± 7.9	6.4 ± 3.7**	16.9 ± 4.7	5.8 ± 3.4**	14.9 ± 5.7
FPA (ng/ml)	48.4 ± 18.8*	23.1 ± 10.1	22.2 ± 9.7*	11.5 ± 5.2	24.4 ± 9.8**	6.6 ± 3.4
D-dimer (μg/ml)	33.1 ± 16.4*	4.1 ± 2.5	21.2 ± 19.8*	5.0 ± 3.4	9.6 ± 3.4**	1.8 ± 0.8
Rewarming phase						
PLT (/mm³)	6.9 ± 1.2**	12.1 ± 4.7	4.8 ± 1.5**	12.8 ± 6.6	6.1 ± 1.4*	12.6 ± 8.5
FPA (ng/ml)	35.5 ± 5.4*	5.0 ± 2.0	57.2 ± 8.8*	4.5 ± 1.4	59.3 ± 8.1*	4.9 ± 1.9
D-dimer (μg/ml)	7.5 ± 3.3*	1.8 ± 0.3	10.5 ± 6.8*	1.9 ± 0.6	13.3 ± 6.4*	2.7 ± 1.1

Entries given as mean ± SD. $n = 24$
PLT, platelet; FPA, fibrino-peptide A
* $P < 0.05$
** $P < 0.01$

in disseminated intravascular coagulopathy (DIC) (Table 24). The background of these pathophysiological changes includes activation of leukocytes and endothelial injury, tissue factor generation, activation of extrinsic pathway of coagulation, systemic microembolus formation, and organ failures. Ventilator respiratory management, pharmacological management for increased coagulopathy, improving oxygen delivery to major organs, antimicrobial therapy for enterobacteria, activation of immune function, fluid resuscitation for maintaining microcirculation, metabolic and nutritional support, prevention of acute renal failure, and management for acute lung injury are major targets of DIC management in the ICU. The management of sepsis and DIC based on a care map is useful (Fig. 93).

Sepsis-associated respiratory failure is one of the most difficult ICU management issues during brain hypothermia treatment. Inadequate ventilation management of air pressure, pressure pattern, tidal volume (V_T), and ventilatory rate can markedly worsen lung injury. The use of low tidal volume (10–15 ml/kg → 5–9 ml/kg), moving away from normal gas-exchange blood values (PaO_2 > 75 mmHg → SaO_2 90% ± 5%, $PaCO_2$ 40 ± 5 mmHg → accept 40–50 mmHg, if other parameters do not achieve normal values, pH 7.4 ± 0.05 → accept ≥37.3), low airway pressure (maintain plateau pressure

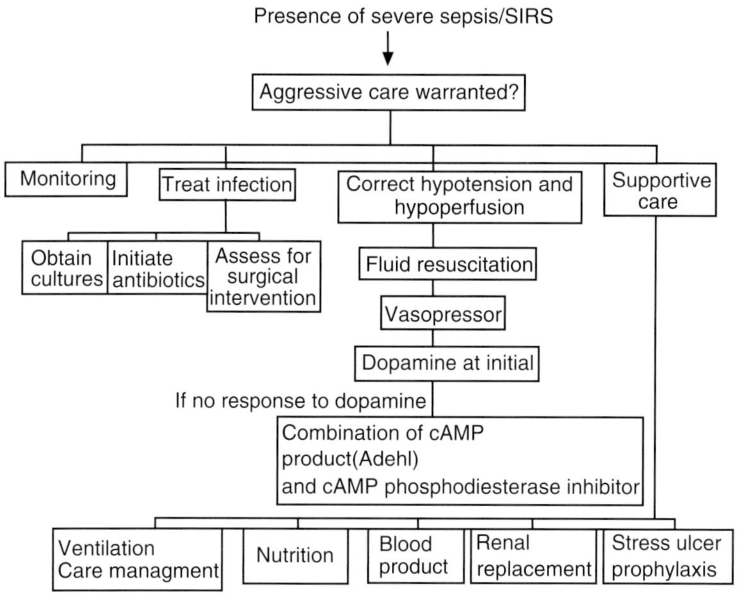

Fig. 93. The care map for sepsis and disseminated intravascular coagulability (DIC)

$\leq$35 cmH_2O), PEEP at about 10–15 cmH_2O with constant $PaCO_2$, and inspiratory/expiratory (I/E) ratio greater than 1, and the new ventilatory and oxygenation technique with management of hemoglobin enzyme are fundamental ventilation management steps. A high airway pressure can easily complicate baro-trauma in infected lungs. The use of effective airway management and respiratory rehabilitation support the ventilation therapy.

Pharmacological management for reduced perfusion pressure is fluid resuscitation (crystalloid and colloids) combined with dopamine administration. If this management is unsuccessful in maintaining stable systemic circulation, combined administration of adehl (cyclic adenosine monophosphate production) and or amurinon (cyclic adenosine monophosphate phosphodiesterase inhibitors), followed by doputamine is recommended. Insulin-resistant hyperglycemia is not activated by this pharmacological blood pressure management.

Based on the known pathogenetic mechanism of DIC, three major treatment strategies can be distinguished: inhibition of systemic activation of coagulation, enhancement of fibrinolysis, and restoration of the relative or absolute deficiencies of natural inhibitors of coagulation. AT-III combined with low molecular weight heparin (danaparoid sodium), tissue factor pathway inhibitor (TFPI), and protein C are effective in preventing the systemic activation of coagulation as well as the proinflammatory response and lethal effects of *E. coli* bacteria.

Adequate tissue oxygenation requires management of oxygen delivery, and oxygen transport with good circulation of the bloodstream. $PaO_2/FiO_2 \geq 300$, $SaO_2 \geq 99\%$, oxygen delivery >700–800 ml/min, Hb $\geq$ 11 g/dl, DPG 12–15 μg/dl, phosphate 3–5 mg/dl, pH $\geq$ 7.3, $PaCO_2$ 32–38 mmHg, $ETCO_2$ 24–28 mmHg, AT-III > 100%, and serum albumin $\geq$ 3.0 mg/dl are indication parameters of oxygenation therapy.

Staphylococcus aureus, fungemia, *E. coli*, *Klebsiella sp.*, *Pseudomonas aeruginosa* and their complications are major causes of sepsis. To determine the choice of antibiotics, the end toxin potentials of antibiotics must be considered for the treatment of DIC and sepsis. For antibiotics that enhance end toxin release, cefataxime, cefazidime, aztreonam, and quinolones are nominated. On the other hand, as inhibitors of end toxin release, the action of aminoglycoside, polymixin, tetracycline, teichoplanin, meropenam, and chloramphenicol has been demonstrated. Aminoglycoside, amphotericin B, arbekacin and vancomycin are easy to use for the management of sepsis without severe renal dysfunction. If renal dysfunction is a complication, the use of cefoperazone, which is metabolized in the liver, is one of the methods of choice. However, these antibiotics do not work under the conditions of severe hypo-albuminemia (serum albumin < 2.5 mg/dl) because of unstable antibiotics in the bloodstream, complication of free bacteria, diarrhea caused by enteral mucous edema and ischemia, and activation of proinflammatory cytokines. Before antimicrobial therapy, care should be taken to ensure that serum albumin is higher than 3.0 g/dl, AT-III is greater than 100%, serum phosphate is 3.0–5.0 mg/dl, serum glucose is 120–140 mg/dl, and there is sufficient oxygen delivery.

Metabolic and nutritional support is also important in the management of DIC and sepsis. After stabilizing

BBB dysfunction and the replacement of serum albumin, ω-3 unsaturated fatty acid enteral nutrition (fibren-HY) can begin, combined with 1% $ZnCl_2$ and glutamine for 3–4 days in cases of CSF/serum albumin ratio lower than 0.01. After the peak time of cytokine production or clinical signs of the disappearance of vascular reaction of conjunctives, amino acid enteral nutrition is recommended. Early enteral nutrition is very successful for the prevention of immune crisis and immunological dysfunction.

Prevention of Hypokalemia

During brain hypothermia, hypopotassemia is one of the common complications in serum electrolytes. The consumption of potassium in the metabolic shift from glucose to lipid metabolism, elimination from intestinal organs, and reduced vasopressin are considered to be causes of hypopotassemia. However, the detailed mechanism of hypopotassemia during brain hypothermia treatment is not get elucidated. Hypopotassemia with potassium levels lower than 3.0 mg/dl can easily introduce cardiac dysfunction, such as arrhythmia, AV block, and elongation of the QT interval. The paresis of intestinal peristalsis is also a serious complication during brain hypothermia treatment. The replacement of potassium by infusion drip is recommended for serum potassium levels lower than 3.0 mg/dl.

Indications to Stop Hypothermia

Indications to halt advanced brain hypothermia include cardiac arrhythmia, elongation of the QT interval to greater than 450 mm/s, hypopotassemia with potassium level lower than 3 mEq/dl, hypo-albuminemia with serum albumin lower than 3.0 g/dl, lymphocytopenia lower than 1000 mm^3, and oxygen delivery less than 500 ml/min. After replacement therapy or stabilization of these pathophysiological changes, advanced brain hypothermia treatment can be restarted. If these abnormal parameters cannot be controlled, brain temperature should be rewarmed by 0.5°–1.0°C and maintained at about 34°–34.5°C. In most cases, the complications associated with hypothermia are recorded at brain tissue temperatures lower than 33°C.

The observation of a J wave on the ECG, which increases at lower body temperature, does not mean the occurrence of cardiac dysfunction. The environment of electrical conduction in cardiac muscle is changed according to the J wave appearance. However, the precise mechanism of the J wave is not known. The cardiac output begins to reduce as the brain tissue temperature falls below 33°C. The other complications of immune crisis, including lymphocytopenia, metabolic imbalanced hyperglycemia, elongation of the QT interval, and muscle metabolic reduction, also progress more rapidly at brain tissue temperatures below 33°C. Therefore, the risk of hypothermia-associated complications is markedly different between mild (34°C) and moderate (32°–33°C) brain hypothermia. This is why brain tissue temperature at 34°C is known as mild brain hypothermia, and brain tissue temperature at 32°–33°C is known as moderate brain hypothermia.

Other complications of hypothermia, such as ventricular fibrillation, hypercalcemia, hyperglycemia, consumption of vitamin A with unstable membrane phosphate metabolism, prolonged muscle relaxation, shivering, and prolonged coagulation time, are recorded as a physiological reactions of brain hypothermia treatment.

The indications and contraindications of brain hypothermia treatment are listed in Table 5 (Chap. 29). If various contraindicated factors, such as shock, arrhythmia, severe hyperglycemia, and cardiac insufficiency, can be managed within 6 h, brain hypothermia treatment can be started with care. In these cases, mild brain hypothermia is recommended initially. After maintenance or stabilization of vital signs and ensuring that oxygen delivery is more than 700–800 ml/min, serum glucose is lower than 180 mg/dl, serum potassium is higher than 3 mEq/dl, there is no arrhythmia, and the QT interval is less than 450 mm/s, more advanced moderate brain hypothermia treatment can progress. The two-step induction is very successful in avoiding the complications of brain hypothermia treatment. The clinical result of the two-step induction is better than that for rapid induction of moderate brain hypothermia.

The Computed Algorithm Management System

In the ICU, severely brain-injured patients are managed with an understanding of the mechanism of brain damage, the systemic responses of cardiopulmonary function, excess release of HPA axis neurohormones, changes of immune function, administration of neuronal oxygenation, and imbalance of glucose metabolism. These management targets are diagnosed by monitoring of cardiopulmonary function using the Swan Ganz catheter, blood gases, laboratory examinations, monitoring of intracranial pathophysiological changes such as ICP, SjO_2, brain tissue oxygen tension, jugular venous temperature, brain tissue temperature, tympanic membrane temperature, and CBF, neuronal function by

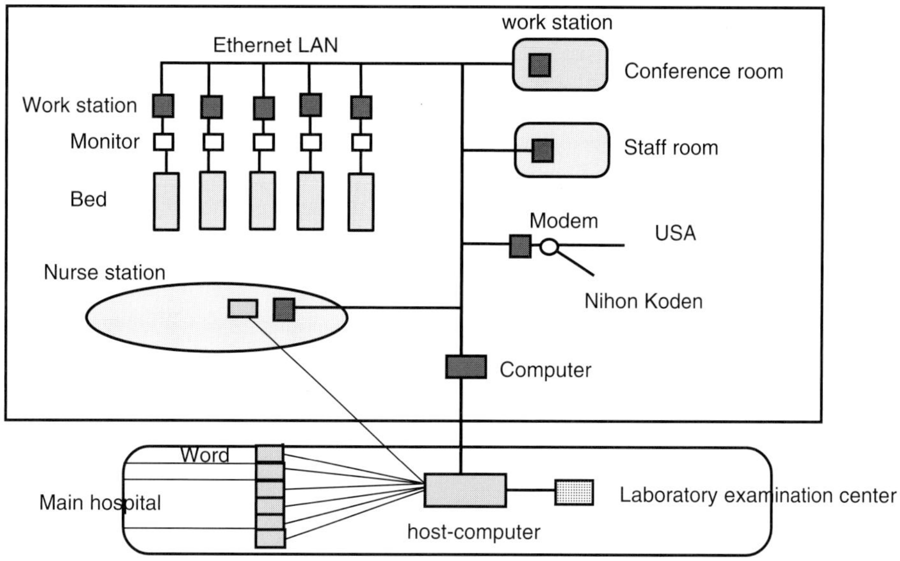

Fig. 94. The block diagram of the computer care management system in the medical center

electroencephalogram (EEG) and brain stem auditory evoked potential, and morphological changes of the brain by computed tomography or magnetic resonance imaging. However, successful treatment of severe brain damage can be obtained by not only understanding the relationships between each brain injury mechanism, but also by a total diagnosis approach to brain damage. The computed total care management system is very useful for understanding the relationships between each brain injury mechanism and total diagnosis of brain damage.

In the ICU management of critically ill patients, team management is the accepted standard. For the success of team care management, real time monitors should be present at the bedside, in the conference room, and also in the staff office. It is preferable that a senior doctor should contribute toward team management and maintain a very high level of medical input throughout the computed care management system. The block diagram of our computed ICU care management system is described in Fig. 94.

The computed ICU care management system opened a new concept for monitoring severely brain-injured patients. The cerebral thermal index with monitoring of SjO_2 is very successful for monitoring changes of CBF and brain metabolism. The computed monitoring of alveolar capillary CO_2 permeability index (end tidal CO_2/(cardiac output × $PvCO_2$) is also useful to diagnose the alveolar permeability.

One of the difficult points of the computed monitoring system is the inclusion of the algorithm care management system. The medical team cannot be at full strength for the entire day, and especially so at midnight. This is because senior medical staff doctor cannot always work at this time. Therefore, the question of how to take perfect care of the patient, even at midnight, is important. Without establishing the management care system, it is difficult to support patients with the most advanced medical management.

Concept of Computed Algorithm Management

Abnormal data, that are recorded by the computer monitoring system, can be identified by automatic flashing on the bedside display. The selection of abnormal flashing data on the computer display brings up seven cards that describe the algorithm management. In this section, the most popular algorithm management cards for brain hypothermia treatment are discussed.

Algorithm for Unstable Brain Tissue Temperature

The contents of the seven algorithm cards contain information about brain tissue temperature, the effect of brain temperature on brain damage, fundamental management of brain tissue temperature, pharmacological treatment to control brain tissue temperature, management of complications that are associated with brain tissue temperature, and recommendations for management of brain tissue temperature. Each of the cards for algorithm management of brain tissue temperature are described in Table 25–33.

Table 25. Algorithm management of brain tissue temperature: information

- Brain temperature (BT) changes by 4 factors
  - Blood temperature (core temperature)
    - Main basic factor of brain temperature
  - BP (CPP)
    - Carrier of core temperature into the brain
  - Brain metabolism (0.5°C)
    - Small factor
  - CBF
    - Carrier and washout factor of brain temperature
- Brain temperature is regulated by CBF washout mechanism
  - Brain thermal pooling (SBP < 90–100 mmHg, reperfusion and >38°C body temperature)
  - BT = jugular venous blood temperature
- Cooling of brain temperature method
  - Cooling blanket method: lower blanket water temperature and change cooling body surface
  - Direct blood cooling method
  - Chilled saline gastric lavage
  - Cooling body by alcohol or steamed water evaporation
  - Cooling CSF
- Unsuccessful cooling of brain tissue temperature
  - Blood temperature is not low enough
  - Blanket is too small
  - Blanket water flow is slow
  - Obese patient (fatty tissue is slow conductor of heat), two-machine cooling method is recommended
  - Body wrapping is not complete
  - Room temperature is high
  - Many heat-generating machines around the bed
  - Bed making is not suitable
  - Infections and high fever
  - Malignant hyperthermia
  - Dehydration

BP, Blood pressure; CPP, cerebral perfusion pressure; CBF, cerebral blood flow; SBP, systolic blood pressure; CSF, cerebrospinal fluid

Table 26. Algorithm management of brain tissue temperature: diagnosis of CBF disturbances and brain metabolism by monitoring of brain tissue temperature, internal jugular venous blood temperature, tympanic membrane temperature, and internal jugular venous O_2 saturation

	CTI	$SjvO_2$
Hypermetabolism	→	↘
Hypometabolism	→	↗
Ischemia	↗	↘
Ischemic hypermetabolism	↑	—↗
Ischemic hypermetabolism	↗	—↘
Nonfilling	<1	↗↘
Luxury perfusion	↘	↗
Recovery	↘	↘

CTI, Cerebral thermal index (brain tissue temperature ÷ tympanic membrane temperature or internal jugular venous blood temperature ÷ tympanic membrane temperature); $SjvO_2$, internal jugular venous blood saturation

Table 27. Algorithm management of brain tissue temperature: pathophysiology

- Mild brain hypothermia (~>34°C of brain tissue temperature)
  - 50% prevention of NO radicals
  - Reduction of catecholamine surge is about 50%. This effect is diagnosed by monitoring of serum hyperglycemia, lactate and 2,3 DPG

Catecholamine surge
ATP ↓→ cAMP
↓
ATP + glycogen → hyperglycemia (>230 mg/dl)
↓
Lactate production and DPG reduction

  - Increase anaerobic metabolism by imbalance of cerebral oxygenation and glucose metabolism
  - Unsuccessful neuroprotection of A10 nervous system
- Rapid or unstable changes between mild and moderate brain hypothermia
  - Difficult to maintain stable $\bar{D}O_2$ > 700 ml/min
  - Unstable brain metabolism
    - >34°C: glucose-dominant metabolism
    - <34°C: lipid-dominant metabolism
  - Unstable immune function
  - Difficult prevention of selective radical attack to the dopamine nervous system
  - No recovery of injured brain and stop progress of secondary brain damage
  - Brain damage will be much worse at rewarming stage

DPG, diphosphoglycerate

Table 28. Algorithm management of brain tissue temperature: basic management

- Stabilize cardiopulmonary functions
  - SPB > 100 mmHg
  - Hb > 12 mg/dl
  - DPG > 14 μmol/ml
  - $\bar{D}O_2$ > 700–800 ml/min
  - K^+ > 3 mEq/dl
- Stabilize autonomic nerve reactions
  - Anesthesia
  - Analgesia
- Increase neuroimmune functions
  - Increase IGF-1, L-arginin infusion
  - Replacement hormone, growth hormone
  - Activate skeletal muscle protein synthesis
- Antipyretics medication
- Technical considerations
  - Alcohol heat evaporation
  - Chilled saline gastric lavage
  - Complete body wrapping and prevent heat conductance to room air
  - Reduce room temperature to 18°C
  - Maintain room air outflow circulation
  - Two cooling machines
  - Direct blood cooling method
  - Ventilator drive with air compressor
  - Limited use of heat-generating medical devices around the bed
  - Combination of isolated cooling of CSF circulation

SBP, Systolic blood pressure; Hb, hemoglobin

Table 29. Algorithm management of brain tissue temperature: medication

Stabilize cardiopulmonary functions
- BP > 100 mmHg, E + dopamine or E + vasopressin
  - E, 8 mg/250 mlD5W (bronchodilatation and increase CO)
  - D, 400 mg/250 mlD5W (increase CO and maintain renal flow)
  - V, 0.1–0.4 U/min (increase CO without ATP consumption)
- $\bar{D}O_2$ > 700–800 ml/min, Doputrex 500 mg/250 mlD5W (increase CO)

Stabilize autonomic nerve reactions
- Anesthesia, midazolam (Dormicum) 10 A (200 mg) + K-free maintenance solution, solita T4-200 ml, 10–20 ml/h drip infusion
- Analgesia, [Fetanest 0.1–0.2 ml/kg/2–3 h + vecuronium (0.02–0.2 mg/kg)] 1–2 day followed by buprenorphine HCl (Lepetan) 0.8 mg(4 A)/day, adult i.v. drip

Prevent hypothalamus edema and increase neuroimmune functions
- Increase IGF-1, L-arginine infusion (one bottle infusion drip/h)
- Steroid hormone, methylpredonisolone 5–30 mg/kg loading followed by a tapering dose

Antipyretics medication
- Aspirin 320–650 mg by rectal suppository every 4–6 h, not to exceed a total daily dose of 3.6 g[a]
- Acetaminophen 325–365 mg po tubing every 4–6 h in adult, or 10 mg/kg every 4 h in children

CO, Cardiac output
[a]Aspirin + acetaminophen every 6 h may be tried if failed at low temperature

Table 30. Algorithm management of brain tissue temperature: complications

Unstable cardiac output and cardiac dysfunction

Unstable metabolic conditions
- Glucose metabolism dominant at ~34°C
- Lipid metabolism dominant at lower than 34°C of brain hypothermia
  - Rapid induction of 32°–33°C brain hypothermia produces hyperglycemia and increases brain tissue glucose and lactate more than 34°C brain hypothermia management. Therefore, 32°–33°C brain hypothermia without correct management of hyperglycemia is much worse than 34°C mild brain hypothermia management

Unstable immune functions
- Rapid reduction of growth hormone below 33°C brain tissue temperature

  ↓

- Reduce CD4 and lymphocytes

Reduce the neuronal protection mechanism of brain hypothermia with ICP elevation, brain edema, glutamate neuroexcitation, dopamine radical attack

No recovery of brain damage and restart brain damage at the rewarming stage

↓

Much worse brain damage

Table 31. Algorithm management of brain tissue temperature: special considerations

Before lowering temperature of blanket water

Two checks ↓
- Cardiopulmonary function is stabilized
- Is brain temperature controllable?

↓

Remove the negative factors and keep cerebral oxygenation

↓

Start basic nursing care plan of algorithm for uncontrolled brain temperature

Table 32. Algorithm management of brain tissue temperature: keywords

Brain tissue temperature
Cooling
Hypothermia

Table 33. Algorithm management of brain tissue temperature: references

1. Iatrou CC, Domaingue CM, Thomas RD, Nye DH (2002) The effect of selective brain cooling on intracerebral temperature during craniotomy. Anaesth Intensive Care 30:167–170
2. Safar P, Behringer W, Bottiger BW, Sterz F (2002) Cerebral resuscitation potentials for cardiac arrest. Crit Care Med 30(4 Suppl):S140–144
3. al-Alousi LM, Anderson RA, Worster DM, Land DV (2002) Factors influencing the precision of estimating the postmortem interval using the triple-exponential formulae (TEF). Part II. A study of the effect of body temperature at the moment of death on the postmortem brain, liver and rectal cooling in 117 forensic cases. Forensic Sci Int 125:231–236
4. Callaway CW, Tadler SC, Katz LM, Lipinski CL, Brader E (2002) Feasibility of external cranial cooling during out-of-hospital cardiac arrest. Resuscitation 52:159–165
5. Yan Y, Tang W (2001) Changes of evoked potentials and evaluation of mild hypothermia for treatment of severe brain injury. Chin J Traumatol 4:8–13
6. Zhu L, Diao C (2001) Theoretical simulation of temperature distribution in the brain during mild hypothermia treatment for brain injury. Med Biol Eng Comput 39:681–687
7. Mustafa S, Thulesius O (2002) Cooling-induced carotid artery dilatation: an experimental study in isolated vessels. Stroke 33:256–260
8. Taylor DL, Mehmet H, Cady EB, Edwards AD (2002) Improved neuroprotection with hypothermia delayed by 6 hours following cerebral hypoxia-ischemia in the 14-day-old rat. Pediatr Res 51:13–19
9. Laptook AR, Shalak L, Corbett RJ (2001) Differences in brain temperature and cerebral blood flow during selective head versus whole-body cooling. Pediatrics 108:1103–1110
10. Felberg RA, Krieger DW, Chuang R, Persse DE, Burgin WS, Hickenbottom SL, Morgenstern LB, Rosales O, Grotta JC (2001) Circulation 104:1799–1804

Table 34. Algorithm management of hypotension: information

Shock: SBP < 90 mmHg Shock index (SI) = pulse ÷ SBP	Bleeding volume →	SI = 1; 1000 ± 250 ml SI = 2; 2000 ± 250 ml SI = 3; 3000 ± 250 ml

Mean BP = [diastolic BP + (SBP – diastolic BP)] ÷ 3
Mean BP = (cardiac output × peripheral resistance) ÷ 80 + central venous pressure
Peripheral resistance = [(Mean BP – central venous pressure) × 80] ÷ cardiac output
CBF autoregulation works under the SBP at 70–170 mmHg, and mean BP at 50–150 mmHg
Brain thermo-pooling occur at BT > 38°C, after reperfusion, SBP < 90–100 mmHg
Catecholamine surges
NE (~1 h) > vasopressin (~2 h) > E (~3 h) > dopamine (more ~3 h)
Masking brain hypoxia—neuronal hypoxia even with normal PaO_2, CBF, CPP, and oxygen delivery
Causes: hemoglobin DPG reduction, brain thermo-pooling, hyperglycemia acidosis (pH < 7.2), blood shift for intestinal organ by dopamine dominant circulation

SBP, Systolic blood pressure; BP, blood pressure; NE, norepinephrine; E, epinephrine

Table 35. Algorithm management of hypotension: diagnosis

	Adult	Children
• Blood volume	65 ml/kg	80 ml/kg
• Pulse	60–90/min	Nursing 120–160/min Infancy 90–140/min School children 75–100/min
• Blood pressure	94–140/62–80 mmHg	New born 60–90/20–60 mmHg Nursing 74–100/50–70 mmHg Infancy 82–100/50–78 mmHg School children 84–120/54–80 mmHg
• Stroke volume	50–120 ml/beat	Newborn 5 ml/beat Infancy 15 ml/beat School children 35 ml/beat
• Cardiac index	2.5–4 l/min m^{-2}	3.5–4 l/min m^{-2}
• SVR	800–1600	800–1600
• PVR	80–240	80–240
• Right atrial pressure	5 mmHg	3 mmHg
• PCWP/LAP	10 mmHg	8 mmHg
• Left atrial pressure	120/10 mmHg	100/6 mmHg
• Aortic pressure	120/80 mmHg	100/6 mmHg

SVR, Systemic vascular resistance; PVR, pulmonary vascular resistance; PCWP/LAP, pulmonaly capillary wedge pressure/left atrium pressure

Algorithm for Low Blood Pressure

The maintenance of blood pressure is very important during brain hypothermia treatment. Dehydration therapy using manitol, reduced serum catecholamines, hyperventilation to reduce brain swelling, AV block by hypothermia, and occult bleeding with multiple trauma are major causes of low blood pressure at the cooling stage. The algorithm management cards for the management of blood pressure are shown in Tables 34–42.

Algorithm for ICP Elevation

The management of ICP is focused on maintaining a pressure lower than 15 mmHg at the cooling stage, although elevation to 20 mmHg is permissible under ICU management. However, ICP elevation can occur as a result of unsuccessful management of brain ischemia, hypoxia, edema, brain thermo-pooling, and vascular engorgement. The prevention or restoration of brain ischemia, hypoxia, brain swelling, and brain thermo-pooling are initial targets of management, and brain hypothermia is one of the methods used to treat these pathophysiological changes. The management of brain hypothermia for the control of ICP does not provide a useful restoration effect. The algorithm management cards for ICP elevation are shown in Tables 43–51.

Algorithm for Pulmonary Infections

The complication of severe pulmonary infection during the cooling stage is a very serious condition for the management of patients. Inadequate oxygen uptake, reduced immune function, cardiac dysfunction, and

Table 36. Algorithm management of hypotension: pathophysiology

1. The maintaining force to CBF
2. Washout the brain temperature (BT)
3. Promote acute brain swelling
• Cerebral perfusion pressure (CPP)
• Lower CPP = MAP – ICP < 80 mmHg
• Tympanic membrane temperature ÷ core temperature < 1.0
↓
Brain ischemia
• ICP 20–25 mmHg: venous stasis
• ICP 25–35 mmHg: CBF disturbances
• ICP 35–45 mmHg: brain swelling
• ICP > 45 mmHg: non or poor filling
Acute brain swelling
Disturbed autoreguration to CBF: SBP < 70 mmHg, >180 mmHg; $PaCO_2$ > 45 mmHg
Brain thermo-pooling (elevation of brain tissue temperature >40°C)
Body temperature >38°C, BP < 90–100 mmHg after reperfusion
Non effect of oxygen inhalation
Low Hb-DPG

Table 37. Algorithm management of hypotension: basic management

Elastic bandaging of extremities
Normal volume replacement
Medication
Stage 1 (brain temperature ~34°C) E → E + vasopressin (within 3 h)
Stage 2 (brain temperature 32°–33°C) E + vasopressin + dobutrex → vasopressin + dobutrex
SBP maintain > 100 mmHg
CPP > 80 mmHg
Hb > 12 mg/dl
Oxygen delivery > 700 ml/min
2,3-DPG > 13 mmol/ml
Serum K^+ > 3 mEq/dl
Serum glucose 120–160 mg/dl

Table 38. Algorithm management of hypotension: medication to increase cardiac output and vascular resistance and provide volume replacement

Dosage	Compatible solution	Incompatible drugs
NE 8 mg/250 ml D5W	Aminophyline	Insulin
Low systemic vascular resistence	Amphotericine B	Lidocaine HCl
	Azathioprine Na	Pentobarbital Na
	Folic acid	Phenobarbital Na
	Furosemide	Sodium bicarbonate
E 2 mg/250 ml D5W or NS	Aminophyline	Pentobarbital Na
Bronchiospasm, anaphylactic, septic, or cardiogenic shock	Amphotericine B	Phenobarbital Na
	Imperiling Na	Propofol
	Azathioprine Na	Sodium bicarbonate
	Lidocaine HCl	Warfarin sodium
D 400 mg/250 ml D5W	Acyclovir Na	Cefoperazone Na
3–10 μg/kg min^{-1} β1 and D effects 10–40 μg/kg min^{-1} via α1 sepsis, cardiogenic shock, renal insufficiency	Alteplase	Chloramphenicol Na succinate
	Amphotericine B	Ganciclovir Na
	Imperiling Na	Gentamicin sulfate
	Azathioprine Na	Propofol
	Cefazolin Na	Sodium bicarbonate
	Cefepime HCl	
Dobutrex	Acyclovir Na	Cefuroxine
500 mg/250 mlD5W	Alteplase	Chroramphenicol
Low cardiac output, cardiogenic shock, congestive heart failure, cardiomyopathy	Aminophyline	Digoxin
	Amphotericine B	Folic acid
	Imperiling Na	Furosemide
	Azathioprine Na	Heparine sodium
	Bumetanide	Penicillin G
	Cefazolin Na	Phenobarbital
	Cefepime HCl	Propofol

D5W, Dextrose 5% in water; NS, NaCl 0.9%; D, dopamine

Table 39. Algorithm management of hypotension: complications

Brain ischemia caused by prolonged hypotension
Worsening at rewarming stage with short duration of hypothermia treatment. Short-duration brain hypothermia stops progression of secondary brain damage. The primary brain damage, with not enough recovered neurons, reprogresses at rewarming stage. The rapid pathophysiological changes by rewarming worsen reprogression of primary brain damage
Difficult moderate brain hypothermia treatment (32°–33°C) caused by unstable cardiac function associated with reduced serum catecholamines. The cardiac output is reduced below brain tissue temperature of 33°C
Easy to reduce the platelets and fall in disseminated intravascular coagulopathy by suppression of liver function

DIC, Disseminated intravascular coagulation

Table 40. Alorithm management of hypotension: special considerations

1. Hypotension is major cause of unsuccessful brain hypothermia treatment and elevation of ICP at rewarming stage
2. Main cause of hypotension is different time window and level of lower brain temperature 3–6h

——————————————→ time

Catecholamine induced cardiomyocontraction and coronary spasm	Blood shift to intestine (bladder temperature > tympanic membrane temperature)
Reduced circulation volume	Reduced CO by moderate brain hypothermia

Management: control BP > 90 mmHg and combination of oxygen management to prevent brain hypoxia

1. Mild brain hypothermia 2. No dehydration therapy 3. Bronchial dilatation with no ATP consumption, intestinal vasodilatation, hypertensive drugs 4. Intermittent elastic bandaging of extremities 5. Flat position	→	1. Moderate hypothermia 2. Increase cardiac output 3. No intestinal vasodilatation hypertensive drugs 4. Increase SVR by elastic bandaging of extremities 5. Flat position depends on ICP elevation

1. Hb > 11–12 mg/dl
2. 2,3-DPG > 14 mmol/ml
3. $\bar{D}O_2$ > 700–800 ml/min
4. Serum glucose 120–150 mg/dl
5. O_2ER 23%–25%
6. Serum K^+ >3 mEq/dl

CO, Cardiac output; ATP, Adenosine triphosphate; SVR, systemic vascular resistance

Table 41. Algorithm management of hypotension: keywords

Hypothermia
Hypotension
Blood pressure

Table 42. Algorithm management of hypotension: references

1. Kitagawa H, Akiyama T, Yamazaki Mori H, Sunagawa H (2002) Effects of moderate hypothermia on in situ cardiac sympathetic nerve endings. Neurochem Int 40:235–242
2. Laussen PC, Murphy JA, Zurakowski D, Sullivan LJ, McGowan FX Jr, Demaso DR (2001) Bispectral index monitoring in children undergoing mild hypothermic cardiopulmonary bypass. Paediatr Anaesth 11:567–573
3. Mori K, Itoh Y, Saito J, Takeyama Y, Kurata Y, Kaneko M, Asai Y, Torigoe T, Dickson EW (2001) Post-resuscitative hypothermic bypass reduces ischemic brain injury in swine. Acad Emerg Med 8:937–945
4. Nakae Y, Fujita S, Namiki A (2001) Isoproterenol enhances myofilament Ca(2+) sensitivity during hypothermia in isolated guinea pig beating hearts. Anesth Analg 93:846–852
5. Chi OZ, Choi YK, Lee DI, Kim YS, Lee I (2001) Intraoperative mild hypothermia does not increase the plasma concentration of stress hormones during neurosurgery. Can J Anaesth 48:815–818
6. Jalan R, Olde Damink SW, Deutz NE, Hayes PC, Lee A (2001) Restoration of cerebral blood flow autoregulation and reactivity to carbon dioxide in acute liver failure by moderate hypothermia. Hepatology 34:50–54
7. Ozaki H, Nagai Y, Tochihara Y (2001) Physiological responses and manual performance in humans following repeated exposure to severe cold at night. Eur J Appl Physiol 84:343–349
8. Xu H, Aibiki M, Seki K, Ogura S, Yokono S, Ogli K (2000) Effects of induced hypothermia on renal sympathetic nerve activity and baroreceptor reflex in urethane-anesthetized rabbits. Crit Care Med 28:3854–3860
9. Weis SJ, Muniz A, Ernst AA, Lippton HL, Nick TG (2000) The effect of prior hypothermia on the physiological response to norepinephrine. Resuscitation 45:201–207
10. Himmelseher S, Pfenninger E (2000) Neuroprotection in neuroanesthesia: current practices in Germany. Anaesthesist 49:412–419
11. Krismer AC, Lindner KH, Kornberger R, Wenzel V, Mueller G, Hund W, Oroszy S, Lurie KG, Mair P (2000) Cardiopulmonary resuscitation during severe hypothermia in pigs: does epinephrine or vasopressin increase coronary perfusion pressure? Anesth Analg 90:69–73
12. Kanstrup IL, Poulsen TD, Hansen JM, Andersen LJ, Bestle MH, Christensen NJ, Olsen NV (1999) Blood pressure and plasma catecholamines in acute and prolonged hypoxia: effects of local hypothermia. J Appl Physiol 87:2053–2058
13. Lesser JB, Koorn R, Vloka JD, Kuroda MM, Thys DM (1999) The interaction of temperature with thiopental and etomidate on extracellular dopamine and glutamate levels in Wistar-Kyoto rats subjected to forebrain ischemia. Acta Anaesthesiol Scand 43:989–998
14. Roscher R, Ingemansson R, Algotsson L, Sjoberg T, Steen S (1999) Effects of dopamine in lung-transplanted pigs at 32 degrees C. Acta Anaesthesiol Scand 43:715–721
15. Weiss SJ, Muniz A, Ernst AA, Lippton HL (1998) The physiological response to norepinephrine during hypothermia and rewarming. Resuscitation 39:189–195
16. Azzam FJ, Fiore AC (1998) Postoperative junctional ectopic tachycardia. Can J Anaesth 45:898–902
17. Sellden E, Lindahl SG (1998) Amino acid-induced thermogenesis to prevent hypothermia during anesthesia is not associated with increased stress response. Anesth Analg 87:637–640
18. De Riva C (1997) Hypoglycaemia unawareness in a young boy with insulin-dependent diabetes mellitus and anti-adrenal medullary antibodies. Diabetes Metab 23:528–532
19. Sellke FW, Tofukuji M, Stamler A, Li J, Wang SY (1997) Beta-adrenergic regulation of the cerebral microcirculation after hypothermic cardiopulmonary bypass. Circulation 96(9 Suppl):II-304–310
20. Roscher R, Ingemansson R, Wetterberg T, Algotsson L, Sjoberg T, Steen S (1997) Contradictory effects of dopamine at 32 degrees C in pigs anesthetized with ketamine. Acta Anaesthesiol Scand 41:1213–1217

Table 43. Algorithm management of ICP elevation: information

- $ICP = \dfrac{\text{brain volume} + \text{CSF} + \text{Blood dume} + \text{mass lesion}}{\text{volume of cranial cavity}}$
- CPP = MABP − ICP
- Normal value: ICP 10–12 mmHg, CPP > 65–75 mmHg
- Brain edema
  - Cytotoxic edema (brain hypoxia)
  - Vasogenic edema (vascular engorgement)
  - Interstitial edema (BBB destruction)
  - Osmotic edema (hypo-albuminemia <2.5 g/dl)

> Brain hypoxia: PaO_2 < 60 mmHg, DPG < 10 mmol/gHb,
> Vascular engorgement: disturbed auto regulation + BP elevation, $PaCO_2$ 45–50 mmHg, and SBP > 180 mmHg are trigger factors
> BBB destruction: CSF/serum albumin ratio (CSAR) > 0.01,
> CSAR > 0.02 severe BBB dysfunction
> Osmotic edema: severe hypo-albuminemia (serum albumin < 2.5 g/dl)

- Water filtration (WF) rate in the brain capillary

WF = K [(vascular pressure-tissue pressure) – (serum osmotic pressure-tissue osmotic pressure)]

Arterial side capillary pressure = 35–40 mmHg
Venous side capillary pressure = 12–20 mmHg
Brain tissue pressure = 8 mmHg
Serum osmotic pressure = 25 mmHg
Tissue osmotic pressure = 5 mmHg

→ Interstitial water is removed to venous root by −7 mmHg pressure

- ICP elevation occurs with brain edema, hydrocephalus, vascular engorgement, mass lesion such as hematoma, and cranial decompression

MABP, Mean arterial blood pressure

Table 44. Algorithm management of ICP elevation: diagnosis

Clinical signs and symptom of ICP elevation	
Headache	
Vomiting	
Disappearance of venous pulsation of eye base → choked disc	
Tympanic membrane temperature is lower than core temperature	
ICP monitor	
CSF ventricular pressure	
Epidural pressure	
Brain tissue pressure	
Calibration of zero point of ICP	
Closed skull	height of III ventricle
Semi closed decompressed external skull bone	height of heart
ICP elevation	more than 20 mmHg
Evaluation of ICP	
Closed skull	all kinds of ICP monitoring are useful
Semi-closed skull bone	CSF ventricular pressure is only available
Effect of atmospheric air pressure	
More than 1010 hPa produces compression of brain	
Less than 1010 hPa activates brain explosion through skull cavity	

Table 45. Algorithm management of ICP elevation: pathophysiology

ICP elevation and pathophysiological changes	
ICP	Pathophysiological changes
20–25 mmHg	Venous stasis, plasma skimming, heterogeneous hypoxia
25–30 mmHg	Disturbances of microcirculation, plasma skimming brain hypoxia, intercompartment pressure difference
30–45 mmHg	CBF disturbances, disturbances of autoregulation herniation
>45 mmHg	Poor filling and nonfilling
Time course	
Acute brain swelling (few seconds)	
Brain edema (peak 24–48 h)	
Severe BBB damage: (CSF albumin/serum albumin ratio > 0.02)	
Serum cytokines (proinflammatory cytokines, helper T-cell induced cytokines, and anti-inflammatory cytokines) directly affect the injured brain tissue	
Herniation	
Brain stem death	
Effect of pathophysiology by original diseases	

Table 46. Algorithm management of ICP elevation: basic management

Direct management of ICP elevation
- Remove hematoma and large external decompression that includes lower temporal lobe
- Head-up position (CPP > 80 mmHg)
- Management of hypo-albuminemia (serum albumin > 3.5 g/dl)
- Hyperosmotic, diuretic therapy
  - Manitol > glycerol (not indicated at hyperglycemia)
- Suppress the CSF production
  - Furosemide, lasix

Management of promoting factors
- Prevent bronchial obstruction
- Lower PEEP (<7 cmH_2O)
- Lower mediastinal pressure (<15 mmHg)
- Prevent abdominal hypertension (<15 mmHg)
  - Urinary catheter, gastric tube, and ileum tube
- $PaCO_2$ 25–35 mmHg

Maintain adequate CPP (80–100 mmHg)
- Elastic bandaging of extremities
- Abdominal aorta balloon catheter

Management of masking brain hypoxia
- SaO_2 > 98%, FiO_2/PaO_2 > 350
- $\bar{D}O_2$ > 700–800 ml/min, DO_2I > 600 ml/min
- pH > 7.3
- DPG 10–15 mmol/gHb
- Gastric pHi > 7.3
- Hb > 11–12 mg/dl
- AT-III > 100%
- $ETCO_2$ 32%–38%

PEEP, Positive endo-expiratory pressure

Table 47. Algorithm management of ICP elevation: medication

Direct pharmacological management of ICP elevation	
Hyperosmotic, diuretic fluid administration	
Manitol and glycerol	
Suppression of CSF production	
Furosemide and lasix	
Anti-edema	Albumin infusion
Prevent IL1, TNF cytokines	
Steroid	Not indicated at hyperglycemia (>180 mg/dl)
Stabilization of ICP	
Anesthesia combination with analgesia	
Midazolum (use at serum albumin > 3.5 g/dl)	
Propofol	
Muscle relaxation	
Maintaine adequate CPP (80–100 mmHg)	
Prevent excess blood shunt to intestine	
Vasopressin > NE	
Management of masking brain hypoxia	
$\bar{D}O_2$ > 800 ml/min	Doptorex + NE
pH > 7.3	$NaHCO_3$
DPG 10–15 μmol/gHb	K_2HPO_4, inosin IV
Gastric pHi > 7.3	AT-III > 100%
Hb > 11–12 mg/dl	Reserved blood (check the DPG and temperature > 32°C)
SBP > 100 mmHg	NE > D > vasopressin > E

Table 48. Algorithm management of ICP elevation: complications

ICP	ICP elevation	
20–25 mmHg	↓	Venous stasis
25–35 mmHg	↓	CBF disturbances Intercompartment pressure difference Microembolus (plasma skimming) AT-III consumption
>35 mmHg	↓	Unconsiousness
	Herniation Brain stem damage	
>45 mmHg	↓	Coma > anisocolia > bilateral pupil dilatation > breathing arrest Poor filling Non filling
	No recovery	

Table 49. Algorithm management of ICP elevation: special considerations

Surgical considerations
- Before surgery: elastic bandage to the legs and, if possible, insert the aorta balloon catheter to prevent brain ischemia
- Surgical position: semi-sitting 30–40 degree head-up position
- Large external decompression
- When brain swelling or not enough brain decompression are observed, other side routine craniotomy should be considered
- Low temperature irrigation saline to prevent brain thermo-pooling
- Normal oxygen delivery and replacement of DPG

ICU management after surgery
- Initial stage (within 3–6 h): prevent masking brain hypoxia and ischemia
  - After vital signstadization, biochemial examination, and neurological examination (loss of opthalmic venous pulsation), midazolam-combined analgesia and anti-muscle relaxant addition, one-shot corticosteroid addition for prevention of proinflammatory cytokines
  - No head-up position, prevent airway obstruction, Hb > 11 g/dl, $PaCO_2$ 34–38 mmHg, SaO_2 > 98%, $ETCO_2$ 32%–39%, SjO_2 65%–75% (SjO_2 < 55%)
  - SBP > 100 mmHg and DPG > 10 mmol/gHb, BT control about at 34°C and CPP > 70% (if BT > 38°C CPP > 80 mmHg), no dehydration fluid resuscitation
  - After Swan Ganz catheter monitor $\bar{D}O_2I$ > 600 ml/min, O_2ER 23%–25%, O_2ER < 18% replacement of DPG, prevent abdominal hypertension, replacement of magnesium
  - ICP < 20 mmHg (Camino ICP senser is not available to external decompressed cases, Spiegel berg ICP or ventricular CSF monitor is recommended)
  - After stabilizing brain oxygenation, BT reduce to 32°C–33°C/5–6 h (if arrythmia and elongation QT > 450 mm/s, BT 34°C)
- Second Stage (after 6–12 h)
  - Serum albumin control at > 3.5 mg/dl (or > 3 mg/dl)
  - ICP 20–25 mmHg (10–15 degree head-up position > manitol addition > fluosemide addition CSF drainage)
  - Prolonged 20–25 mmHg requires CT-scan examination
  - CSF/serum albumin ratio > 0.02 requires high dose of corticosteroid addition and management of systemic cytokine reactions

CT, Computed tomography

Table 50. Algorithm management of ICP elevation: keywords

Hypothermia
ICP
Brain edema

cytokine chemical encephalitis are major clinical issues complicated by severe pneumonia. Cytokine chemical encephalitis is very difficult to manage because this complication involves severe BBB dysfunction, progression of brain edema, and uncontrollable increases in neurotoxic glutamate even with moderate brain hypothermia. Therefore, the complication of pneumonia can cause unsuccessful brain hypothermia management. The management of pneumonia is a key point for the success of brain hypothermia management. In our ICU, the complication of pneumonia was 64% 10 years ago, at the initial stage of brain hypothermia ICU management; however, this complication has reduced to about 5%–8% because of hypothermia-specific infectious management as described in this section. The algorithm management cards for pneumonia are shown in Tables 52–60.

Table 51. Algorithm management of ICP elevation: references

1. Steiner T, Ringleb P, Hacke W (2001) Treatment options for large hemispheric stroke. Neurology 57(5 Suppl 2):S61–68
2. Schneweis S, Grond M, Staub F, Brinker G, Neveling M, Dohmen C, Graf R, Heiss WD (2001) Predictive value of neurochemical monitoring in large middle cerebral artery infarction. Stroke 32:1863–1867
3. Chung C, Gottstein J, Blei AT (2001) Indomethacin prevents the development of experimental ammonia-induced brain edema in rats after portacaval anastomosis. Hepatology 34:249–254
4. Kawai N, Nakamura T, Okauchi M, Nagao S (2000) Effects of hypothermia on intracranial pressure and brain edema formation: studies in a rat acute subdural hematoma model. J Neurotrauma 17:193–202
5. Hayashi N (2000) Brain hypothermia treatment for the management of severe pediatric brain injury. No To Hattatsu 32:122–131
6. Schwab S, Hacke W (1999) Therapy of increased intracranial pressure in space-occupying media infarcts. Z Arztl Fortbild Qualitatssich 93:203–208
7. Schwab S, Schwarz S, Spranger M, Keller E, Bertram M, Hacke W (1998) Moderate hypothermia in the treatment of patients with severe middle cerebral artery infarction. Stroke 29:2461–2466
8. Oriot D, Nassimi A (1998) Intracranial hypertension in the infant: from its physiopathology to its therapeutic management. Arch Pediatr 5:773–782
9. Ichai C, Ciais JF, Grimaud D (1997) The internal environment and intracranial hypertension. Ann Fr Anesth Reanim 16:435–444
10. Arkadopoulos N, Chen SC, Khalili TM, Detry O, Hewitt WR, Lilja H, Kamachi H, Petrovic L, Mullon CJ, Demetriou AA, Rozga J (1998) Transplantation of hepatocytes for prevention of intracranial hypertension in pigs with ischemic liver failure. Cell Transplant 7:357–363
11. Shiozaki T, Sugimoto H, Taneda M, Oda J, Tanaka H, Hiraide A, Shimazu T (1998) Selection of severely head injured patients for mild hypothermia therapy. J Neurosurg 89:206–211
12. Hayashi N (1998) The control of brain tissue temperature and stimulation of dopamine-immune system to the severe brain injury patients. Nippon Rinsho 56:1627–1635
13. Gayle MO, Frewen TC, Armstrong RF, Gilbert JJ, Kronick JB, Kissoon N, Lee R, Tiffin N, Brown T (1989) Venous bulb catheterization in infants and children. Crit Care Med 17:385–388
14. Nordby HK, Nesbakken R (1984) The effect of high dose barbiturate decompression after severe head injury. A controlled clinical trial. Acta Neurochir (Wien) 72:157–166
15. Kassell NF, Peerless SJ, Drake CG, Boarini DJ, Adams HP (1980) Treatment of ischemic deficits from cerebral vasospasm with high dose barbiturate therapy. Neurosurgery 7:593–597

Table 52. Algorithm management of pneumonia: information

Pneumonia is acute infection including alveolar space and interstitial tissue. The type is classified by etiology, infectious pattern, and epidemiology

- Etiology
  - Infectious pneumonia
    - Triggered by immune reduction and respiratory weakness
  - Aspiration pneumonia
    - Two causes: acid gastric juice chemical pneumonia and intestinal bacteria pneumonia, triggered by vomiting
- Infectious pattern
  - Lobular pneumonia
  - Segmental or lobular pneumonia
    - X ray observation
  - Bronchoi pneumonia
  - Interstitial pneumonia
- Epidemiology
  - Pneumococcal pneumonia
    - Most common (60%), about 10% mortality
  - Streptococcus pneumonia
    - 10%–15% of nosocomical pneumonia, 35% mortality
  - Pseudomonas pneumonia
    - Common with aspiration pneumonia
  - Other pathogen
    - *Staphylococcus aureus*, *Hemophilus influenzae*, *Chlamydia pneumoniae*, *Legionella pneumophila*, *Klebsiella pneumoniae*, *Mycoplasma pneumoniae*
  - Influenza virus A pneumonia

Table 53. Algorithm management of pneumonia: diagnosis

Diagnosis is based on the characteristic symptoms combined with an infiltrate on chest X-ray. About 30%–50% of patients have no identifiable pathogen despite clinical signs. The bacterial culture studies of sputum and blood are important.

- Lung
  - CRP: C reactive protein (standard; 100)
    - Pneumococcal pneumonia
  - Gram stain, TB stain
    - TB, Chlamydia, Legionella, Mycoplasma
  - Candidia antibody
    - Lactic coagulation reaction <2. Neutropenia is a danger factor
  - Fungal infection
    - Antibacterial therapy, altered host defense mechanism are common causes. Kelatomycosis is common clinical sign
  - Mycoplasma
    - High incidence in hypothermia by reduced CD4 activity and growth hormone. X-ray: patchy bronchio pneumonia in the lower lobes. Pleura effusion and lobular consideration is not common
  - Virus infection
    - Diffuse interstitial infiltration pattern
- Immune function
  - Lymphocytopenia (<1500 mm^3) shows the reduction of immune function
    - Lymphocyte: T-cell (55–80%) and B-cell (5%–20%) normal
    - Immune function: CD_3 58%–88%, CD_4 25%–55%, CD_8 17%–44%, NK-cell 45 ± 5 (M), 30 ± 5 (F)
- Special consideration of brain hypothermia
  - Growth hormone reduction, CD4 immune suppression
  - Effect of albumin-binding type antibiotics reduced by hypo-albuminemia

Table 54. Algorithm management of pneumonia: pathophysiology

Pneumonia	Danger factor	Injured brain
• $PaO_2 < 60$ mmHg		
• $\bar{D}O_2 < 700$–800 ml/min	Low Hb-DPG →	Neuronal hypoxia
• pH < 7.2		
• Elevation of body temperature	SBP < 100 mmHg →	Thermo-pooling
• Increasing of inflammatory cytokines	BBB destruction →	Cytokines encephalitis
	CSF/serum albumin ratio > 0.01	

Danger signs: immature neutrophils, acute renal failure, albumin < 3 g/dl, Ca > 6 mg/dl, creatinine > 5 mg/dl

Table 55. Algorithm management of pneumonia: basic management

- Clean nasal-oral cavity, trachea and bronchus. Strong aspiration should be delayed
- O_2ER 20%–25%, Hb >11–12 mg/dl, Ht < 40%
- Serum albumin > 3.5 mg/dl
- Gastric lavage, abdominal pressure < 15 mmHg, gastric juice pH < 3
- Gastric wall pHi > 7.3, AT-III > 100%, Ht < 40%
- Immune activation: arginine + arginine + IGF1
- Antibiotic therapy
- Respiratory rehabilitation
- Early skeletal muscle massage and activate protein synthesis by sorbutamol and arginine
- Enteral immune nutrition (glutamine + Arginine + $ZnCl_2$)
- Prevent ventilator associated pneumonia (VAP): high incidence in parasinusitis
  - Early onset VAP
    - Pneumococcus and influenza
  - Late onset VAP
    - MRSA, Pseudomonas, Enterobactor
  - Cuff pressure < 30 cmH_2O
- Management of ventilator

Table 56. Algorithm management of pneumonia: medication

Pneumococcal pneumonia (most common, 5%–25% oral ex)
- Penicillin G (PG) 500000 to 2 million U i.v. every 4–6h > oxacillin 2g i.v. every 4–6h (25% P-resisted) > vancomycin 1g i.v. every 12h. Alternative drugs: cephalosporin (CP), erythromycin (EM), clindamycin (CM). Oral treatment: CM 300mg every 6h. If meningitis is suspected cefotaxime 2g i.v. every 4 to 6h + vancomycin 1g i.v. every 12h

Streptococcal pneumonia
- PG 500000 to 1 million U i.v. every 4 to 6h (or CP + CM)

Staphylococcus aureus (after influenza, 30%–40% serious)
- Penicillinase resistant penicillin: oxacillin or nafcillin 2g i.v. every 4 to 6h (alternate: cephalothin 2g i.v. every 4 to 6h) > vancomycin 1g i.v. every 12h (30%–40% Methicillin resistant strains)

Hemophilia influenza (30% b-lactamase resist)
- Trimethoprim-sulfamethoxazole (TMP-SMX) 20mg/kg per day, cefuroxamine 0.25–1g i.v. every 6h

Fungal pneumonia
- Fluconazole 200–800mg/day > amphotericin B 0.4mg/kg per day prevent: ketoconazole 200mg/day + clotrimazole 10mg every 8h

Legionairres disease
- EM 1g i.v. every 6h start > rifampin 300mg i.v.

Chlamydia pneumonia
- Tetracycline or EM 10–20 days

Carini pneumonia
- TMP-SMX 20mg/kg per day

Steroids effective: high IL1/IL10 and IL1/IL2. Colitis: sulfasalazine 1–3g/day. Immunological replacement: GH, IGF-1, IL10 (iv), early muscle massage, replacement of early enteral globulin

Table 57. Algorithm management of pneumonia: complications

Adult respiratory distress syndrome (ARDS): PaO_2/FiO_2 < 200mmHg, low lung compliance, bilateral diffuse chest infiltration, PCWP < 18mmHg
- Treatment: 1. Avoid risk factors 2. Increase FiO_2, PEEP < 5cmH_2O, keep plateau pressure < 35mmHg, permissive hypercapnia, adequate fluid management, maximize O_2 delivery, avoid MSOF, nutritional support
- Pleuritis: pancreatitis, subphrenics abscess, lymph obstruction, hypo-albuminemia (serum albumin < 2.5mg/dl, TP < 3mg/dl)

Bacterial endocarditis: usually caused by streptococcal infection. Signs: valve dysfunction, hypertrophic cardiomyophathy, arrhythmia
- Treatment: PG 500000 to 1 million U i.v. every 4 to 6h (or CP + CM). P-resistant streptococci: PG 18–20 million U/day i.v. (ampicillin 12g/day i.v. every 4h) + gentamycine 1mg/kg i.v. every for 4–6 weeks

Liver and intestinal congestion: PEEP >10cmH_2O

ICP elevation: CVP and abdominal pressure >25mmHg

Sepsis: SIRS, lactoacidosis, organs dysfunction
- Treatment: 1. Preferable antibiotics 2. Circulation toxins should be neutralized by antibiotics or γ-globulin 3. Circulating cytokines should be neutralized
- Toxic shock: streptococcal toxin is common. Acute renal failure > hypoalbuminemia > hypocalcamia > shock. Clindamycine suppress bacterial toxin. *S. aureus*: flucloxacillin and gentamycin may inhibit toxin product. Intravenous immunoglobulin neutrize toxins in both staphylococcal and streptococcal

Ventilator complications: decrease venous return to the thorax, CO, BP (by high inspiratory pressure, hypovolemia, and muscle weakness)
- Barotraumas: pressure >35cmH_2O (alveoli pressure) and PEEP is insufficient to collapse lungs

Table 58. Algorithm management of pneumonia: special considerations

- Induction stage
  - Clean nasal-oral cavity
  - Gastric lavage
  - Digestive decontamination (levofloxacin (Cravit, 200 mg) + Amphotericin B 100–300 mg) to prevent pseudomonas aspiation pneumonia and enterobacterial translocation
  - Antibiotics (panipenem betamipron (Carbenin 500 mg × 2/day), or second choice: ceftazidinme (Modasin 1 g ×2/day) or clindamycine (Dalacin, 150–300 mg every 6 h)
  - $\bar{D}O_2I$ >600 ml/min, $\bar{D}O_2$ > 700 ml/min
- Cooling stage
  - Nasal-oral cavity management
  - Gastric juice pH < 3.5
  - Prevent abdominal hypertension < 10 mmHg
  - Antibiotics: immipenem cilastain sodium (Tienam 1–2 g/day × 3) > meropenem trihydrate (Meropn, 1.0–2.0 g/day × 4) for enterobacteria, gram-negative bacteria and pseudomonas
  - AT-III > 80%–100% and gastric pHi > 7.3
  - Gastric immune nutrition replacement > nutrition care
  - Ventilator care and urinary care
  - Breathing rehabilitation (alveolar dysfunction, atelectasis)
  - Intermittent elevation of BT from 32°C to 34°C at evening
  - Replacement of ZnCl, arginine with Hb > 11 g/dl (if lymph-cytopenia occurred, BT keep at 34°C + GH + γ-globulin addition)
  - Serum albumin >3.5 mg/dl
  - Low dosage of antidotes
  - O_2ER 23%–25%, 2,3-DPG 15-10 mmol/gHb
- Prerewarming stage
  - Preconditioning: no severe infection, serum glucose < 150 mg/dl, vitamin A >50 mg/dl, lymphocyte >1500/mm^3, serum albumin >3.5 mg/dl (prealbumin >20 mg/dl), Hb >12 g/dl, DPG >10 mmol/gHb, AT-III 100%, platelet 50000–80000, GDC, muscle massage, abdominal pressure <10 mmHg
  - Antibiotics: arbekacin sulfate (Habekacin, 150–200 mg/day × 2) to prevent pseudomonal aerginosa and MRSA infection, + cefozopran hydrochloride (Firstcin 1–2 g/day × 2) for Tienam-resisted acinetobacter and xantomona + fluconazole (Diflucan 100–200 mg/day × 1) for Candida with evidence of β-D-glucan positive reactions)
  - Digestive decontamination for control of clostridium enteritis and MRSA, enteral administration of levofloxacin (Cravit, 200 mg) and amphotericin B (100–300 mg), combined with vancomycin (2–3 g/day ×4–6 times i.v. drip)
  - $\bar{D}O_2$ > 700 ml/min, O_2ER 23%–25%
- Rewarming stage
  - Slow step-up rewarming
  - Prevent rapid shift from lipid to glucose metabolism
  - Control of serum glucose: 140–170 mg/dl
  - O_2ER 23%–25%
  - Management of neuromuscular junction
  - 34–35°C BT keep for 2–3 days and BT > 36°C and then stop muscle relaxant > anesthesia
  - Nutritional management
  - Antibiotics: Habekacin, 150–200 mg/day × 2 to prevent pseudomonal aerginosa and MRSA infection, + cefozopran hydrochloride (Firstcin 1–2 g/day × 2) for Tienam-resisted acinetobacter + fluconazole (Diflucan 100–200 mg/day × 1) for Candida with evidence of β-D-glucan positive reactions

The pulmonary care management is variable at each stage of brain hypothermia treatment

Table 59. Algorithm management of pneumonia: keywords

Hypothermia
Pneumonia
Infection
Sepsis

Table 60. Algorithm management of pneumonia: references

1. Saito T, Otsuka A, Kurashima A, Watanabe M, Aoki S, Harada A (2001) Study of lymphocyte and NK cell activity during mild hypothermia therapy. No Shinkei Geka 29:633–639
2. Matthys D, Verhaaren H, Deryck Y (1995) Fatal pneumonia complicating hypothermia for the treatment of postoperative junctional ectopic tachycardia. Pediatr Cardiol 16:294–296
3. Wetterberg T, Steen S (1992) Combined use of hypothermia and buffering in the treatment of critical respiratory failure. Acta Anaesthesiol Scand 36:490–492. PMID: 1632175 [PubMed—indexed for MEDLINE]
4. Okada M, Nishimura F (1990) Respiratory function and acid-base status in accidental hypothermia assessed by arterial blood gas analysis. Jpn J Med 29:500–505. PMID: 2128523 [PubMed—indexed for MEDLINE]
5. Clardy CW, Edwards KM, Gay JC (1985) Increased susceptibility to infection in hypothermic children: possible role of acquired neutrophil dysfunction. Pediatr Infect Dis 4:379–382. PMID: 2991867 [PubMed—indexed for MEDLINE]
6. El-Radhi AS, Jawad MH, Mansor N, Ibrahim M, Jamil II (1983) Infection in neonatal hypothermia. Arch Dis Child 58:143–145. PMID: 6338837 [PubMed—indexed for MEDLINE]
7. Edlich RF, Lande AJ, Goodale RL, Wangensteen OH (1968) Prevention of aspiration pneumonia by continuous esophageal aspiration during esophagogastric tamponade and gastric cooling. Surgery 64:405–408. No abstract available PMID: 5302564 [PubMed—indexed for MEDLINE]
8. Jones RH, Bourdillon RE, Finn R, Martindale K (1966) Hypothemia associated with pneumonia and acidosis. Postgrad Med J 42:273–275. No abstract available. PMID: 5938611 [PubMed—indexed for MEDLINE]

Algorithm for Malnutrition and Diarrhea

The management of digestive organs is important for maintaining immune function, prevention of infections, and to determine pharmacological medication. The intestine is very sensitive to catecholamine surge, disturbances of microcirculation caused by reduced AT-III, osmotic gap, hypo-albuminemia, fecal impaction, and medication. The algorithm management cards for diarrhea and malnutrition are shown in Tables 61–69.

Algorithm for Renal Insufficiency

Acute renal failure can be categorized as prerenal, postrenal, or renal. In the management of brain hypothermia treatment, prerenal and renal failure are

Table 61. Algorithm management of diarrhea and nutrition: information

- Causes of diarrhea
  - Enterocolitis and MOF
  - Medication-induced diarrhea
    - Antibiotics; 50% have C. difficile toxins
    - Additives: sorbitol, manitol, xylitol
    - Antacids containing magnesium
    - Asthma medication, e.g., thephyline
    - Cardiac medication: quinidine, procaineamide, digoxin
    - Antihypertensive drugs: angiotensin-converting enzyme inhibitors, β-blockers, hydralazine, guanethidine
    - Diuretics: flosemide, thiazides
    - Cholesterol medications
    - Thyroid hormone
    - Gastrointestinal medications: H2-blockers, metaclopramide, misoprostol
  - Enteral feeding and osmotic gap diarrhea
    - Osmotic gap: greater than 100 mOsm/kg and low fecal pH
  - Hypo-albuminemia
    - Serum albumin: <2.5 g/dl make subumucosal oncotic pressure reduce and lead to edema of intestinal mucosa (difficult absorption of feeding)
  - Mesenteric ischemia
    - Diagnose: gastric pHi < 7.3, AT-III < 70%, leukocytopenia, acidosis, venous thrombosis, hypercoaguable state
  - Fecal impaction caused by medications
    - Medications: narcotics, antihypertensives, diuretic, aluminum antacids

Table 62. Algorithm management of diarrhea and nutrition: diagnosis

- Nutrition
  - Metabolic shift occurs from glucose to lipid following brain hypothermia treatment
  - The balance of glucose to lipid metabolism is equal at 34°C
  - Lipid metabolism becomes dominant at 32°–33°C
  - Rapid induction of 33°–34°C produces increasing serum glucose. Unsuccessful care management of catecholamine surge by delayed induction hypothermia also produces stress related-hyperglycemia. Therefore, combination of delayed start of hypothermia and rapid induction of hypothermia produce very dangerous insulin-resistant hyperglycemia
  - Insulin-resistant hyperglycemia induces vasopressin release and activates BBB dysfunction
  - The calorie deficit is not a major issue
  - The lipid metabolism requires vitamin A and growth hormone. The rehabilitation and massage of brown cells are required to maintain energy metabolism during brain hypothermia treatment
  - The management of serum phosphate (3–5 mg/dl) and magnesium (1.5–1.8 mEq/dl) are also effective to control lipid membrane metabolism
- Diagnosis of malnutrition
  - Muscle degradation, edema of leg, ascitis, hypo-albuminemia (<2.5 g/dl), more than 10 weight loss, intestinal mucous membrane edema, pancreatic duct obstruction and prolonged diarrhea are diagnostic criteria

Table 63. Algorithm management of diarrhea and nutrition: pathophysiology

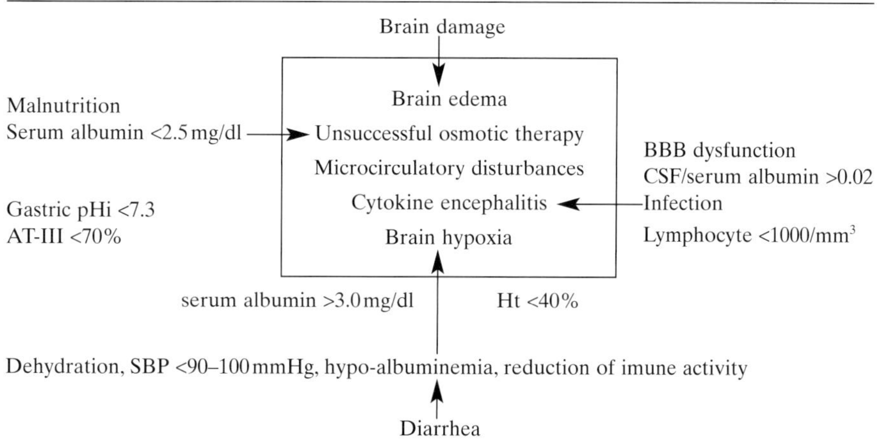

Table 64. Algorithm management of diarrhea and nutrition: basic management

- Remove the causes of diarrhea
  - Antibiotic-associated diarrhea: stop the antibiotics, metronidazole 250 mg pr qi, (severe cases i.v.) > oral, vancomycin 125 mg qid, because high incidence of C. difficile are complicated
- Before feeding care management
  - Serum albumin > 3.5 mg/dl, At-III > 100%, Ht 34%–36%
  - Preliminary feeding: glutamine with arginine (ET)
  - Correct serum electrolytes
  - Management of mesenteric ischemia
- Feeding care management
  - No severe BBB dysfunction (CSF/serum albumin ratio <0.01): early enteral nutrition
  - Severe BBB dysfunction (CSF/serum albumin > 0.01): two-step enteral nutrition
    - First step: saline feed, control of intestinal pressure, $ZnCl_2$
    - Second step (4–5 days later): immune nutrition and then follow with enteral nutrition
  - Management of diarrhea: reduce the feeding volume, isotonic fluid infusion
  - Control of osmotic gap between serum and stool
    - Osmotic gap, → serum Osm–2 (stool Na + K) > 100 mOsm/kg
- Fecal impaction
  - Gentle enema is usually effective
  - DD: diagnose lower anal sphincter pressure

Table 66. Algorithm management of diarrhea and nutrition: complications

Complication	Clinical index
Dehydration and hemoconcentration	Ht > 45%
Acidosis	pH < 7.2, $PaCO_2$ < 23 mmHg
Disturbances of microcirculation	Gastric pHi < 7.3
	SjO_2 < 55%
Organ ischemia and hypoxia	pH < 7.2
	2,3-DPG < 10 μmol/gHb
	SaO_2 > 85%
	Gastric pHi < 7.3
Immune dysfunction	Serum albumin < 2.5 mg/dl
	Total protein < 4.9 g/dl
	Transferin < 140 μg/dl
	Cholesterol < 90 mg/dl
No effect of hyperosmotic therapy for brain edema	Serum albumin < 2.5 mg/dl

Table 68. Algorithm management of diarrhea and nutrition: keywords

Hypothermia
Nutrition
Diarrhea
Bacterial translocation

Table 65. Algorithm management of diarrhea and nutrition: medication

- Treatment of underlying disorder
  - AT-III i.v. infusion
  - Replacement of serum albumin
  - Metronidazole 250 mg i.v.
  - Oral vancomycin 125 mg qid
- Symptomatic treatment
  - Increase intestinal transit time
    - Diphenoxylate 2.5–5 mg tid or qid
    - Codeine phosphate 15–30 mg bid or tid
    - Loperamide hydrochloride 2–4 mg tid or qid
    - Anticholinergics (atropine) can decrease peristalsis
  - Electrolyte fluid replacement
    - Urgent fluid and electrolyte replacement
    - NaCl, KCl, glucose and fluids to counteract acidosis
    - Oral glucose electrolyte solutions
- Malnutrition
  - Immune nutrition
    - Glutamine + arginine + ω2 or 3 food (ET)

Table 67. Algorithm management of diarrhea and nutrition: special considerations

- Prophylactic management for malnutrition and diarrhea
  - Maintain circulation of the digestive organs
    - Ht: 34%–36%
    - AT-III > 100%
    - SBP > 100 mmHg
    - Gastric pHi > 7.3
    - (Serum Osm.) – 2(stool Na + K) < 100 Osm/kg
    - Abdominal pressure or bladder pressure < 10 mmHg
    - Reduce the intestinal luminar pressure through the ileum tube
    - Kinetic therapy
  - Enteral nutrition
    - Early enteral nutrition for patients of CSF/serum albumin < 0.01
      - Saline → immune nutrition (glutamine + arginine + yeast RNA) → honey yogurt
    - Two-step enteral nutrition for patients of CSF/serum albumin > 0.01
      - First step: saline 50 ml to max 150 ml/4 h, and remove retention fluid → repeat for 3–4 days
      - Second stage: honey yogurt
        - Administration method: single administration and remove retention enteral food
        - Dosage: start from 50 ml to max 150 ml/4 h
  - Control of diarrhea
    - Antibiotic-associated diarrhea: stop the antibiotics, metronidazole 250 mg pr qi, (severe case i.v.) > oral, vancomycin 125 mg qid, because high incidence of C. difficile are complicated
    - Management of osmotic gap diarrhea
    - Management of mesenteric ischemia
    - Reduce feeding volume and isotonic fluid infusion

Table 69. Algorithm management of diarrhea and nutrition: references

1. Lichtenstein A, Onuchic LF, Rocha Ados S (1990) Accidental hypothermia: glycemic, hematologic and blood amylase changes. Rev Hosp Clin Fac Med Sao Paulo. 45: 173–177. Review. Portuguese. PMID: 1726374 [PubMed—indexed for MEDLINE]

Table 70. Algorithm management of acute renal failure: information

Clinical conditions associated with rapid, steadily decreasing renal function (azotemia), with or without oliguria
Classification and etiology
- Prerenal type
  - ECF volume depletion: excessive diuresis, hemorrhage, GI loss, transcellular fluid accumulation
  - Low cardiac output: cardiomyopathy, AMI, pulmonary embolism
  - Lower systemic VR: sepsis, liver failure
  - Increase renal VR: liver failure, renal vein thrombosis, cyclosporine
- Renal type
  - Acute tubular injury: ischemia, toxins (aminoglycosides, β-lactam antibiotics, amphotericin, foscarnet, radiocontrast, cyclosporin-B, myoglobinuria, heavy metal, methotrexate)
  - Acute glomerulonephritis: antineutrophil cytoplasmic antibody-associated (cresentic glomerulonephritis, Wagener's GN)
  - Acute tubulointerstitial nephritis: drug reaction (β-lactams, NSAIDs, sulfonamides, phenytoin, allopurinol), pyelonephritis
- Postrenal type
  - Ureteral obstruction and bladder obstruction

Table 72. Algorithm management of acute renal failure pathophysiology

- Prerenal type
  - Oliguria (urine < 500 ml/day)
  - Normal response to ineffective circulating blood volume
- Renal type
  - Renal blood flow reduction, reduced glomerular permeability, tubular obstruction, and hypofiltration

Hypocalcemia
Hyperphosphatemia
Hyperparathyroidism
Reduced calcitriol → Ca deposition in muscle, intestine, and kidneys → Immune dysfunction
↓
Brain edema
Multiple small emboli
Malnutrition
Hemoglobin dysfunction and neuronal hypoxia
Easy infection
Multiple major organ failure

Table 71. Algorithm management of acute renal failure: diagnosis

Index	Prerenal	Renal	Post renal	AGN
U/P osmolarity	>1.5	1–1.5	1–1.5	1–1.5
Urine Na (mmol/l)	<20	40>	40>	<30
Fractional excretion of Na (EF_{Na})	<0.01	>0.04	>0.02	<0.01
Renal failure index (Urine Na ÷ U/P creatinine ratio)	<1	>2	>2	<1

Modest daily rise: serum creatinine, 1–2 mg/dl; urea nitrogen, 10–20 mg/dl. Special considerations to cause: serum creatinine >2 mg/dl→rhabdomyolysis EF_{Na}, Urine Na ÷ U/P creatinine; U/P, urine/plasma ratio; AGN, acute glomerulonephritis

Table 73. Algorithm management of acute renal failure: basic management

Proper maintenance of normal fluid balance, blood volume, and BP
Vasopressor drugs
- Dopamine 1–3 μg/kg min^{-1} i.v.
- Furosemide with manitol or dopamine

Avoid dehydration and ECF depletion
Urography and angiography should be avoided
Dialysis
- Hemodialysis is effective for renal insufficiency; however, for the management of severe brain damage, special consideration is required
- Hyperosmotic management is necessary before the induction of hemodialysis by replacement of albumin and manitol
- All renally excreted substances such as digoxin and antibiotics must be adjusted
- To reduce nitrogen loss, administer i.v. essential amino acids
- Management of hyperphosphatemia
- Management of hyperkalemia
- Management of extra cellular volume, osmolality, acid–base balance, and K balance

Table 74. Algorithm management of acute renal failure: medication

Dopamine
- To increase renal blood flow: 1–3 μg/kg min^{-1} i.v.
- To increase urine output: low dosage 0.5–3 μg/kg min^{-1}
- To increase cardiac output: moderate 5–10 μg/kg min^{-1}
- Max: 40 μg/kg min^{-1}
  - Stimulate receptors primarily in the renal, splanchnic, and coronary vascular beds and increase blood flow

Furosemide
- Typically furosemide is initiated as 20–40 mg by direct intravenous injection over 2 min
- A continuous intravenous infusion of 0.25–0.75 mg/kg h^{-1} for no response to direct injection
- Renal dysfunction requires more than 100 mg initial high doses furosemide
- Compatible drugs: gentamicin sulfate heparin sodium, hydrocortisone sodium succinate, meropenem, tobramycin sulfate

Table 75. Algorithm management of acute renal failure: complications

Brain damage caused by renal failure
Brain edema
Multiple small emboli
Malnutrition of neuronal cells
Neuronal hypoxia by hemoglobin dysfunction
Easy brain infection
Brain damage caused by ARF disease
CBF disturbances by hypovolemia
Disturbance of microcirculation
Severe metabolic acidosis
Neuronal dysfunction by hypocalcemia
Systemic complications
Multiple major organ failure
Easy infection
Immune suppression

Table 76. Algorithm management of acute renal failure: special considerations

Care management
Avoid the causes of acute renal failure
Careful administration of prolonged renal toxic medication
Avoid drugs incompatible with renal function
Acute renal failure should be managed without dialysis for severe brain damage under brain hypothermia only when dialysis is unavailable
Dialysis promotes hypo-albuminemia and brain edema
Dialysis needs preconditioning for replacement of albumin
Dialysis causes the loss of DPG and causes neuronal hypoxia even with normal PaO_2 and oxygen delivery

clinical issues in severely brain-injured patients. Rhabdomyolysis caused by extracellular volume depletion, low cardiac output, low systemic vascular resistance, and increased renal vascular resistance are major causes of acute prerenal failure. Stress-associated hyperglycemia and vasopressin release are trigger factors to reduce the glomerular filtration rate in the acute stage of severe brain damage caused by trauma, stroke, or cardiac-arrested brain ischemia. The causes of acute renal failure are categorized as acute tubular injury, acute glomerulonephritis, acute tubulointerstitial nephritis, and acute vascular nephropathy. During brain hypothermia treatment, drug reaction by antibiotics, hypocalcemia, striated muscle trauma, and radio contrast examination are the main causes of acute renal failure. The algorithm management cards for acute renal failure are shown in Tables 70–78.

Table 77. Algorithm management of acute renal failure: keywords

Severe brain damage
Hypothermia
Acute renal failure
Hemodialysis

Table 78. Algorithm management of acute renal failure: references

1. Hekmat K, Abel M, Zimmermann R, Ruskowski H (1994) Diabetic coma with deep hypothermia. Successful resuscitation with hemofiltration. Anaesthesist 43:750–752. German. PMID: 7840404 [PubMed—indexed for MEDLINE]
2. Pignatelli MG, Comelli LF, Costa P, Pession F, Tesselli L, Poletti G, Di Donato R, Giron GP (1981) Acid-base equilibrium changes during deep hypothermia. Minerva Dietol Gastroenterol 27:395–404. Italian. No abstract available. PMID: 7329580 [PubMed—indexed for MEDLINE]
3. Cancio LC, Wortham WG, Zimba F (1994) Peritoneal dialysis to induce hypothermia in a head-injured patient: case report. Surg Neurol 42:303–307. PMID: 7974124 [PubMed—indexed for MEDLINE]

References

1. Almeida A, Delgado-Esteban M, Bolanos JP, Medina JM (2002) Oxygen and glucose deprivation induces mitochondrial dysfunction and oxidative stress in neurones but not in astrocytes in primary culture. Neurochem 81:207–217
2. Ao H, Moon JK, Tashiro M, Terasaki H (2001) Delayed platelet dysfunction in prolonged induced canine hypothermia. Resuscitation 51:83–90
3. Baker AJ, Zornow MH, Scheller MS, Yaksh TL, Skilling SR, Smullin DH, Larson AA, Kuczenski R (1991) Changes in extracellular concentrations of glutamate, aspatate, glycine, dopamine, serotonin, and dopamine metabolites after transient global ischemia in the rat. J Neurochem 57:1370–1379
4. Billiau A, Vankelecom H (1992) Interferon-γ: general biological properties and effects on the neuro-endocrine axis. In: Bartfai T, Ottoson D (eds) Neuro-immunology of fever. Pergamon, Oxford, New York, Seoul, Tokyo, pp 65–77
5. Boels PJ, Verbeuren TJ, Vanhoutte PM (1985) Moderate cooling depresses the accumulation and the release of newly synthesized catecholamines in isolated canine saphenous veins. Experientia 41:1374–1377
6. Chiolero R, Lemarchand TH, Schutz Y, de Tribolet N, Felber JP, Freeman J, Jequier E (1988) Plasma pituitary hormone levels in severe trauma with or without head injury. J Trauma 28:1368–1374
7. Clifton GL, Miller ER, Choi SC, Levin HS (2002) Fluid thresholds and outcome from severe brain injury. Crit Care Med 30:739–745
8. Corte FD, Mancini A, Valle D, Gallizzi F, Carducci P, Mignani V, De Marinis L (1998) Provocative hypothalamopituitary axis tests in severe head injury: correlation with severity and prognosis. Crit Care Med 26:1419–1426
9. Davila DR, Breif S, Simon J, Hammer RE, Brinster RL, Kelley KW (1987) Role of growth hormone in regulating

T-dependant immune events in aged, nude, and transgenic rodents. J Neurosci Res 18:108–116
10. Dempsey IRJ, Combs DJ, Maley ME, Cowen DE, Roy MW, Donaldson DL (1987) Moderate hypothermia reduces postischemic edema development and leukotriene production. Neurosurgery 21:177–181
11. Dietrich WD, Busto R, Halley M, Valdes I (1990) The importance of brain temperature in alterations of the blood-brain barrier following cerebral ischemia. J Neuropathol Exp Neurol 49:486–497
12. Dorman PJ, Counsell CE, Sanderrock PGA (2000) Recently developed neuroprotective therapies for acute stroke: a qualitative systematic review of clinical trials. In: Prakash A (ed) Acute stroke treatment. Adis, Hong Kong, pp 63–83
13. Dudariev VP, Lanovenko II (1999) Changes in the oxygen-binding properties of the blood in white rats under the influence of hypoxia and its pharmacological correction. *Fiziol Zh* 45:97–103
14. Fedor EJ, Fisher ER, Lee SH, Weitzel WK, Fisher B (1956) Effect of hypothermia upon induced bacteremia. Proc Soc Exp Biol Med 93:510–512
15. Filippi R, Reisch R, Mauer D, Perneczky A (2000) Brain tissue pO_2 related to $SjvO_2$, ICP, and CPP in severe brain injury. Neurosurg Rev 23:94–97
16. Globus MY-T, Busto R, Dietrich WD, Martinez E, Valdes I, Ginsberg MD (1988) Effect on ischemia on the in vivo release of striatal dopamine, glutamate, and γ-aminobutyric acid studied by intracerebral microdialysis. J Neurochem 51:1455–1464
17. Hackl JM, Gottardis M, Wieser C, Rumpl E, Stadler C, Schwarz S, Moukayo R (1991) Endocrine abnormalities in severe traumatic brain injury—a cue to prognosis in severe craniocerebral trauma? Intensive Care Med 17:25–29
18. Han HS, Qiao Y, Karabiyikoglu M, Giffard RG, Yenari MA (2002) Influence of mild hypothermia on inducible nitric oxide synthase expression and reactive nitrogen production in experimental stroke and inflammation. J Neurosci 22:3921–3928
19. Harrington D, Chua TP, Coast AJS (2000) The effect of solbutamol on skeletal muscle in chronic heart failure. Int J Cardiol 73:257–265
20. Hayashi N (1995) Cerebral hypothermia treatment, In: Hayashi N (ed) Cerebral hypothermia treatment. Sogo Igaku, Tokyo, pp 1–105
21. Hayashi N (1997) Combination therapy of cerebral hypothermia, pharmacological activation of the dopamine system, and hormonal replacement in severely brain damaged patients. J Jpn soc Intensive Care Med 4:191–197
22. Hayashi N (1997) Prevention of vegetation after severe head trauma and stroke by combination therapy of cerebral hypothermia and activation of immune-dopaminergic nervous system. Proceedings of the 6th annual meeting of Society for Treatment of Coma 6:133–145
23. Hayashi N (2000) Enhanced neuronal damage in severely brain injured patients by hypothalamus, pituitary, and adrenal axis neuro-hormonal changes. In: Hayashi N (ed) Brain hypothermia. Springer, Berlin Heidelberg New York Tokyo, pp 3–26
24. Hayashi N (2000) The clinical issue and effectiveness of brain hypothermia treatment for severe brain injured patients. In: Hayashi N (ed) Brain hypothermia. Springer, Berlin Heidelberg New York Tokyo, pp 121–151
25. Hayashi N, Hirayama T, Utagawa A (1994) The cerebral thermo-pooling and hypothermia treatment of critical head injury patients. In: Nagai H (ed) Intracranial pressure IX. Springer, Tokyo, pp 589–599
26. Hayashi N, Hirayama T, Utagawa T, Ohata M (1994) Systemic management of cerebral edema based on a new concept in severe head injury patients. Acta Neurochir [Suppl] 60:541–543
27. Hayashi N, Utagawa A, Kinosita K, Izumi T (1999) Application of a novel technique for clinical evaluation of nitric oxide-induced free radiacal reactions in ICU patients. Cell Mol Neurobiol 19:3–17
28. Kagawa M, Nagao S, Bemana I (1996) Arginine vasopressin receptor antagonists for treatment of vasogenic brain edema: an experimental study. J Neurotrauma 13:273–279
29. Kossmann T, Hans V, Lenzlinger PM, Csuka E, Stsahel PF, Trentz O, Morgani-Kossmann MC (1996) Analysis of immune mediator production following traumatic brain injury. In: Schlag G, Redel H, Traber D (eds) Shock, sepsis and organ failure. Springer, Berlin Heidelberg New York pp 263–297
30. Leibowitz SF (1999) Macronutrients and brain peptides: what they do and how they respond. In: Berthoud HR, Seeley RJ (eds) Neural and metabolic control of macronutrient intake. CRC, Boca Raton, pp 389–406
31. Leibowiz SF, Sladek C, Spencer L, Temple D (1988) Neuropeptide Y, epinephrine and norepinephrine in the paraventricular nucleus: stimulation of feeding and the release of corticosterone, vasopressin and glucose. Brain Res Bull 21:905–912
32. Lin TW, Kuo YS (1996) Acute pulmonary oedema following administration of vasopressin for control of massive GI tract haemorrhage in a major burn patient. Burns 22:73–75
33. Lindley RI (2000) Drug therapy for acute ischemic stroke: risks versus benefits. In: Prakash A (ed) Acute stroke treatment. Adis, Hong Kong, pp 53–62
34. MacIntosh TK (1994) Neurological sequele of traumatic brain injury: therapeutic implications. Cerebrovasc Brain Metab Rev 6:109–162
35. McClain CJ, Hennig B, Ott L, Goldblum S, Young AB (1988) Mechanisms and implications of hypoalbuminemia in head-injured patients. J Neurosurg 69:386–392
36. Pasko SA, Volosheniuk TG (1990) Disordered phosphorus metabolism and its correction in the acute period of severe craniocerebral trauma. Zh Vopr Neirokhir Im NN Burdenko 3:14–16
37. Poca MA, Sahuquillo J, Arribas M, Baguena M, Amoros S, Rubio E (2002) Fiberoptic intraparenchymal brain pressure monitoring with the Camino V420 monitor: reflections on our experience in 163 severely head-injured patients. J Neurotrauma 19:439–448

38. Sahuquillo J, Amoros S, Santos A, Poca. MA (2000) Does an increase in cerebral perfusion pressure always mean a better oxygenated brain? A study in head-injured patients. Acta Neurochir [Suppl] 76:457–462
39. Schwarz S, Georgiadis D, Aschoff A, Schwab S (2002) Effects of body position on intracranial pressure and cerebral perfusion in patients with large hemispheric stroke. Stroke 33:497–501
40. Silvka A, Coben G (1985) Hydroxyl radical attack on dopamine. J Biol Chem 260:15466–15472
41. Suarez JI (2001) Treatment of acute brain edema. Rev Neurol 32:275–281
42. Triolo AJ, Osterholm JL, Alexander GM, Bell RD, Frazer GD (1990) Local cerebral glucose metabolism after global ischemia: treatment by ventriculocisternal perfusion with a fluorocarbon emulsion. Neurosurgery 26:487–488
43. Valeri CR, Cassidy G, Khuri S, Feingold H, Ragno G, Altschule MD (1987) Hypothermia-induced reversible platelet dysfunction. Ann Surg 205:175–181

45. Timing of Rewarming

Clinical Issues for Management of Rewarming

The major issues of rewarming during intensive care unit (ICU) management of brain hypothermia are the metabolic shift from lipid to glucose, increasing serum lactate, induction of proinflammatory cytokines, vascular engorgement, heat production, alteration of blood–brain barrier (BBB) function, bloodflow metabolic gap, hyperdynamic microcirculation, and increasing serum catecholamine levels. However, in cases of short duration of mild brain hypothermia (24h at 34°–35°C), the rewarming clinical issues as described above are not serious [2]. Complication at the rewarming stage is more frequently observed in prolonged brain hypothermia treatment. Complication at the rewarming stage is variable and depends on the duration and severity of hypothermia, the degree of control of hypothalamus-pituitary-adrenal (HPA) axis neurohormonal dysfunction, presence of hyperglycemia and hemoglobin dysfunction, complication of pneumonia, degree of recovery from brain damage, and the progression of the brain injury mechanism [2]. To succeed in rewarming from prolonged brain hypothermia treatment, the management of these complications, preconditioning for rewarming stress, and allowing an adaptation time for stress during rewarming are important management techniques. Important preconditioning steps before rewarming are:

Recovery from systemic infections
Treatment of hypo-albuminemia (serum albumin >3.0mg/dl)
Stabilization of immune function (lymphocyte >1500/mm^3)
No rapid activation of glucose metabolism (serum glucose control at 120–150mg/dl)
Sufficient oxygen delivery with normal hemoglobin (Hb) function (Hb > 12mg/dl, 2,3-diphosphoglycerate 10–15mmol/gHb, pH > 7.3, potassium phosphate 3–5mg/dl, O_2ER 23%–25%)
Management of antithrombin-III >100%

After successful preconditioning, the indications for rewarming should be considered. Evidence of neuronal recovery in the injured brain tissue, no intracranial pressure (ICP) elevation (<20mmHg), no evidence of systemic infection, and stable neurohormonal function are especially important at the rewarming stage.

The duration of brain hypothermia is one of the important factors in determining the success of treatment. Short-duration brain hypothermia for the control of brain edema is not enough to allow recovery from severe brain injury. Such treatment can only stop the progression of secondary brain damage and reprogression of the secondary brain injury mechanism occurs with rewarming. Unsuccessful brain hypothermia treatment and rewarming are made much worse by the crucial metabolic shift from lipid to glucose, cytokine activation, ·NO radical formation, vascular engorgement, and energy crisis. Therefore, the timing of rewarming is one of the key points for the success of brain hypothermia treatment. Without recovery from the brain injury mechanism, rewarming is very dangerous. Before starting rewarming, evidence of recovery from brain damage or at least signs of recovery are important for the success of rewarming. However, unnecessarily prolonged brain hypothermia also produces severe systemic infection associated with reduced immune activity, hypo-albuminemia with liver dysfunction, and prolonged lipid-dominant metabolism [1]. The combined complications of pneumonia and severe hypo-albuminemia are, especially dangerous at the rewarming stage. Severe hypo-albuminemia produces worsening of BBB dysfunction. Increased cytokines in the bloodstream because of infection are able to permeate the damaged BBB and produce cytokine encephalitis [1,2]. The progression of brain edema and uncontrollable increases of neurotoxic glutamate occur in injured brain tissue.

Unstable systemic circulation and cardiopulmonary dysfunction are further complications caused by rapid increases of serum catecholamines. The serum catecholamines are very sensitive to temperature [2]. Overly rapid rewarming produces hyperdynamic hemometabolism, activates glucose metabolism, and also causes unstable cardiac function with rapid increases in serum epinephrine. The precise control of serum hyperglycemia before rewarming is also very important.

Determining the duration of brain hypothermia is best performed by examining the severity of brain damage, evidence for neuronal recovery, and the presence of complications such as systemic infection, uncontrollable hyperglycemia, cardiopulmonary dysfunction, and immune dysfunction.

The Indication of Rewarming

The indication of rewarming is an important factor that partly determines the success of brain hypothermia treatment. As a minimum, evidence of recovery of the injured brain tissue or at least signs of recovery, with well-organized control of ICP lower than 20 mmHg, are required. Recording of the θ wave on the background of the δ wave in trended electroencephalogram, no ICP elevation, SjO_2 control at 60%–75%, and no brain swelling on the computed tomography scan are basic signs of neuronal recovery [2]. The presence of these recovery signs suggest the possibility of rewarming without worsening of brain damage.

Another criteria of rewarming is no evidence of severe BBB dysfunction such as the cerebrospinal fluid (CSF)/serum albumin ratio greater than 0.01, no hypo-albuminemia (serum albumin <3.0–3.5 mg/dl), and no severe hyperglycemia (serum glucose >180 mg/dl). The elevation of brain tissue temperature produces vascular engorgement and increases the intravascular pressure. Vascular engorgement under the condition of BBB dysfunction produces progression of interstitial brain edema. Severe hypo-albuminemia produces reduced intravascular osmotic pressure and promotes brain edema. ICP elevation occurs with rewarming because of vascular engorgement and progression of brain edema. However, the occurrence of ICP elevation by the simple reason of vascular engorgement with controlled BBB function (CSF/serum albumin ratio <0.01) is not a big issue. The background of ICP elevation including worsening of brain edema, suggests no indication of rewarming [2].

Unstable function of albumin-binding antibiotics, intestinal mucous membrane edema, and difficult enteral nutrition because of diarrhea, immune suppression, and ease of infection are also clinical issues of severe hypo-albuminemia. The metabolic shift from lipid to glucose is a specific phenomenon of rewarming during hypothermia. The hypoglycemia at the metabolic shift from lipid to glucose is a dangerous condition during the rewarming stage. However, severe hyperglycemia also produces increased brain tissue lactate. Therefore, the precise management of serum glucose between 130 and 150 mg/dl is indicated at the rewarming stage. The details of the indications of rewarming are summarized in Table 79.

Table 79. Indication of rewarming

Recovery of pathophysiology
θ wave on trend EEG
ICP < 20 mmHg,
No brain swelling on CT
SjO_2 60%–75%
No severe BBB dysfunction
CSF/serum albumin < 0.01
No hypoalbuminemia
Serum albumin > 3.0 mg/dl
No severe hyperglycemia
Serum glucose < 150 mg/dl
Temporary rewarming to mild hypothermia
Cardiopulmonary dysfunction
Systolic BP < 90 mmHg
QT > 450 mm/s, arrythmia
Severe infections
Lymphocytes < 1000 mm^3
Prolonged hyperglycemia
Hyperglycemia > 180 mg/dl

EEG, Electroencephalogram; CT, computed tomography

References

1. Hayashi N (2000) Enhanced neuronal damage in severely brain injured patients by hypothalamus, pituitary, and adrenal axis neuro-hormonal changes. In: Hayashi N (ed) Brain hypothermia. Springer, Berlin Heidelberg New York Tokyo, pp 3–26
2. Hayashi N (2000) The clinical issue and effectiveness of brain hypothermia treatment for severe brain injured patients. In: Hayashi N (ed) Brain hypothermia. Springer, Berlin Heidelberg New York Tokyo, pp 121–151

46. Preconditioning for Rewarming

Preconditioning for rewarming means the premanagement required to prevent various complications during the rewarming stage [5,6]. Without suitable management, safe rewarming is difficult. The treatment of hyperglycemia, hypo-albuminemia, blood–brain barrier (BBB) dysfunction, respiratory dysfunction, and complication of infection are especially important [4–6].

Management of Serum Glucose

Hyperglycemia with serum glucose level more than 230 mg/dl and hypoglycemia with serum glucose lower than 100 mg/dl are dangerous complications at the rewarming stage [5,6].

Hyperglycemia

The systemic metabolic shift from lipid to glucose occurs at the rewarming stage [5,6]. The metabolic balance between lipid and glucose metabolism occurs at a core temperature of about 34°C (Fig. 80, Chap. 43). The elevation of brain tissue temperature above 34°C activates the glucose metabolism with consumption of serum glucose. The rate of glucose consumption is variable and depends on the duration of hypothermia, complications of infection, and the rewarming speed. The most important point is coupling of the glucose metabolism to cerebral blood flow (CBF). The slight increase of serum glucose (150–180 mg/dl) at the rewarming stage does not produce serious complications. However, severe hyperglycemia with serum glucose above 220–230 mg/dl stimulates the hypothalamus appetite center and activates the neural feedback mechanism of macronutrient intake and vasopressin release [8,10,11,16,17]. Increasing cerebral cytokines and damage of the BBB are negative events. If hyperglycemic acidosis occurs, reduction of hemoglobin enzyme 2,3-diphosphoglycerate (DPG) concentration, increasing brain tissue glucose and lactate, and neuronal hypoxia progress at the rewarming stage and result in unsuccessful brain hypothermia treatment [5,6]. The management of severe hyperglycemia and serum pH are especially important before rewarming.

The administration of insulin is the management strategy for severe hyperglycemia. However, at the same time, insulin does not work very well because muscle weakness results in reduced glucose consumption. The liver hypofunction associated with prolonged hypothermia also produces a reduction in the expenditure of serum glucose. The release of growth hormone during rewarming also activates hyperglycemia [6]. Without management before rewarming, the management of hyperglycemia can become very difficult at the rewarming stage. The increase of serum catecholamines by rapid rewarming, muscle weakness with prolonged hypothermia, and administration of gluco-corticoid to prevent brain edema are also negative factors for the control of hyperglycemia [1,5,6,8,11,17]. The mechanism of insulin-resistant hyperglycemia is summarized in Fig. 14 (Chap. 22).

The management method for insulin-resistant hyperglycemia is summarized in Table 16 (Chap. 43). At the rewarming stage, glucose consumption does not increase immediately and prolonged hyperglycemia can occur. Metabolic imbalance of the systemic circulation is recorded at the initial rewarming stage. Therefore, at the early stage of rewarming, serum glucose should be around 120–140 mg/dl, and should then be increased gradually to around 140–160 md/dl at the rewarming temperature zone of 35°–36°C [6]. Administration of insulin, no administration of glucocorticoid, and management of muscle weakness are important for the control of hyperglycemia during preconditioning. The replacement of potassium phosphate, magnesium chloride, and arginine, and physiological rehabilitation of muscle weakness and kinetic therapy are effective in activating the uptake of serum glucose into the skeletal muscles and preventing hyperglycemia at the rewarming stage [6].

Replacement of Serum Albumin

Hypo-albuminemia is a high-incidence complication in severely brain-injured patients that undergo prolonged brain hypothermia treatment [6,13]. Hypo-albuminemia with serum albumin lower than 2.5 g/dl produces many nonphysiological conditions at the rewarming stage. Ease of infection with loss of immune activity, progression of brain edema caused by BBB dysfunction, difficult enteral nutrition because of intestinal mucous edema, unstable pharmacological function of antibiotics (albumin-binding type), and ease of infectious free bacteria translocation are major clinical issues of severe hypo-albuminemia (Fig. 60, Chap. 42) [6]. Therefore, the management of hypo-albuminemia by maintaining serum albumin above 3.0–3.5 mg/dl is a very important part of preconditioning for rewarming.

The management of hypo-albuminemia is not easy. The replacement of serum albumin is not successful in most severely brain-injured patients. This is because the replaced serum albumin can easily pass the injured vascular intimae. The replaced albumin can extravasate into the third space under the conditions of BBB dysfunction in the injured brain tissue. The complication of infection in major organs also produces the same situation. As a result, hypo-albuminemia is not corrected and can markedly worsen brain edema and pneumonia at the rewarming stage [6]. The administration of anti-inflammatory medicines for vascular injury is also necessary for the management of hypo-albuminemia. The preliminary management of vascular inflammation and maintenance of microcirculation in the injured brain and infected organs are useful to prevent excess loss of serum albumin. The replacement of antithrombin-III (AT-III) to more than 100% of serum AT-III is useful for the management of vascular endothelium inflammation and to maintain the microcirculation [6].

There are two approaches for the management of hypo-albuminemia. One is enteral nutrition and the other is replacement of serum albumin. Enteral nutrition is not recommended in severely brain-injured patients at the early stage of cooling because enteral nutriton includes neurotoxic glutamate and can easily pass through the damaged BBB. Early enteral nutrition is only indicated in cases of slight BBB dysfunction such as those with a cerebrospinal fluid (CSF)/serum albumin ratio less than 0.01. The BBB dysfunction subsides after 4–5 days in most cases with management of mild hypothermia and pharmacological treatment. The later stages of cooling is the preferred timing for enteral nutrition in severely brain-injured patients.

Management of BBB Dysfunction

Many lipid-soluble substrates, such as psychoactive drugs, diazepam, iodoantipyrine, nicotine, and ethanol, and many gases, such as oxygen, carbon dioxide, and nitrogen, can easily permeate the BBB. In contrast, polar molecules such as glutamate and catecholamines enter the brain slowly [1,9,14]. Uptake in the brain of phenobarbital, propofol, and midazolame is lower than predicted from lipid solubility data because of binding to the plasma proteins. However, severe damage of the BBB can allow neurotoxic glutamate, proinflammatory cytokines, and dopamine into the injured brain tissue [6].

The severity of BBB dysfunction is diagnosed into four categories: severe BBB dysfunction (CSF/serum albumin >0.02), moderate BBB dysfunction (CSF/serum albumin 0.02–0.01), mild BBB dysfunction (CSF/serum albumin 0.007–0.01), and normal BBB function (CSF/serum albumin <0.007). Severe and moderate BBB dysfunction are major factors for brain edema, complicate cytokine encephalitis with pneumonia, and promote the release of neurotoxic glutamate (Fig. 55, Chap. 39). BBB dysfunction occurs as a result of many factors such as direct vascular injury, inflammation of vascular endothelium, malnutrition, overproduction of proinflammatory cytokines, abnormal serum hypo-osmolarity, and hypo-albuminemia [9,14].

Multiple approaches to the management of BBB dysfunction such as treatment of vascular inflammation with AT-III, management of serum hypo-osmolarity by replacement of albumin, and the control of the source of BBB dysfunction are all useful [6]. In the brain tissue, the BBB is not observed in a specific area. The pituitary gland, median eminence, area postrema, preoptic recess, paraphylsis, pineal gland, and endothelium of the choroid plexus are not specific BBB areas. In this area, many substances with high lipid solubility may move across the BBB by simple diffusion [9]. Therefore, management of increasing neurotoxic substrates in the bloodstream must occur before rewarming.

Management of Respiratory Muscle Weakness

Prolonged brain hypothermia treatment produces muscle weakness and can easily cause the complications of pulmonary atelectasis, pneumonia, and immune dysfunction as shown in Fig. 95. The reduction of alanine, glutamate, IGF-1, and growth hormone are common complications in severe brain injury and prolonged brain hypothermia treatment [6,15]. Furthermore,

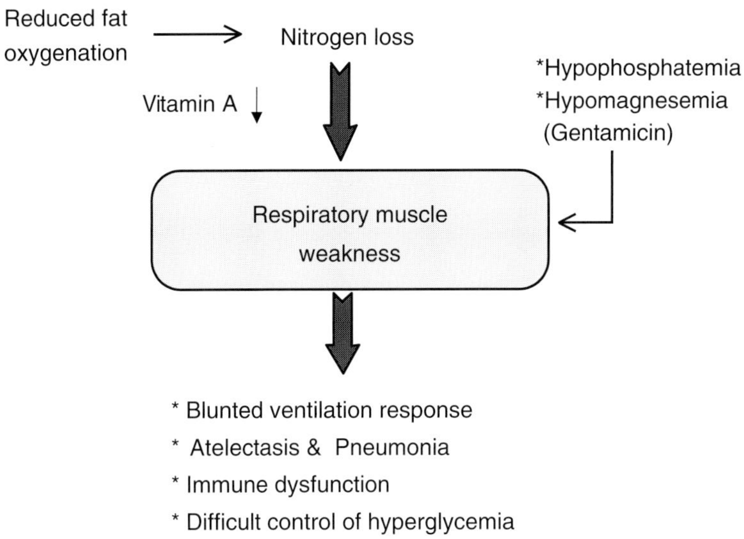

Fig. 95. Nutritional considerations for muscle weakness during brain hypothermia treatment

reduced fat oxygenation, nitrogen loss, hypophosphatemia, and hypomagnesium can cause respiratory muscle weakness. This respiratory muscle weakness not only produces the respiratory weakness, but also produces immune dysfunction because the muscle is the major organ to produce the energy source of lymphocyte immune cells. The treatment of respiratory muscle weakness includes pharmacological treatment, nutritional management, kinetic therapy, and respiratory rehabilitation [3,6].

Pharmacological Treatment of Muscle Weakness

Promotion of protein synthesis in the respiratory muscles with growth hormone, arginine, salbutamol, and glutamine is basic treatment [3,6]. Growth hormone, arginine, and glutamate, are also useful to increase the immune activity and promote lipid metabolism while under hypothermic conditions. Sulbutamol is effective for respiratory recovery by increasing respiratory muscle protein synthesis, prevention of bronchial spasm, and bronchial dilatation. To prevent muscle weakness, the normal control of serum phosphate at 3.0–5.0 mg/dl and serum magnesium at 1.04–1.08 mEq/l are also essential management steps. Administration of amurinone is recommended to prevent protein catabolism in muscles [6].

Rehabilitation of Muscle Weakness

Kinetic therapy is mechanical management to address respiratory muscle weakness. Prolonged bed rest without movement or massage of the body and extremities promotes the release of calcium from bone marrow and results in calcium deposits in respiratory muscle, intestinal organs, and the kidneys [6]. Respiratory muscle weakness progressively develops without pharmacological management, nutritional consideration, and kinetic therapy. During brain hypothermia treatment, massage is very important. Massage to prevent muscle weakness activates protein synthesis in muscle, maintains the energy source of immune cells, prevents thrombosis, and reduces the likelihood of pulmonary microcirculatory disturbances. The massage of subcutaneous brown cells in the neck, subaxillary, and upper back is specifically effective in activating the lipid metabolism and maintaining the energy source of adenosine triphosphate (ATP) without producing lactate under hypothermic conditions [6]. As rehabilitation of pulmonary function, management of respiratory movement, massage of respiratory muscles, and tapping or vibration stimulation of the upper back to prevent alveolus collapse are also necessary.

Nutritional Considerations

Vitamin A deficit, which is diagnosed by observation of the xerophthalmus, will produce activation of nitrogen loss with reduced fat oxygenation. The replacement of vitamin A is also important to stabilize ATP metabolism and phosphate metabolism in cell membranes. This management is particularly important for the control of hemoglobin function under brain hypothermia conditions. Therefore, we prefer the management of vitamin A above at least 50 μg/dl [6].

Enteral administration of amino acid nutrition is very successful in the prevention of respiratory muscle weakness. However, in cases of severe BBB damage, early enteral and parenteral nutrition is not recommended because the neurotoxic glutamate concentration will increase by two to three times with enteral and parenteral amino acid nutrition. We cannot neglect the possibility of neurotoxic glutamate passing through the BBB into the damaged brain tissue. In well-organized BBB function with CSF/serum albumin ratio lower than 0.01, microdialysis studies suggested no evidence of serum glutamate passing into the brain tissue [6]. Monitoring of the CSF/serum albumin ratio is recommended before starting enteral nutrition.

Prevention of Systemic Infections

There are many causes of the high incidence of infection during brain hypothermia treatment. The causes of severe infections during brain hypothermia treatment are [2,6]:

1. Unstable management of hypothalamus–pituitary–adrenal (HPA) axis neuro-endocrinological dysfunctions
2. Reduced immune function
3. Poor management of oxygen and glucose metabolism
4. Undesirable administration of antibiotics
5. Inadequate nutritional management

In severe brain damage caused by trauma, stroke, or cardiac arrest, HPA axis stress-associated hyperglycemia is unavoidable. However, early management of stress-associated hyperglycemia is not easy, as described in Chaps. 22 and 23.

Severe hyperglycemia with serum glucose level above 230 mg/dl promotes infection by stimulation of pro-inflammatory cytokines and vasopressin release [6,7]. These changes stimulate the neuropeptide Y receptors in the vascular walls in major the organs, brain, lungs, and heart [6–8,10–12]. These hyperglycemia-specific microcirculation disturbances complicate the increased vascular permeability and vascular wall inflammation [6,7]. At the rewarming stage, poor management of hyperglycemia can promote the complications of lung edema and pulmonary infection [6]. If the management of BBB function is not adequate as shown by a CSF/serum albumin ratio greater than 0.01, increased cytokines can easily permeate the BBB and promote cytokine encephalitis at the rewarming stage [6]. Worsening of brain edema and neurotoxic brain damage occurs at the rewarming stage. Therefore, as part of hyperglycemia management, serum glucose should be carefully controlled at 120–140 mg/dl before rewarming [6].

Preconditioning befor the start of rewarming requires [6]:

No severe infection
Serum phosphate 3–5 mg/dl
Serum magnesium >1.2 mEq/dl
Serum glucose <150 mg/dl
Vitamin A >50 mg/dl
Lymphocytes >1500 mm^3
Serum albumin >3.5 mg/dl (prealbumin >20 mg/dl)
Hemoglobin (Hb) >12 mg/dl
DPG >10 mmol/gHb
AT-III >100%
Platelet count 50 000–80 000/cu mm
Digastrics decontamination
Muscle massage
Abdominal pressure <10 mmHg

The early enteral administration of nonabsorbable hypothermia-active antibiotics, such as levofloxacin (Cravit, 200 mg) and amphotericin B (100–300 mg) combined with vancomycin 2–3 g/day × 4–6 times i.v. drip) is recommended as digestive decontamination therapy during preconditioning for rewarming. Gram-negative Staphylococcus, *Pseudomonas aeruginosa*, methicillin resistant *Staphylococcus aureus* (MRSA), Tienam resistant Acinetobacter and *Candida albicans* are recorded as high incidence causes of infection during hypothermia treatment. To prevent these bacterial infections, use of arbekacin sulfate (Habekacin, 150–200 mg/day ×2) to prevent Pseudomonal aerginosa and MRSA infection, and cefozopran hydrochloride (Firstcin 1–2 g/day ×2) for Tienam resistant Acinetobacter and fluconazole (Diflucan 100–200 mg/day ×1) for Candida with evidence of β-D-glucan positive reactions is recommended before rewarming [6].

The delivery of sufficient oxygen ($\bar{D}O_2$ > 700–800 ml/min, O_2ER 23%–25%), is also effective in preventing infections at the rewarming stage. In the management of infection at the cooling stage, the control of serum albumin higher than 3.5 mg/dl is especially important because hypo-albuminemia produces serious immune dysfunction via intestinal mucous edema, pancreatic dysfunction, difficult early enteral nutrition with diarrhea, unstable antibacterial function of albumin-binding antibiotics, increasing free bacteria, and likely occurrence of pulmonary edema. Therefore, management of hypo-albuminemia must be carefully controlled at the rewarming stage.

References

1. Dietrich WD, Busto R, Halley M, Valdes I (1990) The importance of brain temperature in alterations of

the blood–brain barrier following cerebral ischemia. J Neuropathol Exp Neurol 49:486–497
2. Fedor EJ, Fisher ER, Lee SH, Weitzel WK, Fisher B (1956) Effect of hypothermia upon induced bacteremia. Proc Soc Exp Biol Med 93:510–512
3. Harrington D, Chua TP, Coast AJS (2000) The effect of solbutamol on skeletal muscle in chronic heart failure. Int J Cardiol 73:257–265
4. Hayashi N (1995) Cerebral hypothermia treatment. In: Hayashi N (ed) Cerebral hypothermia treatment. Sogo Igaku, Tokyo, pp 1–105
5. Hayashi N (1997) Prevention of vegetation after severe head trauma and stroke by combination therapy of cerebral hypothermia and activation of immunedopaminergic nervous system. Proc Soc Treat Coma 6:133–145
6. Hayashi N (2000) The clinical issue and effectiveness of brain hypothermia treatment for severe brain injured patients. In: Hayashi N (ed) Brain hypothermia. Springer, Berlin Heidelberg New York Tokyo, pp 121–151
7. Kagawa M, Nagao S, Bemana I (1996) Arginine vasopressin receptor antagonists for treatment of vasogenic brain edema: an experimental study. J Neurotrauma 13:273–279
8. Kow LM, Pfaff DW (1986) Vasopressin excites ventromedial hypothalamus glucose-responsive neurons in vitro. Physiol Behav 37:153–158
9. Laterra J, Goldstein GW (2000) Ventricular organization of cerebrospinal fluid: blood brain barrier, brain edema, and hydrocephalus. In: Kandel ER, Schwartz JH, Jessell TM (eds) Principles of neural science. McGraw-Hill, New York, pp 1288–1294
10. Leibowitz SF (1999) Macronutrients and brain peptides: what they do and how they respond. In: Berthoud HR, Seeley RJ (eds) Neural and metabolic control of macronutrient intake. CRC, Boca Raton, pp 389–406
11. Leibowiz SF, Sladek C, Spencer L, Temple D (1988) Neuropeptide Y, epinephrine and norepinephrine in the paraventricular nucleus: stimulation of feeding and the release of corticosterone, vasopressin and glucose. Brain Res Bull 21:905–912
12. Lin TW, Kuo YS (1996) Acute pulmonary oedema following administration of vasopressin for control of massive GI tract haemorrhage in a major burn patient. Burns 22:73–75
13. McClain CJ, Hennig B, Ott L, Goldblum S, Young AB (1988) Mechanisms and implications of hypoalbuminemia in head-injured patients. J Neurosurg 69:386–392
14. Pardridge WM (1997) Blood-brain barrier transport mechnisms. In: Welch KMA, Caplan LR, Reise DJ, Siesjo BK, Weir B (eds) Cerebrovascular disease. Academic, New York, pp 21–25
15. Payne LC, Obal F Jr, Opp MR, Krueger JM (1999) Stimulation and inhibition of growth hormone secretion by IL1: the involvement of growth hormone. Neuroendoclinology 56:118–123
16. Stanley BG (1993) Neuropeptide Y in multiple hypothalamic sites controls eating behavior, endocrine, and autonomic system for body energy balance. In: Colmers WF, Wahlestedt C (eds) Biology of neuropeptide Y and related peptide. Humana Press, Totowa, NJ, pp 457–509
17. Temple DL, Leibowitz SF (1994) The neuropeptide Y system (hypothalamus) has a dense concentration of glucocorticoide (type II) receptors that mediate carbon hydrate intake. J Neuroendocrinol 6:479–501

47. Management of Rewarming

The Technique of Rewarming

The technique of rewarming differs for mild and moderate brain hypothermia treatments.

Rewarming From Mild Brain Hypothermia

There are two types of rewarming technique. One is the control of blanket water temperature, and the second is the reduction of the body cooling area by removing the blanket sheet from the patient in a step-wise fashion [8,9,11]. The rewarming speed should be selected with consideration of many factors, such as prolonged hypothermia, complication of cardiopulmonary dysfunction, presence of systemic infection, neuronal recovery levels, and difficulty in controlling hyperglycemia [9,11]. Slow and careful rewarming is recommended for patients who have these clinical issues. The rewarming from mild hypothermia at 34°C after less than 48 h duration is not difficult. The use of careful and constant slow rewarming (0.4°C/h) should be successful. On the other hand, the management of rewarming from brain hypothermia prolonged more than 48 h or moderate brain hypothermia requires an adaptation time of 1–2 days to allow the metabolic shift from lipid to glucose at a brain tissue temperature of 35°–36°C [8,9,11].

At a brain tissue temperature of 34°C, the metabolic balance between glucose and lipid metabolism becomes about even [8,11]. This balance of metabolism mechanisms does not change immediately at the rewarming stage. The adaptation time for the metabolic shift from lipid to glucose during rewarming is part of the technique of careful and slow rewarming.

Rewarming From Moderate Brain Hypothermia

Two step rewarming is recommended for rewarming from moderate brain hypothermia. As a first step, the blanket water temperature should be elevated very slowly (0.1°C/h) from 23°–24°C to about 28°C. When the brain tissue temperature is elevated to 34°C, the warming of the blanket water temperature should be stopped and maintained at 28°–29°C for 1 day as shown in Fig. 96. This procedure produces a temporary stoppage of rewarming at a brain tissue temperature of 35°C for 1–2 days. This time is referred to as an adaptation time for recovery to normothermia [11]. The spontaneous elevation of brain tissue temperature occurs at the end of the adaptation time according to cerebral blood flow (CBF) and metabolism. To prevent rapid elevation of brain tissue temperature after the adaptation time, the blanket water temperature should be reduced very slowly from 28°C to 25°–26°C as shown in Fig. 96. This temporary stoppage of rewarming (1–2 days) at a brain temperature of 34°–35°C produces good physiological adaptation to the changes of metabolic shift from lipid to glucose, increasing serum potassium, vascular engorgement, hyperdynamic circulation, increasing serum catecholamines, production of cytokines, consumption of antithrombin-III (AT-III), and activation of fibrinolysis [2,11].

However, these physiological responses must be treated with care during the adaptation time of the rewarming stage. After these various pathophysiological changes are controlled, rewarming can recommence for elevation of brain tissue temperature up to 36°–37°C. Without this slow step-by-step procedure, acute brain swelling with vascular engorgement and oxygen deficit with rapidly increasing glucose metabolism will occur [8,11]. If the complication of systemic infection was not controlled and blood–brain barrier (BBB) dysfunction is sever [10] (shown as cerebrospinal fluid (CSF)/serum albumin ratio higher than 0.01–0.02), undesirable cytokine encephalitis will occur because of cytokine infiltration into injured brain tissue and the brain hypothermia treatment will fail [9,11].

For rewarming to succeed, continuous monitoring of brain tissue temperature or jugular venous blood temperature is effective [8]. As an alternate monitor to evaluate brain tissue temperature, the tympanic membrane temperature is also useful.

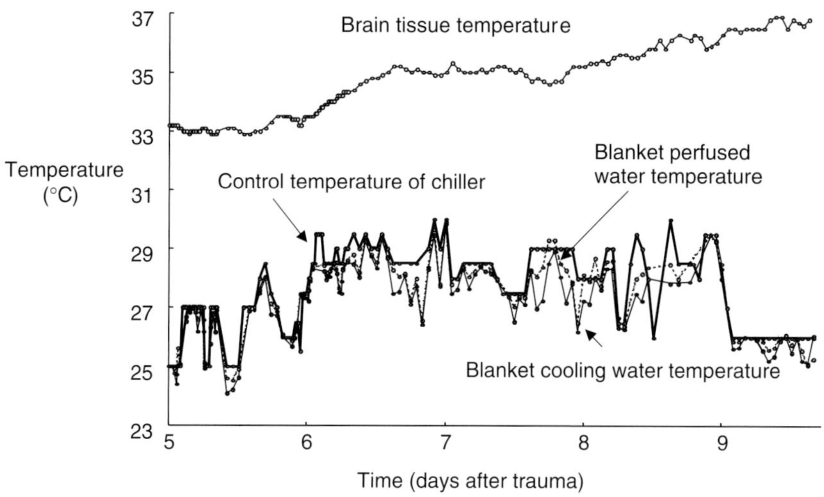

Fig. 96. Changes of brain tissue temperature and blanket cooling water temperature

For rewarming after the adaptation stage, different techniques can be used. Rewarming can be achieved by control of the blanket water temperature, by reducing the cooling area by removing the cooling blanket stepwise from the patient's body and legs, or by a combination of these techniques. The maintenance of blanket water temperature at around 26°–27°C for 1–2 days produces spontaneous normothermia. Reducing the cooling area at the same time produces undesirable rapid rewarming of the brain tissue. Therefore, the technique of reducing the cooling area is only indicated in cases with no serious complications such as pneumonia during the cooling stage, or in patients not seriously brain injured. The stable slow rewarming process after the adaptation stage is especially important in cases of severely brain-injured patients of Glasgow Come Scale Score (GCS) 4–5 [8–11].

If stable rewarming fails and intracranial pressure (ICP) is elevated more than 25 mmHg, the brain tissue temperature should be immediately reduced to 34°C. In this case, rewarming can be retried after stabilization of brain swelling and control of ICP to lower than 15 mmHg. The step-by-step rewarming process and allowance of an adaptation time for physiological changes during rewarming are very important techniques for the success of brain hypothermia treatment.

Monitoring at the Rewarming Stage

Monitoring of Brain Tissue Temperature and Jugular Venous Blood Temperature

Continuous monitoring of brain tissue temperature is very useful for the management of rewarming, however, the meaning of brain tissue temperature is different according to the location of measurement. This requires an explanation of brain tissue temperature in detail to understand the pathophysiological changes in the injured brain during rewarming.

The localized tissue temperature is affected by many factors including blood temperature (core temperature), heat production by localized tissue metabolism, retention of local microcirculation, and the temperature circumstance of particular organs [8,10]. The deep brain tissue temperature and white matter temperature are a little higher than the surface brain tissue temperature or the cortical brain tissue temperature because of lower washout radiation capacity of localized brain tissue temperature with low CBF. In normal conditions, these differences of localized brain tissue temperature are about 0.1°–0.3°C. However, the difference between cortical and white matter brain temperature may increase to about 0.2°–0.7°C because of reduced localized CBF. The deep brain tissue and white matter can undergo a thermo-pooling phenomenon more easily than the surface cortical brain tissue because of CBF disturbances [10]. These localized CBF disturbances are easy to diagnose by monitoring the differences between the ventricular CSF temperature and the cortical brain tissue temperature, and also indirectly by monitoring the internal jugular venous blood temperature. This is because the ventricular CSF temperature reflects the deep brain tissue temperature rather than the surface temperature, and the jugular venous blood temperature reflects the mean brain tissue temperature. In our series of clinical studies of severe brain trauma, the ventricular temperature was elevated by up to 0.7°C higher than the jugular venous blood temperature [8–11].

The difference in ventricular CSF temperature and tympanic membrane temperature is also an indirect parameter of CBF disturbance. Ventricular CSF

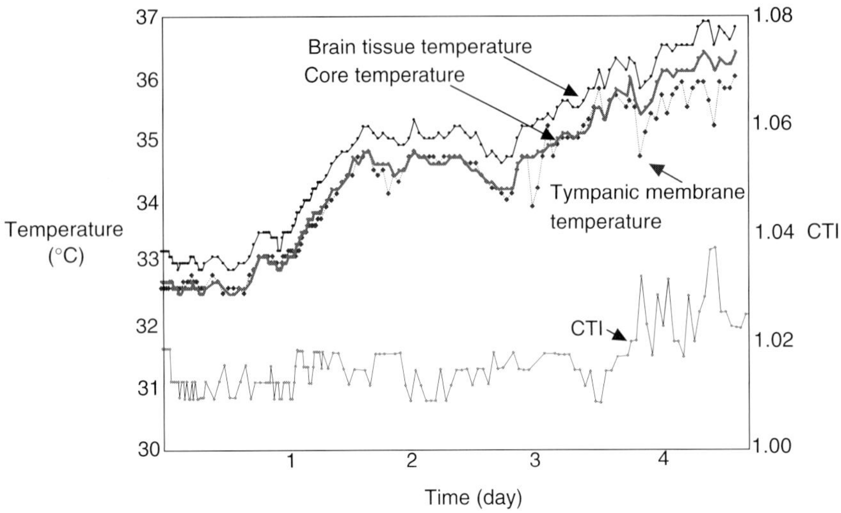

Fig. 97. Cerebral blood flow disturbances with vascular engorgement and heat retention at the rewarming stage. Cerebral thermal index (*CTI*) is defied as brain tissue temperature/tympanic membrane temperature

temperature higher than tympanic membrane temperature suggests a CBF disturbance associated with reduced cerebral venous outflow. The difference between the jugular venous blood temperature and the tympanic membrane temperature suggests CBF disturbance indirectly. Brain tissue temperature (internal jugular venous blood temperature) higher than tympanic membrane temperature suggests brain thermopooling associated with cerebral outflow CBF disturbance at the rewarming stage (Fig. 97) [8–10]. However, progressively lower temperatures for both parameters suggest the dangerous complication of poor filling. Understanding the meanings of ventricular temperature, cortical brain tissue temperature, white matter temperature, and jugular venous blood temperature is very useful for diagnosis of CBF disturbance and precise management of rewarming.

Elevated brain tissue temperature is washed out by the CBF. Therefore, the internal jugular venous blood temperature elevates with elevation of the brain tissue temperature at the rewarming stage. The cortical blood flow is higher than white matter CBF by about 4–5 times. Therefore, jugular venous blood temperature more closely reflects the cortical brain temperature rather than the deep white matter temperature [8]. As an alternate monitor of brain tissue temperature, the internal jugular venous blood temperature is more accurate than tympanic membrane temperature, core temperature, and bladder temperature. These localized temperature changes are correlated to each other because the systemic circulating blood temperature is the main component of these localized temperatures. However, in cases of nonfilling and poor filling of cerebral circulation, the jugular venous blood temperature is not similar to the brain tissue temperature. This is because in internal jugular venous blood is contaminated by external venous blood. In this case, the internal jugular venous blood temperature is difficult to use as an alternate monitor of brain tissue temperature.

Tympanic Membrane Temperature

The continuous monitoring of tympanic membrane temperature is much more useful than intermittent measurement. The tympanic membrane temperature indirectly provides information about carotid circulation into the brain. The difference between the right and left tympanic membrane temperature is less than 0.8°C in nonpathological conditions. A difference of more than 0.8°C between the right and left tympanic membrane temperature suggests the presence of unilateral CBF disturbances [10]. Vasospasm and cerebral thrombosis produce elevation of the tympanic membrane temperature of about 0.6°C higher than the noninjured side. This is because the internal carotid blood flow is obstructed in the cranium and shifts to the external carotid blood flow. The tympanic membrane is fed by external carotid blood flow. The progressive elevation of brain and jugular venous blood temperature with reduced difference between the jugular venous blood temperature and tympanic membrane temperature are typical signs of cerebral vasospasm (Fig. 98). The continuous or computed monitoring of this localized temperature is very useful for diagnosis of intracranial or extracranial CBF disturbances.

The tympanic membrane temperature can also provide information about the distribution of the systemic circulation. In a physiological condition, the tympanic membrane temperature is always higher than rectal and bladder temperature. However, in cases of severe CBF disturbance, the bladder and rectal tem-

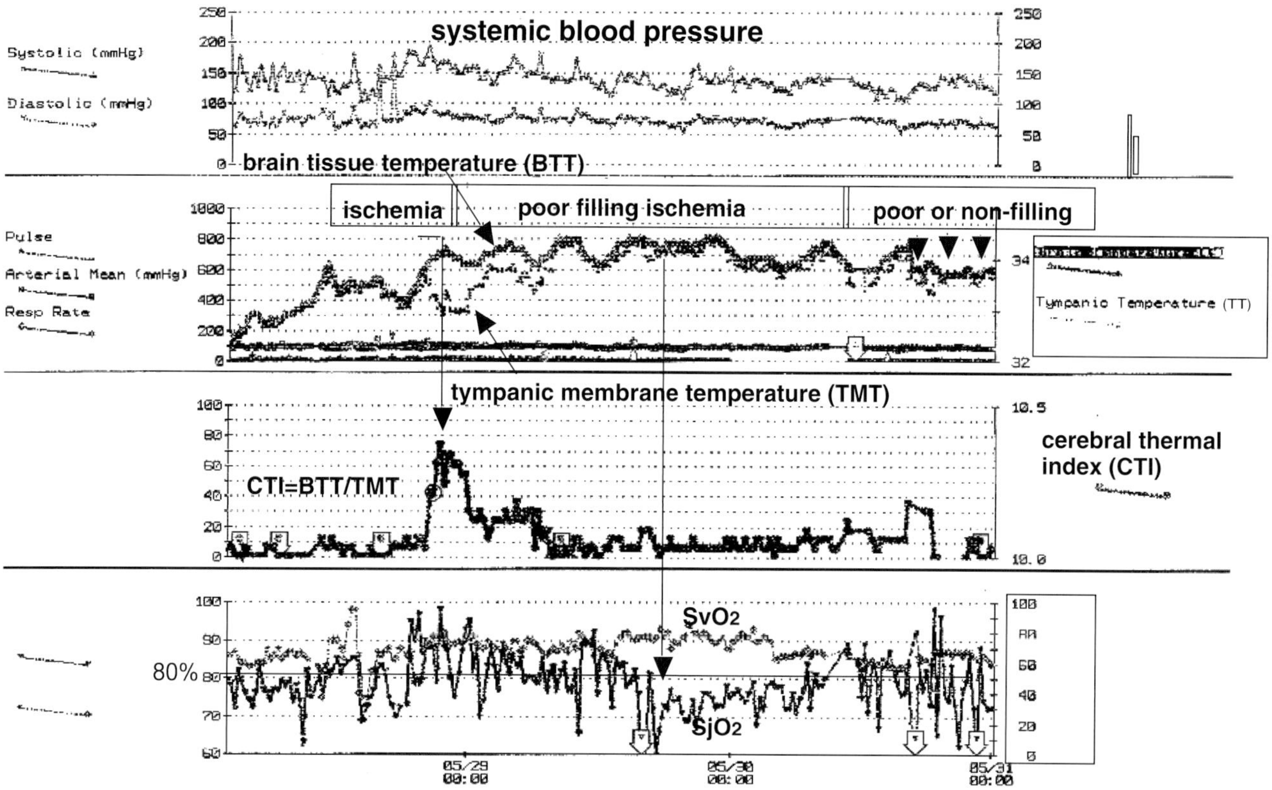

Fig. 98. Cerebral hemodynamic changes at the rewarming stage. Cerebral vasospasm was evaluated by dissociation of brain tissue temperature (BTT) and tympanic membrane temperature (TMT), that follows the progressive fluctuating elevation of MTT and TMT. The BTT becomes equal to TMT when cerebral thermo-pooling reaches the teminal stage of brain metabolism

peratures are higher than the tympanic membrane temperature. A tympanic membrane temperature/bladder temperature ratio less than 0.96 suggests a blood shift to the intestinal organs rather than cerebral circulation [8,10].

Bladder Temperature

The bladder temperature is not the same as the brain tissue temperature; however, its changes correlate simultaneously to changes in brain tissue temperature. The monitoring of bladder temperature and tympanic membrane temperature are useful for evaluation of blood shift of the systemic circulation into the abdominal side rather than cerebral circulation. The elevation of bladder temperature above the tympanic membrane temperature indirectly suggests severe CBF disturbance.

In a complication of cystitis, localized bladder inflammation produces increased heat production in the bladder and, simultaneously, inflammatory cytokines and pyrogen increase the blood temperature of the systemic circulation. Therefore, elevated bladder temperature provides information about systemic circulation into the bladder.

The brain tissue temperature/bladder temperature ratio (or brain tissue temperature – bladder temperature difference) indirectly suggests the conditions of blood distribution into the brain and bladder. A ratio higher than 1.0 suggests a normal flow pattern. However, in conditions of blood flow shift to the abdominal side caused by dopamine dominant circulation, the brain tissue temperature/bladder temperature ratio reduces to less than 1.0. This phenomenon can be monitored in severely reduced CBF and also in systemic circulation maintained by dopamine. The continuous monitoring of bladder temperature and brain tissue temperature (or jugular venous blood temperature), simultaneously, is very useful to diagnose the blood shift into the abdominal side from cerebral circulation [8].

Therefore, the previously held concept that, normal blood pressure, normal cerebral perfusion pressure (CPP) [5] and normal ICP [12] are sufficient to evaluate the maintenance of cerebral circulation is not correct. The blood shift to the intestinal organs in systemic circulation is also necessary to evaluate the cerebral circulation. The critical value of brain tissue temperature/bladder temperature ratio to diagnose the presence of severe CBF disturbance is less than 0.96. Lower than 0.96 suggests serious CBF disturbance.

In cases of intestinal organ ischemia, the bladder temperature reduces and therefore increases the core temperature/bladder temperature ratio above 1.0 at the rewarming stage. This information is very useful to determine the possible start time for enteral nutrition. The combination monitors of bladder temperature, brain temperature, core temperature, bladder pressure, and gastric pHi are very useful to indirectly diagnose the intestinal digestive organ circulation.

Saturation of Internal Jugular Venous Blood Oxygen

Rewarming is indicated with the evidence of neuronal recovery or at least signs of recovery in injured brain tissue. The simultaneous monitoring of the internal jugular venous blood temperature and the saturation of internal jugular venous blood oxygen (SjO_2) is very useful to evaluate the recovery of the neuronal oxygen metabolism and circulation [6,10,14]. The SjO_2 changes dynamically by three factors, one of which is cerebral circulation. Low values of SjO_2, lower than 50%–55%, suggest the reduction of CBF. Reduced cerebral oxygen consumption produces high values of SjO_2 of more than 80%. The increasing of SjO_2 can theoretically be interpreted as a result of increased CBF; however; increased CBF and reduced oxygen consumption are unusual pathophysiological changes. Therefore, SjO_2 of more than 80% suggests reduced oxygen expenditure in most cases. The normal value of SjO_2 is about 60%–70%. SjO_2 at 55%–60% suggests the interplay of reduced CBF and increased cerebral oxygen metabolism. SjO_2 70%–80% suggests the compensation of high flow to the reduced cerebral oxygen metabolism. However, precise diagnosis of CBF changes and cerebral oxygen metabolism should decided by analysis of SjO_2, cerebral thermal index (CTI) defined as the jugular blood temperature/tympanic membrane temperature ratio, and the tympanic membrane temperature/bladder temperature ratio (Table 14, Chap. 42). During the rewarming stage, SjO_2 should be controlled at 60%–75%.

Intracranial Pressure

ICP elevation can occur because of many reasons at the rewarming stage. The most serious ICP elevation at the rewarming stage is caused by progression of brain edema in injured brain tissue [12]. Short duration of hypothermia, insufficient recovery, complication of infection without management of BBB dysfunction, and progression of chemical encephalitis are major causes of brain edema [10]. To avoid these complications, the rewarming criteria are important. Evidence of recovery or at least signs of moving toward restoration on the trend EEG, no ICP elevation, no signs of brain swelling on computed tomography (CT), $JvO_2 < 80\%$, and management of CSF/serum albumin ratio less than 0.01, serum albumin greater than 3.5 mg/dl, and control of serum glucose at 120–140 mg/dl are important [11].

As reasons for ICP elevation, the overproduction of carbon dioxide can occur with a rapid shift from lipid- to glucose-dominant metabolism. We have observed prolonged ICP elevation of about 30–35 mmHg for 1 week without neurological damage. The reason for no neurological damage even with 30–35 mmHg ICP elevation for 1 week is unclear. The control of glucose metabolism and neuronal oxygenation that includes management of hemoglobin function might be more effective than control of ICP elevation [11]. ICP elevation can be easily controlled by hyperventilation rather than using manitol administration at the rewarming stage. However, $PaCO_2$ lower than 25 mmHg should be avoided to prevent cerebral ischemia by vasoconstriction.

Atmospheric Pressure

Changes of atmospheric pressure affect the autonomic nervous function and also directly affect the brain tissue compression of externally decompressed patients. The mechanical compressive pressure for externally decompressed brain tissue is higher than 1010 hPa. However, at atmospheric pressure less than 1010 hPa, the brain tissue pressure becomes higher than the external atmospheric pressure and can cause the brain to shift toward the externally decompressed area (Fig. 72, Chap. 42). This specific brain shift can cause a small laceration in the deep brain. With approaching bad weather, and especially with significant drops in atmospheric pressure, protective preliminary management of brain edema and ICP elevation with manitol administration should prevent these complications. Therefore, with bad weather approaching and the likelihood of atmospheric pressure lower than 1010 hPa, rewarming is not recommended. If rewarming cannot escape bad weather, careful intensive care unit (ICU) management for ICP elevation and brain edema are necessary. The administration of high osmotic agents, replacement of albumin, control of AT-III to more than 100%–130%, administration of furosemide to reduce CSF production, maintenance of oxygen delivery above 700–800ml/min, and use of the head-up position are important [9,11].

Biochemical Monitoring

Many pathophysiological reactions occur at the rewarming stage after prolonged hypothermia. The metabolic shift from lipid to glucose, increasing serum catecholamines and hyperdynamic circulation, vascular engorgement, increasing cardiac output, circulation and oxygen metabolic gap, activation of fibrinolysis more than coagulation, and activation of proinflammatory cytokines are the main changes [9,11]. These rewarming-specific pathophysiological changes can easily complicate brain swelling and worsen infections. To take care of these clinical issues, biochemical analysis for serum glucose, serum albumin, serum phosphate and magnesium, AT-III or protein C, TAT and DD-dimer, PaO_2/FiO_2 ratio, pH, and oxygen delivery are required.

Management of ICP Elevation at the Rewarming Stage

The management of ICP at the rewarming stage is one of the key points for the a success of brain hypothermia treatment. Two types of ICP elevation are recorded. One is acute brain swelling and the other is the progression of brain edema. The background of these two ICP elevation mechanisms are different [12]. When ICP elevation is recorded at the rewarming stage, the causes of ICP elevation must be made clear as soon as possible.

Prevention of Acute Brain Swelling

Acute brain swelling that occurs at the rewarming stage is caused by vascular engorgement, hypercapnia ($PaCO_2 > 45$–50mmHg), mediastinal hypertension, and abdominal hypertension higher than 20–25mmHg. All of these ICP elevation mechanisms occur by extacranial lesions [3]. Therefore, the prognosis is not as bad as for complications arising from brain edema. Control of $PaCO_2$ below 40mmHg, 15° head-up position [13], removal of enteral gases, continuous urinary drainage, and prevention of airway obstruction are recommended treatments for acute brain swelling [11]. Prolonged bed rest and hypo-albuminemia can easily complicate venous stasis at the peripheral extremities. The resultant venous thrombosis and leg swelling can complicate pulmonary micro-emboli and conceal pulmonary dysfunction [9,11,15]. Reduced AT-III also activates the formation of micro-emboli in the peripheral circulation. The massage of peripheral extremities, control of serum albumin at more than 3.5g/dl by replacement, and maintenance of more than 100% of AT-III are important ICU measures to prevent acute brain swelling at the rewarming stage. Good neuronal oxygenation and precise management of serum glucose at 120–140mg/dl are the most important ICU strategies for the management of acute brain swelling. We have experienced many cases with good neurological outcomes because of good management of neuronal oxygenation and hyperglycemia even with elevation of ICP at 30–35 mmHg for sereral days by vascular engorgement.

Prevention of Brain Edema

ICP elevation caused by brain edema is a serious complication at the rewarming stage and is different to acute brain swelling. The background to worsening brain edema depends on the type of rewarming procedure. In cases of brain hypothermia treatment of short duration without recovery from brain damage, rewarming worsens brain edema and cause ICP elevation [11]. The temporarily stopped mechanism of brain damage reprogresses with rewarming. The overlap of the reprogression of the brain injury mechanism and rewarming-associated stress reactions worsens the overall condition [9,11]. For treatment of this ICP elevation, the brain tissue temperature should be reduced to 34°C, oxygen delivery maintained, hyperglycemia controlled [1], hypo-albuminemia controlled by replacement of albumin to give CSF/serum albumin ratio less than 0.01, and hyperosmotic therapy for brain edema [9,11].

Another clinical issue of brain edema at the rewarming stage is the complication of pulmonary infection combined with BBB dysfunction [8,11]. The combination of BBB dysfunction with systemic infection produces the serious complication of ICP elevation at the rewarming stage. In most cases, these complications result in unsuccessful brain hypothermia treatment because of uncontrollable increases of neurotoxic glutamate with cytokine encephalitis in the brain tissue. Other causes of infection at the cooling and rewarming stages are the inadequate control of HPA axis neurohormonal abnormality, immune dysfunction, intestinal management, hypo-albuminemia, nutritional management, and poor selection of antibiotics [8].

As treatment, stabilization of BBB function by administration of anti-inflammatory agents and replacement of serum albumin are useful with management of infection [11]. The management of infection during the rewarming stage is similar to that used during preconditioning and is described in Chap. 46.

Management of Systemic Circulation and Metabolism During Rewarming

At the rewarming stage, the pattern of blood flow changes to hyperdynamic circulation with increased cardiac output, peripheral vascular dilatation, and increased serum dopamine concentration [2,11]. The rewarming-specific circulation increases in the intestinal organs initially. At this stage, unnecessary dehydration therapy for the prevention of brain edema without control of hypo-albuminemia produces severe disturbances of microcirculation in all organs. The intestinal digestive organ is especially sensitive to ischemia and hypo-albuminemia. Severe hypo-albuminemia (serum albumin <2.5 mg/dl) and unnecessary manitol dehydration therapy cause difficult enteral nutrition because of diarrhea and intestinal organ ischemia. To prevent these complications and stabilize the systemic circulation, normovolemic fluid resuscitation is the first choice. The management of the reduced inorganic phosphate, management of the osmotic gap between serum and stool such as [serum Osm – 2 (stool Na + K) > 100 mOsm/kg], and careful management of serum glucose at 120–150 mg/dl are important.

The maintenance of oxygen delivery is not difficult in hyperdynamic circulation at the rewarming stage. However, oxygen metabolism cannot increase with increasing systemic circulation. At the initial time of rewarming, glucose and oxygen metabolisms are still low compared with hyperdynamic circulation. This discrepancy between metabolism and circulation could limit the rate of rewarming.

Hyper-metabolism, and increased oxygen demand and glucose consumption occur at the late stage of rewarming. At this time, spontaneous breathing management activates oxygen demand and glucose consumption by hyperventilation. Neuronal hypoxia develops in this case with rewarming. Sufficient oxygen delivery with pulmonary ventilation control under anesthesia, analgesia, and muscle relaxation is strongly recommended until rewarming is finished [9,11].

Unsuccessful control of hyperglycemia with serum glucose higher than 230 mg/dl produces 2,3-diphosphoglycernte (DPG) reduction so that the release of oxygen from binding hemoglobin becomes difficult [10]. Therefore, this complication produces neuronal hypoxia even with normal control of oxygen delivery and oxygen inhalation. Precise management of serum pH, hyperglycemia, and hypo-albuminemia is important.

Management of Pulmonary Infection at Rewarming Stage

Infection control is more important at the cooling and preconditioning stages than at rewarming time. This is because pulmonary infection observed at the rewarming stage started at the cooling or preconditioning stage [9,11]. The management of pulmonary infection at the rewarming stage is not much different to preconditioning care. The background of pulmonary infection at the rewarming stage includes reduced immune activity. Prolonged bed rest, swelling of the legs caused by hypo-albuminemia, and reduced AT-III level can easily cause micro-embolus formation in the pulmonary circulation. Uncontrolled severe hyperglycemia also stimulates vasopressin release, and stimulates the neuropeptide Y receptor in pulmonary circulation. Poor ICU management at the cooling stage results in a difficult infection control at the rewarming stage.

The special considerations for management of infection that are required at the rewarming stage are the control of hypo-albuminemia, prevention of rapidly increasing serum catecholamines, selection of appropriate antibiotics, management of intestinal digestive organs, administration of enteral nutrition, management of BBB dysfunction, and support of immune function [9,11].

Severe hypo-albuminemia produces intestinal mucous edema and pulmonary interstitial edema. These specific hypo-albuminemia conditions and malnutrition cause pancreatic duct obstruction, intestinal organ ischemia, bacterial translocation, and immune lymphocytopenia. Rapid rewarming produces increased serum catecholamine levels. Catecholamine surge is a serious complication because it contributes to progression of metabolic hyperglycemia, metabolic acidosis, reduction of hemoglobin DPG, slow release of bound oxygen from hemoglobin, stimulation of neuropeptide Y receptors hypothalamus appetite center, release of vasopressin by the feedback mechanism of neural control of macronutrient hyperglycemia, and worsening of BBB function by vasopressin release [9,11]. To prevent these catecholamine-associated complications, very slow step-wise rewarming and well-organized anesthesia is recommended until the end of rewarming. The management of infection is summarized in Fig. 91 (Chap. 44).

Antibiotics are selected by evidence of sensitivity to cultured bacteria. However, the efficacy of antibiotics

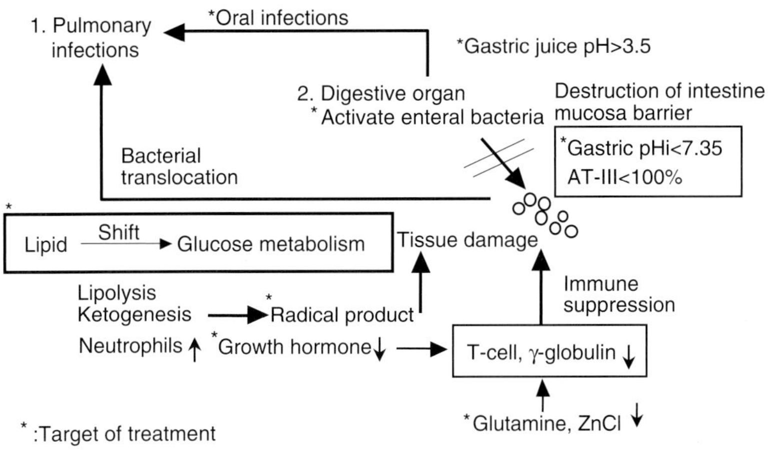

Fig. 99. Promotion of infection at the rewarming stage

is also influenced by the level of serum albumin, liver function, and renal function. As causes of bacterial infection, gram-negative Staphylococcus, *Candida albicans*, *Pseudomonas aerginosa* and Tienam resistant Acinetobacter are the major bacteria responsible for systemic infections at the rewarming stage. To prevent of these complications, enteral administration of levofloxacin (Cravit, 200 mg) and amphotericin B (100–300 mg) combined with vancomycin (2–3 g/day × 4–6 times i.v. drip) is recommended as digestive de-contamination therapy. As an another intravenous administration of antibiotics, the combination of arbekacin sulfate (Habekacin, 150–200 mg/day × 2) to prevent Pseudomonas and methceillin infection, cefozopran hydrochloride (Firstcin 1–2 g/day × 2) resistant for Tienam resistant Acinetobacter and fluconazole (Diflucan 100–200 mg/day × 1) for Candida (evidence of β-D-glucan positive reactions) is useful chemotherapy (see critical path).

Suitable fluid resuscitation, replacement of albumin, control of AT-III, replacement of serum phosphate and magnesium, and control of hyperglycemia are important management needs. However, well-organized preconditioning management before starting rewarming is more successful to prevent these complications.

Prolonged moderate brain hypothermia can produce reduced immune function because of reduced growth hormone level, and muscle weakness from reduced microcirculation and limited muscle rehabilitation [4,11]. Severe lymphocytopenia with lymphocytes less than 1000/mm^3 is an indication of immune dysfunction. The replacement of growth hormone (or arginine that is an activator of growth hormone), potassium phosphate, and serum magnesium, the use of muscle rehabilitation, prevention of peripheral edema, and the use of intermittent moderate brain hypothermia is prophylactic management during rewarming.

Nutritional Considerations at the Rewarming Stage

Figure 99 shows the mechanism of infection at the rewarming stage. The management of nutrition at the rewarming stage requires the replacement of an energy source of calories, maintenance of energy for immune cells, stabilization of intestinal digestive organs, and maintenance of nutritional conditions [9,11]. However, for nutritional management to succeed at the rewarming stage, pretreatment for severe BBB dysfunction is necessary. This is because neurotoxic glutamate will increase by about two to three times with enteral and parenteral amino acid nutrition. In well-organized BBB with CSF/serum albumin ratio lower than 0.01, microdialysis studies suggested that serum glutamate did not pass into the brain tissue and no worsening of brain edema occurred. However, in cases of severe BBB damage as shown by CSF/serum albumin ratio greater than 0.01–0.02, the neurotoxic glutamate can pass the BBB with enteral and parenteral nutrition and promote serious chemical brain damage. The preliminary management of BBB dysfunction with replacement of serum albumin to higher than 3.5 mg/dl, with anti-inflammatory medicine for the vascular wall such as AT-III and protein C, and administration of a radical scavenger such as Radicut are useful to avoid nutritional complications at the rewarming stage [9,11].

The control of BBB dysfunction, (CSF/serum albumin ratio lower than 0.01) followed by enteral administration of amino acid is very successful in preventing respiratory muscle weakness [9,11]. Respiratory muscle protein metabolism can be maintained at the rewarming stage by replacement of glutamine and arginine in combination with pharmacological treatment, phosphate, magnesium, vitamin A, and sulbutamol [7,11].

References

1. Almeida A, Delgado-Esteban M, Bolanos JP, Medina JM (2002) Oxygen and glucose deprivation induces mitochondrial dysfunction and oxidative stress in neurones but not in astrocytes in primary culture. Neurochem 81: 207–217
2. Bioch M (1967) Cerebral effects of rewarming following prolonged hypothermia: significance for the management of severe cranio-cerebral injury and acute pyrexia. Brain 90:769–784
3. Birman H, Haq A, Hew E, Aberman A (1984) Continuous monitoring of mixed venous oxygen saturation in hemodynamically unstable patients. Chest 86:753–756
4. Davila DR, Breif S, Simon J, Hammer RE, Brinster RL, Kelley KW (1987) Role of growth hormone in regulating T-dependant immune events in aged, nude, and transgenic rodents. J Neurosci Res 18:108–116
5. Feng H, Huang G, Gao L, Tan H, Liao X (2000) Effect of intracranial pressure and cerebral perfusion pressure on outcome prediction of severe traumatic brain injury. Chin J Traumatol 3:226–230
6. Filippi R, Reisch R, Mauer D, Perneczky A (2000) Brain tissue pO_2 related to $SjvO_2$, ICP, and CPP in severe brain injury. Neurosurg Rev 23:94–97
7. Harrington D, Chua TP, Coast AJS (2000) The effect of solbutamol on skeletal muscle in chronic heart failure. International J of Cardiology 73:257–265
8. Hayashi N (1995) Cerebral hypothermia treatment. In: Hayashi N (ed) Cerebral hypothermia treatment. Sogo Igaku, Tokyo, pp 1–105
9. Hayashi N (1997) Prevention of vegetation after severe head trauma and stroke by combination therapy of cerebral hypothermia and activation of immune-dopaminergic nervous system. Proc Soc Treat Coma 6:133–145
10. Hayashi N (2000) Enhanced neuronal damage in severely brain injured patients by hypothalamus, pituitary, and adrenal axis neuro-hormonal changes. In: Hayashi N (ed) Brain hypothermia. Springer, Berlin Heidelberg New York Tokyo, pp 3–26
11. Hayashi N (2000) The clinical issue and effectiveness of brain hypothermia treatment for severe brain injured patients. In: Hayashi N (ed) Brain hypothermia. Springer, Berlin Heidelberg New York Tokyo, pp 121–151
12. Langfitt TW (1969) Intracranial pressure. Clin Neurosurg 16:436–471
13. Schwarz S, Georgiadis D, Aschoff A, Schwab S (2002) Effects of body position on intracranial pressure and cerebral perfusion in patients with large hemispheric stroke. Stroke 33:497–501
14. Sheinberg M, Kanter MJ, Robertson CS, Contant CF, Narayan RK, Grossman RG (1992) Continuous monitoring of jugular venous oxygen saturation in head-injury patients. J Neurosurg 76:212–217
15. Valeri CR, Cassidy G, Khuri S, Feingold H, Ragno G, Altschule MD (1987) Hypothermia-induced reversible platelet dysfunction. Ann Surg 205:175–181

V. Prevention of Memory Disturbances and Vegetative State

48. Clinical Issues in the Management of Unconsciousness and Vegetative State Patients

Unconsciousness is diagnosed by the lack of response to verbal, painful and other external stimulation [7]. Lesions include brainstem reticular formations, whole brain mantle cortex, and interconnection brain between the cortices and reticular formation. However, after use of brain hypothermia treatment that includes treatment for stress-associated hypothalamus–pituitary–adrenal (HPA) axis neurohormonal dysfunction [4], many herniated patients, who would previously have been considered to have a low chances of survival using intracranial pressure (ICP)-oriented treatment, have survived [2,5]. In this group, we have observed many patients whose recoveries are difficult to explain and understand by the previous diagnostic method of the Glasgow Coma Scale (GCS) [7].

Although patients appear to be in a coma and do not respond to external stimulation, some patients are aware of stimulation and events that occur around the bedside [1–3,5,6]. After recovered, the patients say [I am sleeping with good feeling, however, many peoples say that open eyes and speak same things. But I cannot open eyes and difficult to make response. However, why I must open eyes? I am sleeping very comfortable. Few days later, I understand reason of why I am staying here. I am brain injured patients or cardiac arrested patients and now I am receiving medical treatment. However, still I cannot open eyes and difficult make a response to verbal and painful stimulation]. Who can say this patient is coma? However GCS diagnostic evaluation suggests the coma.

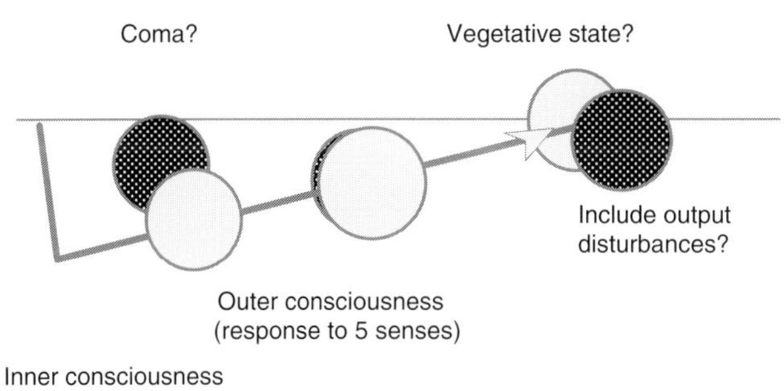

Fig. 100. Dissociation of inner and outer consciousness and output disturbances

For a long time, we have diagnosed consciousness by monitoring responsiveness to external stimulation [7]. However, human consciousness is not simple. There are two types of consciousness. One is responsive consciousness to external stimulation, and the other is inner consciousness relating to emotion, feelings of love, memory, thought, judgement, anger, and volition [1–5]. In most cases of severe brain damage, both forms of consciousness will be damaged simultaneously. However, damage of the outer consciousness without damage of the inner consciousness can produce dissociation of outer and inner consciousness (Fig. 100). More severe damage to the outer consciousness than the inner consciousness produces coma; however, many patients understand their own situation as described by recovered patients. On the other hand, damage of the inner consciousness that is more severe than that to the outer consciousness produces patients that open their eyes by outer stimulation and yet provide no emotional response. Is this situation that of the vegetative state? Where is the center of inner consciousness? What kind of mechanism occurs in selective damage of the inner consciousness? How can the responsiveness of the inner consciousness be diagnosed? If these questions can be answered, new approaches could be developed for the management of vegetation.

References

1. Hayashi N (1997) Combination therapy of cerebral hypothermia, pharmacological activation of the dopamine system, and hormonal replacement in severely brain damaged patients. J Jpn Soc Intensive Care Med 4:191–197
2. Hayashi N (1997) Prevention of vegetation after severe head trauma and stroke by combination therapy of cerebral hypothermia and activation of immune-dopaminergic nervous system. Proc Soc Treat Coma 6:133–145
3. Hayashi N (1999) The brain hypothermia therapy for prevention of vegetation after severe brain injury. (In Japanese) Nippon Geka Gakkai Zasshi 100:443–448
4. Hayashi N (2000) Enhanced neuronal damage in severely brain injured patients by hypothalamus, pituitary, and adrenal axis neuro-hormonal changes. In: Hayashi N (ed) Brain hypothermia. Springer, Berlin Heidelberg New York Tokyo, pp 3–26
5. Hayashi N (2000) The clinical issue and effectiveness of brain hypothermia treatment for severe brain injured patients. In: Hayashi N (ed) Brain hypothermia. Springer, Berlin Heidelberg New York Tokyo, pp 121–151
6. Hayashi N, Hirayama T, Utagawa T, Ohata M (1994) Systemic management of cerebral edema based on a new concept in severe head injury patients. Acta Neurochir [Suppl] 60:541–543
7. Teasdale G, Jennett B (1974) Assessment of coma and impaired consciousness. A practical scale. Lancet 2:81–84

49. The New Concept of Unconsciousness and Mechanism of Vegetation

Damage to the dopamine A10 central nervous system can easily result in damage to intelligence, personality, and cause memory disturbances [12,20]. In previous clinical reports about effective pharmacological treatment of the vegetative state, memory, cognition, and aphasia were associated with the replacement of dopamine. These reports are summarized in Table 80. All of these reports suggest interrelationships between the dopamine nervous system and vegetation [2–6,10,14–18].

The dopamine A10 nervous system works as part of the neuronal function affecting emotion, feelings of love, memory, thought, judgement, anger, and volition (Fig. 34, Chap. 26). Therefore, I hypothesize that damage to the dopamine A10 nervous system will trigger vegetation or mental retardation [8,11–13,20]. Baker et al. [1] demonstrated that dopamine release occurs with reduced dihydroxyphenylacetic acid (DOPAC) in ischemic brains in rabbits (Fig. 101). The extracellular dopamine released from the injured dopamine nervous system reacts with oxygen to produce hydrogen peroxide and quinine [1,19]. Hydrogen peroxide can easily convert to neurotoxic $\cdot OH^-$ radicals (Fig. 33, Chap. 26). Therefore, the release of dopamine from injured neurons causes selective radical damage to the dopamine nervous system in the central nervous system (Fig. 102) [7,9,10,12].

Simple management for selective radical attack of the dopamine nervous system is the prevention of dopamine release and control of $\cdot NO$ radicals in the acute stage. The early induction of brain hypothermia at 33°–34°C is useful for preventing dopamine release [9,12]. Pharmacological treatment such as metoclopramide also prevents dopamine release from the hypothalamus. Administration of radical scavengers is another approach to prevent selective damage to the dopamine A10 nervous system in the acute stage [9,12]. As an additional phenomenon, release of brain tissue dopamine suppresses the release of prolactin and thyroid hormones [21]. To prevent secondary immune dysfunction and sick euthroid syndrome as an additional complication of dopamine release, replacement of prolactin and thyroid hormone is important at the acute stage.

In the chronic stage, severe cases cannot make a full recovery of consciousness. The functional recovery of the dopamine A10 nervous system is important for recovery of inner consciousness at the chronic stage [11,12]. As a method of replacement of cerebral dopamine, the combination of pharmacological treatment such as levodopa (300–400 mg/day), amantadine (100–200 mg × 3/day) or parlodel (2.5–20 mg/day), and administration of estrogen (Estraderm TTS 1 patch/day) is effective. Median nerve intermittent electrical stimulation (20 s on, 50 s off, 10–20 mA, 30 pulses/s, duration time 300 m/s) is also effective [7,9,10,12].

For the recovery of neurons in the primarily injured brain tissue, prolonged brain hypothermia lasting more than 48 h is considered indispensable. The clinical results of these treatments in severely brain-injured patients (Glasgow Coma Score <6) revealed good recovery and an extremely low incidence of vegetation. The initial purpose of brain hypothermia treatment is to provide sufficient cerebral oxygen supply within 3–6 h after insult with stabilization of systemic circulation. Oxygen delivery that is higher than 700–800 ml/min is very important for mild or moderate brain hypothermia treatment to succeed and provide a recovery from serious neuronal conditions in primarily injured brain tissue. After 6 h, brain hypothermia is very effective in preventing secondary pathophysiological changes in injured neurons. However, brain hypothermia has a third beneficial mechanism: prevention of vegetation by reducing excess release of cerebral dopamine from injured brain tissue. In previous studies of the vegetative state, the effectiveness of pharmacological activation of dopamine and electrical stimulation of the central nervous system to increase the cerebrospinal fluid (CSF) dopamine has been reported [12,13]. Low levels of dopamine and luteinizing hormone (LH) in the jugular venous blood were also recorded in prolonged vegetation. Following brain hypothermia, the jugular venous blood dopamine decreased and strongly correlated to lowering of the brain tissue temperature (Fig. 32, Chap. 26). From these results, I hypothesize that the dopamine nervous system plays an important role in vegetation, and low brain tissue temperature can

Table 80. Effectiveness of pharmacological treatment of severe brain injury and vegetative state patients in the chronic stage

Arousal ⟶	Activity ⟶	Memory, cognition ⟶	Aphasia
L-dopa (Chandra 1978)	Amphetamine (Hill 1944, Feeney 1985)	Vasopressin (Sahgal 1984)	Bromcriptine (Crisman 1988)
Sinemet (L-dopa/carbidopa): (Lal 1988, Haig 1990)	Tricyclic antidepressant (amitriptyline, imipramine) (Mysiw 1987)	Amphetamine, methylphenidate (Ritalin), magnesium pemolate (Cylert) (Glenn 1986)	
Amphetamine, methylphenidate (Ritalin), magnesium pemolate (Cylert) (Glenn 1986)		Amantadine and bromcriptine (Gualtieri 1989)	
Amantadine (Gualtieri 1989)		Hydergine (Markstein 1989)	

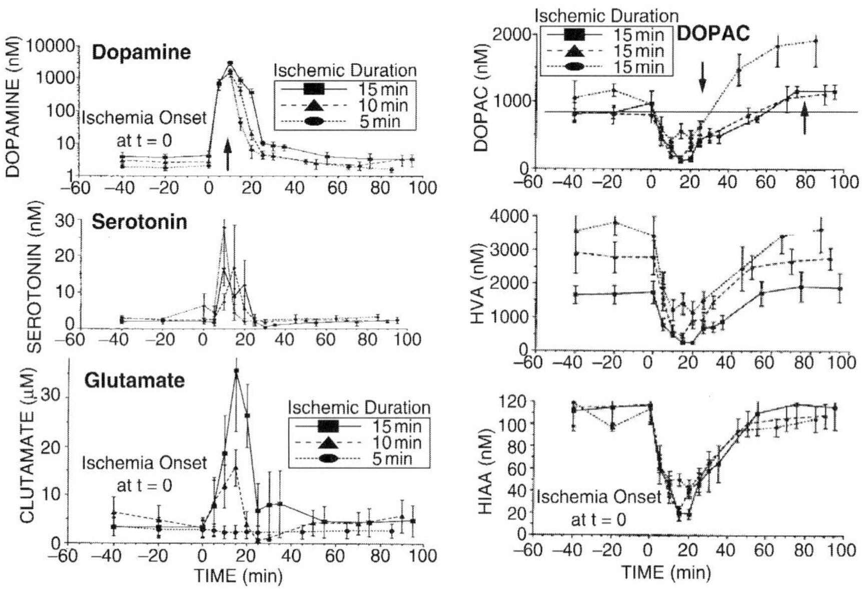

Fig. 101. Changes in extracellular concentrations of glutamate, aspartate, glycine, dopamine, serotonin, and dopamine metabolites after transient global ischemia in the rabbit brain. Baker et al. (1991) J Neurochem

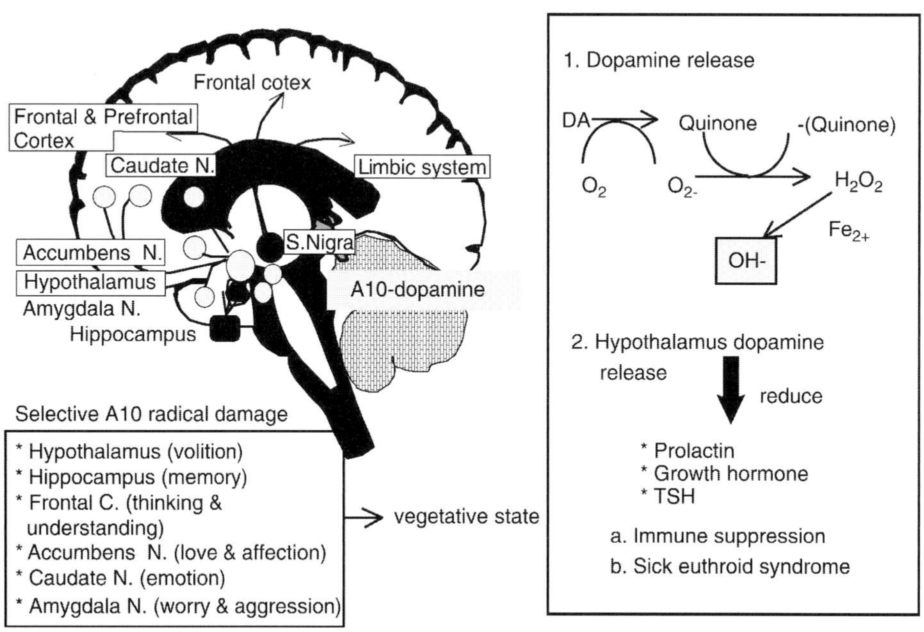

Fig. 102. Schema of selective radical damage of the dopamine A10 nervous system and the complicated fall into vegetation with immune suppression and sick euthroid syndrome. TSH, thyroid stimulating hormone

Table 81. Management of dopamine A10 nervous system in severely brain-injured patients

1. Acute stage: prevent dopamine release and use radical scavengers
Prevent dopamine release in hypothalamus by administration of metoclopramide
Brain hypothermia: 32°–34°C, prevent cerebral dopamine release and radical attack to the dopamine A10 nervous system
Replacement of prolactin and thyroid hormone
Administration of radical scavengers
2. Chronic stage: activate dopamine A10 nervous system
Cerebral dopamine replacement therapy
Pharmacological treatment: levodopa (300–400 mg/day), amantadine (100–200 mg/day)
Uptake of cerebral dopamine, estrogen (Estraderm TTS patch 2 mg/day)
Median nerve stimulation: 10–20 mA 20 s on 30 s off, 30 pulse/s, duration time 300 ms
Music therapy

prevent excitatory neuronal death within the dopamine nervous system.

The low incidence of vegetation in brain hypothermia patients is not only due to prevention of intracellular secondary injury, but also due to reduction of excess leakage of dopamine from injured brain tissue. We observed 5 of 28 cases (18%) return to an ordinary lifestyle from the vegetative state, while others retained neuronal deficits caused by the original brain disease. However, in all these patients, intelligence and personality were maintained after 3 months. Therefore, as a late treatment after brain hypothermia, cerebral dopamine therapy is necessary in severely brain-injured patients.

Our clinical trials of pharmacological activation of dopamine synapses with combination of amantadine, estraderm patches, and increasing CSF dopamine by intermittent stimulation of the median nerve, have been revealed as very effective for neuronal recovery and prevention of vegetation (Table 81) [9,12]. We must focus on the protection of specific parts of the nervous system to prevent vegetation and not only on the general management of neuronal recovery in the primarily injured brain tissue. One of the difficult points is that the dopamine nervous system includes motor and emotional function. The question of how to diagnose the reversibility of the emotional center of the dopamine A10 nervous system requires further investigation.

References

1. Baker AJ, Zornow MH, Scheller MS, Yaksh TL, Skilling SR, Smullin DH, Larson AA, Kuczenski R (1991) Changes in extracellular concentrations of glutamate, aspatate, glycine, dopamine, serotonin, and dopamine metabolites after transient global ischemia in the rat. J Neurochem 57:1370–1379
2. Chandra B (1978) Treatment of disturbances of consciousness caused by measles encephalitis with Levodopa. Eur Neurol 17:265–270
3. Crisman LM, Childs A, Wilcox RE, Barrow N (1988) The effect of bromocriptine on speech dysfunction in patients with diffuse brain injury (akinetic mutism). Clin Neuropharmacol 11:462–466
4. Galski T, Krotenberg R (1989) The usefulness of Hydergine on cognition in patients with traumatic head injury. Arch Phys Med Rehabil 70:A-12
5. Glenn MB (1986) CNS stimulants: applications for traumatic brain injury. J Head Trauma Rehabil 1:74–76
6. Gualtieri CT, Chandler M, Coons TB, Brown LT (1989) Amantadine: a new clinical profile for traumatic brain injury. Clin Neuropharmacol 12:258–270
7. Haig AJ, Ruess LM (1990) Recovery from vegetative state of six months duration associated with Sinemet (levodopa/carbidopa). Arch Phys Med Rehabil 71:1081–1083
8. Hayashi N (1997) Combination therapy of cerebral hypothermia, pharmacological activation of the dopamine system, and hormonal replacement in severely brain damaged patients. J Jpn Sco Intensive Care Med 4:191–197
9. Hayashi N (1997) Prevention of vegetation after severe head trauma and stroke by combination therapy of cerebral hypothermia and activation of immune-dopaminergic nervous system. Proc Soc Treat Coma 6:133–145
10. Hayashi N (1999) The brain hypothermia therapy for prevention of vegetation after severe brain injury. (In Japanese) Nippon Geka Gakkai Zasshi 100:443–448
11. Hayashi N (2000) Enhanced neuronal damage in severely brain injured patients by hypothalamus, pituitary, and adrenal axis neuro-hormonal changes. In: Hayashi N (ed) Brain hypothermia, Springer, Berlin Heidelberg New York Tokyo, pp 3–26
12. Hayashi N (2000) The clinical issue and effectiveness of brain hypothermia treatment for severe brain injured patients. In: Hayashi N (ed) Brain hypothermia. Springer, Berlin Heidelberg New York Tokyo, pp 121–151
13. Hayashi N, Hirayama T, Utagawa T, Ohata M (1994) Systemic management of cerebral edema based on a new concept in severe head injury patients. Acta Neurochir [Suppl] 60:541–543
14. Hill D (1944) Amphetamine in psychopathic states. Br J Addiction 44:50–54
15. Lal S, Merbtiz CP, Grip JC (1990) Modification of function in head-injured patients with sinemet. Brain Inj 2:225–233
16. Markstein R (1989) Pharmacological approaches in the treatment of senile dementia. Eur Neurol 29 Suppl 3:33–41. Moore RY, Bhatnagar RK, Heller A (1971) Anatomical and chemical studies of a nigro-neostriatal projection in the cat. Brain Res 30:119–135
17. Mysiw WJ, Jackson RD (1987) Tricyclic antidepressant therapy after traumatic brain injury. J Head Trauma Rehabil 2:34–42

18. Sahgal A (1984) A critique of the vasopressin-memory hypothesis. Psychopharmacology 83:215–228
19. Silvka A, Coben G (1985) Hydroxyl radical attack on dopamine. J Biol Chem 260:15466–15472
20. Simon H, Le Moal M, Stinus L, Calas A (1979) Anatomical relationships between the ventral mesencephalic tegmentum-A10 region and the locus coeruleus as demonstrated by anterograde and retrograde tracing technique. J Neural Trans 44:77–86
21. Zis AP, McGarvey KA, Clark CM, Lam RW, Adams SA (1992) The role of dopamine in seizure-induced prolactin release in humans. Convuls Ther 8:126–130

50. Diagnosis of Reversibility of the Vegetative State

The dopamine A10 nervous system is a major part of the emotional center [1,6]. Therefore, emotional stimulation by live music therapy could release dopamine from the hypothalamus A10 nervous system and also suppress the pituitary function. This physiological reaction can be monitored by the increased cerebrospinal fluid (CSF) dopamine and reduced CSF prolactin as signs of an active dopamine A10 nervous system (Fig. 103). No observation of increasing CSF dopamine/prolactin ratio suggests no function of the hypothalamus dopamine A10 nervous system. We have studied the reliability of this diagnostic method for the evaluation of the dopamine A10 nervous function. The monitoring of CSF dopamine/prolactin ratio was very useful to determine the responsiveness of the dopamine A10 nervous system (Fig. 103). As a very impressive sign of the effect of emotional music stimulation on the vegetative patient, increased CSF dopamine/prolactin ratio was more sensitive when the patient was held rather than just listening to the music. The reversibility of the vegetative state was determined by simultaneous increases of CSF dopamine/prolactin ratio and the cortical neuronal responsive marker, CSF norepinephrin and dopamine as shown in Fig. 104 by music stimulation (Fig. 105). This clinical evidence suggests that the dopamine A10 nervous system is a major part of the inner consciousness and is a very important management target for the prevention of vegetation in severely brain-injured patients [2–5].

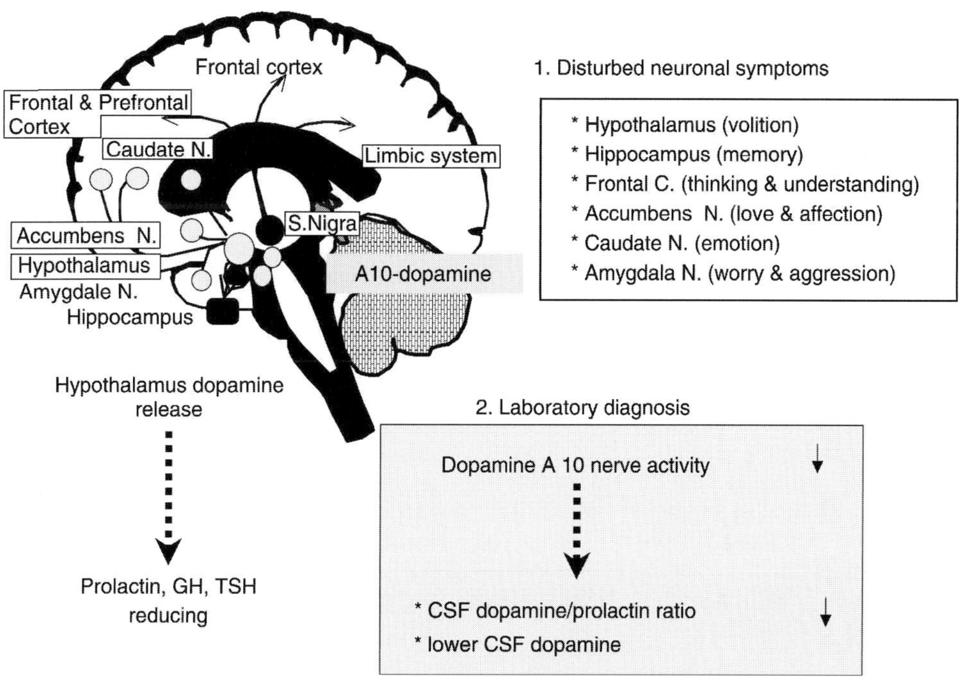

Fig. 103. Schema for the diagnosis of dopamine A10 nervous activity

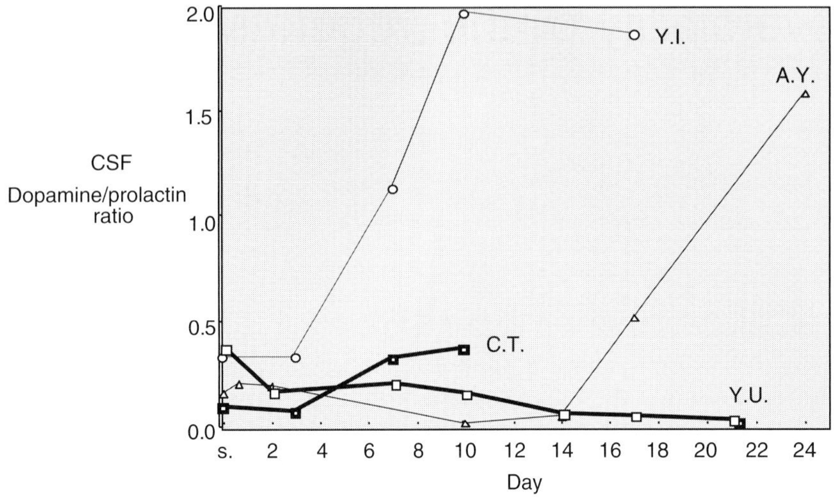

Fig. 104. Diagnosis of the A10 nervous system response in vegetative patients after dopamine replacement therapy. Thin line, effective treatment; thick line, ineffective treatment

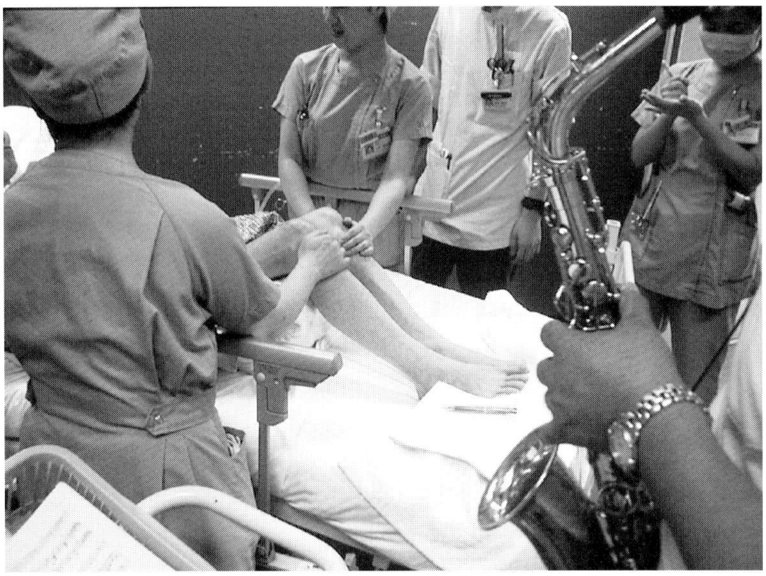

Fig. 105. Music therapy for stimulation of the dopamine A10 nervous system

References

1. Creutz LM, Kritzer MF (2002) Estrogen receptor-beta immunoreactivity in the midbrain of adult rats: regional, subregional, and cellular localization in the A10, A9, and A8 dopamine cell groups. J Comp Neurol 446:288–300
2. Hayashi N (1997) Prevention of vegetation after severe head trauma and stroke by combination therapy of cerebral hypothermia and activation of immune-dopaminergic nervous system. Poc Soc Treat Coma 6:133–145
3. Hayashi N (1999) The brain hypothermia therapy for prevention of vegetation after severe brain injury. (In Japanese) Nippon Geka Gakkai Zasshi 100:443–448
4. Hayashi N (2000) Enhanced neuronal damage in severely brain injured patients by hypothalamus, pituitary, and adrenal axis neuro-hormonal changes. In: Hayashi N (ed) Brain hypothermia. Springer, Berlin Heidelberg New York Tokyo, pp 3–26
5. Hayashi N (2000) The clinical issue and effectiveness of brain hypothermia treatment for severe brain injured patients. In: Hayashi N (ed) Brain hypothermia. Springer, Berlin Heidelberg New York Tokyo, pp 121–151
6. Simon H, Le Moal M, Stinus L, Calas A (1979) Anatomical relationships between the ventral mesencephalic tegmentum-A10 region and the locus coeruleus as demonstrated by anterograde and retrograde tracing technique. J Neural Trans 44:77–86

51. Management of Complicated Neuronal Dysfunction: Emotion, Memory, Cognition, and Behavior

Emotion, memory, cognition, and behavior make up many parts of brain function. Therefore, the management of these complicated neuronal issues are different to the management of focal neuronal signs such as hemiparesis, visual disturbances, and hearing disturbances.

Mechanism of Emotional Disturbance

Also part of the limbic system, the amygdala plays an important role in emotional function. The Yakovlev circuit [6], that consists of the amygdaloid nucleus, hypothalamus ventromedial nucleus, thalamus dorsal medial nucleus, anterior temporal lobe cortex, and orbital face cortex of the frontal lobe, is the main part of emotion neuronal function. This emotional Yakovlev circuit functions with connections to the dopamine A10 nervous system. Interestingly, these neurons are sensitive to many hormones, such as estrogen, catecholamines, adrenocorticotropic hormone (ACTH), and thyroid stimulating hormone (TSH) [2,3,5,7–11]. The destruction of the Yakovlev circuit releases catecholamines and ACTH into the systemic circulation and inversely reduces the serum TSH and gonadotropin. Therefore, many posttraumatic emotionally depressed patients show low values of serum thyroid hormones. The replacement of thyroid hormone, is effective for recovery from emotional depression.

Mechanism of Memory, Cognition, and Behavior Disturbances

Memory, cognition, and behavior are highly associated with the Papez circle [8], which is a circuit of the hippocampus, cingulate gyrus, fornix, anterior thalamus, and mamillary nucleus. This circuit is also connected to the dopamine A10 nervous system as previously described as a center of inner consciousness and maintenance of interagency.

Much information from the visual, auditory, and sensory systems are initially brought into the hippocampus. This information is kept as short-term memory and is checked against past memory in the cortex. The integrated information is then translated into the Papez circuit and the dopamine A10 nervous system. Human memory, cognition, and behavior are decided and established throughout this information mechanism. Damage to memory, cognition, and behavior are produced by diffuse brain injury, severe brain hypoxia, and severe brain ischemia that includes the Papez circuit.

Management of Emotion, Memory, Cognition, and Behavior Disturbances

The management of complicated neuronal dysfunction, which includes that of emotion, memory, cognition, and behavior, are summarized in the following sections.

Neuronal Environment Management

Maintaining the cerebral perfusion pressure, cerebral blood flow, microcirculation, and normal intracranial pressure is important with control of systemic circulation.

Maintain Neuronal Homeostasis

Sufficient oxygen delivery, prevention of anemia, maintenance of hemoglobin function, prevention of hyperglycemia, and normal control of serum phosphate, magnesium, and serum glucose are recommended management steps [2,3].

Activation of Injured Neuronal Function

Combination of dopamine replacement therapy and thyroid hormone replacement therapy is advised. This

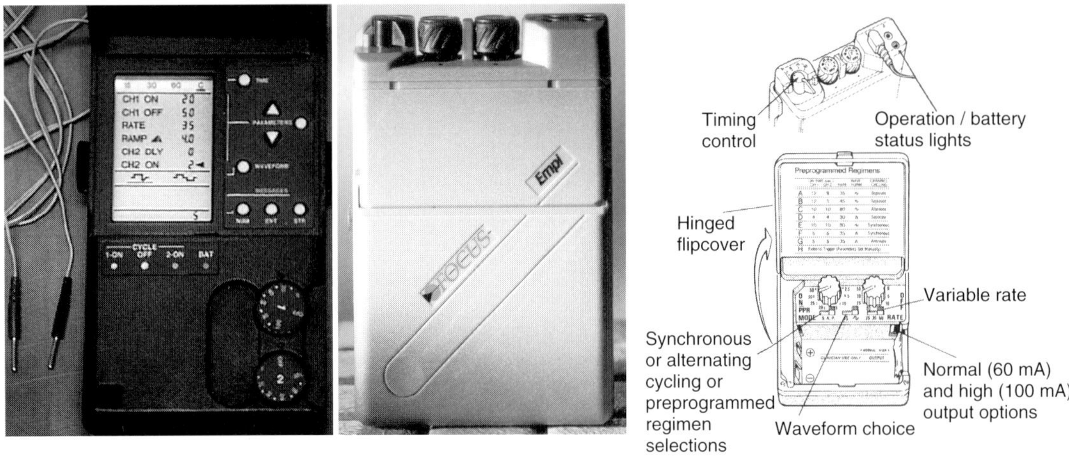

Fig. 106. Median nerve stimulation (Edwin Cooper method) for activation of dopamine A10 nerve system. Application pattern: 20 s on, 50 s off, 10–20 mA, 30 pulses/s duration time 30 ms

neurohormonal replacement therapy is very effective in improving attention and communication. The combination of dopamine replacement therapy is [1–4]:

Pharmacological treatment: levodopa (300–400 mg/day), amantadine (100–200 mg/day) and parodel (10–15 mg/day)
Uptake of cerebral dopamine: estrogen (Estraderm TTS patch 2 mg/day)
Median nerve stimulation: 10–20 mA/20 s on 30 s off, 30 pulse/s, duration time 300 m/s (Fig. 106).
Music therapy

References

1. Hayashi N (1997) Combination therapy of cerebral hypothermia, pharmacological activation of the dopamine system, and hormonal replacement in severely brain damaged patients. J Jpn Soc Intensive Care Med 4:191–197
2. Hayashi N (1997) Prevention of vegetation after severe head trauma and stroke by combination therapy of cerebral hypothermia and activation of immune-dopaminergic nervous system. Proc Soc Treat Coma 6:133–145
3. Hayashi N (2000) The clinical issue and effectiveness of brain hypothermia treatment for severe brain injured patients. In: Hayashi N (ed) Brain hypothermia. Springer, Berlin Heidelberg New York Tokyo, pp 121–151
4. Hayashi N, Hirayama T, Utagawa T, Ohata M (1994) Systemic management of cerebral edema based on a new concept in severe head injury patients. Acta Neurochir [Suppl] 60:541–543
5. Hruska RE, Silbergeld EK (1980) Estrogen treatment enhances dopamine receptor sensetivity in the rat striatum. Eur J Pharmacol 61:397–400
6. Livingston KE, Escobar A (1971) Anatomical bias of the limbic system concept: a proposed reorientation. Arch Neurol 24:17–21
7. MacIntosh TK, Hayes R, DeWitt D, Agura V, Faden AI (1987) Endogenous opioids may mediate secondary damage after experimental brain injury. Am J Physiol 258:565–574
8. Papez JW (1937) A proposed mechanism of emotion. Arch Neurol Psych 38:725–743
9. Sahgal A (1984) A critique of the vasopressin-memory hypothesis. Psychopharmacology 83:215–228
10. Simon H, Le Moal M, Stinus L, Calas A (1979) Anatomical relationships between the ventral mesencephalic tegmentum-A10 region and the locus coeruleus as demonstrated by anterograde and retrograde tracing technique. J Neural Trans 44:77–86
11. Zis AP, McGarvey KA, Clark CM, Lam RW, Adams SA (1992) The role of dopamine in seizure-induced prolactin release in humans. Convuls Ther 8:126–130

52. Surgical Management After Brain Hypothermia Treatment to Prevent Vegetation and Memory Disturbance

The analysis of neurotransmitters in the cerebrospinal fluid (CSF) provides much information about neuronal function and CBF disturbances. The neurotransmitter levels in the cortex such as those of dopamine, norepinephrine, and serotonin will be changed in the CSF by damage to brain tissue. However, the background and meaning of CSF neurotransmitters are not simple. We have recorded two types of neuronal dysfunction with changes of CSF neurotransmitters [1]. One is very low levels of neurotransmitters in the CSF and the other is high levels in the CSF of vegetative patients. Reduced neurotransmitter levels in CSF at the vegetative state can be explained as a result of massive neuronal loss or reduced neuronal activity. Some patients in this group could respond to neurotransmitter replacement therapy. The reversibility of vegetative patients is diagnosed with simultaneous increases of the CSF dopamine/prolactin ratio and CSF neurotransmitter level as described in Chap. 50.

Vegetative patients that have increased neurotransmitters in the CSF are not expected to respond to dopamine replacement therapy. As a mechanism of increasing neurotransmitters in the CSF, disturbances of cerebral microcirculation and retention of CSF circulation are possible. Accumulated neurotransmitters in the brain tissue may confuse the neuronal synaptic functions. Prolonged difficult control of CSF outflow produces this interstitial accumulation of neurotransmitters. We have observed many cases of unexpected good recovery from severe diffuse brain injury in patients with prolonged CSF retention. The effectiveness of a ventriculo–abdominal shunt in normal pressure hydrocephalus is well known. To explain the effectiveness of a ventriculo–abdominal shunt in normal pressure hydrocephalus, synaptic confusion by accumulated neurotransmitters in the interstitial brain tissue by disturbance of CSF circulation is plausible. From this hypothesis, an active ventriculo–abdominal shunt or CSF drainage is recommended from the acute stage.

Reference

1. Hayashi N (2000) The clinical issue and effectiveness of brain hypothermia treatment for severe brain injured patients. In: Hayashi N (ed) Brain hypothermia. Springer, Berlin Heidelberg New York Tokyo, pp 121–151

53. Indications and Criteria for Dopamine Replacement Therapy

In severely brain-injured patients such as those with a Glasgow Coma Scale score (GCS) less than 5, unconsciousness does not lead to recovery soon after brain hypothermia treatment. Patients that open their eyes with external stimulation, offer no emotional response, and show no understanding of verbal stimulation have poor prognosis [1]. Vegetative patients require dopamine replacement therapy. The indications for dopamine replacement therapy are:

Persistent coma
Vegetative state
Expressive response around eye and mouth after tapping stimulation
Low cerebrospinal fluid (CSF) dopamine level
Response of CSF dopamine/prolactin ratio to treatment

Dopamine replacement therapy needs at least 3–4 weeks [2]. The treatment of vegetation is very difficult in most cases. The indications for dopamine replacement therapy do not mean it will be successful, rather they suggests the possibility of recovery.

The effectiveness of dopamine replacement therapy can be evaluated after 1 week, even with no neurological recovery signs, with the presence of simultaneous increasing of CSF dopamine and CSF dopamine/prolactin ratio (Fig. 104, Chap. 50). If no response of these CSF dopamine parameters is observed after 3 weeks of combined dopamine replacement therapy, clinical recovery from the vegetative state is not expected.

High concentration of CSF dopamine suggests no response to cerebral dopamine replacement therapy. The mechanism of dopamine replacement therapy is stimulation or activation of dopamine neuronal functions. However, high concentration of CSF dopamine suggests excessive release of dopamine from injured neurons and difficulty of washout from CSF. The overaccumulation of dopamine in extracellular space could produce the synaptic confusion and poor neuronal function. In these cases, the removal of excess interstitial dopamine by ventricular peritoneal shunting and maintenance of cerebral microcirculation are recommended. Currently, there is no evidence of neuronal recovery in areas of high concentration of CSF dopamine.

References

1. Hayashi N (1997) Combination therapy of cerebral hypothermia, pharmacological activation of the dopamine system, and hormonal replacement in severely brain damaged patients. J Jpn Soc Intensive Care Med 4:191–197
2. Hayashi N (2000) The clinical issue and effectiveness of brain hypothermia treatment for severe brain injured patients. In: Hayashi N (ed) Brain hypothermia. Springer, Berlin Heidelberg New York Tokyo, pp 121–151

VI. Specific Consideration for Disease: Cardiac Arrest, Occlusive Cerebral Stroke, and Subarachnoid Hemorrhage

54. Brain Hypothermia After Resuscitation from Cardiopulmonary Arrest

A recent clinical trial of brain hypothermia for post-resuscitation management of cardiopulmonary arrest (CPA) patients demonstrated the effectiveness of the treatment [3,14,17,18]. The concept and mechanism of hypothermia are similar to those in experimental animal studies, such as the prevention of brain edema and free radical reactions after reperfusion, and management of brain hypoxia [2,3,17,20,21]. However, the brain injury mechanism after cardiac arrest in humans is not similar to that in anesthetized experimental animal models [7,8,13]. Stress to the hypothalamus–pituitary–adrenal (HPA) axis [4] and excess neurohormonal reactions [15,16] after cardiac arrest produces brain injury mechanisms that were not observed in anesthetized experimental animal models [11,12]. Insulin-resistant hyperglycemia associated with epinephrine surge [7,9–11] and slow release of bound oxygen from hemoglobin [5,11] that produces ineffective oxygen inhalation are major issues at the acute stage after resuscitation from cardiac arrest (Fig. 107). The slow release of oxygen from binding hemoglobin because of reduced hemoglobin 2,3-diphosphoglycerate (DPG) is a big issue for neuronal oxygenation [11]. Our clinical study of the time window of DPG changes after cardiac arrest showed that a 50% reduction occurs after 20min and DPG is reduced by 70% 30min after cardiac arrest (Fig. 108). This means oxygen inhalation and oxygen delivery are ineffective even with normal control of PaO_2, cerebral blood flow (CBF), and oxygen delivery. The management of these stress-associated brain injury mechanisms under hypothermia, special consideration for management of cardiac arrest, the new technique of brain hypothermia, and sophisticated criteria for brain hypothermia treatment could provide more successful clinical results than previous management [7–13].

Special Consideration of Brain Hypothermia Treatment for Cardiopulmonary Arrest

The brain ischemia and brain hypoxia that occur after resuscitation from cardiac arrest are variable [1]. This is because cardiac arrest is diagnosed by no pulsation of the carotid artery, breathing arrest, and deep coma. However, no pulsation of the carotid artery does not mean complete cardiac arrest and includes ventricular tachycardia (VT) or complete cardiac arrest with 0–60mmHg of systolic blood pressure [1]. The duration of cardiac arrest is also important because prolonged brain hypoxia and energy crisis affect the reversibility of injured neurons. In addition, DPG, the oxygen releasing factor of hemoglobin, decreases over time after cardiac arrest (Fig. 108). Our clinical studies showed almost no DPG at 50–60min after cardiac arrest. This results in ineffective oxygen inhalation and difficulty in supplying oxygen to neurons in the brain tissue. These factors also affect the cardiac reversibility and original cardiac disease. The cardiac function after resuscitation is also variable, and can be stable or unstable. From this background, there are two approaches of brain hypothermia treatment for neuronal restoration after cardiac arrest [13].

One brain hypothermia treatment is for patients with stable cardiopulmonary function after early cardiac massage, sufficient oxygen inhalation, and easily reversible cardiac disease. The other brain hypothermia treatment occurs under the control of cardiopulmonary function with percutaneous cardiopulmonary support system (PCPS) for patients that have difficulty tolerating the overload on the postresuscitated cardiac function to maintain the cerebral circulation. These patients require a short resting of the cardiac function to keep energy for cardiac recovery [13,18]. The PCPS supports the cardiac function during the resting time [12,18,19].

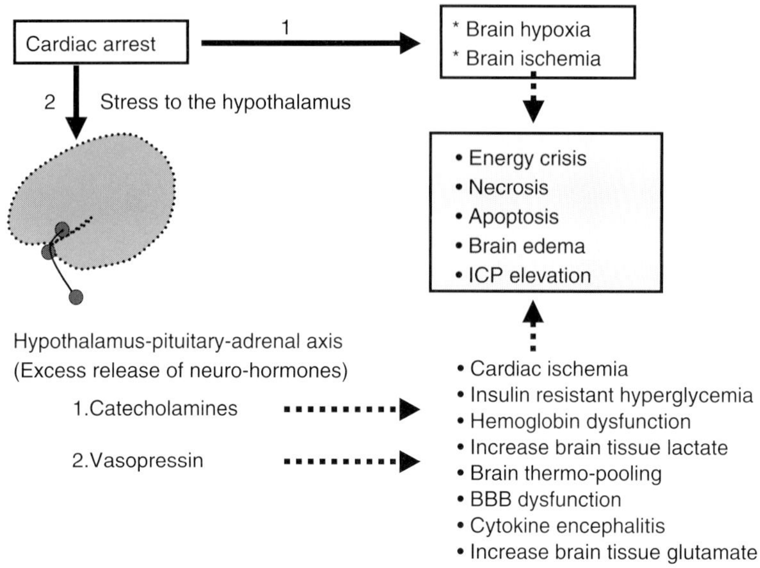

Fig. 107. Mechanism of brain damage after cardiac arrest

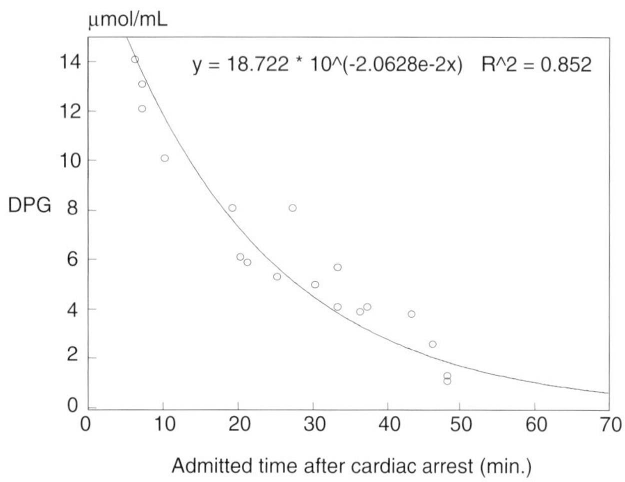

Fig. 108. Time window for changes in serum glucose and hemoglobin 2,3-diphosphoglycerate (DPG) after cardiac arrest

Neuronal Restoration and Management of Cardiopulmonary Function During Brain Hypothermia

The difficulty of brain hypothermia treatment for CPA patients is the management of stable cardiac functions. The presence of cardiac disease and reduced serum catecholamines caused by hypothermia are negative factors for continuing brain hypothermia treatment. Therefore, stable blood pressure without pharmacological treatment after resuscitation is a very important prerequisite for the introduction of brain hypothermia treatment for CPA patients. To fulfill this requirement a temporary balloon catheter is introduced into the abdominal aorta and inflated intermittently or incompletely to maintain coronary and cerebral circulation. The technique is similar to the management of severe brain injury as described previously [12]. However, the recommended brain temperature is about 34°C. If the systemic circulation is stable and serum glucose is 120–140 mg/dl, moderate brain hypothermia can begin. The reduction of serum glucose consumption occurs because of the metabolic shift from glucose to lipid that occurs under mild hypothermia. Poor management of stress-associated HPA axis neurohormonal abnormality also produces severe hyperglycemia. Without management of hyperglycemia, further increases in brain tissue glucose and lactate will occur under moderate brain hypothermia [10,12].

The management of hemoglobin dysfunction is also important for neuronal restoration after resuscitation from CPA [13]. Many patients are admitted to hospital about 20–30 min after cardiac arrest. Our clinical studies of hemoglobin DPG after CPA showed unexpectedly low values of 5%–50% of normal levels. This complication suggests the presence of masking neuronal hypoxia, even with normal PaO_2 and sufficient oxygen delivery, because hemoglobin-bound oxygen is difficult to release into the brain tissue with reduced DPG [11]. There is no direct DPG replacement management method. Normalization of DPG at the acute stage requires careful control of serum glucose at 120–140 mg/dl, management of serum pH above 7.3, inorganic phosphate at more than 3.0 mg/dl, and management of serum magnesium [12].

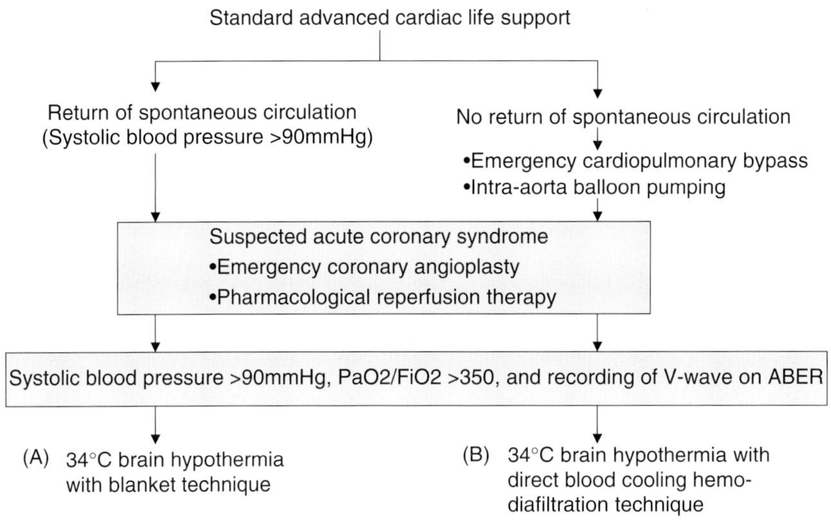

Fig. 109. Care plan for cerebral resuscitation after cardiac arrest

Rewarming should only be started with evidence of neuronal recovery, such as pupil light reflex, recording of α wave on trend electroencephalogram (EEG), and 60%–75% SjO_2. In postresuscitation patients after cardiac arrest, the brain tissue is not damaged directly as in brain trauma and cerebral stroke patients. Therefore, the duration of brain hypothermia is shorter than for brain trauma and stroke patients. A duration of 12–72h is recommended in most cases.

Neuronal Restoration Using Percutaneous Cardiopulmonary Support System During Brain Hypothermia

The maintenance of CBF after cardiac arrest is difficult with prolonged VT or ventricular fibrillation (VF) without some response to electrical defibrillation [6]. Probably, such patients require resting of cardiac function during brain and cardiac resuscitation. To overcome this difficult situation, the hypoxic damaged brain and ischemic heart are managed by maintenance of oxygenation and metabolic substrates using PCPS initially. After that, brain tissue temperature can be reduced to 34°C by directly cooling the blood. A pacemaker maintains the cardiac beat. The block diagram of this treatment is presented in Fig. 50 (Chap. 35). However, without recovery of cardiac infarction, brain resuscitation and social recovery cannot be expected. Cardiac ischemia caused by thrombosis of the coronary artery is managed with percutaneous transluminal coronary angioplasty (PTCA) under PCPS management. Figure 109 shows the care plan for cerebral resuscitation after cardiac arrest. The precise control of hyperglycemia (Fig. 110), hemoglobin dysfunction (Fig. 108), oxygen delivery, lipid metabolism, neuronal excitation, hypo-albuminemia, immune dysfunction, neurohormonal abnormality, intravascular coagulability, and brain edema are important during this treatment (Fig. 107) [12,13]. Restoration therapy for the hypoxic brain and ischemic heart uses similar techniques to those used for severe brain trauma, as described earlier.

Cardiac arrest longer than 1–2h was considered to be a contraindication for further treatment. However, we have experienced three dramatic recovery cases by this combination brain hypothermia treatment [13]. These patients suffered cardiac arrest for 3–5 days; however, all of these patients recovered without neuronal deficit. The effectiveness of this treatment can be diagnosed by the appearance of the pupil light reflex between 2 and 24h after treatment.

The amazing neuronal recoveries from prolonged cardiac arrest were observed in the cases of a 65-year-old man with acute myocardial infarction, a 23-year-old woman with hypertrophic cardiomyopathy, and a 40-year-old woman with myocarditis. The specific cardiac diseases were not recorded. The criteria for induction of this combination therapy of PCPS, cardiac beat control by pacemaker, and brain hypothermia management are the presence of a bystander for cardiac massage, early oxygenation, control of serum pH greater than 7.3, and control of serum glucose to less than 180mg/dl. The maintenance of systolic blood pressure higher than 90mmHg, PaO_2/FiO_2 greater than 350, and the presence of a V-wave on the auditory brain stem evoked potential after PTCA are also favored.

The preparation of heparinized catheterization is required for this treatment. Therefore, this treatment is not suitable for hemorrhagic brain damage such as

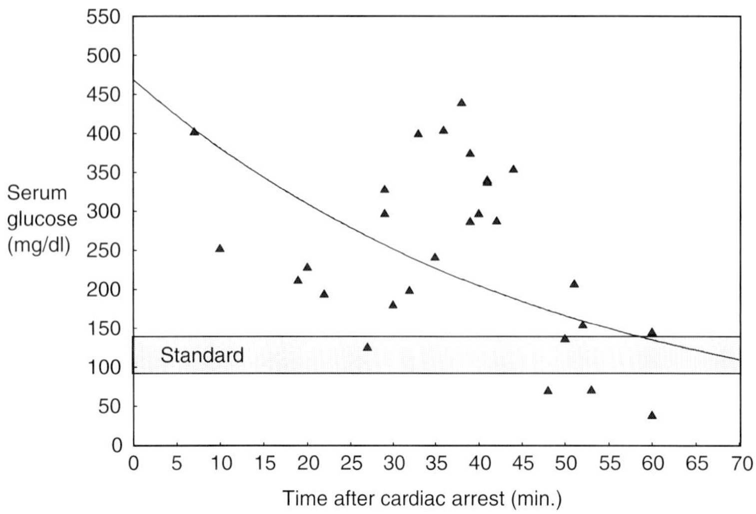

Fig. 110. Sequential changes of hypothalamus-pituitary-adrenal axis stress-associated hyperglycemia after cardiac arrest

head trauma, or subarachnoid hemorrhage. Neuronal restoration for occlusive stroke patients and postresuscitation cardiac arrest patients are indicated for this treatment.

References

1. American Heart Association (2002) Guidelines 2000 for cardiopulmonary resuscitation and emergency cardiovascular care. Circulation 102:1–383
2. Baker AJ, Zornow MH, Scheller MS, Yaksh TL, Skilling SR, Smullin DH, Larson AA, Kuczenski R (1991) Changes in extracellular concentrations of glutamate, aspartate, glycine, dopamine, serotonin, and dopamine metabolites after transient global ischemia in the rat. J Neurochem 57:1370–1379
3. Bernard SA, Gray TW, Buist MD, Jones BM, Silvester W, Gutteridge G, Smith K (2002) Treatment of comatose survivors of out-of-hospital cardiac arrest with induced hypothermia. N Engl J Med 346:557–563
4. Corte FD, Mancini A, Valle D, Gallizzi F, Carducci P, Mignani V, De Marinis L (1998) Provocative hypothalamopituitary axis tests in severe head injury: correlation with severity and prognosis. Crit Care Med 26:1419–1426
5. Dudariev VP, Lanovenko II (1999) Changes in the oxygen-binding properties of the blood in white rats under the influence of hypoxia and its pharmacological correction. Fiziol Zh 45:97–103
6. Gussak I, Chaitman BR, Kopecky SL, Nerbonne JM (2000) Rapid ventricular repolarization in rodents: electrocardiographic manifestations, molecular mechanisms, and clinical insights. J Electrocardiol 33:159–170
7. Hayashi N (1995) Cerebral hypothermia treatment. In: Hayashi N (ed) Cerebral hypothermia treatment. Sogo Igaku, Tokyo, pp 1–105
8. Hayashi N (1996) Advance of cerebral hypothermia treatment. J Critical Med 8:295–300
9. Hayashi N (1997) Combination therapy of cerebral hypothermia, pharmacological activation of the dopamine system, and hormonal replacement in severely brain damaged patients. J Jpn Soc Intensive Care Med 4:191–197
10. Hayashi N (1997) Prevention of vegetation after severe head trauma and stroke by combination therapy of cerebral hypothermia and activation of immune-dopaminergic nervous system. Proc Soc Treat Coma 6: 133–145
11. Hayashi N (2000) Enhanced neuronal damage in severely brain injured patients by hypothalamus, pituitary, and adrenal axis neuro-hormonal changes. In: Hayashi N (ed) Brain hypothermia. Springer, Berlin Heidelberg New York Tokyo, pp 3–26
12. Hayashi N (2000) The clinical issue and effectiveness of brain hypothermia treatment for severe brain injured patients. In: Hayashi N (ed) Brain hypothermia. Springer, Berlin Heidelberg New York Tokyo, pp 121–151
13. Hayashi N, Nagso K, Utagawa A, Sakurai A (2001) The push back of life edge from cardiac death by combination therapy with percutaneous cardiopulmonary support and brain hypothermia treatment in cardiac arrested patients. Cardiovasc Med Surg 3:68–77
14. Holzer M, Cerchiari E, Martens P, Roine R, Strez F (2002) Mild therapeutic hypothermia to improve the neurologic outcome after cardiac arrest. N Engl J Med 346:549–555
15. Leibowitz SF (1999) Macronutrients and brain peptides: what they do and how they respond. In: Berthoud HR, Seeley RJ (eds) Neural and metabolic control of macronutrient intake. CRC, Boca Raton, pp 389–406
16. Leibowiz SF, Sladek C, Spencer L, Temple D (1988) Neuropeptide Y, epinephrine and norepinephrine in the paraventricular nucleus: stimulation of feeding and the release of corticosterone, vasopressin and glucose. Brain Res Bull 21:905
17. Leonov Y, Sterz F, Safar P, Radovsky A, Oku K, Tisherman S, Stezoski SW (1990) Mild cerebral hypother-

mia during and after cardiac arrest improves neurologic outcome in dogs. J Cereb Blood Flow Metab 10:57–70
18. Nagao K, Hayashi N, Kanmatsuse K, Arima K, Ohtsuki J, Kikushima K, Watanabe I (2000) Cardiopulmonary cerebral resuscitation using emergency cardiopulmonary bypass, coronary reperfusion therapy and mild hypothermia in patients with cardiac arrest outside the hospital. J Am Coll Cardiol 36:776–783
19. Okamoto K, Nagao K, Miki T, Nitobe E, Arima K, Hayashi N (2000) New hypothermia method using blood-cooling system: Monan and Kanem method. In: Hayashi N (ed) Brain Hypothermia. Springer, Berlin Heidelberg New York Tokyo, pp 203–212
20. Safar P, Behringer W, Bottiger BW, Sterz F (2002) Cerebral resuscitation potentials for cardiac arrest. Crit Care Med 30:S140–144
21. Silvka A, Coben G (1985) Hydroxyl radical attack on dopamine. J Biol Chem 260:15466–15472
22. Vassallo SU, Delaney KA, Hoffman RS, Slater W, Goldfrank LR (1999) A prospective evaluation of the electrocardiographic manifestations of hypothermia. Acad Emerg Med 6:1121–1126

55. Brain Hypothermia for Occlusive Cerebral Stroke

The mechanism of brain damage caused by occlusive cerebral stroke is different with acute onset and chronic progression. The harmful stress-associated neurohormonal reactions of the hypothalamus–pituitary–adrenal (HPA) axis and hyperglycemia [8–10] are only observed at the acute onset of large cerebral infarction (Table 82). In this group, a higher incidence of complete cerebrovascular obstruction (CVO) than incomplete CVO was recorded. However, in cases of slow onset, incomplete occlusive cerebral stroke or small cerebral infarction are most common and stress-associated hyperglycemia is not recorded. The intensive care unit (ICU) management strategy is different in these two groups.

Consideration of Brain Hypothermia for Acute Onset of Cerebral Infarction

The acute onset of cerebral infarction is mainly produced by complete CVO. Without early recanalization, the neurological prognosis is poor. Neuroprotection in the ischemic and hypoxic injured brain, recanalization with angioplasty, anticoagulation, thrombolysis and hemodilution, and prevention of secondary brain damage caused by HPA axis neurohormonal abnormality are major treatments for the acute onset of severe cerebral infarction [1,6,11]. The requirement for additional management for atrial fibrillation and cardiac infarction was observed at 53% and 35%, respectively, in acute onset type. The complications of atrial fibrillation and cardiac infarction in slow onset of cerebral infarction were 50% and 25%, respectively (see Table 82). Additional management targets were not much different in both groups. However, hyperglycemia that is an indirect consequence of stimulation of the HPA axis [9] was observed at high incidence (86%) in the acute onset type, and at 14% in the slow onset type. The mean serum glucose level during stress-associated hyperglycemia was 257 mg/dl in the acute onset type. Severe hyperglycemia that is produced by catecholamine surge, is accompanied by anaerobic metabolism in the injured brain tissue, active vasopressin release, changes of vascular permeability in the brain and lungs, hemoglobin dysfunction caused by reduced 2,3-diphosphoglycerate (DPG) levels, and ineffective oxygen inhalation [9]. The reduced hemoglobin DPG level produces neuronal hypoxia because of the difficult release of oxygen from binding hemoglobin, even with normal PaO_2 and sufficient oxygen delivery [9]. These human-specific pathophysiological changes were not described in studies of anesthetized animals. Hyperglycemia associated with catecholamine surge progresses within about 3–5 min after insult. Therefore, as an initial treatment for the acute onset of cerebral occlusive stroke, sufficient neuronal oxygenation, suitable administration of metabolic substrates, control of brain thermo-pooling, careful control of serum pH between 7.34 and 7.40, and management of harmful stress-associated hyperglycemia are necessary before the start of anti-brain edema therapy [10].

The management of harmful stress-associated hyperglycemia is not easy because of insulin resistance. The early induction of brain hypothermia is very effective to prevent this pathophysiology and catecholamine surge [10]. However, induction of brain hypothermia cannot always start immediately after insult. Therefore, severe hyperglycemia associated with HPA axis stress is unavoidable. The early management of HPA axis neurohormonal abnormality, control of hyperglycemia, control of serum pH, careful management of immune dysfunction, control of lipid metabolism, activation of muscle metabolism, stabilization of systemic circulation, replacement of albumin, magnesium, inorganic phosphate, and antithrombin-III (AT-III), control of cerebral blood flow (CBF) with hemodilution, and prevention of brain edema under brain hypothermia are the initial treatments for occlusive cerebral stroke [10]. However, without recanalization of occluded cerebral vessels, the progression of cerebral infarction will markedly reduce expectations of recovery. If hypoxic neurons in the ischemic brain tissue can survive by combination of the various management strategies described above with brain hypothermia [1,3–5,7] until the recanalization of occluded cerebral vessels, the patient may survive.

A typical case that was effectively treated by this strategy of management with brain hypothermia is presented. A 75-year-old man was diagnosed with brain stem infarction. He initially complained of difficult speech and vertigo. One hour later, he complained of sudden onset of left hemiparesis and then fell into a coma. The patient was admitted to hospital 30 min later. Vital signs were unstable and hyperglycemia (serum glucose 230 mg/dl) was recorded. However, computed tomography showed no abnormal signs. Magnetic resouance imaging (MRI) suggested the possibility of brain stem infarction. Localized pontine edema was recorded as shown in Fig. 111. Cerebral angiographic study suggested complete occlusion of the vertebral artery. Intravascular angioplasty was immediately attempted. However, unfortunately, the balloon catheter could not be inserted at the vascular occlusion because of severe vertebral artery sclerosis. Systemic administration of urokinase (240 000 U) and replacement of AT-III (>100%) were carried out under brain hypothermia treatment at 33°–34°C. Triple H therapy (hypertensive (systolic blood pressure >130–140 mmHg), hypervolemic, and hemodilusion) was continued with combination of low molecular weight dextran L and 24 000 U urokinase (drip). Five days later, prompt papillary reactions were observed and recovery of auditory evoked potential was recorded. Rewarming started 6 days after insult. Clinical recovery was observed step by step. Two months later, no neurological deficit was recorded. The neuronal death of the brain stem was excluded after 5 days of brain hypothermia treatment. The angiogram and MRI studies at 5 days are presented in Fig. 111.

Table 82. Background of occlusive cerebral stroke

	Acute onset	Slow onset
Onset		
Cases	17 (59%)	12 (41%)
Recurrence	9 (53%)	5 (41%)
First onset	8 (47%)	7 (59%)
Complicated disease		
Atrial fibrillation	9 (53%)	6 (50%)
Acute myocardial infarction	6 (35%)	3 (25%)
Diabetes mellitus	5 (29%)	3 (25%)
Insulin-resistant hyperglycemia (serum glucose > 180 mg/dl)		
Hyperglycemia	86%	14%
Mean serum glucose	257.8 mg/dl	133.8 mg/dl
Early admission		
0–6 h	6 (35%)	0 (0%)

Slow Onset of Cerebral Infarction

The brain injury mechanism and systemic neurohormonal immune responses following the slow onset of cerebral occlusive stroke are completely different to

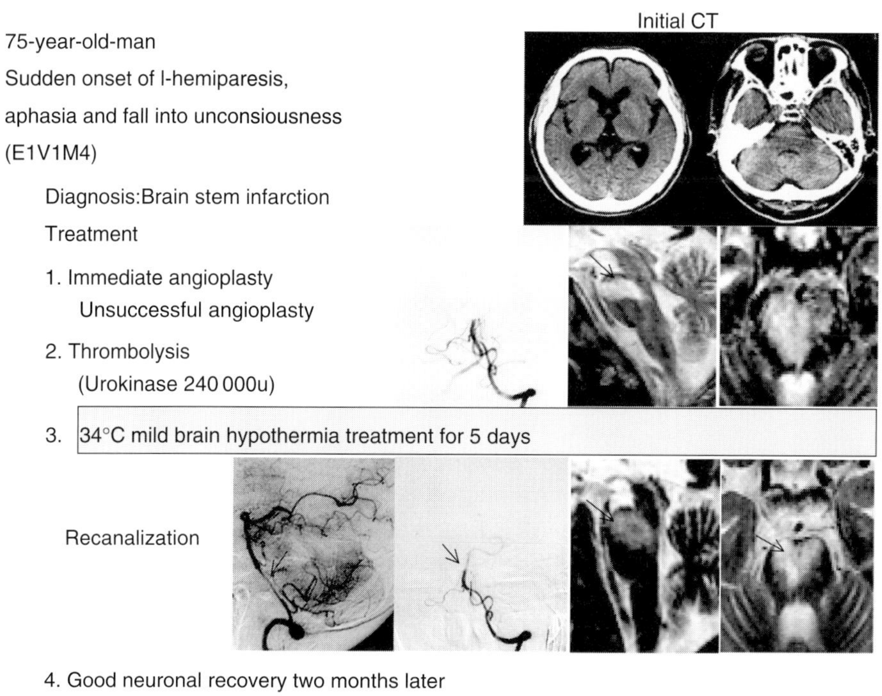

Fig. 111. Brain stem infarction

Table 83. National institute of health stroke scale

Item	Name	Response
1a	Consciousness	0 = Alert 1 = Not alert, arousable 2 = Not alert, obtunded 3 = Unresponsive
1b	Questions	0 = Answers both correctly 1 = Answers one correctly 2 = Answers neither correctly
1c	Commands	0 = Performs both tasks correctly 1 = Performs one task correctly 2 = Performs neither tasks
2	Gaze	0 = Normal 1 = Partial gaze palsy 2 = Total gaze palsy
3	Visual fields	0 = No visual loss 1 = Partial hemianopsia 2 = Compete hemianopsia 3 = Bilateral hemianopsia
4	Facial palsy	0 = Normal 1 = Minor paralysis 2 = Partial paralysis 3 = Complete paralysis
5	Motor arm a. Left b. Right	0 = No drift 1 = Drift before 10 s 2 = Falls before 10 s 3 = No effort against gravity 4 = No movement
6	Motor leg a. Left b. Right	0 = No drift 1 = Drift before 5 s 2 = Falls before 5 s 3 = No effort against gravity 4 = No movement
7	Ataxia	0 = Absent 1 = One limb 2 = Two limbs
8	Sensory	0 = Normal 1 = Mild loss 2 = Severe loss
9	Language	0 = Normal 1 = Mild aphasia 2 = Severe aphasia 3 = Mute or global aphasia
10	Dysarthria	0 = Normal 1 = Mild 2 = Severe
11	Extinction, inattention	0 = Normal 1 = Mild 2 = Severe

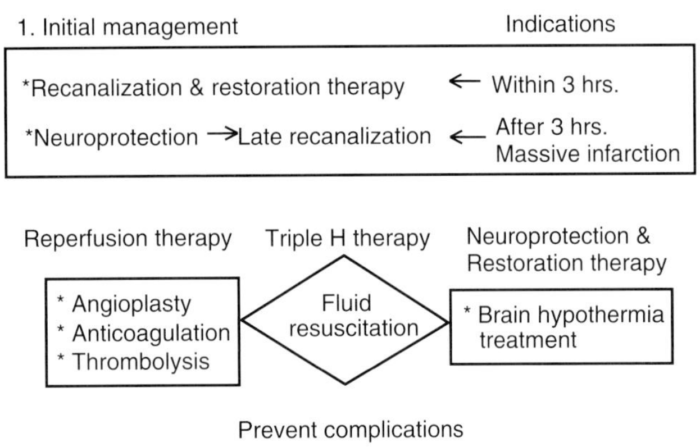

Fig. 112. Strategies for management of ischemic brain stroke

those for the acute onset of cerebral infarction. In slow onset of cerebral infarction, harmful stress-associated hyperglycemia is only recorded in 14% of cases compared with 86% in cases of acute onset of cerebral stroke, as described in Table 82. The mean value of serum glucose was 134 mg/dl in the slow onset and 258 mg/dl in the acute onset type. In slow onset of cerebral infarction, no signs of catecholamine surge-associated hyperglycemia, neuronal hypoxia, vasopressin release, or proliferation of cytokines in systemic circulation have been recorded. Therefore, pathophysiological changes of occlusive cerebral stroke are very similar to those in anesthetized experimental animal models [2,7]. Neuronal hypoxia in injured brain tissue caused by reduced hemoglobin DPG, hyperglycemia-associated increases of lactate in the brain, and vasopressin-related blood–brain barrier (BBB) dysfunction are not major clinical issues in the slow onset of cerebral infarction. The management of slow onset brain ischemia and brain infarction should be focused on recanalization in cases without severe BBB dysfunction (shown as cerebrospinal fluid (CSF)/serum albumin ratio <0.01) or if the NIH Stroke Scale (Table 83) is less than 20. Severe BBB dysfunction (CSF/serum albumin ratio >0.02) does not indicate recanalization therapy because hemorrhagic infarction may occur by reflow. As methods for recanalization, angioplasty by intravascular surgery, thombolysis with tissue plasminogen activator (tPA) (100 mg/1–2 h i.v.) or urokinase (240 000 U/day drip), oral intake of antiplatelet (aspirin 300 mg/day) and ticlopidine hydrochloride (Panaldine 200 mg/day), and triple H therapy are recommended. Neuronal oxygenation and maintenance of adequate metabolic substrates under the control of brain tissue hypothermia provide effective neuroprotection in the ischemic brain. The slow progression of secondary brain damage such as brain edema, intracranial pressure elevation (peak time is between 24 and 48 h), and tissue necrosis caused by radical attack are important during brain hypothermia treatment. To manage slow onset brain infarction, brain tissue temperature control at around 34°C, replacement of serum albumin to higher than 3.5 g/dl, maintenance of microcirculation combined with triple H therapy, thrombolytic therapy using tPA, antivascular inflammation therapy with 100%–140% AT-III, and administration of anticerebral ischemic medications, as shown in Table 18 (Chap. 43) are important. Figure 112 shows the strategies for management of ischemic brain stroke.

References

1. Almeida A, Delgado-Esteban M, Bolanos JP, Medina JM (2002) Oxygen and glucose deprivation induces mitochondrial dysfunction and oxidative stress in neurones but not in astrocytes in primary culture. J Neurochem 81: 207–217
2. Benveniste H, Jorgensen MB, Sandberg M, Christensen T, Hagberg H, Diemer NH (1989) Ischemic damage in hippocampal CA1 is dependent on glutamate release and intact innervation from CA3. J Cereb Blood Flow Metab 9:629–639
3. Busto R, Dietrich WD, Globus MY-T, Ginsberg MD (1989) Postischemic moderate hypothermia inhibits CA1 hippocampal ischemic neuronal injury. Neurosci Lett 101:299–304
4. Connolly JE, Boyd RJ, Calvin JW (1962) The protective effect of hypothermia in cerebral ischemia: experimental and clinical applications by selective brain cooling in the human. Surgery 52:15–24
5. Dietrich WD, Busto R, Halley M, Valdes I (1990) The importance of brain temperature in alterations of the blood-brain barrier following cerebral ischemia. J Neuropathol Exp Neurol 49:486–497
6. Dorman PJ, Counsell CE, Sanderrock PGA (2000) Recently developed neuroprotective therapies for acute stroke: a qualitative systematic review of clinical trials. In: Prakash A (ed) Acute stroke treatment. Adis, Hong Kong, pp 63–83
7. Han HS, Qiao Y, Karabiyikoglu M, Giffard RG, Yenari MA (2002) Influence of mild hypothermia on inducible nitric oxide synthase expression and reactive nitrogen production in experimental stroke and inflammation. J Neurosci 22:3921–3928
8. Hayashi N (1997) Prevention of vegetation after severe head trauma and stroke by combination therapy of cerebral hypothermia and activation of immune-dopaminergic nervous system. Proc Soc Treat Coma 6:133–145
9. Hayashi N (2000) Enhanced neuronal damage in severely brain injured patients by hypothalamus, pituitary, and adrenal axis neuro-hormonal changes. In: Hayashi N (ed) Brain hypothermia. Springer, Berlin Heidelberg New York Tokyo, pp 3–26
10. Hayashi N (2000) The clinical issue and effectiveness of brain hypothermia treatment for severe brain injured patients. In: Hayashi N (ed) Brain hypothermia. Springer, Berlin Heidelberg New York Tokyo, pp 121–151
11. Lindley RI (2000) Drug therapy for acute ischemic stroke: risks verusus benefits. In: Prakash A (ed) Acute stroke treatment. Adis, Hong Kong, pp 53–62

56. Special Consideration of Brain Hypothermia Treatment for Subarachnoid Hemorrhage

Clinical Issues of Subarachnoid Hemorrhage

Brain hypothermia treatment is very effective for severe head trauma [13,15,17,19], postresuscitation of cardiac arrest [18,30], brain hypoxia [30], and occlusive cerebral stroke [9,11,30]. However, the effectiveness of brain hypothermia treatment for subarachnoid hemorrhage (SAH) is still controversial. The reason for the ineffectiveness of brain hypothermia treatment for SAH is the difficulty in controlling cerebral vasospasm under brain hypothermia. The diffuse vascular narrowing of cerebral vasospasm produces severe cerebral ischemia that is difficult to treat even with brain hypothermia management (Fig. 113). However, there are many questions about the relationships between the progression of cerebral vasospasm and brain hypothermia. The worsening of vasospasm by brain hypothermia, delayed progression of cerebral vasospasms during brain hypothermia, worsening of vasospasms after rewarming, good prognosis even with presence of diffuse vascular narrowing (Fig. 114), and poor prognosis without severe vasospasm are major clinical issues. Recent clinical studies using microdialysis [4] provided answers to these questions and also demonstrated a new brain injury mechanism [14] in severe SAH. Without understanding these clinical issues, brain hypothermia treatment for severe SAH is unsuccessful.

Worsening of Vasospasm by Brain Hypothermia

The reasons for worsening of vasospasm by brain hypothermia are delayed induction of brain hypothermia and difficulty in controlling stress-associated hyperglycemia [15]. Most SAH occurs in the neighborhood of the hypothalamus. The SAH accidental event produces much more stimulation of the hypothalamus–pituitary–adrenal (HPA) axis than other neuronal disease. Therefore, excess release of vasopressin and catecholamines [14] occur immediately and severely. This reaction produces very high incidence of catecholamine surge-associated insulin-resistant hyperglycemia (Fig. 17, Chap. 22). Severe hyperglycemia (serum glucose >230 mg/dl) stimulates neuropeptide Y receptors of the appetite center of the hypothalamus and again activates the release of vasopressin by the neural feedback mechanism of macronutrient control [3,8,22–24,36,37]. This SAH-specific release of excess vasopressin produces various pathophysiological conditions [14,21,22,27,32]. Vasopressin is an antidiuretic hormone and a very strong vasoconstrictor of cerebral vessels and in the lungs [20,25]. Pulmonary edema, blood-brain barrier (BBB) dysfunction, brain edema, cerebral blood flow (CBF) disturbances, increasing brain tissue lactate, and worsening of brain edema are negative events. In the management of this HPA axis neurohormonal reaction, the delayed induction of brain hypothermia has much difficulty in controlling insulin-resistant hyperglycemia and neurohormonal abnormality at the initial stage [15]. A mistake at this point is rapid induction of brain hypothermia to lower than 34°C at later than 3 h after SAH. The stress to the HPA axis produces insulin-resistant hyperglycemia [19]. Simultaneously, hypothermia lower than 34°C produces the metabolic shift from glucose to lipid metabolism [12,13,15]. This metabolic change that is specific to moderate hypothermia activates the hyperglycemia further because of reduced glucose consumption. Recent clinical studies using microdialysis and cerebrospinal fluid (CSF) biochemical analysis in severely brain-injured patients with SAH, trauma, and cardiac arrest demonstrated that excess release of vasopressin produced BBB dysfunction and promoted the production of proinflammatory cytokines interleukin1 (IL1) and IL6 (Fig. 3, Chap. 22). Therefore, hyperglycemia with SAH results in increasing brain tissue lactate, excess release of vasopressin, and associated brain injury mechanisms such as BBB dysfunction, brain edema, CBF disturbances, activated proinflammatory cytokines, and pulmonary edema [14,25].

To prevent these negative events after SAH, early induction of brain hypothermia to 34°C, and precise control of hyperglycemia [15], hypo-albuminemia

58-year-old-man

Clinical diagnosis: Left-internal carotid posterior communicating aneurysm with thin subdural hematoma, H&C: grade 5.

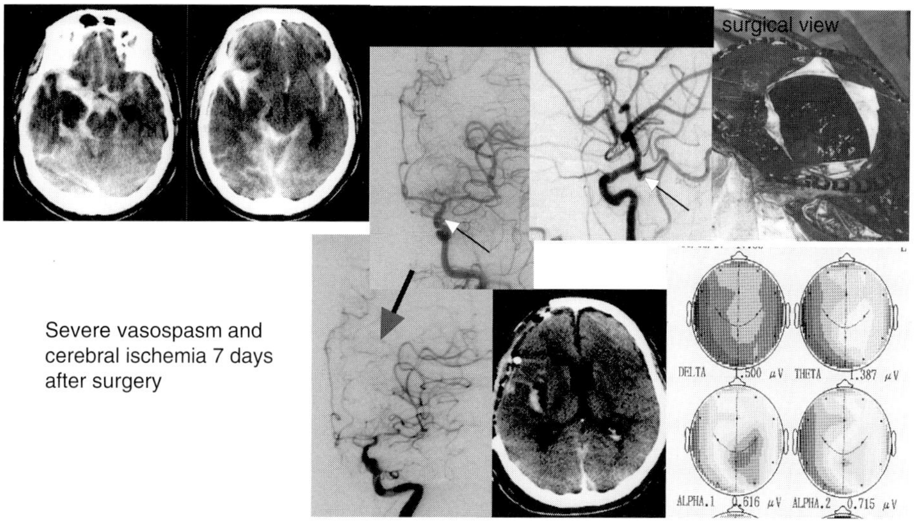

Fig. 113. Severe subarachnoid hemorrhage and delayed vasospasm after ruptured aneurysm

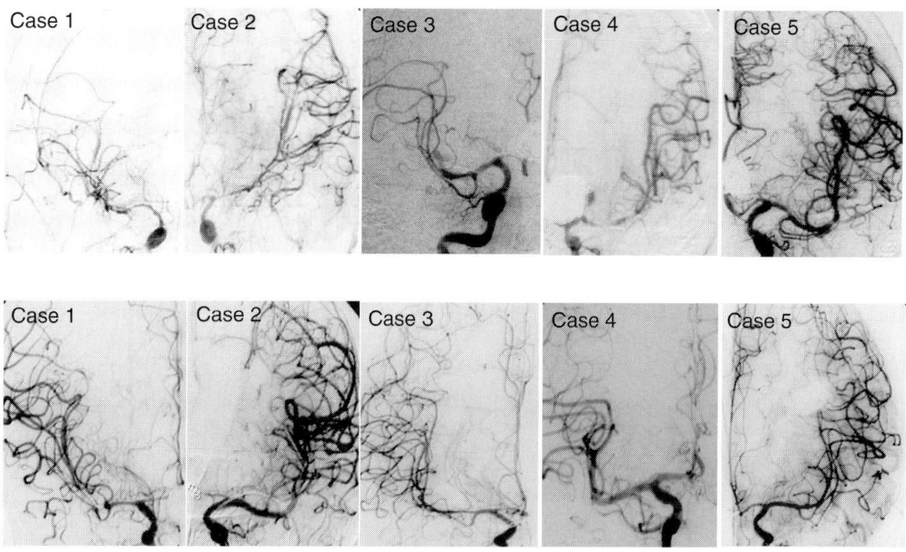

Fig. 114. Contrasting types of prognosis with diffuse narrowing of cerebral vasospasm after cerebral subarachnoid hemorrhage. *Upper panel*, poor prognosis; *lower panel*, good prognosis

[15,28], and dehydration [7], and careful induction of moderate brain hypothermia (32°–33°C) are important. Moderate brain hypothermia is not indicated without successful management of hyper glycemia.

Delayed Vasospasm and Worsening of Cerebral Vasospasm by Rewarming

The hemolytic chemical factors and meta-hemoglobin are considered to be trigger factors of vasospasm. However, the vasospasmic functions of these biochemical factors in CSF are also prevented under hypothermia conditions. The very strong vasodilating action of NO is also prevented under hypothermia [11,17]. The presence of vasospasmogenic factors in CSF during brain hypothermia treatment produces delayed vasospasm and worsening of cerebral vasospasm at the rewarming stage. To prevent these complications, removal of the vasoconstrictive chemical substances by CSF drainage is strongly recommended in brain hypothermia treatment for SAH.

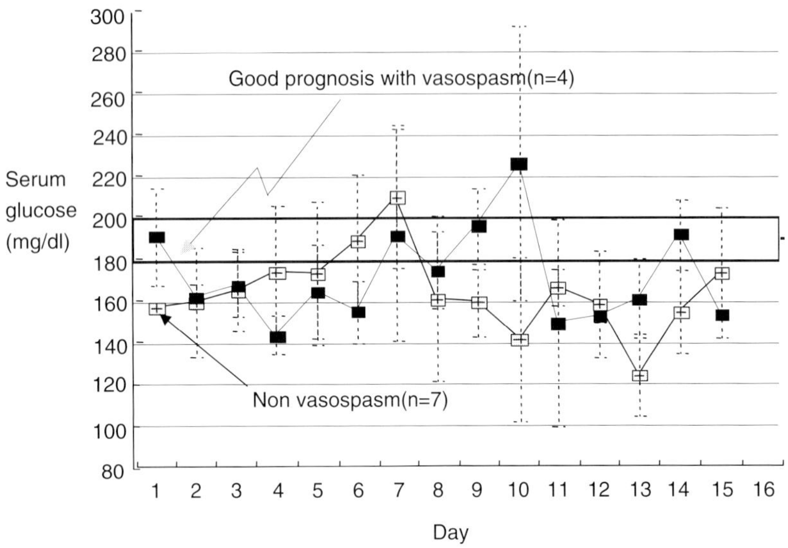

Fig. 115. Sequential changes of stress-associated hyperglycemia in cases of no cerebral vasospasm and cases with good prognosis even with diffuse narrowing cerebral vasospasm. Each group shows the indirect parameter of hypothalamus-pituitary-adrenal axis neurohormonal reaction. Hyperglycemia is not severe

Good Prognosis Even With Diffuse Narrowing Cerebral Vasospasm

Brain hypothermia is a very neuroprotective environment for ischemic and hypoxic cerebral insults. Well-organized management of hyperglycemia [15], correction of hemoglobin dysfunction [10,15,29], prevention of BBB dysfunction (CSF/serum albumin ratio <0.01), and no complication of infection during brain hypothermia produces good clinical prognosis even with cerebral vasospasm as shown in Fig. 114.

Poor Prognosis With or Without Severe Vasospasm

The complication of severe vasospasm produces poor prognosis because of brain ischemia. However, there are many cases that show poor prognosis without severe cerebral vasospasms. The main event of cerebral vasospasm occurs from about 2–3 days after SAH. Before the vasospasm, the presence of another very strong brain damage mechanism could be speculated. New brain injury mechanisms in SAH must be investigated for the success of brain hypothermia treatment.

New Brain Injury Mechanism After Subarachnoid Hemorrhage

Brain edema is another factor that promotes secondary brain damage. However, the time window for the occurrence of cerebral vasospasm and the peak time for progression of brain edema are not very different. The existence of good prognosis and bad prognosis in cases of severe cerebral vasospasm is difficult to explain by the previous concept. We have studied this question and have introduced a new concept of brain injury mechanism that includes direct brain damage and harmful stress-associated HPA axis neurohormonal dysfunction as previously described. The catecholamine surge-associated hyperglycemia is more common in SAH than in trauma or occlusive cerebral stroke (Fig. 7, Chap. 22).

The clinical prognosis and the interaction between cerebral vasospasm and hyperglycemia associated with HPA-axis neurohormonal dysfunction were studied. Severe SAH patients were divided into three groups: type I ($n = 8$), no vasospasm with good prognosis; type II ($n = 11$), diffuse vasospasm with poor prognosis; and type III ($n = 4$), diffuse vasospasm with good to mild disability prognosis. The sequential changes in hyperglycemia were studied in each group for 2 weeks. The type I group showed no hyperglycemia upon admission and the serum glucose level was below 180 mg/dl. The mean value of persistent hyperglycemia was 159 mg/dl as shown in Fig. 115. One week later, serum glucose increased to more than 180 mg/dl, temporarily for 2 days; however; hyperglycemia was not severe throughout the 2 weeks.

The type II and type III groups showed HPA axis neurohormonal dysfunction-associated hyperglycemia in all cases upon admission to the hospital (Fig. 116). No difference in the severity of hyperglycemia was recorded between the type II and type III groups at admission time. The mean values of serum glucose in the type II and type III groups were 189 mg/dl and 192 mg/dl, respectively. However, the sequential changes of hyperglycemia overtime were completely different. Hyperglycemia was difficult to control in the type II group while hyperglycemia was easy to control in the

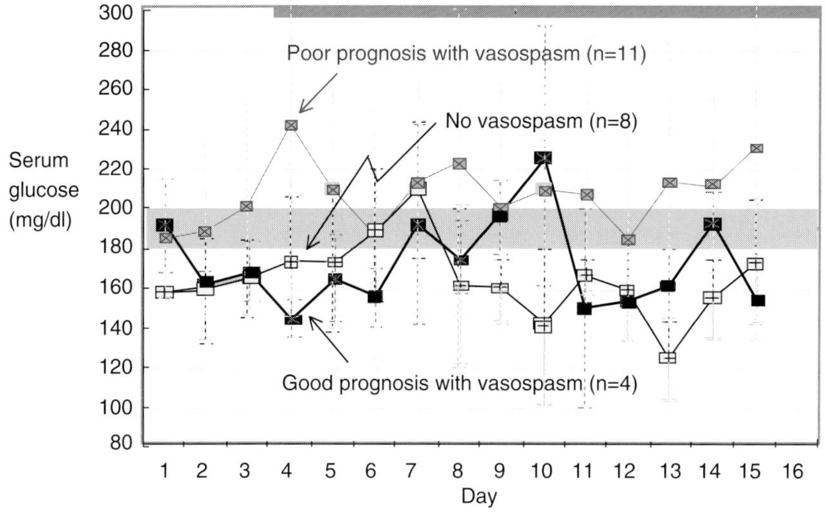

Fig. 116. Two types of hypothalamus-pituitary-adrenal axis stress reactions after severe cerebral vasospasm. Severe stress-associated hyperglycemia was recorded in cases with poor prognosis and was not observed in the cases with good prognosis

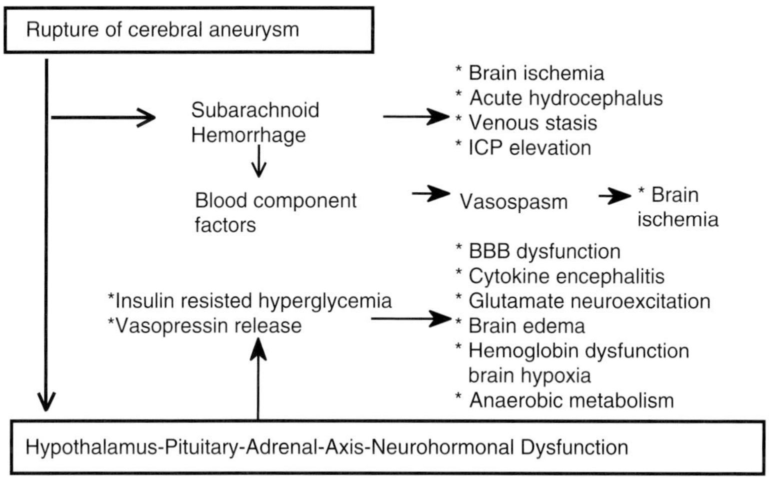

Fig. 117. Schema of pathophysiology in the brain tissue after ruptured cerebral aneurysm

type III group. The important point is that uncontrollable severe hyperglycemia occurred before the start of the cerebral vasospasm and continued for more than 2 weeks (Fig. 116).

These data suggested that, in SAH, harmful stress to the HPA axis occurs very rapidly and is more severe than other head trauma such as cerebral infarction. This is because SAH occurs in the neighborhood of the hypothalamus. The brain damage mechanism and pathophysiology after severe SAH is summarized in Fig. 117. From these results, HPA axis neurohormonal dysfunction associated-hyperglycemia, excess release of vasopressin, BBB dysfunction, cytokine encephalitis, hemoglobin-associated brain hypoxia, and anaerobic brain metabolism are speculated to occur before the progression of vasospasm.

The brain injury mechanisms after SAH are summarized as three pathophysiologies. One is SAH directly associated with pathophysiological changes such as brain hypoxia [1], brain edema, free radical reactions [2,11], neuroexcitation [2,24], acute hydrocephalus, and cerebral venous outflow collapse. Another is vasospasm associated with brain ischemia and infarction, and a third is associated with HPA axis neurohormonal dysfunction-associated hyperglycemia [12–14], hemoglobin dysfunction [14], neuronal hypoxia, worsening of BBB dysfunction by excess release of vasopressin [14,20], and increasing of brain tissue glucose and lactate. The peak time of cerebral vasospasm is between 2 and 14 days; however, HPA axis neurohormonal dysfunction occurs within 5 min and continues for 4–7 days. Therefore, in SAH, harmful stress-associated HPA axis neurohormonal dysfunction could be occurring much more severely than in other brain trauma.

Considerations of Brain Hypothermia Treatment for Subarachnoid Hemorrhage

Early Induction of Brain Hypothermia and Control of HPA Axis Stimulation

It is impossible to completely prevent harmful stress-associated hyperglycemia because it occurs so rapidly, within 3–5 min. This is especially so when aneurysm rupture occurs very close to the hypothalamus and pituitary gland. Stimulation of the HPA axis occurs very severely and very rapidly. Therefore, the intensive care unit management should be focused on the prevention of HPA axis stimulation-associated hyperglycemia [14], neuronal hypoxia caused by hemoglobin dysfunction [14,17,34], and cardiopulmonary dysfunction [15] caused by catecholamine surge [5] as soon as possible. The management of CBF disturbance, intracranial pressure (ICP) elevation, and brain edema become possible after these treatments. Early induction of brain hypothermia and control of brain tissue temperature at around 33°–34°C prevent the catecholamine surge trigger factor.

Control of Insulin-Resistant Hyperglycemia and Hemoglobin Dysfunction

The prevention of excess release of epinephrine into the bloodstream is important for suppression of hyperglycemia. Our clinical studies using microdialysis demonstrated that epinephrine specifically triggers the metabolic shift from glycogen to glucose (Fig. 23, Chap. 22; 71, Chap. 44). These metabolic changes are produced systemically mainly by HPA axis stress reactions (Fig. 15, Chap. 22). Without early control of serum epinephrine release with mild hypothermia (34°–35°C), administration of insulin for the control of hyperglycemia will not succeed. However, overly rapid lowering of the brain tissue temperature to about 32°–33°C, produces more difficult control of hyperglycemia, as described previously, because of reduced glucose consumption by the metabolic shift from glucose to lipid [15]. The clinical issue of this management is the difficulty in slowing the cooling and control of the HPA axis associated-hyperglycemia. This stress-related hyperglycemia is, commonly, insulin resistant. Severe hyperglycemia is caused by glycogenolysis with epinephrine release, reduced insulin production because of catecholamine surge, reduced insulin sensitivity by released adrenal–cortical hormones, and low glucose consumption by muscle wastage. Severe hyperglycemia (serum glucose >230 mg/dl) produces vasopressin release by the feedback mechanism of neural control of macronutrient intake [24,36,37]. The implication of vasopressin release for positive or negative effects for brain damage is not completely understood. Our preliminary clinical studies using microdialysis techniques suggested an antidiuretic effect, changes of the BBB function, induction of proinflammatory cytokines (IL1 and IL6) in CSF space, promotion of pulmonary edema, and worsening of cerebral vasospasm in the ruptured aneurysm. Therefore, early management of stress-associated hyperglycemia is one of the important points if SAH patients are to survive with brain hypothermia treatment.

Severe hyperglycemia combined with a serum pH lower than 7.2 is a serious threat to hemoglobin function. Hemoglobin enzyme, 2,3-diphosphoglycerate (DPG) dramatically decreases and causes slow release of oxygen from binding hemoglobin [15]. In these conditions, normal PaO_2, sufficient oxygen delivery, and high values of jugular oxygen saturation do not provide adequate neuronal oxygenation. Ineffective oxygen inhalation in severe SAH patients occurs because of stress to the HPA axis [14]. These stress-associated human-specific pathophysiological changes result in poor prognosis for ruptured cerebral aneurysm (Fig. 118). In the management of DPG reduction, effective administration of potassium phosphate has been reported. To stabilize the cell membrane of red cells, management of serum phosphate at 3–5 mg/dl, serum magnesium at 1.2–1.8 mEq/dl, and vitamin A greater than >50 mg/dl are required at least. These management steps are also effective for the prevention of respiratory muscle weakness and pulmonary infection. SAH stress-associated hyperglycemia can be controlled by multifaceted treatment for these pathophysiological changes.

Washing the Clot of Basal Cistern and Continuous CSF Drainage

The hemorrhaged blood in CSF contains many vasoactive chemical substances. Massive SAH complicates the high incidence of vasospasm. This vasospasm after SAH has been considered to be prevented by nitric oxide radical reactions. Nitric oxide has, however, biphasic effects to SAH patients. The positive effect is the prevention of vasospasm while the negative effects are neural cell membrane damage and BBB dysfunction.

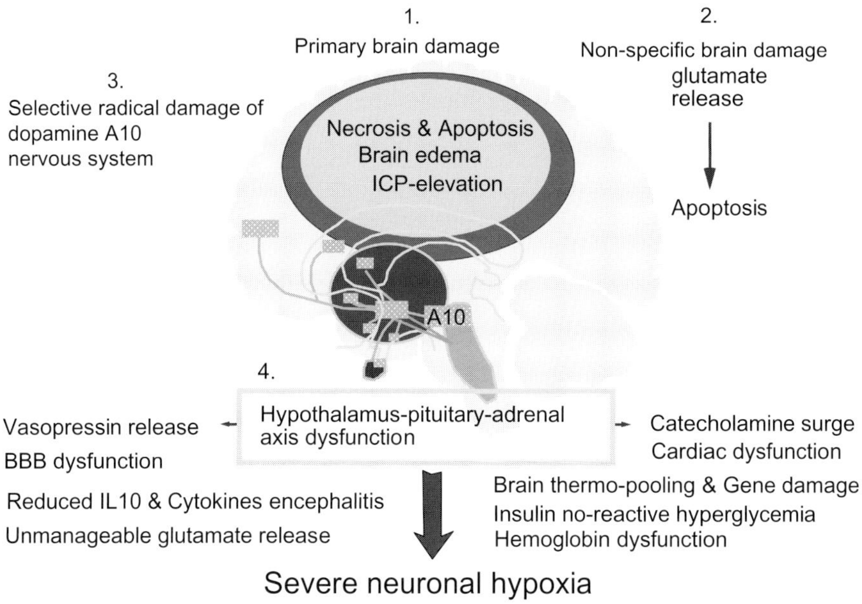

Fig. 118. Mechanism of brain damage after severe subarachnoid hemorrhage

Because brain hypothermia prevents NO radical production [11,17], severe vasospasms may progress more easily and severely if the theory of NO control of vasospasm is correct. To prevent this complication, washing the clot in the CSF of the basal cistern and continuous CSF drainage is strongly recommended during brain hypothermia treatment for SAH patients. The washout of SAH around the basal cistern is important during surgery. Opening of the basal cistern can be achieved by cutting the Liliequist membrane. Washout of the CSF clot in the basal cistern with chilled saline is also effective to cool the hypothalamus directly and is effective in preventing of selective radical attack of the dopamine A10 nervous system and excess HPA axis neurohormonal reactions [15]. Continuous CSF drainage is also effective for minimizing the complication of cerebral vasospasms and management of damage to the dopamine A10 nervous system.

Management of Cerebral Vasospasm

Direct management for cerebral vasospasm is not yet established. Angioplasty by intravascular balloon catheter combined with anticoagulant (heparin 2000–5000 U bolus injection) is designed for use during brain hypothermia treatment. However, this approach is only effective in most cases if the treatment is of short duration and not persistent. Washout of the trigger factors for vasospasm in SAH, management of neuroprotection for the ischemic brain using hypothermia that includes control of hemoglobin dysfunction, hyperglycemia, disturbed microcirculation, hypo-albuminemia, direct oxygen administration, and control of selective NO radical attack to the dopamine A10 nervous system are important treatment [6,13,15,26].

References

1. Almeida A, Delgado-Esteban M, Bolanos JP, Medina JM (2002) Oxygen and glucose deprivation induces mitochondrial dysfunction and oxidative stress in neurones but not in astrocytes in primary culture. J Neurochem 81: 207–217
2. Baker AJ, Zornow MH, Scheller MS, Yaksh TL, Skilling SR, Smullin DH, Larson AA, Kuczenski R (1991) Changes in extracellular concentrations of glutamate, aspartate, glycine, dopamine, serotonin, and dopamine metabolites after transient global ischemia in the rat. J Neurochem 57:1370–1379
3. Beck B (2000). Quantitative and macronutrient-related regulation of hypothalamic neuropeptide Y, galanin and neurotensin. In: Berthoud HR, Seeley RJ (eds) Neural and metabolic control of macronutrient intake. pp 455–464, CRC Press, Boca Raton New York Washington DC
4. Binnert C, Tappy L (2002) Microdialysis in the intensive care unit: a novel tool for clinical investigation or monitoring? Curr Opin Clin Nutr Metab Care 5:185–188
5. Boels PJ, Verbeuren TJ, Vanhoutte PM (1985) Moderate cooling depresses the accumulation and the release of newly synthesized catecholamines in isolated canine saphenous veins. Experientia 41:1374–1377
6. Clark LC Jr, Spokane RB, Hoffmann RE, Sudan R, Homan MM, Maloney AC, Jacobs SJ, Stroup TL, Winston PE (1988) Polarographic cerebral oxygen availability,

fluorocarbon blood levels and efficacy of oxygen transport by emulsions. Biomater Artif Cells Artif Organs 16: 375–393
7. Clifton GL, Miller ER, Choi SC, Levin HS (2002) Fluid thresholds and outcome from severe brain injury. Crit Care Med 30:739–745
8. Corte FD, Mancini A, Valle D, Gallizzi F, Carducci P, Mignani V, De Marinis L (1998) Provocative hypothalamopituitary axis tests in severe head injury: correlation with severity and prognosis. Crit Care Med 26:1419–1426
9. Dempsey IRJ, Combs DJ, Maley ME, Cowen DE, Roy MW, Donaldson DL (1987) Moderate hypothermia reduces postischemic edema development and leukotriene production. Neurosurgery 21:177–181
10. Dudariev VP, Lanovenko II (1999) Changes in the oxygen-binding properties of the blood in white rats under the influence of hypoxia and its pharmacological correction. Fiziol Zh 45:97–103
11. Han HS, Qiao Y, Karabiyikoglu M, Giffard RG, Yenari MA (2002) Influence of mild hypothermia on inducible nitric oxide synthase expression and reactive nitrogen production in experimetal stroke and inflammation. J Neurosci 22:3921–3928
12. Hayashi N (1995) Cerebral hypothermia treatment. In: Hayashi N (ed) Cerebral hypothermia treatment. Sogo Igaku, Tokyo, pp 1–105
13. Hayashi N (1997) Prevention of vegetation after severe head trauma and stroke by combination therapy of cerebral hypothermia and activation of immune-dopaminergic nervous system. Proc Soc Treat Coma 6:133–145
14. Hayashi N (2000) Enhanced neuronal damage in severely brain injured patients by hypothalamus, pituitary, and adrenal axis neuro-hormonal changes. In: Hayashi N (ed) Brain hypothermia. Springer, Berlin Heidelberg New York Tokyo, pp 3–26
15. Hayashi N (2000) The clinical issue and effectiveness of brain hypothermia treatment for severe brain injured patients. In: Hayashi N (ed) Brain hypothermia. Springer, Berlin Heidelberg New York Tokyo, pp 121–151
16. Hayashi N, Hirayama T, Utagawa T, Ohata M (1994) Systemic management of cerebral edema based on a new concept in severe head injury patients. Acta Neurochir [Suppl] 60:541–543
17. Hayashi N, Utagawa A, Kinosita K, Izumi T (1999) Application of a novel technique for clinical evaluation of nitric oxide-induced free radical reactions in ICU patients. Cell Mol Neurobiol 19:3–17
18. Hayashi N, Nagso K, Utagawa A, Sakurai A (2001) The push back of life edge from cardiac death by combination therapy with percutaneous cardiopulmonary support and brain hypothermia treatment in cardiac arrested patients. Cardiovasc Med Surg 3:68–77
19. Jiang JY, Lyeth BG, Kapasi MZ, Jenkins LW, Povlishock JT (1992) Moderate hypothermia reduces blood–brain barrier disruption following traumatic brain injury in the rat. Acta Neuropathol (Berl) 84:495–500
20. Kagawa M, Nagao S, Bemana I (1996) Arginine vasopressin receptor antagonists for treatment of vasogenic brain edema: an experimental study. J Neurotrauma 13:273–279
21. Kossmann T, Hans V, Imhof HG, Stocker R, Grob P, Trentz O, Morgani-Kossmann MC (1995) Intrathecal and serum interleukin-6 and acute-phase response in patients with severe traumatic brain injuries. Shock 4:311–317
22. Kow LM, Pfaff DW (1986) Vasopressin excites ventromedial hypothalamus glucose-responsive neurons in vitro. Physiol Behav 37:153–158
23. Leibowitz SF (1999) Macronutrients and brain peptides: what they do and how they respond. In: Berthoud HR, Seeley RJ (eds) Neural and metabolic control of macronutrient intake. CRC Boca Raton, pp 389–406
24. Leibowiz SF, Sladek C, Spencer L, Temple D (1988) Neuropeptide Y, epinephrine and norepinephrine in the paraventricular nucleus: stimulation of feeding and the release of corticosterone, vasopressin and glucose. Brain Res Bull 21:905–912
25. Lin TW, Kuo YS (1996) Acute pulmonary oedema following administration of vasopressin for control of massive GI tract haemorrhage in a major burn patient. Burns 22:73–75
26. Lindley RI (2000) Drug therapy for acute ischemic stroke: risks verusus benefits. In: Prakash A (ed) Acute stroke treatment. Adis, Hong Kong, pp 53–62
27. MacIntosh TK, Hayes R, DeWitt D, Agura V, Faden AI (1987) Endogenous opioids may mediate secondary damage after experimental brain injury. Am J Physiol 258:E565–574
28. McClain CJ, Hennig B, Ott L, Goldblum S, Young AB (1988) Mechanisms and implications of hypoalbuminemia in head-injured patients. J Neurosurg 69:386–392
29. Morgan TJ, Koch D, Morris D, Clague A, Purdie DM (2001) Reduced red cell 2,3-diphosphoglycerate concentrations in critical illness without decreased in vivo P50. Anaesth Intensive Care 29:479–483
30. Nagao K, Hayashi N, Kanmatsuse K, Arima K, Ohtsuki J, Kikushima K, Watanabe I (2000) Cardiopulmonary cerebral resuscitation using emergency cardiopulmonary bypass, coronary reperfusion therapy and mild hypothermia in patients with cardiac arrest outside the hospital. J Am Coll Cardiol 36:776–783
31. Nilsson OG, Saveland H, Boris-Moller F, Brandt L, Wieloch T (1996) Increased levels of glutamate in patients with subarachnoid haemorrhage as measured by intracerebral microdialysis. Acta Neurochir Suppl 67:45–47
32. Payne LC, Obal F Jr, Opp MR, Krueger JM (1992) Stimulation and inhibition of growth hormone secretion by IL1: the involvement of growth hormone. Neuroendoclinology 56:118–123
33. Rosomoff HL (1959) Protective effects of hypothermia against pathological processes of the nervous system. Ann NY Acad Sci 80:475–486
34. Sahuquillo J, Amoros S, Santos A, Poca MA (2000) Does an increase in cerebral perfusion pressure always mean a better oxygenated brain? A study in head-injured patients. Acta Neurochir Suppl 76:457–462
35. Silvka A, Coben G (1985) Hydroxyl radical attack on dopamine. J Biol Chem 260:15466–15472

36. Stanley BG (1993) Neuropeptide Y in multiple hypothalamic sites controls eating behavior, endocrine, and autonomic system for body energy balance. In: Colmers WF, Wahlestedt C (eds) Biology of neuropeptide Y and related peptide. Humana Press, Totowa, NJ, pp 457–509
37. Temple DL, Leibowitz SF (1994) The neuropeptide Y system (hypothalamus) has a dense concentration of glucocorticoide (type II) receptors that mediate carbon hydrate intake. J Neuroendocrinol 6:479–501

VII. Clinical Outcome of Brain Hypothermia Treatment

57. Severe Brain Trauma

Marion et al. [16] and Clifton et al. [4] reported the effectiveness of hypothermia, 32°C for 48h, for severe brain injury in 1993. The hypothermia treatment was focused on neuroprotection, such as prevention of brain edema, prevention of free radical reactions, tolerance of brain hypoxia caused by reduced oxygen consumption, and prevention of intracranial pressure (ICP) elevation [1–3,6,7,17–19]. However, in 2001, negative effects of hypothermia treatment (32°C for 48h) were reported from a multi-trial study by Clifton et al. [5]. This is because the concept of restoration therapy for dying neurons in injured brain tissue, that includes management of hypothalamus–pituitary–adrenal (HPA) axis-associated hemoglobin dysfunction [9] and neuronal hypoxia [8,10,11], control of increasing brain tissue lactate with metabolic shift from glucose to lipid [11], control of brain thermo-pooling [12–14], management of catecholamine surge-associated insulin-resistant hyperglycemia, consideration of short-duration hypothermia worsening at the rewarming stage [11], management of growth hormone-reduced immune dysfunction [11], selective radical attack to the dopamine A10 nervous system [10], and complication of cytokine encephalitis with pulmonary infections [15], was not included. The high incidence of pulmonary infection (about 60%) is a big issue for the success of brain hypothermia treatment. The increase of serum interleukin1 (IL1) and IL6 cytokines under the condition of damaged blood-brain-barrier (BBB) cerebrospinal fluid (CSF)/serum albumin ratio more than 0.01 produces an uncontrollable increase in brain tissue glutamate even with brain hypothermia (32°–34°C).

We have opened a new concept of brain hypothermia treatment after identifying the brain thermo-pooling phenomenon in severe brain injury in 1994. After that, many brain injury mechanisms were found in severely brain-injured patients associated with stress to the HPA axis and the hypothalamus–pituitary–thyroid axis that were not observed in anesthetized experimental brain-injured animal models. Many negative effects of hypothermia and associated management techniques developed in our intensive care unit (ICU) [9,11] have been demonstrated. Clinical results are still under development.

We have focused on the effect of brain hypothermia treatment for critically ill patients with a Glasgow Coma Scale score (GCS) less than 6. We have used two emergency medical centers in Tokyo. Nihon University Emergency and Critical Care Medical Center in Itabashi Hospital and Nihon University Emergency Medical Center in Surugadai Hospital. The ICU management system is the same in the two hospitals. A randomized study of the effectiveness of brain hypothermia treatment in one hospital is, ethically, very difficult. Brain hypothermia treatment was performed in 99 cases of severe brain injury with GCS less than 6 at Itabashi Hospital. Normothermia treatment (36°–37°C) was used for 64 cases with GCS less than 6 at Surugadai Hospital [11]. The efficacy of brain hypothermia was related to the severity of brain injury as indicated by the Glasgow Coma Scale on admission. The patients with initial GCS of 3 did not benefit from brain hypothermia treatment except for two that cardiac arrested during surgery because of uncontrollable massive hemorrhage and basal skull fracture. These two cases were GCS 4 with bilateral subdural hematoma upon admission and fell to GCS 3 during surgery after 10 and 15min by cardiac arrest. However, in cases of GCS 4, 5, and 6, clinical benefit was observed as shown in Fig. 119 and Table 84. Among these patients with higher scores, 29% in GCS 4, 26% in GCS 5, and 34% in GCS 6 in the brain hypothermia group had a good outcome. In the normothermia group with previous-concept treatment, good outcome was limited, 4% in GCS 4, 7% in GCS 5, and 6% in GCS 6. The effectiveness of brain hypothermia treatment for severely brain-injured patients was impressive.

An interesting observation from our brain hypothermia treatment was that memory, intelligence, and personality were not specifically disturbed after brain hypothermia. It appears that in the acute stage, the dopamine A10 nervous system is protected from ·NO radical attack because of the prevention of excess release of dopamine by the early induction of

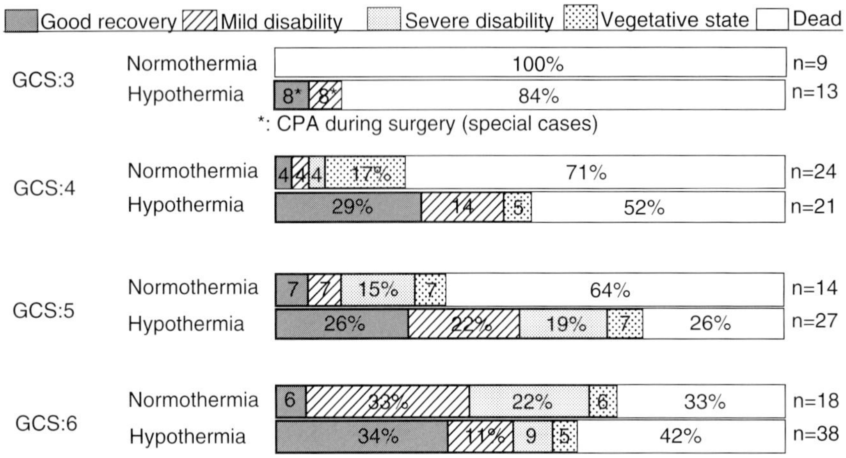

Fig. 119. Difference in clinical prognosis 3 months after normothermia treatment (65 cases at Nihon University Surugadai Hospital) and moderate brain hypothermia treatment (99 cases at Nihon University Itabashi Hospital). The effectiveness of brain hypothermia treatment for severe brain trauma is much better than normothermia treatment, even with Glasgow Coma Scale score (GSC) less than 6

Table 84. Clinical prognosis of traumatic severe brain injury 3 months later with moderate brain hypothermia and normothermia treatment

Glasgow outcome score \ Glasgow coma score	3		4		5		6	
	Hypothermia	Normothermia	Hypothermia	Normothermia	Hypothermia	Normothermia	Hypothermia	Normothermia
1. Death	11 (84%)	9 (100%)	11 (52%)	17 (71%)	7 (26%)	9 (64%)	16 (42%)	6 (33%)
2. Vegetative state	—	—	1 (5%)	4 (17%)	2 (7%)	1 (7%)	2 (5%)	1 (6%)
3. Severe disability	—	—	—	1 (4%)	5 (19%)	2 (15%)	3 (9%)	4 (22%)
4. Moderate disability	1* (8%)	—	3 (14%)	1 (4%)	6 (22%)	1 (7%)	4 (11%)	6 (33%)
5. Mild or no disability	1* (8%)	—	6 (29%)	1 (4%)	7 (26%)	1 (7%)	13 (34%)	1 (6%)
Total	13	9	21	24	27	14	38	18

*, complicated cardiac arrest during surgery

hypothermia in combination with pharmacological treatment of metoclopramide [11,14].

However, many severely brain-injured patients cannot recover soon after brain hypothermia management. In these cases, cerebral dopamine replacement therapy is necessary. The combination of pharmacological treatment by administration of levodopa (300–400 mg/day), amantadine (100–200 mg/day) and parodel (10–15 mg/day), patches of estrogen, and intermittent electrical stimulation of the peripheral median nerve for 3–4 weeks are successful. The responsiveness of dopamine replacement therapy can be diagnosed by monitoring the increase of CSF dopamine/CSF prolactin ratio (Fig. 103, Chap. 50). Emotional stimulation by holding the patient and listening to music is also effective to stimulate dopamine A10 nervous system. Forty percent of patients in a vegetative state showed clinical benefits from the combination of cerebral dopamine replacement therapy. We have observed good recovery from vegetation (18%) back to a useful lifestyle, memory, personality, and intelligence. The quality of neuronal recovery does not stop 3 months after trauma, and continues for several years. Therefore, even after brain hypothermia treatment, clinical recovery can be expected for 2–4 years with cerebral dopamine replacement therapy and neurological rehabilitation.

References

1. Busto R, Globus MY-T, Dietrich WD, Martines E, Valdes I, Watson DB, Ginsberg MD (1989) Effect of mild hypothermia on ischemia-induced release of neurotransmitters and free fatty acids in rat brain. Stroke 20:904–910
2. Cardell M, Boris MF, Wieloch T (1991) Hypothermia prevents the ischemia-induced trans-location and inhibition of protein kinase C in the rat striatum. J Neurochem 57:1814–1817
3. Chopp M, Welch KMA, Tidwell CD, Knight R, Helpern JA (1988) Effect of mild hyperthermia on recovery of metabolic function after global cerebral ischemia in cats. Stroke 19:1521–1525
4. Clifton GL, Allen S, Barrodale P, Plenger P, Berry J, Koch S, Fletcher J, Hayes RL, Choi SC (1993) A phase II study of moderate hypothermia in severe brain injury. J Neurotrauma 10:263–271

5. Clifton GL, Miller ER, Choi SC, Levin HS, McCauley S, Smith KR Jr, Muizelaar JP, Wagner FC Jr, Marion DW, Luerssen TG, Chesnut RM, Schwartz M (2001) Lack of effect of induction of hypothermia after acute brain injury. N Engl J Med 344:556–563
6. Connolly JE, Boyd RJ, Calvin JW (1962) The protective effect of hypothermia in cerebral ischemia: experimental and clinical applications by selective brain cooling in the human. Surgery 52:15–24
7. Dietrich WD, Halley M, Valdes I, Busto R (1991) Interrelationships between increased vascular permeability and acute neuronal damage following temperature controlled brain ischemia in rats. Acta Neuopathol 81:615–625
8. Dudariev VP, Lanovenko II (1999) Changes in the oxygen-binding properties of the blood in white rats under the influence of hypoxia and its pharmacological correction. Fiziol Zh 45:97–103
9. Hayashi N (1997) Prevention of vegetation after severe head trauma and stroke by combination therapy of cerebral hypothermia and activation of immune-dopaminergic nervous system. Proc Soc Treat Coma 6:133–145
10. Hayashi N (2000) Enhanced neuronal damage in severely brain injured patients by hypothalamus, pituitary, and adrenal axis neuro-hormonal changes. In: Hayashi N (ed) Brain hypothermia. Springer, Berlin Heidelberg New York Tokyo, pp 3–26
11. Hayashi N (2000) The clinical issue and effectiveness of brain hypothermia treatment for severe brain injured patients. In: Hayashi N (ed) Brain hypothermia. Springer, Berlin Heidelberg New York Tokyo, pp 121–151
12. Hayashi N, Hirayama T, Utagawa T, Ohata M (1994) Systemic management of cerebral edema based on a new concept in severe head injury patients. Acta Neurochir [Suppl] 60:541–543
13. Hayashi N, Hirayama T, Utagawa A (1994) The cerebral thermo-pooling and hypothermia treatment of critical head injury patients. In: Nagai H (ed) Intracranial pressure IX. Springer, Berlin Heidelberg New York Tokyo, pp 589–599
14. Hayashi N, Kinoshita K, Shibuya T (1997) The prevention of cerebral thermo-pooling, damage of A10 nervous system, and free radical reactions by control of brain tissue temperature in severely brain injured patients. In: Teelken AW (ed) Neurochemistry. Plenum, New York, pp 97–103
15. Holzer M, Cerchiari E, Martens P, Roine R, Strez F (2002) Mild therapeutic hypothermia to improve the neurologic outcome after cardiac arrest. N Engl J Med 346:549–555
16. Marion DW, Obrist WD, Carlier PM, Penrod LE, Darby JM (1993) The uses of moderate therapeutic hypothermia for patients with severe head injuries: a preliminary report. J Neurosurg 79:354–362
17. Marion DW, Penrod LE, Kelsey SF, Obrist WD, Kochanek PM, Palmer AM, Wisniewski SR, Dokosky ST (1997) Treatment of traumatic brain injury with moderate hypothermia. N Engl J Med 336:540–546
18. Rosomoff HL, Holaday DA (1954) Cerebral blood flow and cerebral oxygen consumption during hypothermia. Am J Physiol 179:85–88
19. Rosomoff HL (1959) Protective effects of hypothermia against pathological processes of the nervous system. Ann NY Acad Sci 80:475–486

58. Cardiac Arrest

Brain resuscitation after cardiopulmonary resuscitation has a poor prognosis [1]. The clinical results from our medical center without using brain hypothermia treatment showed, good recovery in 6 of 187 cases (3.2%), and mortality in 166 of 187 cases (88.8%) (Table 85). The other 8% of cases were mild disability 2.7%, severe disability 1.1%, and vegetative state 4.3%. The clinical results were largely unsuccessful with poor outcomes. However, recent clinical treatments have been recently developed for cardiopulmonary arrest (CPA) [2,4–6].

The difficult points for patients to survive are the progressive hemoglobin dysfunction with ineffective oxygen inhalation and the difficulty in maintaining the systemic circulation after cardiopulmonary resuscitation (Fig. 108, Chap. 54). We have introduced the percutaneous cardiopulmonary support system (PCPS) to maintain cerebral circulation after cardiopulmonary resuscitation [3,5]. Advanced clinical results were not clearly obtained by introducing PCPS treatment. Good recovery was observed in 3 of 33 cases (9.1%) and mortality occurred in 29 of the 33 cases (87.8%). Mild disability was recorded in 1 case (3.0%). No patients survived with severe disability or vegetative state in the PCPS treated group. The ineffectiveness of PCPS for cardiopulmonary arrest suggested that maintenance of cerebral blood flow (CBF) is not enough for neuronal resuscitation after cardiac arrest.

The combination of PCPS and mild brain hypothermia management was supported with the insertion of a pacemaker to control arrhythmia and percutaneous transluminal coronary angioplasty (PTCA) to prevent cardiac infarction after stabilization of vital signs following PCPS. The rate of good recovery improved to be 10 in 50 cases (20%) and mortality was reduced to 38 in 50 (76%). Mild disability was recorded in 2 cases (4%) and there were no patients with severe disability or vegetation. In this treatment, there were 3 cases of unexpected neuronal recovery even with prolonged cardiac arrest for 3–5 days. All data were obtained without classification of cardiac-arrested patients. The age range was 20–75 years. The initial cardiac massage was performed at 5–15 min after cardiac arrest. The patients included various cardiac arrest types: stand still, ventricular fibrillation, and ventricular tachycardia.

The recent clinical advantage for the management of cardiac arrests is the classification of cardiac arrests and assessment of entry criteria for management using brain hypothermia treatment. The effectiveness of hypothermia for treatment of cardiac arrest was recently reported by Bernard et al. [2] and group studies with Holzer (Austria), Cerchiari (Italy), Martens (Belgium), Roine (Finland), and Strez (Austria) [4]. The entry criteria for inclusion were witnessed cardiac arrest, ventricular fibrillation or nonperfusing ventricular tachycardia as the initial cardiac rhythm, a presumed cardiac origin of the arrest, an age of 18–75 years, an estimated interval of 5–15 min from the patient's collapse to the first attempt at resuscitation by emergency medical personnel, and an interval of no more than 60 min from collapse to restoration of spontaneous circulation. The patients were excluded if they met any of the following criteria: a tympanic membrane temperature below 30°C on admission, drug-induced cardiac arrest, pregnancy, evidence of hypotension (mean ABP < 60 mmHg) for more than 30 min after the return of spontaneous circulation, or evidence of hypoxia (SaO_2 < 85%) for more than 15 min after the return of spontaneous circulation.

The management method was very simple. After spontaneous circulation with cardiopulmonary resuscitation, the body was cooled to 32°–34°C within 4 h after cardiac arrest and hypothermia was continued for 24 h under anesthesia, analgesia, and muscle relaxation. Management for stress-associated HPA axis neurohormonal abnormality, neuronal hypoxia, insulin-resistant hyperglycemia, and the negative effects of hypothermia such as increasing brain tissue lactate, incomplete neurological recovery and BBB dysfunction were not included. However, the clinical results were better than those of the normothermia group. In clinical studies by Bernard et al. [2], normal or minimal disability outcomes were recorded in 15 of 43 cases (34.8%) in the hypothermia group and in 7 of 34 cases (20.5%) in the normothermia group. The mortality was 51.2% and 67.6%, respectively. In studies by Holzer et al. [4], favor-

Table 85. Clinical results of cardiopulmonary-arrested patients without entry criteria

	n	Age (years)	Prognosis				
			GR	MD	SD	VS	D
Previous CPNR	187	65.0	6 (3.2%)	5 (2.7%)	2 (1.1%)	8 (4.3%)	166 (88.8%)
PCPS	33	37.7	3 (9.1%)	1 (3.0%)	0 (0%)	0 (0%)	29 (87.8%)
PCPS + hypothermia	50	62.3	10 (20%)	2 (4.0%)	0 (0%)	0 (0%)	38 (76.0%)
Total	270	550	19 (7.3%)	8 (2.9%)	2 (0.7%)	8 (2.9%)	233 (86.3%)

GR, Good recovery; MD, mild disability; SD, severe disability; VS, vegetative state; D, death; CPNR, cardiopulmonary neuronal resuscitation; PCPS, percutaneous cardiopulmonary support system

Table 86. Clinical results of resuscitation for cardiac arrest

Course	*n*	Prognosis				
		Good recovery and mild disability (%)	Moderate disability (%)	Severe disability (%)	Vegetative state (%)	Death (%)
A	29	13 (44.8%)	0 (0%)	1 (3.4%)	9 (31.1%)	6 (20.7%)
B	23	12 (52.2%)	1 (4.3%)	0 (0%)	2 (8.7%)	8 (34.8%)
Total	52	25 (48.1%)	1 (1.9%)	1 (1.9%)	11 (21.2%)	4 (26.9%)

A, Return of spontaneous circulain, emergency coronary angioplasty, and 34°C brain hypothermia; B, No return of spontaneous circulation, emergency cardiopulmonary bypass, intra-aorta balloon pumping, emergency coronary angioplasty and 34°C brain hypothermia, see Fig. 109

able neurological outcome was recorded in 75 of 136 cases (55%) in the hypothermia group and in 54 of 137 cases (39%) in the normothermia group. Death occurred in 56 of 137 cases (41%) and in 76 of 138 cases (55%), respectively.

We have studied the effectiveness of brain hypothermia treatment for cardiac-arrested patients in two groups. Group A (29 cases) was treated with mild brain hypothermia (34°C) with the blanket technique and group B (23 cases) was treated with the direct blood-cooling hemodiafiltration technique as described in Chap. 54. The triage and entry criteria are described in Fig. 109 (Chap. 54). The criteria for induction of brain hypothermia and the strategy are different to those in the European studies. Our entry criteria included more severely injured patients than in the reports of Bernard et al. [2] and Holzer et al. [4] because our criteria did not include returning to spontaneous circulation.

The difference in the clinical results of the two groups was not large. Group B showed low incidence of vegetation. In group A, normal or minimal disability outcomes were recorded in 13 of 29 cases (44.8%). The incidence of severe disability, vegetative state, and death were recorded in 1 of 29 (3.4%), 9 of 29 (31.1%), and 6 of 29 cases (20.7%), respectively. In group B, good recovery or minimal disability was recorded in 12 of 23 cases (52.2%), a little better than group A. Moderate disability, vegetative state, and death were recorded in 1 of 23 (4.3%), 2 of 23 (8.7%), and 8 of 23 cases (34.8%), respectively. The combined clinical result of brain hypothermia treatment for cardiac arrest was 48.1% with good recovery, 1.9% with moderate disability, 1.9% of with severe disability, 21.2% in the vegetative state, and 26.9% resulting in death. Brain hypothermia treatment for postresuscitation of cardiac arrest is effective (Table 86) in our ICU.

References

1. American Heart Association (2002) Guidelines 2000 for cardiopulmonary resuscitation and emergency cardiovascular care. Circulation 102:1–383
2. Bernard SA, Gray TW, Buist MD, Jones BM, Silvester W, Gutteridge G, Smith K (2002) Treatment of comatose survivors of out-of-hospital cardiac arrest with induced hypothermia. N Engl J Med 346:557–563
3. Hayashi N, Nagso K, Utagawa A, Sakurai A (2001) The push back of life edge from cardiac death by combination therapy with percutaneous cardiopulmonary support and brain hypothermia treatment in cardiac arrested patients. Cardiovasc Med Surg 3:68–77
4. Holzer M, Cerchiari E, Martens P, Roine R, Strez F (2002) Mild therapeutic hypothermia to improve the neurologic outcome after cardiac arrest. N Engl J Med 346:549–555
5. Nagao K, Hayashi N, Kanmatuse K, Arima K, Ohtuki J, Kikushima K, Watanabe I (2000) Cardiopulmonary cerebral resuscitation using emergency cardiopulmonary bypass, coronary perfusion therapy and mild hypothermia in patients with cardiac arrest outside the hospital. J Am Coll Cardiol 36:776–783
6. Safar P, Behringer W, Bottiger BW, Sterz F (2002) Cerebral resuscitation potentials for cardiac arrest. Crit Care Med 30:S140–144

VIII. Clinical Protocol for Application of Brain Hypothermia

59. Critical Path of Brain Hypothermia Treatment

Standard management for severely brain-injured patients does not exist because the pathophysiological changes that occur do not follow one pattern. The critical path of brain hypothermia treatment is difficult to determine because additional management of complications from hypothermia are required. Therefore, the critical path, which is based on previous concepts, is not introduced for brain hypothermia treatment. However, if a critical path of brain hypothermia treatment can be developed, many severely brain-injured patients could be managed more effectively and survival could be improved in many hospitals.

The difficult points to standardize in brain hypothermia treatment of severe and critical brain damage include the different time course of secondary brain damage between patients, the ease of treating various complications (caused not only by severe brain damage but also by poor management of hypothermia), and limited information about pharmacological action at 32°–34°C. The management plans to cope with the different time courses of secondary brain damage between patients, should use a phase care management style. The short duration of brain hypothermia stops the progression of secondary brain damage and does not provide restoration. In such cases, reprogression of brain damage occurs at the rewarming stage and overlaps with rewarming stress. The phase care management style must cover variable-length management until signs of recovery are observed. The complications that affect the reversibility of brain damage also affect phase care management. However, management of complications cannot be included in the standard phase care management because complications do not occur in all patients. Special considerations for essential management targets that must be achieved at each phase are required. Standard management of each phase also must be included in this system. As a technique, computed critical path management may succeed in these issues. To cover the problem of limited pharmacological information and to adapt to developing medical treatment, computed intensive care unit (ICU) management is successful.

Critical Path Care Plan for Management of Brain Hypothermia Treatment

Combination of standard care management and algorithm care management is a basic concept for treatment of severely brain-injured patients who show variable brain injury mechanisms, different time courses, many complications, and no response to management. The total design of a critical path for brain hypothermia treatment for severe brain damage is presented in Table 87. The total management course is divided into six stages: first induction stage, second induction stage, cooling stage, preconditioning for rewarming, rewarming stage, and posthypothermia stage. The standard management for each stage includes a care plan, orders, intervention, intravenous medication, brain monitoring, and systemic care monitors. The content of each of these parts can be retrieved from the bedside computer display. The management targets of each stage are listed in the total care management plan as shown in Table 87. If these management targets are not achieved, the algorithm management method for each management target appears on the computer display after clicking on the name of the target.

Stage Care Plan

The concept of brain hypothermia treatment and ICU techniques are described in detail in other parts of this book. This discussion summarizes the contents of standard care and algorithm care methods for each stage. Management of the induction stage is divided into two steps: induction of mild brain hypothermia to 34°C (induction stage 1) and induction of moderate brain hypothermia at 32°–33°C (induction stage 2).

Table 87. Outline of the critical path of brain hypothermia treatment

Stage	Stage 1 Induction 1	Stage 2 Induction 2	Stage 3 Cooling	Stage 4 Preconditioning	Stage 5 Rewarming	Stage 6 Posthypothermia
Duration	3 h	6 h	3–7 days	1–2 days	1–2 days	3–4 weeks
Algorithm of management targets	Stabilize vital signs Shivering Catecholamine surge Neuronal hypoxia Hyperglycemia 34°C brain temperature Dopamine release Radical reaction	Mild or moderate hypothermia? Serum glucose < 160 mg/dl $\bar{D}O_2$ > 700 ml/min Hemoglobin dysfunction AT-III > 100% Hypopotassemia SBP > 100 mmHg Fluid resuscitation	Intermittent hypothermia ICP < 15 mmHg Brain edema AT-III > 100% Serum albumin > 3.5 mg/dl Immune dysfunction Prevent infection Activate lipid metabolism	Evidence of neuronal recovery No severe infection CSF/serum albumin < 0.01 Serum glucose 120–140 mg/dl Enteral nutrition Recover immune function Activate lipid metabolism	Step by step rewarm Adaptation time Serum glucose 130–150 mg/dl $\bar{D}O_2$ > 700 ml/min O_2ER 23%–35% $PaCO_2$ 32–36 mmHg Serum pH 7.3–7.4 Serum phosphate > 3 mg/dl Serum Mg^+ > 1.3 mmol/dl Replacement vitamin A Infection control	A10-Dopamine replacement therapy Restoration therapy of vegetation Neurorehabilitation
Standard management						
Order						
Basic care plan	①	①	①	①	①	①
Care order	②	②	②	②	②	②
Intervention	③	③	③	③	③	③
IV medication	④	④	④	④	④	④
Monitor						
Brain monitor	⑤	⑤	⑤	⑤	⑤	⑤
Systemic care monitor	⑥	⑥	⑥	⑥	⑥	⑥

Induction Stage 1

Standard Management

Stage 1.1. Basic Care Plan

Start brain hypothermia within 3h after insult, maintain the systolic blood pressure greater than 100mmHg, evaluate Glasgow Coma Scale (GCS) less than 8 for surgical indication, rapid management of stress-associated hyperglycemia, maintain hemoglobin function with control of serum pH, phosphate, and magnesium, prevent catecholamine surge, neuronal oxygenation, prevent enterobacterial infection, and suppress hypothalamus dopamine release.

Stage 1.2. Care Order

Systolic blood pressure (SBP): control at 120–160mmHg by fluid resuscitation.

SBP >170mmHg hypertension: drip the antihypertensive drug, diltiazem hydrochloride (Helvesser), 250mg, diluted with 100ml saline at 2ml/h.

Blood gases: PaO_2 >100mmHg, PaO_2/FiO_2 ratio >350, $PaCO_2$ 34–38mmHg.

Urine: maintain at 0.5ml/kg^{-1}.

Serum glucose: control serum glucose at 120–140mg/dl by drip of rapid-action insulin (Humarin R), 50U diluted with 100ml saline.

Administration speed: start from 2ml/h and then slow down to 1ml/h after serum glucose becomes lower than 200mg/dl.

Serum potassium: control at 3.5–4.5mEq/l by drip of KCl 1A, diluted with 80ml saline. Replacement speed 40ml/h for serum K^+ <2.0mEq/l, 20ml/hour for serum K^+ 1.2–2.5mEq/l, 15ml/h for serum K^+ 2.6–3.0mEq/l, 10ml/h for serum K^+ 23.1–3.05mEq/l, and 5ml/h for serum K^+ 3.6–34.0mEq/l.

Stage 1.3. Intervention

Bronchial intubation and ventilator care management.
Fluid resuscitation by central venous catheterization.
Catheter insertion for monitoring arterial blood gases.
Insertion of naso–gastric tube.
Insertion of Foley catheter for urinary drainage.
Monitoring of electrocardiogram (ECG).
Biochemical analysis.

Blood type.
X-ray examination.
Gastric lavage with digastrics decontamination (one-shot enteral administration of nonabsorbable antibiotics: levofloxacin (Cravit, 200 mg) + amphotericin B 100–300 mg as described in Stage 1.4.).

Stage 1.4. Intravenous Medication

Fluid resuscitation: 7% Acetic acid Ringer solution (Veen F) and Saline Hess solution at induction stage, except hypoglycemia. The replacement of potassium phosphate, vitamin A, vitamin B, Mg^{++}, 5% albumin, and antithrombin-III (AT-III) are recommended.
Crush induction of anesthesia: midazolam 0.15–0.25 mg/kg h^{-1} anesthesia, combined with pancuronium 0.05 mg/kg h^{-1} muscle relaxation, and buprenorphine 1.0–2.0 mg/kg h^{-1} analgesia. Propofol is much better for unstable cardiopulmonary function than midazolam. At the beginning of the induction stage, propopfol is preferred.
Management of aspiration pneumonia: first choice is panipenem beta amipron (Carbenin 500 mg × 2/day), second choice is ceftazidime (Modasin 1 g × 2/day) or clindamycine (Dalacin, 150–300 mg per 6 h) + one-shot enteral administration of nonabsorbable antibiotics: levofloxacin (Cravit, 200 mg) + amphotericin B 100–300 mg to prevent Pseudomonas aspiration pneumonia and enteral bacterial translocation.

Stage 1.5. Brain Monitoring and Management

Computed brain monitoring: tympanic membrane temperature/core temperature >1.0, internal jugular venous blood temperature/tympanic membrane temperature >1.0, ventricular cerebrospinal fluid (CSF) temperature/internal jugular venous blood temperature >1.0, ventricular CSF temperature/bladder temperature >1.0.
Intracramial pressure (ICP) <20 mmHg.
Microdialysis monitoring.
SjO_2 >60%.
Cerebral perfusion pressure (CPP) >80 mmHg.
Trend electroencephalogram (EEG).
Auditory brain stem evoked response (ABER).

Stage 1.6. Monitoring and Management of Systemic Hemodynamic Changes

SBP >100 mmHg.
Monitoring of ECG for arrhythmia, ST changes, and QT interval <450 mm/s.
Right flowing catheter monitoring of cardiac output (CO).
Cardiac index (CI).
Oxygen delivery ($\bar{D}O_2$) >700 ml/min $\bar{D}O_2I$ > 500.
Oxygen extraction ratio (O_2ER) 22%–26%.
Bladder pressure <15 mmHg.
Gastric pHi >7.3.
Intestinal luminar pressure <15 mmHg.
Biochemical examinations: serum glucose, AT-III, hemoglobin, serum albumin, troponin I, CPK, GOT, GPT, Ht, hemoglobin A1C, serum osmolarity, creatinine.

Stage 1 Algorithm Management

Stabilize vital signs: elastic bandaging of extremities, normal volume replacement, medication, maintain SBP >100 mmHg, CPP >80 mmHg, Hb >12 mg/dl, oxygen delivery >800 ml/min, 2,3-diphosphoglycerate (DPG) >13 µmol/ml. Serum K^+ >3 mEq/dl, serum glucose 120–140 mg/dl.
Shivering: midazolam anesthesia 0.15–0.25 mg/kg h^{-1}, combined with pancuronium muscle relaxant 0.05 mg/kg h^{-1}, and buprenorphine analgesia 1.0–2.0 mg/kg h^{-1}.
Catecholamine surge: control of catecholamine surge by control of brain tissue temperature at 34°C, administration of metoclopramide.
Neuronal hypoxia: PaO_2/FiO_2 ratio >350, hemoglobin DPG: 12–14 µmol/ml, oxygen delivery >700 ml/min, CPP >80 mmHg, AT-III >100%.
Hyperglycemia: administration of insulin with control of serum phosphate and magnesium, 7% acetate Ringer solution, steroid contraindicated, activate respiratory muscle metabolism with salbutamol.
Rapid induction of mild brain hypothermia: combination of blanket cooling method and gastric lavage with chilled saline, alcohol heat evaporation, complete body wrapping and insulation from room air, reduce room temperature to 18°C, maintain room air outflow circulation, two cooling machines, remove heat generating medical devices from the bedside.
Dopamine release: early induction of brain hypothermia and administration of metoclopramide.
Prevention of radical reaction: early induction of mild brain hypothermia and continue to moderate brain hypothermia, control of Hb >11 g/dl, administration of vitamins E and C.

Induction Stage 2

Standard Management

Stage 2.1. Basic Care Plan

Select mild or moderate brain hypothermia. Internal jugular venous temperature, ventricular CSF temperature, tympanic temperature, core temperature, and bladder temperature should be monitored simultaneously.

Stabilize vital signs for induction to moderate brain hypothermia. SBP >100 mmHg, treat hypokalemia, ensure no arrhythmia, QT-interval <450 mm/s, serum glucose 120–140 mg/dl are diagnostic criteria.
Brain monitoring. SjO_2 65%–80%, ICP <20 mmHg.

Stage 2.2. Care Order

SBP: control at 120–160 mmHg by fluid resuscitation.
SBP >170 mmHg hypertension: drip antihypertensive drug diltiazem hydrochloride (Helvesser), 250 mg, diluted with 100 ml saline, 2 ml/h. Complication of bradycardia (HR <50 bpm): nicardipine hydrochloride (Perdipin) 2–5 µg/kg min^{-1}.
Blood gases: PaO_2 >100 mmHg, PaO_2/FiO_2 ratio >350, $PaCO_2$ 35 mmHg.
Urine volume: more than 0.5 ml/kg h^{-1}.
Serum glucose: 120–140 mg/dl by drip of rapid-action insulin (Humarin R) 50 U diluted with 100 ml saline. Administration speed: start at 2-ml/h and slow to 1 ml/h after serum glucose falls below 200 mg/dl.
Serum potassium: control at 3.5–4.5 mEq/l by drip of KCl 1A, diluted with 80 ml saline. Replacement speed: 40 ml/h for serum K^+ <2.0 mEq/l, 20 ml/h for serum K^+ 1.2–2.5 mEq/l, 15 ml/h for serum K^+ 2.6–3.0 mEq/l, 10 ml/h for serum K^+ 23.1–3.05 mEq/l, and 5 ml/h for serum K^+ 3.6–34.0 mEq/l.

Stage 2.3. Intervention

Ventilator management.
Ventricular drainage.
ICP monitoring.
SjO_2 monitoring.
Cardiac output and O_2ER.
Body weight.
Blood gases.
Microdialysis monitoring.

Stage 2.4. Intravenous Medication

Fluid resuscitation: 7% Acetic acid Ringer solution (Veen F) + H_2 receptor antagonist (Zantac 50 mg/A) + metoclopramide (Prinmperan) 1A + panthenol (Pantol 500 mg × 2).
Maintenance fluid: actit solution 500 ml + carbazochrome sodium sulfonate (Adona) 50 ml + tranexamic acid (Transamin S) 1A + hemocoagulase (Reptilase-S 1A proteolysis enzyme) (drip).
Enzyme inhibitor: ulinastatin (Miraclid) 300 000 unit/day + maintenance fluid (T4-solution) 400 ml (drip).
Proteolysis enzyme: gabexate mesilate (FOY) 1500–2000 mg + maintenance fluid (T4-solution) 200 ml (drip).
Antiepileptic phenytoin–phenobarbital (Aleviatin) 250 mg + saline 20 ml (i.v.), flush saline 20 ml, Aleviatin 125 mg + saline 20 ml (i.v.).
Adsorbed tetanus toxoid 0.5 ml (IM) + human antitetanus immunoglobulin 250 IU (i.m.).
Anesthesia: midazola (20A) + maintenance fluid (T4-soution) 160 ml drip 1 ml/h, combined drip with pancuronium bromide (Myoblock) 20A+T4-solution 160 ml, and buprenophine hydrochloride (Lepetan) 3–5A + saline 100 ml.
Heparin calcium (Hepacarin) 5000 U + saline 100 ml drip, 5 ml/h to prevent complication of SjO_2 monitoring.
Blood transfusion for Hb <10 mg/dl.

Stage 2.5. Brain Monitoring and Management

CPP >80 mmHg.
ICP <20 mmHg.
SjO_2 70%–80%.
Trend EEG.
ABER.
Care management of ICP >20 mmHg:

1. Prevent venous stasis by management of neck position, mediastinal pressure, abdominal hypertension, full stomach, and bladder pressure.
2. Diagnose the effectiveness of CSF drainage by changes in ICP during 3 min open/close drainage.
3. Continuous CSF drainage.
4. Manage hypercapnia.
5. Replacement of serum albumin to 3.5 mg/dl.
6. Head-up position.
7. Management of hyperglycemia and serum electrolytes.
8. Control of blood pressure.
9. Administration of manitol 100 ml/30–60 min.

Stage 2.6. Monitoring and Management of Systemic Homodynamic Changes

CI >2.2.
$\bar{D}O_2I$ >500.
$\bar{V}O_2I$ >125.
O_2ER 22%–26%.
SVRI 1800–2500.
PAWP >8–12 mmHg.
Care management of cardiac disturbances:

1. Preload disturbances: administration of crystalloid, colloid, diuretics, and dopamine 1–3 µg/ml min^{-1}.
2. Contraction disturbances: administration of dobutrex and/or PDE-III inhibitor.
3. After load disturbances: administration of noradrenalin and/or Ca blocker.
4. Electric imbalance: Na, K, Mg, IP, and Ca.

Neuronal oxygenation:

1. PaO_2/FiO_2 >300–350.
2. Manage neck position.
3. Check the correct position of intubation tube.
4. Control mechanical ventilation volume 10–15 ml/kg, PEEP 3–5 cm H_2O, auto-sigh 20–25 ml/kg.
5. Management of red blood cells: Hb >11 mg/dl, DPG 12–14 µmol/ml, inorganic phosphate >3.0 mg/dl.

Laboratory examinations: blood gases analysis every 2 h, complete blood cell count, serum glucose, serum albumin, IP, Mg, AT-III, D-dimer, α2-PI, SFMC, PF1+2, APC, and platelet aggregation.

MRSA bacterial analysis.

Gastrointestinal examination and management: gastric juice from N/G tube <200 ml/day.

Stage 2 Algorithm Management

Serum glucose <160 mg/dl:

1. Early brain hypothermia (33°–34°C) induction within 3 h after brain damage. Catecholamine surge-associated hyperglycemia should be minimized.
2. Replacement of insulin.
3. No administration of cortisol.
4. Activate protein synthesis of muscle by administration of arginine, salbutamol, clenbuterol, glutamine.
5. Inhibit protein catabolism: amurinone.
6. Rehabilitation and kinetic therapy.

DO_2 >700 ml/min and SBP >100 mmHg: fluid resuscitation, administration of norepinephrine + doptorex. Elastic bandaging of extremities. Temporary insertion of abdominal balloon catheter into the abdominal aorta.

Hemoglobin dysfunction: control of serum pH >7.3. Serum glucose 120–140 mg/dl. AT-III >100%. Serum inorganic phosphate 3–5 mg/dl. Serum magnesium 1.4–1.8 mEq/l. Serum albumin >3.5 mg/dl. Vitamin A 50–100 mg/dl.

AT-III >100%: replacement of serum albumin.

Hypokalemia: control K^+ at 3.5–4.5 mEq/l by drip of KCl 1A, diluted with 80 ml saline. Replacement speed: 40 ml/h for serum K^+ <2.0 mEq/l, 20 ml/h for serum K^+ 1.2–5 mEq/l, 15 ml/h for serum K^+ 2.6–3.0 mEq/l, 10 ml/h for serum K^+ 23.1–3.05 mEq/l, and 5 ml/h for serum K^+ 3.6–34.0 mEq/l.

Cooling Stage (Stage 3)

Standard Management

Stage 3.1. Basic Care Plan

The major targets of ICU management at the cooling stage are: restoration of injured brain tissue, maintenance of neuronal oxygenation and metabolic balance, maintenance of lipid metabolism, management of ICP and brain edema, careful management of BBB function, control of immune dysfunction, maintenance of neurohormonal function, nutritional consideration, and prevention of infections.

Stage 3.2. Care Order

SBP: control at 120–160 mmHg by fluid resuscitation.

SBP >170 mmHg hypertension: drip antihypertensive diltiazem hydrochloride (Helvesser) 250 mg, diluted with 100 ml saline at 2 ml/h. With complication of bradycardia (HR <50 bpm), change to nicardipine hydrochloride (Perdipin) 2–5 µg/kg min^{-1}.

Blood gases: PaO_2 >100 mmHg, PaO_2/FiO_2 ratio >350, $PaCO_2$ 35 mmHg.

Urine volume: more than 0.5 ml/kg h^{-1}.

Serum glucose: 120–140 mg/dl by drip of rapid-action insulin (Humarin R): 50 U diluted with 100 ml saline. Administration speed: start with 2 ml/h and slow to 1 ml/h after serum glucose falls below 200 mg/dl.

Serum potassium: control at 3.5–4.5 mEq/l by drip of KCl 1A, diluted with 80 ml saline. Replacement speed: 40 ml/h for serum K^+ <2.0 mEq/l, 20 ml/h for serum K^+ 1.2–2.5 mEq/l, 15 ml/h for serum K^+ 2.6–3.0 mEq/l, 10 ml/h for serum K^+ 23.1–3.05 mEq/l, and 5 ml/h for serum K^+ 3.6–34.0 mEq/l.

Stage 3.3. Intervention

Ventilator management.

Ventricular drainage.

ICP monitoring.

SjO_2 monitoring.

Cardiac output and O_2ER.

Insert ileum gastric tube.

Determine indication for kinetic therapy using dyna care bed.

Microdialysis monitoring.

Stage 3.4. Intravenous Medication

Fluid resuscitation: 7% Acetic acid Ringer solution (Veen F) + H_2 receptor antagonist (Zantac 50 mg/A) + metoclopramide (Prinmperan) 1A + panthenol (Pantol 500 mg × 2).

Maintenance fluid: combination of physiosol-3 500 ml, amicaliq 500 ml, and hicaliq 500 ml (drip).

Administration of vitamins C and E, and $ZnCl_2$.

Enzyme inhibitor: ulinastatin (Miraclid) 300000 U/day + maintenance fluid (T4-solution) 400 ml (drip).

Proteolysis enzyme: gabexate mesilate (FOY) 1500–2000 mg + maintenance fluid (T4-solution) 200 ml (drip).

Vitamin kit: vitamin C 500 mg, vitamin B1 50 mg, vitamin B2 20 mg, vitamin 6 20 mg (i.v.).

Antepileptic phenytoin–phenobarbital (Aleviatin) 250 mg + saline 20 ml (i.v.), flush saline 20 ml, Aleviatin 125 mg + saline 20 ml (i.v.).

Antibiotics: immipenem cilastain sodium (Tienam 1–2 g/day × 3) > meropenem trihydrate (Meropn, 1.0–2.0 g/day × 4) for enterobacteria, gram-negative bacteria, and pseudomonas.

Anesthesia: midazolam (20A) + maintenance fluid (T4-solution) 160 ml drip 1 ml/h, combined drip with pancuronium bromide (Myoblock) 20A+T4-solution 160 ml, and buprenophine hydrochloride (Lepetan) 3–5A + saline 100 ml.

Heparin calcium (Hepacarin) 5000 U + saline 100 ml drip, 5 ml/h to prevent complication of SjO_2 monitoring.

Blood transfusion for Hb >10 mg/dl.

Stage 3.5. Brain Monitoring and Management

CPP >80 mmHg, ICP <20 mmHg, SjO_2 70%–80%, monitoring of trend EEG, ABER, brain tissue temperature, internal jugular venous blood temperature, tympanic membrane temperature, core temperature, bladder temperature, and CT.

Stage 3.6. Monitoring and Management of Systemic Homodynamic Changes

CI >2.2.

$\bar{D}O_2I$ >500.

$\bar{V}O_2I$ >125.

O_2ER 22%–26%.

SVRI 1800–2500.

PAWP >8–12 mmHg.

Care management of cardiac disturbances:

1. Preload disturbances: administration of crystalloid, colloid, diuretics, and dopamine 1–3 μg/ml min^{-1}.
2. Contraction disturbances: administration of dobutrex and/or PDE-III inhibitor.
3. After load disturbances: administration of noradrenalin and/or Ca blocker.
4. Electric imbalance: Na, K, Mg, IP, and Ca.

Neuronal oxygenation:

1. PaO_2/FiO_2 >300–350.
2. Manage neck position.
3. Check the correct position of intubation tube.
4. Controlled mechanical ventilation volume 10–15 ml/kg, PEEP 3–5 cm H_2O, auto-sigh 20–25 ml/kg.
5. Management of red blood cells: Hb >11 mg/dl, DPG 12–14 μmol/ml, inorganic phosphate >3.0 mg/dl.

Water balance: intake/output each 8 h.

Laboratory examinations: blood gases analysis every 2 h, complete blood cell count, serum glucose, serum albumin, IP, Mg, AT-III, D-dimer, α2-PI, SFMC, PF1+2, APC, and platelet aggregation.

MRSA bacterial analysis.

Gastrointestinal examination and care management: gastric juice from N/G tubes <200 ml/day, abdominal X-ray, nutritional consideration with management of BBB dysfunction (CSF/serum albumin ratio <0.01), and special enteral care management. Cetraxate hydrochloride (Neuer-S), L-glutamine (Glumin-S), Antibiotic-resistent lactic acid bacteria (Biofermin-R), potassium permanganate, and Daiken Tyutou are enteral management drugs.

Stage 3 Algorithm Management

Intermittent hypothermia: prolonged brain hypothermia, below 32°–33°C, produces a reduction of pituitary hormones. Deficiency of growth hormone and thyroid hormones causes an unavoidable depletion of immune function. To prevent this complication, intermittent control of brain tissue temperature between 32°C and 34°C is a very useful management technique. The temporary elevation of brain tissue temperature is recommended at 1800–2200 hours because physiological growth hormone is naturally released at this time. The detailed techniques are described previously in this book.

Brain edema and control of ICP <15 mmHg: ICP elevation to more than 20 mmHg produces venous stasis and disturbances of microcirculation. To prevent microcirculation disturbance, CSF drainage, head-up position, reduction of abdominal pressure and mediastinal pressure, prevention of hypo-albuminemia, administration of hyperosmotic solution, manitol, and reduction of CSF production by acetazolamide (Diamox) are prescribed management.

AT-III >100%: peripheral vascular stasis is one of the complications of the cooling stage of brain hypothermia. Prolonged bed rest, peripheral vascular contraction, subcutaneous edema caused by the complication of hypo-albuminemia, complication of infection, and consumption of AT-III by severe brain damage are causes of reduced AT-III. Lower than 80%–90% of AT-III is critical and promotes the systemic disturbance of microcirculation and development of inflammation of vascular intimae. Our clinical studies suggest the management of AT-III affects to prognosis and success of brain hypothermia treatment.

Serum albumin >3.5 mg/dl: prolonged hypothermia promotes synthesis of protein and albumin. Increasing cytokines produces hypo-albuminemia. In severely brain-injured patients, rapid development of hypo-albuminemia is a big clinical issue. Progression of brain edema, ineffective manitol hyperosmotic diuretics for brain edema, complication of pulmonary edema, intestinal mucous edema, pancreatic duct obstruction caused by intestinal wall edema, immune dysfunction, bacterial translocation, unstable pharmacological function of protein-binding drugs, increased free bacteria and ease of infection are major complications of hypo-albuminemia. Therefore, replacement of albumin and nutritional consideration for hypo-albuminemia are important management strategies during the cooling stage of brain hypothermia treatment.

Immune dysfunction: reduced growth hormone levels and energy crisis in lymphocytes are major causes of immune dysfunction during brain hypothermia treatment. The reduction of growth hormone is unavoidable with prolonged moderate brain hypothermia because the temperature of the pituitary gland is also lowered. Glutamine is the energy source for lymphocytes and is produced in lung tissue and skeletal muscles. This glutamine is expended by lymphocytes in the intestinal digestive organs. Therefore, muscle hypometabolism, pulmonary infection, and mucous edema in the digestive organ caused by hypo-albuminemia also produce immune dysfunction. Administration of arginine, salbutamol, and growth hormone are effective in maintaining immune function because of stimulation of protein synthesis in skeletal muscles and promotion of the lipid metabolism which is the main metabolism under hypothermia.

Prevention of infection: Complication with severe infection during the cooling stage causes the failure of brain hypothermia treatment. Increased serum pro-inflammatory cytokines can permeate the damaged BBB and produce cytokine encephalitis with uncontrollable increases of neurotoxic glutamate in injured brain tissue. Therefore, as management of infection during brain hypothermia treatment, the killing of bacteria, activation of immune function, the management of BBB (CSF/serum albumin ratio <0.01), management of serum albumin (>3.5 mg/dl), no activation of vasopressin release by neural control of the feedback mechanism to hyperglycemia, maintenance of protein synthesis in skeletal muscles, and administration of bacteria-sensitive non-protein-binding antibiotics are indicated. The intermittent control of brain tissue temperature at 32°–33°C, administration of arginine, and rehabilitation of skeletal muscles are also effective to increase the immune function. The choice of systemic administration of antibiotics and digestive decontamination antibiotics therapy was described previously in this book.

Activation of lipid metabolism: brain hypothermia below 34°C produces metabolic shift from glucose to lipid metabolism. The lipid metabolism requires vitamin A and adequate growth hormone for energy metabolism without lactate production. Excessive replacement of growth hormone produces hyperglycemia. Therefore, careful monitoring of serum glucose is important for replacement therapy of growth hormone and arginine.

Preconditioning for Rewarming (Stage 4)

Standard Management

Stage 4.1. Basic Care Plan

Rewarming can occur after exact diagnosis of some form of recovery. The recording of a θ wave on the background of the δ wave in trend EEG, no ICP elevation, SjO_2 control at 60%–75%, and no brain swelling on CT scan are basic signs of neuronal recovery. To succeed in rewarming from brain hypothermia treatment, various preconditioning managements are necessary.

Stage 4.2. Care Order

Rewarming from brain hypothermia, especially prolonged treatment below 34°C, produces various physiological changes such as metabolic shift from lipid to glucose, vascular engorgement, increased metabolic activity, activated cytokine production, increase in ·NO radicals, increased serum cytokines, uncoupling of bloodflow and metabolism in major organs, and oxygen demand in the brain tissue. Before rewarming, preconditioning management is recommended for adaptation or prevention of negative effects to the brain by these physiological changes. No severe infection, lymphocytes >1500/mm^3, T-H (CD4) lymph >55%, serum glucose 120–140 mg/dl, prealbumin >20 mg/dl, serum albumin >3.5 mg/dl, vitamin A >50 mg/dl, Hb >12 g/dl, O_2ER 23%–25%, AT-III >100%, and gastric pHi >7.35 are the major targets for preconditioning care. The success of care management ensures no trouble during rewarming.

Stage 4.3. Intervention

EEG (recovery from δ wave to θ wave or recording of α wave), ABR, brain CT (no signs of brain swelling or severe brain edema), ICP <20 mmHg, CPP >70–80 mmHg are basic management.

Prevention of systemic infection at the rewarming stage is another important management step in this stage. Digestive decontamination for control of clostridium enteritis and MRSA by enteral administration of levofloxacin (Cravit, 200 mg) and amphotericin B (100–300 mg), combined with vancomycin (2–3 g/day ×

4–6 times i.v. drip) is useful prophylactic management for rewarming stage infection.

Stage 4.4. Intravenous Medication

Maintenance fluid: combination of physiosol-3 500 ml, amicaliq 500 ml, 7% acetic acid Ringer solution (Veen F) and hicaliq 500 ml (drip). Calorie increases with monitoring of serum glucose.
Administration of vitamins C and E, and $ZnCl_2$.
Enzyme inhibitor: ulinastatin (Miraclid) 300 000 U/day + maintenance fluid (T4-solution) 400 ml (drip).
Proteolysis enzyme: gabexate mesilate (FOY) 1500–2000 mg + maintenance fluid (T4-solution) 200 ml (drip).
Antiepileptic: phenytoin–phenobarbital, Aleviatin 125 mg + saline 20 ml (i.v.), prepare the flush saline 20 ml.
Antibiotics: arbekacin sulfate (Habekacin, 150–200 mg/day × 2) to prevent pseudomonal aerginosa and MRSA infection, + cefozopran hydrochloride (Firstcin 1–2 g/day × 2) for Tienam resistant Acinetobacter and xantomona + fluconazole (Diflucan 100–200 mg/day × 1) for Candida with evidence of β-D-glucan-positive reactions).
Anesthesia: midazola (20A) + maintenance fluid (T4-soution) 160 ml drip 1 ml/h, combined drip with pancuronium bromide (Myoblock) 20A+T4-solution 160 ml, and buprenophine hydrochloride (Lepetan) 3–5A + saline 100 ml.
Heparin calcium (Hepacarin) 5000 U + saline 100 ml drip, 5 ml/h to prevent complication of SjO_2 monitoring.
Blood transfusion for Hb <10 mg/dl.

Stage 4.5. Brain Monitoring and Management

CPP >80 mmHg, ICP <20 mmHg, SjO_2 70%–80%, trend EEG (recovery from δ wave to θ wave or recording of α wave), ABER, brain CT (no signs of brain swelling or severe brain edema or CT).

Stage 4.6. Monitoring and Management of Systemic Homodynamic Changes

CI >2.2.
$\bar{D}O_2I$ >500.
$\bar{V}O_2I$ >125.
O_2ER 22%–26%.
SVRI 1800–2500.
PAWP >8–12 mmHg.
Management of cardiac disturbances:
1. Preload disturbances: administration of crystalloid, colloid, diuretics, and dopamine 1–3 $\mu g/ml\,min^{-1}$.
2. Contraction disturbances: administration of dobutrex and/or PDE-III inhibitor.
3. After load disturbances: administration of noradrenalin and/or Ca blocker.
4. Electric imbalance: Na, K, Mg, IP, and Ca.

Neuronal oxygenation:
1. PaO_2/FiO_2 >300–350.
2. Manage neck position.
3. Check the correct position of intubation tube.
4. Controlled mechanical ventilation volume 10–15 ml/kg, PEEP 3–5 cmH_2O, auto-sigh 20–25 ml/kg.
5. Management of red blood cells: Hb >11 mg/dl, DPG 12–14 μmol/ml, inorganic phosphate >3.0 mg/dl.

Water balance: intake/output every 8 h.
Laboratory examinations: $PaCO_2$ 32–36 mmHg, serum glucose 120–150 mg/dl, serum albumin >3.5 mg/dl, IP >3 mg/dl, AT-III >120%, D-dimer.
Gastrointestinal examination and management: gastric juice from N/G tubes <200 ml/day, abdominal X-ray, nutritional consideration for management of BBB dysfunction (CSF/serum albumin ratio <0.01), and special enteral care management. Cetraxate hydrochloride (Neuer-S), L-glutamine (Glumin-S), antibiotic-resistant lactic acid bacteria (Biofermin-R), potassium permanganate, and Daiken Tyutou are enteral management drugs. The management of digastrics decontamination with nonabsorbable and hypothermia-active antibiotics levofloxacin (Cravit, 200 mg) and amphotericin B (100–300 mg) combined with intravenous drip administration of vancomycin (2–3 g/day × 4–6 times) are indicated for prevention of systemic infection.

Stage 4 Algorithm Management

Evidence of neuronal recovery: the big issue at rewarming is reprogression of brain injury mechanism that was stopped at the cooling stage. Without evidence of neuronal recovery or at least signs of recovery, rewarming makes the condition much worse. If neuronal recovery was not diagnosed by monitoring of ICP, SjO_2, EEG, and CSF biochemical changes, the cooling stage should be extended for a few more days. Management is same as Standard Management, Stage 4.1. Basic Care Plan, Stage 4.2. Care Order, Stage 4.3. Intervention, Stage 4.4. Intravenous Medication, Stage 4.5. Brain Monitoring, Stage 4.6. Monitoring and Management of Systemic Homodynamic Changes, and Algorithm Management. No signs of brain edema or other complications on the CT examination are also useful to diagnose neuronal recovery.
No severe infection and CSF/serum Albumin <0.01: the elevation of body temperature by rewarming stimulates the activity of serum cytokines. Increased serum cytokines can easily permeate the damaged BBB. This serious complication causes the failure of brain hypothermia treatment at the rewarming stage. Therefore, management of severe pulmonary infection and management of BBB dysfunction (CSF/

serum albumin ratio <0.01) must be achieved before rewarming. The actual management method is described previously in this book.

Serum glucose 120–140 mg/dl: Administration of insulin with control of serum phosphate and magnesium, 7% acetate Ringer solution, contraindicated steroid, activate respiratory muscle metabolism by salbutamol.

Enteral nutrition: the management of nutrition at the rewarming stage requires the replacement of an energy source of calories, feed to immune cells, stabilization of the intestinal digestive organ, and maintenance of nutritional conditions. The management of BBB dysfunction is also important because neurotoxic glutamate increases about two to three times with enteral and parenteral amino acid nutrition. In well-organized BBB with CSF/serum albumin ratio lower than 0.01, microdialysis studies provided no evidence of serum glutamate passing into the brain tissue and no evidence of worsening brain edema. Preliminary management of BBB dysfunction with replacement of serum albumin to higher than 3.5 mg/dl, anti-inflammatory medicine for the vascular wall such as AT-III and protein C, and radical scavenger such as Radicut are useful to avoid nutritional complications at the rewarming stage. The replacement of serum albumin is very effective for the control of intestinal mucous membrane edema and prevention of diarrhea caused by enteral nutrition. Preliminary feeding (with glutamine and arginine), correct serum electrolytes, control of the osmotic gap (serum Osm—2 (stool Na + K) >100 mOsm/kg) and management of mesenteric ischemia are also useful before feeding management. Two actual enteral nutrition courses are prepared. One uses saline immune nutrition (glutamine + arginine + yeast RNA) with administration of honey yogurt, and control of BBB function at CSF/serum albumin ratio lower than 0.01. The other is two-step enteral nutrition with CSF/serum albumin 0.01–0.02. First step: saline 50 ml to max 150 ml/4 h, and remove retention fluid, repeat for 3–4 days. Second stage: administration of honey yogurt (50 ml to max 150 ml/4 h). The detailed techniques are described in Chap. 44. The combination of enteral nutrition with honey yogurt and arginine is very effective for stimulation of lipid metabolism without production of lactate.

Rewarming Stage (Stage 5)

Standard Management

The metabolism shift from lipid to glucose occurs with rewarming. This metabolic shift also produces the uncoupling between blood flow and metabolism. The patterns of these changes are variable with duration and level of hypothermia. Brain hypothermia at 32°C produces predominant lipid metabolism (about 80%) and glucose metabolism is reduced to about 20%. This metabolic balance, however, is about even at a brain tissue temperature of 34°–35°C. At 36°C, glucose metabolism is dominant (90%–95%) over lipid metabolism. Therefore, short-duration brain hypothermia at 34°C does not need prolonged adaptation time, and careful slow rewarming is possible. However, prolonged moderate brain hypothermia requires very slow rewarming that includes adaptation times for the metabolic shift and uncoupling of blood flow and metabolism.

Stage 5.1. Basic Care Plan

Rewarming from mild brain hypothermia can be performed with increases of brain tissue temperature of 0.1°C/h, as shown in Fig. 96 (Chap. 47). However, rewarming from 32°–33°C requires an adaptation time for uncoupling between metabolic changes and blood flow at 34°–35°C for about 1–2 days. These techniques are described in Chap. 97.

Stage 5.2. Care Order

SBP: control at 120–160 mmHg by fluid resuscitation.

SBP >170 mmHg hypertension: drip antihypertensive drug diltiazem hydrochloride (Helvesser) 250 mg, diluted with 100 ml saline at 2 ml/h. With the complication of bradycardia (HR <50 bpm), change to nicardipine hydrochloride (Perdipin) 2–5 μg/kg min^{-1}.

Blood gases: PaO_2 >100 mmHg, PaO_2/FiO_2 ratio >350, $PaCO_2$ 35 mmHg.

Urine volume: more than 0.5 ml/kg h^{-1}.

Serum glucose: 120–140 mg/dl by drip of rapid-action insulin (Humarin R) 50 U diluted with 100 ml saline. Administration speed: start at 2 ml/h and slow to 1 ml/h after serum glucose falls below 200 mg/dl.

Serum potassium: control at 3.5–4.5 mEq/l by drip of KCl 1A, diluted with 80 ml saline. Replacement speed: 40 ml/h for serum K^+ <2.0 mEq/l, 20 ml/h for serum K^+ 1.2–2.5 mEq/l, 15 ml/h for serum K^+ 2.6–3.0 mEq/l, 10 ml/h for serum K^+ 23.1–3.05 mEq/l, and 5 ml/h for serum K^+ 3.6–34.0 mEq/l.

Stage 5.3. Intervention

Change ileus tube to ED tube. Digestive decontamination for control of clostridium enteritis and MRSA by enteral administration of levofloxacin (Cravit, 200 mg) and amphotericin B (100–300 mg), combined with vancomycin (2–3 g/day × 4–6 times i.v. drip) is useful prophylactic management of rewarming stage infections.

Stage 5.4. Intravenous Medication

Maintenance fluid: hicaliq-1 700 ml + amizet XB 300 ml +10% NaCl 2A + zantac 20A + panrol 500 mg × 2 (drip).

Administration of vitamins B, C, and E, and $ZnCl_2$.

Proteolysis enzyme: gabexate mesilate (FOY) 1500–2000 mg + maintenance fluid (Solita T4-solution) 200 ml (drip).

Antiepileptic: phenytoin–phenobarbital, Aleviatin 125 mg + saline 20 ml (i.v.), prepare flush saline 20 ml.

Change antibiotics: arbekacin sulfate (Habekacin, 150–200 mg/day ×2) to prevent pseudomonal aerginosa and MRSA infection, + cefozopran hydrochloride (Firstcin 1–2 g/day ×2) for Tienam-resistant Acinetobacter and xantomona + fluconazole (Diflucan 100–200 mg/day ×1) for Candida with evidence of β-D-glucan-positive reactions).

Anesthesia: midazolam (20A) + maintenance fluid (T4-soution) 160 ml drip 1 ml/h, combined drip with pancuronium bromide (Myoblock) 20A+T4-solution 160 ml, and buprenophine hydrochloride (Lepetan) 3–5A + saline 100 ml.

Heparin calcium (Hepacarin) 5000 U + saline 100 ml drip, 5 ml/h to prevent complication of SjO_2 monitoring.

Stage 5.5. Brain Monitoring and Management

ICP <25 mmHg, SjO_2 60%–75%, CPP >80 mmHg, ABER, and CT.

Stage 5.6. Monitoring and Management of Systemic Homodynamic Changes

CI >2.2, $\bar{D}O_2I$ >500, $\bar{V}O_2I$ >125, O_2ER 22%–26%, SVRI 1800–2500, PAWP >8–12 mmHg

Management of cardiac disturbances

1. Preload disturbances: administration of crystalloid, colloid, diuretics, and dopamine 1–3 μg/ml min^{-1}.
2. Contraction disturbances: administration of dobutrex and/or PDE-III inhibitor.
3. After load disturbances: administration of noradrenalin and/or Ca blocker.
4. Electric imbalance: Na, K, Mg, IP, and Ca.

Neuronal oxygenation

1. PaO_2/FiO_2 >300–350.
2. Manage neck position.
3. Check the correct intubation tube position.
4. Controlled mechanical ventilation volume 10–15 ml/kg, PEEP 3–5 cmH_2O, auto-sigh 20–25 ml/kg.
5. Management of red blood cells: Hb >11 mg/dl, DPG 12–14 μmol/ml, inorganic phosphate >3.0 mg/dl.

Water balance: intake/output every 8 h (two times/day).

Laboratory examinations: $PaCO_2$ 32–36 mmHg, serum glucose 120–150 mg/dl, serum albumin >3.5 mg/dl, IP >3 mg/dl, AT-III >120%, D-dimer platelet.

Gastrointestinal examination and management: gastric juice from N/G tube abdominal X-ray, nutritional consideration for management of BBB dysfunction (CSF/serum albumin ratio <0.01), and special enteric care management. Cetraxate hydrochloride (Neuer-S), L-glutamine (Glumin-S), antibiotic-resistant lactic acid bacteria (Biofermin-R), potassium permanganate, and Daiken Tyutou are enteric management drugs. The management of digastrics decontamination with nonabsorbable and hypothermia-active antibiotics [combination of levofloxacin (Cravit, 200 mg) and amphotericin B (100–300 mg), combined intravenous drip of vancomycin, 2–3 g/day × 4–6 times)] and administration of enteric nutrition are indicated to prevent systemic infections.

Stage 5 Algorithm Management

The control of brain tissue temperature: rewarming from short-duration brain hypothermia is not difficult; however, rewarming from prolonged brain hypothermia produces many negative effects on the injured brain tissue. Step-wise rewarming to 34°C and then an adaptation time of 1–2 days is very successful for rewarming from prolonged moderate brain hypothermia treatment. After that, the cooling blanket is removed from the body piece by piece over 1–2 days. This careful rewarming technique for prolonged brain hypothermia treatment is one of the key points for success of brain hypothermia treatment.

Prevention of hyperglycemia: administration of insulin by drip is useful for the control of hyperglycemia. In this stage, growth hormone to increase the immune activity is not recommended because this makes control of hyperglycemia difficult because of increasing serum glucose. Microdialysis studies suggest that control of serum glucose at 130–150 mg/dl is effective.

Oxygen metabolism: the oxygen demand increases during the rewarming stage. The control of oxygen delivery over 700 ml/min, PaO_2/FiO_2 >350, and O_2ER at 23%–35% are fundamental. To maintain hemoglobin function, the control of $PaCO_2$ 32–36 mmHg, serum pH 7.3–7.4, serum phosphate >3 mg/dl, and serum Mg^{++} >1.3 mmol/dl are also important. The major pitfall of oxygen management at the rewarming stage is the early management of spontaneous breathing without sufficient oxygen delivery and control of hemoglobin dysfunction. Spontaneous breathing is effective to avoid pulmonary atelectasis; however, oxygen demand also increases. Spontaneous breathing can cause brain hypoxia with poor oxygen delivery and hemoglobin DPG reduction. This is the last pitfall of unsuccessful brain hypothermia treatment. Ventilator breathing management should be used until the end stage of rewarming under anesthesia, analgesia, and muscle relaxation.

Infectious control: the worsening of infection at the rewarming stage is rare with good management of preconditioning. The management technique to control infection is very different as previously described. Infectious control during the cooling stage, algorithm management method for infection control, and management at the preconditioning stage have reduced the complication of pneumonia to less than 10% in our ICU. The complication of severe pulmonary infection with severe BBB damage (CSF/serum albumin >0.01–0.02) produces chemical cytokine encephalitis. The complication of severe infection during brain hypothermia indicates failure of the treatment. Careful management of infection during brain hypothermia treatment is important.

Posthypothermia Stage (Stage 6)

Standard Management

Damage of the dopamine A10 nervous system produces memory disturbance, emotional disturbance, and vegetation. Released dopamine from the dopamine nervous system produces neurotoxic·OH^- radicals after reaction with oxygen and then causes selective damage of the dopamine nervous system. This concept to the selective damage of the dopamine nervous system was hypothesized for a long time. Hypothermia is very effective in preventing the release of dopamine from the dopamine A10 nervous system. Recent clinical studies of the dopamine A10 nervous function support this hypothesis.

Stage 6.1. Basic Care Plan

The management techniques to prevent the release of dopamine at the acute stage was discussed in the algorithm management section and in Chap. 44. In this discussion, restoration therapies for the dopamine A10 nervous system in the chronic stage are presented. The various neuronal injury patterns in the dopamine A10 nervous system can be considered in vegetative patients. Many neurons in the dopamine A10 nervous system died and cannot recover from the vegetative state. No functioning of the dopamine A10 nervous system, however, remaining dopamine very resistant to the management of CBF and brain metabolism. Synaptic confusion in the dopamine A10 nervous system is caused by retention of neurotransmitters in interstitial space, reduced metabolic substrates for production of synaptic dopamine, and feeble dopamine synapses and so dopamine A10 neurons are thought to be causes of dopamine A10 nervous system malfunction. The replacement of metabolic substrates of dopamine neurotransmitters, pharmacological and electrophysiological stimulation of the dopamine A10 nervous system, increasing activity of the dopamine A10 nervous system by hormonal therapy, and monitoring of the dopamine A10 nervous system responsiveness are basic treatments for the restoration of vegetative patients after brain hypothermia treatment.

Stage 6.2. Care Order

SBP: control at 120–160 mmHg by fluid resuscitation.
Blood gases: PaO_2 >100 mmHg, PaO_2/FiO_2 ratio >350, $PaCO_2$ 35 mmHg.
Urine volume: more than 0.5 ml/kg h^{-1}.
Serum glucose: 120–140 mg/dl by drip of rapid-action insulin (Humarin R): 50 U diluted with 100 ml saline.
Serum potassium 3.5–4.5 mEq/l.
Serum magnesium >1.0 mmol/l.
Serum inorganic phosphate 2.5–4.5 mg/dl.
Prolactin: male 2–18 ng/ml, female 2–30 ng/ml.
T4-throxin: free 0.8–1.8 ng/dl, total 4.5–12 μg/dl.
Estron: male 29–81 pg/ml, female 40–150 pg/ml.

Stage 6.3. Intervention

Electrical median nerve stimulation for 3 weeks: 10–20 mA, 20 s on, 30 s off, 30 pulse/s, duration time 300 ms.
Emotional stimulation: music therapy.

Stage 6.4. Medication

Intracerebral dopamine replacement therapy: levodopa (300–400 mg/day), amantadine (100–200 mg/day) and parodel (10–15 mg/day).
Estrogen (Estraderm TTS patch 2 mg/day) patch therapy.
Antiepileptic therapy.
Replacement of vitamin B.

Stage 6.5. Brain Monitoring

CSF neurotransmitter analysis: dopamine, norepinephrine, and serotonin.
Responsiveness of dopamine A10 nervous system: increasing of CSF dopamine/CSF prolactin ratio after treatment.
EEG, CT, MRI, Xe-CBF, somatosensory evoked potential (extend N20 position or disappearance of N20) and visual evoked potential (extend the P300 300 ms positive wave).

Stage 6.6. Monitoring and Management of Systemic Homodynamic Changes

SBP >100 mmHg, O_2ER 22%–26%.
Management of cardiac function.
Electric imbalance: Na, K, Mg, IP, and Ca.

Neuronal oxygenation: PaO_2/FiO_2 >300–350, Hb >11 g/dl, DPG 12–14 μmol/ml, inorganic phosphate >3.0 mg/dl.

Water balance: Ht <40.

Laboratory examinations: serum glucose 120–150 mg/dl, serum albumin >3.5 mg/dl, AT-III >120%.

Stage 6 Algorithm Management

Dopamine replacement therapy: dopamine replacement therapy provides support for the non-functioning dopamine A10 nervous system. The responsiveness of the dopamine A10 nervous system can be diagnosed by the increased CSF dopamine/prolactin ratio even with no neurological response. Our clinical research suggested that the CSF dopamine/prolactin ratio increased between 3 and 14 days after music emotional stimulation and recorded neuronal recovery from vegetation. No patients recovered from vegetation without response of the CSF dopamine/prolactin ratio. Effective stimulation of the dopamine A10 nervous system includes pharmacological dopamine replacement therapy, estrogen patch therapy, median nerve stimulation, and music therapy. The big responses of the CSF dopamine/prolactin ratio to emotional body contact and music therapy were impressive. However, more effective methods for activation of the dopamine A10 nervous system are still under research.

Restoration therapy for vegetation: In the chronic stage, response of the dopamine A10 nervous system shown as increased CSF dopamine/prolactin ratio is an essential factor for successful neuronal recovery from vegetation. However, cortical neuronal response is also important for restoration from vegetation. Our preliminary clinical studies of neurotransmitter response using music therapy suggested that increased CSF epinephrine and homovanillic acid, and small responses of CSF alanine, glutamine, and 5-hydroxyindoleacetic acid suggest good prognosis for recovery from the vegetative state. However, large increases of CSF alanine, glutamine, and 5-hydroxyindoleacetic acid are negative indicators for vegetation therapy. It was surprising that the release of neurotoxic neurotransmitters was recorded in response to emotional music stimulation in cases of poor prognosis for recovery from vegetation. Response of the dopamine A10 nervous system and dopamine and nor-epinephrine-releasing neurons, and slight responses of neurotoxic transmitter-releasing neurons are important factors for recovery from vegetation. The mechanism of prolonged brain damage and the responsiveness of neurotoxic transmitter release to emotional stimulation must be considered further. Intracerebral dopamine replacement therapy and suppression of the neuronal activity that releases glutamate, alanine, and 5-hydroxyindoleacetic acid is an area of future treatment.

Neurorehabilitation: the early planning of neurorehabilitation is very important. However, this book does not discuss neurorehabilitation therapy.

60. Closing Remarks

For a long time, the management targets for treatment of severe brain injury have been misunderstood. There is no doubt of the effectiveness of hypothermia treatment for ischemic brain insults in animal studies, as described in chapter 1. However, in clinical studies, the effects of hypothermia were dissimilar to those observed in previous animal studies. Essentially, the results of hypothermia treatment in experimental animal studies and in clinical results are different. The reason for this difference is very simple: the brain injury mechanisms in experimental animal models and in severely traumatized brain-injured patients are different.

The systemic pathophysiological changes caused by stress-associated hypothalamus–pituitary–thyroid–adrenal axis neurohormonal reactions are not observed to a significant degree in anesthetized experimental animal models. Preliminary anesthesia minimizes this reaction to injury. Therefore, the symptoms and complications that occur in clinical patients, such as insulin-resistant hyperglycemia, activated glutamate neurotoxicity, reduction of hemoglobin 2,3-diphosphoglycerate and slow release of bound oxygen from hemoglobin in injured brain tissue, limited effect of oxygen inhalation, blood–brain barrier dysfunction associated with vasopressin release, delayed neuronal restoration by suppression of estrogen, and brain thermo-pooling, are not observed in anesthetized experimental animal models.

For a long time, the control of cerebral blood flow and intracranial pressure (ICP), prevention of brain edema and free radical reactions, and reduction of brain metabolism by hypothermia and barbiturate pharmacological therapies have been major treatments for severely brain-injured patients. The use of hypothermia is very successful for neuroprotection by reducing oxygen consumption, vascular engorgement, free radical reactions and the progression of brain edema. However, previous hypothermia treatment methods were not enough to prevent the brain injury mechanism of hypothalamus–pituitary–thyroid–adrenal axis neurohormonal reactions. Hypothermia is one of the environmental treatments for neuronal restoration. The precise control of brain tissue temperature, early induction of brain hypothermia to prevent catecholamine surge, control of insulin-resistant hyperglycemia, management of hemoglobin dysfunction, and management of the negative effects of hypothermia are important. Without understanding these stress-associated brain injury mechanisms, poorly coordinated brain hypothermia treatment is unavoidable.

ICP-oriented brain hypothermia treatment has also been reported. However, ICP-oriented brain hypothermia treatment is not successful in severely brain-injured patients because ICP elevation occurs as result of worsening neuronal hypoxia and metabolic imbalance. The initial management is the prevention of neuronal hypoxia and control of metabolic imbalance rather than control of ICP. ICP-oriented brain hypothermia treatment is a form of neuroprotection therapy rather than neuronal restoration therapy.

The use of brain hypothermia is not all beneficial and some negative effects are also recorded. Metabolic shift from glucose to lipid metabolism, immune suppression associated with reduced growth hormone levels, the complications of systemic infection, unstable cardiopulmonary circulation caused by reduced catecholamine, and rewarming stress are negative effects of brain hypothermia treatment. For the success of brain hypothermia treatment, ingenious management techniques are required. Therefore, simple brain cooling management is not adequate for restoration of dying neurons in severely brain-injured patients. The detailed techniques for brain hypothermia treatment are described in Chap. 2.

The new findings of the effectiveness of brain hypothermia treatment for prevention of vegetation and diagnostic methods to determine emotional responsiveness during the vegetative state are demonstrated in this book. This information will be very helpful to open the door for the management of vegetation in severe brain damage. Recent experimental studies have focused on the effectiveness of sex hormones. In this book, estrogen replacement therapy was described for the prevention of vegetation by activation of cerebral dopamine uptake, for the benefit of cell plasticity, stimulation of mitogen remyelinzation, and to protect apoptosis. However, experimental studies have demonstrated the effectiveness of estrogen at the acute stage including the reuptake of lactate in neurons, reduced neuron excitation, increased expression of the anti-apoptotic factor bcl-2, and activation of the mitogen-activated protein kinase pathway. The better prognosis in women over that in men is not doubted in severe brain injury. More studies about estrogen therapy for the acute stage of neuronal restoration therapy are required.

The concept of brain hypothermia treatment has changed three times with new findings of brain injury mechanism over the past 11 years. Brain hypothermia treatment is still in the developmental phase. The effectiveness of brain hypothermia treatment has been ascertained not only in severe brain trauma, but also in cardiac-arrested patients. Understanding of stress-associated neurohormonal brain hazards, the mechanism of brain hypothermia treatment, and the negative effects of brain hypothermia will see this treatment adopted for cerebral stroke patients.

In this book, the critical path of brain hypothermia treatment was demonstrated. This critical path is focused toward severe traumatic brain injury. However, this critical path could be used for acute stroke, and cardiac arrested patients with modification. It is my hope that this book will provide guidance for management of severe brain trauma, stroke, hypoxia, and postresuscitation of cardiac arrest and help to obtain good clinical results.

Appendix. Critical Pathway of Brain Hypothermia Treatment

1. Mild brain hypothermia treatment (34°C)

   Indication: GCS 6–9, unstable vital signs, insulin-resistant hyperglycemia
   Induction: within 3–6 h
   Duration: 2–7 days

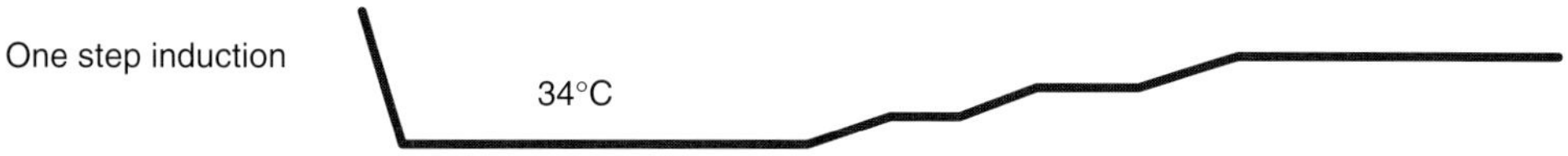

2. Moderate brain hypothermia treatment (32°–33°C)

   Indication: GCS 6–4, hemiated patient after controled vital signs and hyperglycemia
   Induction: within 3–4 h
   Duration: 4–14 days

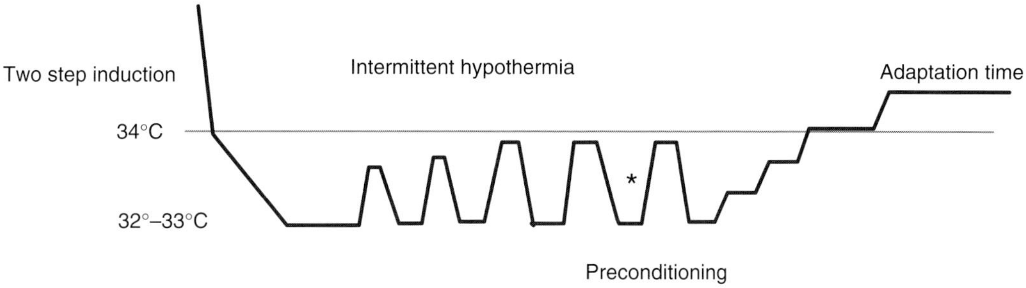

Contraindication
- Severity: GCS=3, brain death
- Pathophysiology: shock, MOF, severe infections, cardiac insufficiency, arrhythmia
- Disease: uncontrollable subarachnoid hemorrhage
- Time: >6 h, >24 h (time dependent)
- Age: ?

Outline of the critical path of brain hypothermia treatment

Stage	Stage 1 Induction 1	Stage 2 Induction 2	Stage 3 Cooling	Stage 4 Preconditioning	Stage 5 Rewarming	Stage 6 Post hypothermia
Duration	3h	6h	3–7 days	1–2 days	1–2 days	3–4 weeks
Algorithm of Management Targets	Stabilize vital signs Shivering Catecholamine surge Neuronal hypoxia Hyperglycemia 34°C brain temperature Dopamine release Radical reaction	Mild or moderate hypothermia? Serum glucose <160mg/dl DO_2 >700ml/min Hemoglobin dysfunction AT-III >100% Hypopotassemia SBP > 100mmHg Fluid resuscitation	Intermittent hypothermia ICP <15mmHg Brain edema AT-III >100% Serum albumin >3.5mg/dl Immune dysfunction Prevent infection Activate lipid metabolism	Evidence of neuronal recovery No severe infection CSF/serum albumin <0.01 Serum glucose 120–140mg/dl Enteral nutrition Recover immune function Activate lipid metabolism	Step by step rewarm Adaptation time Serum glucose 130–150mg/dl $\bar{D}O_2$ >700ml/min O_2ER 23–35 $PaCO_2$ 32–36mmHg Serum pH 7.3–7.4 Serum Phosphate >3mg/dl Serum Mg^+ >1.3mmol/dl Replacement vitamin A Infection control	A 10-Dopamine replacement therapy Restoration therapy of vegetation Neurorehabilitation
Standard Management Order						
Basic care plan	①	①	①	①	①	①
Care order	②	②	②	②	②	②
Intervention	③	③	③	③	③	③
IV medication	④	④	④	④	④	④
Monitor						
Brain monitor	⑤	⑤	⑤	⑤	⑤	⑤
Systemic care monitor	⑥	⑥	⑥	⑥	⑥	⑥

Stage 1.1.

Basic care plan:

- Start brain hypothermia within 3h after insult.
- Maintain the systolic blood pressure > 100 mmHg.
- Evaluate GCS < 8 and surgical indication.
- Rapid management of stress-associated hyperglycemia.
- Maintain hemoglobin function with control of serum pH, phosphate, and magnesium.
- Prevent catecholamine surge.
- Neuronal oxygenation.
- Prevent enterobacterial infection.
- Suppress hypothalamus dopamine release.

Stage 1.2.

Care order:

- Systolic blood pressure (SBP): control at 120–160 mmHg by fluid resuscitation.
- SBP > 170 mmHg hypertension: drip the antihypertensive drug, diltiazem hydrochloride (Helvesser), 250 mg, diluted with 100 ml saline at 2 ml/h.
- Blood gases: PaO_2 > 100 mmHg, PaO_2/FiO_2 ratio > 350, $PaCO_2$ 34–38 mmHg.
- Urine: maintain at 0.5 ml/kg h^{-1}.
- Serum glucose: control serum glucose at 120–140 mg/dl by drip of rapid – action insulin (Humarin R), 50 U diluted with 100 ml saline.
  * Administration speed: start from 2 ml/h and then slow down to 1 ml/hour after serum glucose becomes lower than 200 mg/dl.
- Serum potassium: control at 3.5–4.5 mEq/l by drip of KCl 1A, diluted with 80 ml saline.
  * Replacement speed 40 ml/h for serum K^+ < 2.0 mEq/l.
  * 20 ml/h for serum K^+ 1.2–2.5 mEq/l.
  * 15 ml/h for serum K^+ 2.6–3.0 mEq/l.
  * 10 ml/h for serum K^+ 23.1–3.05 mEq/l.
  * 5 ml/h for serum K^+ 3.6–34.0 mEq/l.

Stage 1.3.

Intervention:

- Bronchial intubation and ventilator care management.
- Fluid resuscitation by central venous catheterization.
- Catheter insertion for monitoring arterial blood gases.
- Insertion of naso-gastric tube.
- Insertion of Foley catheter for urinary drainage.
- Monitoring of ECG.
- Biochemical analysis.
- Blood type.
- X-ray examination.
- Gastric lavage.
- Digastrics decontamination.
  * One shot enteral administration of nonabsorbable antibiotics: levofloxacin (Cravit, 200 mg) + amphotericin B, 100–300 mg.

Stage 1.4.

Intravenous medication:

- Fluid resuscitation: 7% Acetic acid Ringer solution (Veen F) and Saline Hess solution at induction stage, except hypoglycemia. The replacement of potassium phosphate, vitamin A, vitamin B, Mg^{++}, 5% albumin, and AT-III are recommended.
- Crush induction of anesthesia: midazolam 0.15–0.25 mg/kg h^{-1} anesthesia, combined with pancuronium 0.05 mg/kg h^{-1} muscle relaxation, and buprenorphine 1.0–2.0 mg/kg h^{-1} analgesia. Propofol is much better for unstable cardiopulmonary function than midazolam. At the beginning of the induction stage, propopfol is preferred.
- Management of aspiration pneumonia: first choice is panipenem betamipron (Carbenin 500 mg × 2/day), second choice is ceftazidime (Modasin 1 g × 2/day) or clindamycine (Dalacin, 150–300 mg per 6 h) + one-shot enteral administration of nonabsorbable antibiotics: levofloxacin (Cravit, 200 mg) + Amphotericin B, 100–300 mg to prevent Pseudomonas aspiration pneumonia and enteral bacterial translocation.

Stage 1.5.

Brain monitoring and management:

- Computed brain monitoring:
  * Tympanic membrane temperature/core temperature > 1.0.
  * Internal jugular venous blood temperature/tympanic membrane temperature > 1.0.
  * Ventricular CSF temperature/internal jugular venous blood temperature > 1.0.
  * Ventricular CSF temperature/bladder temperature > 1.0.
- ICP < 20 mmHg.
- Microdialysis monitoring.
- SjO_2 > 60%.
- CPP > 80 mmHg.
- Trend EEG.
- Auditory brain stem evoked response (ABER).

Stage 1.6.

Monitoring and management of systemic hemodynamic changes:

- SBP > 100 mmHg
- Monitoring of ECG for arrhythmia, ST changes, and QT interval < 450 mm/s.
- Right flowing catheter monitoring of cardiac output (CO).
- Cardiac index (CI).
- Oxygen delivery > 700 ml/min.
- Oxygen extraction ratio (O_2ER) 22%–26%.
- Bladder pressure < 15 mmHg.
- Gastric pHi > 7.3.
- Intestinal luminar pressure < 15 mmHg.
- Serum glucose and hemoglobin A1C.
- AT-III.
- Hemoglobin.
- Serum albumin.
- Troponin I and CPK.
- GOT and GPT.
- Ht.
- Serum osmolarity.
- Creatinine.

Stage 1. Algorithm management

- Stabilize vital signs: elastic bandaging of extremities, normal volume replacement, medication, maintain SBP > 100 mmHg, CPP > 80 mmHg, Hb > 12 mg/dl, oxygen delivery > 800 ml/min., 2,3-DPG > 13 μmol/ml.
- Serum K^+ > 3 mEq/dl, serum glucose 120–140 mg/dl.
- Shivering: midazolam anesthesia 0.15–0.25 mg/kg h^{-1} combined with pancuronium muscle relaxant 0.05 mg/kg h^{-1}, and buprenorphine analgesia 1.0–2.0 mg/kg h^{-1}.
- Catecholamine surge: control of catecholamine surge by control of brain tissue temperature at 34°C, administration of metoclopramide.
- Neuronal hypoxia: PaO_2/FiO_2 ratio > 350, hemoglobin DPG: 12–14 μmol/ml, oxygen delivery > 700 ml/min, CPP > 80 mmHg, AT-III > 100%.
- Hyperglycemia: administration of insulin with control of serum phosphate and magnesium.
- 7% acetate Ringer solution.
- Steroid contraindicated.
- Activate respiratory muscle metabolism with albutamol.
- Rapid induction of mild brain hypothermia: combination of blanket cooling method and gastric lavage with chilled saline, alcohol heat evaporation, complete body wrapping and insulation from room air, reduce room temperature to 18°C, maintain room air outflow circulation, two cooling machines, remove heat generating medical devices from the bedside.
- Dopamine release: early induction of brain hypothermia and administration of metoclopramide.
- Prevention of radical reaction: early induction of mild brain hypothermia and continue to moderate brain hypothermia.
- Control of Hb > 11 mg/dl, administration of vitamins E and C.

Stage 2.1.

Basic care plan:

- Select mild or moderate brain hypothermia.
- Monitor internal jugular venous temperature.
- Monitor ventricular CSF temperature.
- Monitor tympanic temperature.
- Monitor core temperature.
- Monitor bladder temperature.
- Stabilize vital signs for induction to moderate brain hypothermia.
- SBP > 100 mmHg.
- Treat hypokalemia.
- Ensure no arrhythmia.
- QT-interval < 450 mm/s on ECG.
- Serum glucose 120–140 mmHg.
- Brain monitoring, SjO2 65%–80%.
- ICP < 20 mmHg.

Stage 2.2.

Care order:

- Systolic blood pressure (SBP): 120–160 mmHg by fluid resuscitation.
- SBP > 170 mmHg hypertension: drip antihypertensive drug diltiazem hydrochloride (Helvesser), 250 mg, diluted with 100 ml saline at 2 ml/h.
- Complication of bradycardia (HR < 50 bpm): nicardipine hydrochloride (Perdipin) 2–5 μg/kg min^{-1}.
- Blood gases: $PaO_2 > 100$ mmHg, PaO_2/FiO_2 ratio > 350, $PaCO_2$ 35 mmHg.
- Urine volume: more than 0.5 ml/kg h^{-1}.
- Serum glucose: 120–140 mg/dl by drip of rapid-action insulin (Humarin R) 50 U diluted with 100 ml saline.
  * Administration speed: start at 2 ml/h and slow to 1 ml/h after serum glucose falls below 200 mg/dl.
- Serum potassium: control at 3.5–4.5 mEq/l by drip of KCl 1A, diluted with 80 ml saline.
  * Replacement speed: 40 ml/h for serum $K^+ < 2.0$ mEq/l.
  20 ml/h for serum K^+ 1.2–2.5 mEq/l.
  15 ml/h for serum K^+ 2.6–3.0 mEq/l.
  10 ml/h for serum K^+ 23.1–3.05 mEq/l.
  5 ml/h for serum K^+ 3.6–34.0 mEq/l.

Stage 2.3.

Intervention:

- Ventilator management.
- Ventricular drainage.
- ICP monitoring.
- SjO_2 monitoring.
- Monitoring cardiac output and O_2ER.
- Body weight.
- Blood gases.
- Microdialysis monitoring.

Stage 2.4.

Intravenous medication:

- Fluid resuscitation: 7% Acetic acid Ringer solution (Veen F) + H_2 receptor antagonist (Zantac 50 mg/A) + metoclopramide (Prinmperan) 1A + panthenol (Pantol 500 mg × 2).
- Maintenance fluid: actit solution 500 ml + carbazochrome sodium sulfonate (Adona) 50 ml + tranexamic acid (Transamin S) 1A + hemocoagulase (Reptilase-S 1A proteolysis enzyme) (drip).
- Enzyme inhibitor: ulinastatin (Miraclid) 300 000 unit/day + maintenance fluid (T4-solution) 400 ml (drip).
- Proteolysis enzyme: gabexate mesilate (FOY) 1500–2000 mg + maintenance fluid (T4-solution) 200 ml (drip).
- Antiepileptic phenytoin-phenobarbital (Aleviatin) 250 mg + saline 20 ml (i.v.), flush saline 20 ml, Aleviatin 125 mg + saline 20 ml (i.v.).
- Adsorbed tetanus toxoid 0.5 ml (i.m.) + human antitetanus immunoglobulin 250 IU (i.m.).
- Anesthesia: midazola (20A) + maintenance fluid (T4-soution) 160 ml drip 1 ml/h^{-1} combined drip with pancuronium bromide (Myoblock) 20A + T4-solution 160 ml, and buprenophine hydrochloride (Lepetan) 3-5A + saline 100 ml.
- Heparin calcium (Hepacarin) 5000 U + saline 100 ml drip, 5 ml/h to prevent complication of SjO_2 monitoring.
- Blood transfusion for Hb < 10 mg/dl.

Stage 2.5.

Brain monitoring and management:

- CPP > 80 mmHg.
- ICP < 20 mmHg.
- SjO_2: 70%–80%.
- Trend EEG.
- ABER.

Care management of ICP

(1) Prevent venous stasis by management of neck position, mediastinal pressure, abdominal hypertension, full stomach, and bladder pressure.
(2) Diagnose the effectiveness of CSF drainage by changes in ICP during 3 min open/close drainage.
(3) Continuous CSF drainage.
(4) Manage hypercapnia.
(5) Replacement of serum albumin to 3.5 mg/dl.
(6) Head-up position.
(7) Management of hyperglycemia and serum electrolytes.
(8) Control of blood pressure.
(9) Administration of manitol 100 ml/30–60 min.

Stage 2.6.

Monitoring and management of systemic homodynamic changes: CI > 2.2, DO_2I > 500, VO_2I > 125, O_2ER 22–26%, SVRI 1800–2500, and PAWP > 8–12 mmHg.

- Management of cardiac disturbances:
  (1) Preload disturbances: administration of crystalloid, colloid, diuretics, and dopamine 1–3 $\mu g/ml\,min^{-1}$.
  (2) Contraction disturbances: administration of dobutrex and/or PDE-III inhibitor.
  (3) After load disturbances: administration of noradrenalin and/or Ca blocker.
  (4) Electric imbalance: Na, K, Mg, IP, and Ca.
- Neuronal oxygenation:
  (1) PaO_2/FiO_2 > 300–350.
  (2) Manage neck position.
  (3) Check the correct position of intubation tube.
  (4) Control mechanical ventilation volume 10–15 ml/kg, PEEP 3–5 cmH_2O, auto-sigh 20–25 ml/kg.
  (5) Management of red blood cells: Hb > 11 mg/dl, DPG 12–14 μmol/ml, inorganic phosphate > 3.0 mg/dl.
- Laboratory examinations: blood gas analysis every 2 h, complete blood cell count, serum glucose, serum albumin, IP, Mg, AT-III, D-dimer, α2-PI, SFMC, PF1+2, APC, and platelet aggregation.
- MRSA bacterial analysis.
- Gastrointestinal examination and management: gastric juice from N/G tube < 200 ml/day.

Stage 2. Algorithm management

- Serum glucose < 160 mg/dl:
  1. Early brain hypothermia (33°–34°C) induction within 3 h after brain damage. Catecholamines surge-associated hyperglycemia should be minimized.
  2. Replacement of insulin.
  3. No administration of cortisol.
  4. Activate protein synthesis of muscle by administration of arginine, salbutamol, clenbuterol, glutamine.
  5. Inhibit protein catabolism: amurinone.
  6. Rehabilitation and kinetic therapy.
- $\bar{D}O_2 > 700$ ml/min and SBP > 100 mmHg:
  1. Fluid resuscitation, administration of norepinephrine + doptorex.
  2. Elastic bandaging of extremities.
  3. Temporary insertion of abdominal balloon catheter into the abdominal aorta.
- Hemoglobin dysfunction:
  1. Control of serum pH > 7.3.
  2. Serum glucose 120–140 mg/dl.
  3. Serum inorganic phosphate 3–5 mg/dl and magnesium 1.4–1.8 mEq/l.
  4. Serum albumin > 3.5 mg/dl, vitamin A 50–100 mg/dl.
- AT-III > 100%: replacement of serum albumin.
- Hypokalemia: control K^+ at 3.5–4.5 mEq/l by drip of KCl 1A, diluted with 80 ml saline.

  Replacement speed: 40 ml/h for serum $K^+ < 2.0$ mEq/l.
  20 ml/h for serum K^+: 1.2–2.5 mEq/l.
  15 ml/h for serum K^+: 2.6–3.0 mEq/l.
  10 ml/h for serum K^+: 23.1–3.05 mEq/l.
  5 ml/h for serum K^+: 3.6–34.0 mEq/l.

Stage 3.1.

Basic care plan:

- Restoration of injured brain tissue.
- Maintaining neuronal oxygenation.
- Metabolic balance.
- Maintaining lipid metabolism.
- Management of ICP and brain edema.
- Careful management of BBB function.
- Control of immune dysfunction.
- Maintaining neurohormonal function.
- Nutritional consideration.
- Prevention of infections.

The major target of ICU management at the cooling stage are:

Stage 3.2.

Care order:

- Systolic blood pressure (SBP): control between at 120–160 mmHg by fluid resuscitation.
- SBP > 170 mmHg hypertension: drip antihypertensive drug diltiazem hydrochloride (Helvesser), 250 mg, diluted with 100 ml saline at 2 ml/h.
  Complication of bradycardia (HR < 50 bpm): nicardipine hydrochloride (Perdipin) 2–5 µg/kg min^{-1}.
- Blood gases: $PaO_2 > 100$ mmHg, PaO_2/FiO_2 ratio > 350, $PaCO_2$ 35 mmHg.
- Urine volume: more than 0.5 ml/kg h^{-1}.
- Serum glucose: 120–140 mg/dl by drip of rapid-action insulin (Humarin R): 50 U diluted with 100 ml saline.
  * Administration speed: start with 2 ml/h and slow to 1 ml/h after serum glucose becomes lower than 200 mg/dl.
- Serum potassium: control at 3.5–4.5 mEq/l by drip of KCl 1A, diluted with 80 ml saline.
  * Replacement speed: 40 ml/h for serum K^+ < 2.0 mEq/l.
  * 20 ml/h for serum K^+ 1.2–2.5 mEq/l.
  * 15 ml/h for serum K^+ 2.6–3.0 mEq/l.
  * 10 ml/h for serum K^+ 23.1–3.05 mEq/l.
  * 5 ml/h for serum K^+ 3.6–34.0 mEq/l.

Stage 3.3.

Intervention:

- Ventilator management.
- Ventricular drainage.
- ICP monitoring.
- SjO_2 monitoring.
- Monitoring of cardiac output and O_2ER.
- Insert ileum gastric tube.
- Kinetic therapy using dyna care bed.
- Microdialysis monitoring.

Stage 3.4.

Intravenous medication:

- Fluid resuscitation: 7% Acetic acid Ringer solution (Veen F) + H2 receptor antagonist (Zantac 50 mg/A) + metoclopramide (Prinmperan) 1A + panthenol (Pantol 500 mg × 2).
- Maintenance fluid: combination of physiosol-3 500 ml, Amicaliq 500 ml, and Hicaliq 500 ml (drip).
- Administration of vitamins C and E, and $ZnCl_2$.
- Enzyme inhibitor: ulinastatin (Miraclid) 300 000 U/day + maintenance fluid (T4-solution) 400 ml (drip).
- Proteolysis enzyme: gabexate mesilate (FOY) 1500–2000 mg + maintenance fluid (T4-solution) 200 ml (drip).
- Vitamin kit: vitamin C 500 mg, vitamin B1 50 mg, vitamin B2 20 mg, vitamin 6 20 mg (i.v.).
- Antiepileptic medicine: phenytoin-phenobarbital (Aleviatin) 250 mg + saline 20 ml (i.v.), flush saline 20 ml, Aleviatin 125 mg + saline 20 ml (i.v.).
- Antibiotics: immipenem cilastain sodium (Tienam 1–2 g/day × 3) > meropenem trihydrate (Meropn, 1.0–2.0 g/day × 4) for enterobacteria, gram-negative bacteria, and pseudomonas.
- Anesthesia: midazolam (20A) + maintenance fluid (T4-solution) 160 ml drip 1 ml/h, combined drip with pancuronium bromide (Myoblock) 20A + T4-solution 160 ml, and buprenophine hydrochloride (Lepetan) 3-5A + saline 100 ml.
- Heparin calcium (Hepacarin) 5000 U + saline 100 ml drip, 5 ml/h to prevent complication of SjO_2 monitoring.
- Blood transfusion for Hb > 10 mg/dl.

Stage 3.5.

Brain monitoring and management:

- CPP > 80 mmHg.
- ICP < 20 mmHg.
- SjO_2 70%–80%.
- Trend EEG.
- ABER.
- CT.
- Brain tissue temperature.

Stage 3.6.

Monitoring and management of systemic homodynamic changes: CI > 2.2, $\bar{D}O_2I > 500$, $\bar{V}O_2I > 125$, O_2ER 22%–26%, SVRI 1800–2500, and PAWP > 8–12 mmHg.

- Management of cardiac disturbances:
  (1) Preload disturbances: administration of crystalloid, colloid, diuretics, and dopamine 1–3 μg/ml min^{-1}.
  (2) Contraction disturbances: administration of dobutrex and/or PDE-III inhibitor.
  (3) After load disturbances: administration of noradrenalin and/or Ca blocker.
  (4) Electric imbalance: Na, K, Mg, IP, and Ca.
- Neuronal oxygenation:
  (1) $PaO_2/FiO_2 > 300–350$.
  (2) Manage neck position.
  (3) Check the correct position of intubation tube.
  (4) Controlled mechanical ventilation volume 10–15 ml/kg, PEEP 3–5 cmH_2O, auto-sigh 20–25 ml/kg.
  (5) Management of red blood cells: Hb > 11 g/dl, DPG 12–14 μmol/ml, inorganic phosphate >3.0 mg/dl.
- Water balance: intake/output each 8 hours.
- Laboratory examinations: blood gases analysis every 2 h, complete blood cell count, serum glucose, serum albumin, IP, Mg, AT-III, D-dimer, α2-PI, SFMC, PF1 + 2, APC, and platelet aggregation.
- MRSA bacterial analysis.
- Gastrointestinal examination and care management: gastric juice from N/G tubes <200 ml/day, abdominal X-ray, nutritional consideration with management of BBB dysfunction (CSF/serum albumin ratio <0.01), and special enteral care management. Cetraxate hydrochloride (Neuer-S), L-glutamine (Glumin-S), Antibiotic-resistent lactic acid bacteria (Biofermin-R), potassium permanganate, and Daiken Tyutou are enteral management drugs.

Stage 3. Algorithm management

1. **Intermittent hypothermia**: prolonged brain hypothermia, below 32°–33°C, produces a reduction of pituitary hormones. Deficiency of growth hormone and thyroid hormones causes an unavoidable depletion of immune function. To prevent this complication, intermittent control of brain tissue temperature between 32°C and 34°C is a very useful management technique. The temporary elevation of brain tissue temperature is recommended at 1800–2200 hours because physiological growth hormone is naturally released at this time. The detailed techniques are described previously in this book.
2. **Brain edema and control of ICP < 15 mmHg**: ICP elevation to more than 20 mmHg produces venous stasis and disturbances of microcirculation. To prevent microcirculation, CSF drainage, head-up position, reduction of abdominal pressure and mediastinal pressure, prevention of hypo-albuminemia, administration of hyper-osmotic solution, manitol, and reduction of CSF production by acetazolamide (Diamox) are prescribed management.
3. **AT-III > 100%**: peripheral vascular stasis is one of the complications of the cooling stage of brain hypothermia. Prolonged bed rest, peripheral vascular contraction, subcutaneous edema caused by the complication of hypo-albuminemia, complication of infection, and consumption on of AT-III by severe brain damage are causes of reducted of AT-III. Lower than 80%–90% of AT-III is critical and promotes the systemic disturbance of microcirculation and development of inflammation of vascular intimae. Our clinical studies suggest the management of AT-III affects to prognosis and success of brain hypothermia treatment.
4. **Serum albumin >3.5 mg/dl**: prolonged hypothermia promoter synthesis of protein and albumin. Increasing cytokines produces hypo-albuminemia. In severely brain-injured patients, rapid development of hypo-albuminemia is a big clinical issue. Progression of brain edema, ineffective manitol hyperosmotic diuretics for brain edema, complication of pulmonary edema, intestinal mucous edema pancreatic duct obstruction caused by intestinal wall edema, immune dysfunction, bacterial translocation, unstable pharmacological function of protein-binding drugs, increased free bacteria and ease of infection are major complications of hypo-albuminemia. Therefore, replacement of albumin and nutritional consideration for hypo-albuminemia are important management strategies during the cooling stage of brain hypothermia treatment.
5. **Immune dysfunction**: reduced growth hormone levels and energy crisis in lymphocytes are major causes of immune dysfunction during brain hypothermia treatment. The reduction of growth hormone is unavoidable with prolonged moderate brain hypothermia because the temperature of the pituitary gland is also lowered. Glutamine is the energy source for lymphocytes and is produced in lung tissue and skeletal muscles. This glutamine is expended by lymphocytes in the intestinal digestive organs. Therefore, muscle hypometabolism, pulmonary infection, and mucous edema in the digestive organ caused by hypo-albuminemia also produce immune dysfunction. Administration of arginine, salbutamol, and growth hormone are effective in maintaining immune function because of stimulation of protein synthesis in skeletal muscles and promotion of the lipid metabolism which is the main metabolism under hypothermia.
6. **Prevention of infection**: complication with severe infection during the cooling stage causes the failure of brain hypothermia treatment. Increased serum proinflammatory cytokines can permeate the damaged BBB and produce cytokine encephalitis with uncontrollable increases of neurotoxic glutamate in injured brain tissue. Therefore, as management of infection during brain hypothermia treatment, the killing of bacteria, activation of immune function, the management of BBB (CSF/serum albumin ratio <0.01), management of serum albumin (>3.5 g/dl), no activation of vasopressin release by neural control of the feedback mechanism to hyperglycemia, maintenance of protein synthesis in skeletal muscles, and administration of bacteria-sensitive non-protein-binding antibiotics are indicated. The intermittent control of brain tissue temperature at 32°–33°C, administration of arginine, and rehabilitation of skeletal muscles are also effective to increase the immune function. The choice of systemic administration of antibiotics and digestive decontamination antibiotics therapy was described previously in this book.
7. **Activation of lipid metabolism**: brain hypothermia below 34°C produces metabolic shift from glucose to lipid metabolism. The lipid metabolism requires vitamin A and adequate growth hormone for energy metabolism without lactate production. Excessive replacement of growth hormone produces hyperglycemia. Therefore, careful monitoring of serum glucose is important for replacement therapy of growth hormone and arginine.

Stage 4.1.

Basic care plan:

Rewarming can occur after exact diagnosis of some form of recovery. The recording of a θ wave on the background of the δ wave in trend EEG, no ICP elevation, SjO_2 control at 60%–70%, and no brain swelling on CT scan are basic signs of neuronal recovery. To succeed in rewarming from brain hypothermia treatment, various preconditioning managements are needed.

Stage 4.2.

Care order:

Rewarming from brain hypothermia, especially prolonged treatment below 34°C, produces various physiological changes such as metabolic shift from lipid to glucose, vascular engorgement, increased of metabolic activity, activated cytokine production, increase in ·NO radicals, increased serum cytokines, uncoupling of bloodflow and metabolism in major organs, and oxygen demand in the brain tissue. Before rewarming, preconditioning management is recommended for adaptation or prevention of negative effects to the brain by these physiological changes. The major targets for preconditioning care are:

- No severe infection.
- Lymphocytes >1500/mm^3.
- T-H (CD4) lymph >55%.
- Serum glucose 120–140 mg/dl.
- Prealbumin >20 mg/dl.
- Serum albumin >3.5 mg/dl.
- Vitamin A >50 mg/dl.
- Hb > 12 mg/dl.
- O_2ER 23%–25%.
- AT-III > 100%.
- Gastric pHi > 7.35.

The success of management ensures no trouble during rewarming.

Stage 4.3.

Intervention:

- EEG (recovery from δ wave to θ wave or recording of α wave).
- ABR.
- Brain CT (no signs of brain swelling or severe brain edema).
- ICP (<20 mmHg).
- CPP (>70–80 mmHg).
- Prevention of systemic infection by combined administration of antibiotics:
  (1) Digestive decontamination: control of clostridium enteritis and MRSA by enteral administration of levofloxacin (Cravit, 200 mg) and Amphotericin B, 100–300 mg.
  (2) Combined with vancomycin for (2–3 g/day × 4–6 times i.v. drip) is useful prophylactic management for rewarming stage infection.

Stage 4.4.

Intravenous medication:

- Maintenance fluid: combination of physiosol-3 500 ml, amicaliq 500 ml, 7% acetic acid Ringer solution (Veen F) and hicaliq 500 ml (drip). Calorie increases with monitoring of serum glucose.
- Administration of vitamins C and E, and $ZnCl_2$.
- Enzyme inhibitor: ulinastatin (Miraclid) 300 000 U/day + maintenance fluid (T4-solution) 400 ml (drip).
- Proteolysis enzyme: gabexate mesilate (FOY) 1500–2000 mg + maintenance fluid (T4-solution) 200 ml (drip).
- Antiepileptic phenytoin-phenobarbital, Aleviatin 125 mg + saline 20 ml (i.v.), prepare the flush saline 20 ml.
- Antibiotics: arbekacin sulfate (Habekacin, 150–200 mg/day × 2) to prevent pseudomonal aerginosa and MRSA infection, + cefozopran hydrochloride (Firstcin 1–2 g/day × 2) for Tienam resistant Acinetobacter and xantomona + fluconazole (Diflucan 100–200 mg/day × 1) for Candida with evidence of β-D-Glucan-positive reactions).
- Anesthesia: midazola (20A) + maintenance fluid (T4-soution) 160 ml drip 1 ml/h, combined drip with pancuronium bromide (Myoblock) 20A + T4-solution 160 ml, and buprenophine hydrochloride (Lepetan) 3–5A + saline 100 ml.
- Heparin calcium (Hepacarin) 5000 U + saline 100 ml drip, 5 ml/h to prevent complication of SjO_2 monitoring.
- Blood transfusion for Hb < 10 mg/dl.

Stage 4.5.

Brain monitoring and management:

- CPP > 80 mmHg.
- ICP > 20 mmHg.
- SjO_2 70%–80%.
- Trend EEG (recovery from δ wave to θ wave or recording of α wave).
- ABER.
- Brain CT (no signs of brain swelling, severe brain edema or ICP elevation).

Stage 4.6.

Monitoring and management of systemic homodynamic changes:
CI > 2.2, $\bar{D}O_2I > 500$, $\bar{V}O_2I > 125$, O_2ER 22%–26%, SVRI 1800–2500, and PAWP > 8–12 mmHg.

- Management of cardiac disturbances:
  (1) Preload disturbances: administration of crystalloid, colloid, diuretics, and dopamine 1–3 μg/ml min^{-1}.
  (2) Contraction disturbances: administration of dobutrex and/or PDE-III inhibitor.
  (3) After load disturbances: administration of noradrenalin and/or Ca blocker.
  (4) Electric imbalance: Na, K, Mg, IP, and Ca.
- Neuronal oxygenation:
  (1) $PaO_2/FiO_2 > 300–350$.
  (2) Manage neck position.
  (3) Check the correct position of intubation tube.
  (4) Controlled mechanical ventilation volume 10–15 ml/kg, PEEP 3–5 cmH_2O, auto-sigh 20–25 ml/kg.
  (5) Management of red blood cells: Hb > 11 mg/dl, DPG 12–14 μmol/ml, inorganic phosphate >3.0 mg/dl.
- Water balance: intake/output every 8 hours.
- Laboratory examinations: PaCO2 32–36 mmHg, serum glucose 120–150 mmHg, serum albumin >3.5 mg/dl, IP > 3 mg/dl, AT-III > 120%, D-dimer.
- Gastrointestinal examination and management:
  (1) Gastric juice from N/G tubes <200 ml/day.
  (2) Abdominal X-ray.
  (3) Nutritional consideration for management of BBB dysfunction (CSF/serum albumin ratio <0.01).
  (4) Special enteral care management.
    * Cetraxate hydrochloride (Neuer-S), L-glutamine (Glumin-S), antibiotic-resistant lactic acid bacteria (Biofermin-R), potassium permanganate, and Daiken Tyutou are enteral management drugs.
    * The management of digastrics decontamination with nonabsorbable and hypothermia-active antibiotics levofloxacin (Cravit, 200 mg) and amphotericin B, 100–300 mg, combined with intravenous drip administration of Vancomycin (2–3 g/day × 4–6 times) are indicated for prevention of systemic infections.

Stage 4. Algorithm management

1. **Evidence of neuronal recovery**: the big issue at rewarming is reprogression of brain injury mechanism that was stopped at the cooling stage. Without evidence of neuronal recovery or at least signs of recovery, rewarming makes the condition much worse. If neuronal recovery was not diagnosed by monitoring of ICP, SjO_2, EEG, and CSF biochemical changes, the cooling stage should be extended for a few more days. Management is same as Standard Management, Stage 4.1. Basic Care Plan, Stage 4.2. Care Order, Stage 4.3. Intervention, Stage 4.4. Intravenous Medication, Stage 4.5. Brain Monitoring, Stage 4.6. Monitoring and Management of Systemic Homodynamic Changes, and Algorithm Management. No signs of brain edema or other complications on the CT examination are also useful to diagnose neuronal recovery.
2. **No severe infection and CSF/serum Albumin <0.01**: the elevation of body temperature by rewarming stimulates the activity of serum cytokines. Increased serum cytokines can easily permeate the damaged BBB. This serious complication causes the failure of the brain hypothermia treatment at the rewarming stage. Therefore, management of severe pulmonary infection and management of BBB dysfunction (CSF/serum albumin ratio lower than 0.01) must be achieved before rewarming. The actual management method is described previously in this book.
3. **Serum glucose** 120–140 mg/dl: administration of insulin with control of serum phosphate and magnesium, 7% acetate Ringer solution, contraindicated steroid, activate respiratory muscle metabolism by salbutamol.
4. **Enteral nutrition**: the management of nutrition at the rewarming stage requires the replacement of an energy source of calories, feed to immune cells, stabilization of the intestinal digestive organ, and maintenance of nutritional conditions. The management of BBB dysfunction is also important because neurotoxic glutamate increases about two to three times with enteral and parenteral amino acid nutrition. In well-organized BBB with CSF/serum albumin ratio lower than 0.01, microdialysis studies provided no evidence of serum glutamate passing into the brain tissue and no evidence of worsening brain edema.

   Preliminary management of BBB dysfunction with replacement of serum albumin to higher than 3.5 g/dl, anti-inflammatory medicine for the vascular wall such as AT-III and protein C, and radical scavenger such as Radicut are useful to avoid nutritional complications at the rewarming stage. The replacement of serum albumin is very effective for the control of intestinal mucous membrane edema and prevention of diarrhea caused by enteral nutrition. Preliminary feeding (with glutamine and arginine), correct serum electrolytes, control of the osmotic gap (serum Osm − 2 (stool Na + K) > 100 mOsmk/kg) and management of mesenteric ischemia are also useful before feeding management.

   Two actual enteral nutrition courses are prepared. One uses saline immune nutrition (glutamine + arginine + yeast RNA) with administration of honey yogurt, and control of BBB function at CSF/serum albumin ratio lower than 0.01. The other is two-step enteral nutrition with CSF/serum albumin 0.01–0.02. First step: saline 50 ml to max 150 ml/4 h, and remove retention fluid repeat for 3–4 days. Second stage: administration of honey yogurt (50 ml to max 150 ml/4 h). The detail techniques are described earlier in this book. The combination of enteral nutrition with honey yogurt and arginine is very effective for stimulation of lipid metabolism without production of lactate.

Stage 5.1.

Basic care plan:

- Rewarming from mild brain hypothermia can be performed with increases of brain tissue temperature of 0.1°C/h.
- However, rewarming from 32°–33°C requires an adaptation time for uncoupling between metabolic changes and blood flow at 34°–35°C for about 1–2 days.

Stage 5.2.

Care order:

- Systolic blood pressure (SBP): control between at 120–160 mmHg by fluid resuscitation.
- SBP > 170 mmHg hypertension: drip the antihypertensive drug, diltiazem hydrochloride (Helvesser), 250 mg, diluted with 100 ml saline at 2 ml/h.
  Complication of bradycardia (HR < 50 bpm): nicardipine hydrochloride (Perdipin) 2–5 μg/kg min^{-1}.
- Blood gases: PaO_2 > 100 mmHg, PaO_2/FiO_2 ratio >350, $PaCO_2$ 35 mmHg.
- Urine volume: more than 0.5 ml/kg h^{-1}.
- Serum glucose: 120–140 mg/dl by drip of rapid-action insulin (Humarin R) 50 U diluted with 100 ml saline.
  * Administration speed: start at 2 ml/h and slow to 1 ml/h after serum glucose becomes lower than 200 m g/dl.
- Serum potassium: control at 3.5–4.5 mEq/l by drip of KCl 1A, diluted with 80 ml saline.
  * Replacement speed: 40 ml/h for serum K^+ < 2.0 mEq/l.
  * 20 ml/h for serum K^+ 1.2–2.5 mEq/l.
  * 15 ml/h for serum K^+ 2.6–3.0 mEq/l.
  * 10 ml/h for serum K^+ 23.1–3.05 mEq/l.
  * 5 ml/h for serum K^+ 3.6–34.0 mEq/l.

Stage 5.3.

Intervention:

- Change ileus tube to ED tube.
- Digestive decontamination for control of clostridium enteritis and MRSA by enteral administration of levofloxacin (Cravit, 200 mg) and amphotericin B (100–300 mg).
- Combine with vancomycin (2–3 g/day × 4–6 times i.v. drip) is useful prophylactic management of rewarming stage infections.

Stage 5.4.

Intravenous medication:

- Maintenance fluid: hicaliq-1 700 ml + amizet XB 300 ml + 10% NaCl 2A + zantac 20A + panrol 500 mg × 2 (drip).
- Administration of vitamins B, C, and E, and $ZnCl_2$.
- Proteolysis enzyme: gabexate mesilate (FOY) 1500–2000 mg + maintenance fluid (Solita T4-solution) 200 ml (drip).
- Antiepileptic phenytoin-phenobarbital, Aleviatin 125 mg + saline 20 ml (i.v.), prepare the flush saline 20 ml.
- Change the antibiotics: arbekacin sulfate (Habekacin, 150–200 mg/day × 2) to prevent pseudomonal aerginosa and MRSA infection, + cefozopran hydrochloride (Firstcin 1–2 g/day × 2) for Tienam-resistant Acinetobacter and xantomona + fluconazole (Diflucan 100–200 mg/day × 1) for Candida with evidence of β-D-glucan positive reactions).
- Anesthesia: midazolam (20A) + maintenance fluid (T4-soution) 160 ml drip 1 ml/h, combined drip with pancuronium bromide (Myoblock) 20A + T4-solution 160 ml, and buprenophine hydrochloride (Lepetan) 3–5A + saline 100 ml.
- Heparin calcium (Hepacarin) 5000 U + saline 100 ml drip, 5 ml/h for prevent to complication SjO_2 monitoring.

Stage 5.5.

Brain monitoring and managment:

- ICP < 25 mmHg.
- SjO_2 60%–75%.
- CPP > 80 mmHg.
- ABER.
- CT.

Stage 5.6.

Monitoring and management of systemic homodynamic changes: CI > 2.2, $\bar{D}O_2I > 500$, $\bar{V}O_2I > 125$, O_2ER 22%–26%, SVRI 1800–2500, and PAWP > 8–12 mmHg.

- Management of cardiac disturbances:
  (1) Preload disturbances: administration of crystalloid, colloid, diuretics, and dopamine 1–3 μg/ml min^{-1}.
  (2) Contraction disturbances: administration of dobutrex and/or PDE-III inhibitor.
  (3) After load disturbances: administration of noradrenalin and/or Ca blocker.
  (4) Electric imbalance: Na, K, Mg, IP, and Ca.
- Neuronal oxygenation:
  (1) $PaO_2/FiO_2 > 300$–350.
  (2) Manage neck position.
  (3) Check correct intubation tube position.
  (4) Controlled mechanical ventilation volume 10–15 ml/kg, PEEP 3–5 cmH_2O, auto-sigh 20–25 ml/kg.
  (5) Management of red blood cells: Hb > 11 mg/dl, DPG 12–14 μmol/mL, inorganic phosphate >3.0 mg/dl.
- Water balance: intake/output every 8 hours (two times/day).
- Laboratory examinations: $PaCO_2$: 32–36 mmHg, serum glucose 120–150 mg/dl, serum albumin >3.5 mg/dl, IP > 3 mg/dl, AT-III > 120%, D-dimer, platelet.
- Gastro-intestinal examination and care management:
  (1) Gastric juice from N/G tube abdominal X-ray, nutritional consideration for management of BBB dysfunction (CSF/serum albumin ratio <0.01).
  (2) Special enteric care management. Cetraxate hydrochloride (Neuer-S), L-glutamine (Glumin-S), antibiotic-resistant lactic acid bacteria (Biofermin-R), potassium permanganate, and Daiken Tyutou are enteric management drugs.
  (3) The management of digastrics decontamination with nonabsorbable and hypothermia-active antibiotics (combination of levofloxacin (Cravit, 200 mg) and amphotericin B, 100–300 mg).
  (4) Combined intravenous drip of vancomycin (2–3 g/day × 4–6 times) and administration of enteric nutrition are indicated to prevent systemic infections.

Stage 5. Algorithm management

- **The control of brain tissue temperature**: rewarming from short-duration brain hypothermia is not difficult, however, rewarming from prolonged brain hypothermia produces many negative effects on the injured brain tissue. Step wise rewarming to 34°C and then an adaptation time of 1–2 days is very successful for rewarming from prolonged moderate brain hypothermia treatment. After that, the cooling blanket is remove from the body piece by piece over 1–2 days. This careful rewarming technique for prolonged brain hypothermia treatment is one of the key points for success of brain hypothermia treatment.
- **Prevention of hyperglycemia**: administration of insulin by drip is useful for the control of hyperglycemia. In this stage, growth hormone to increase the immune activity is not recommended, because this makes control of hyperglycemia difficult because of increasing serum glucose. Microdialysis studies suggest that control of serum glucose at 130–150 mg/dl is effective.
- **Oxygen metabolism**: the oxygen demand increases during the rewarming stage. The control of oxygen delivery over 700 ml/min, $PaO_2/FiO_2 > 350$, and O_2ER 23%–35% are fundamental. To maintain hemoglobin function, the control of $PaCO_2$ 32–36 mmHg, serum pH 7.3–7.4, serum phosphate >3 mg/dl, and serum $Mg^+ > 1.3$ mmol/dl are also important. The major pitfall of oxygen management at the rewarming stage is the early management of spontaneous breathing without sufficient oxygen delivery and control of hemoglobin dysfunction. Spontaneous breathing is effective to avoid pulmonary atelectasis, however, oxygen demand also increases. Spontaneous breathing can cause brain hypoxia with poor oxygen delivery and hemoglobin DPG reduction. This is the last pitfall of unsuccessful brain hypothermia treatment. Ventilator breathing management should be used until the end stage of rewarming under anesthesia, analgesia, and muscle relaxation.
- **Infectious control**: the worsening of infection at the rewarming stage is rare with good management of preconditioning. The management technique to control infection is very different as previously described. Infectious control during the cooling stage, algorithm management method for infection control, and management at the preconditioning stage have reduced the complication of pneumonia to less than 10% in our ICU. The complication of severe pulmonary infection with severe BBB damage (CSF/serum albumin >0.01–0.02) produces chemical cytokine encephalitis. The complication of severe infection during brain hypothermia indicates failure of the treatment. Careful management of infection during brain hypothermia treatment is important.

Stage 6.1.

Basic care plan:

The basic treatments for the restoration of vegetative patients after brain hypothermia treatment are:

- The management techniques to prevent the release of dopamine at the acute stage was discussed in the algorithm care management section and earlier in this book.
- The major restoration therapy for vegetation is the management of the dopamine A10 nervous system. The various neuronal injury patterns in the dopamine A10 nervous system can be considered in vegetate patients:
  (1) No functioning of the dopamine A10 nervous system, however, remaining dopamine very resistant to the management of CBF and brain metabolism.
  (2) Synaptic confusion in the dopamine A10 nervous system is caused by retention of neurotransmitters in interstitial space.
  (3) Reduced metabolic substrates for production of synaptic dopamine.
  (4) Feeble dopamine synapses.
- The replacement of metabolic substrates of dopamine neurotransmitters could be through:
  (1) Pharmacological replacement.
  (2) Electrophysiological stimulation of the dopamine A10 nervous system.
  (3) Increasing activity of the dopamine A10 nervous system by hormonal therapy, and monitoring of the dopamine A10 nervous system responsiveness.

Stage 6.2.

Care order:

- Systolic blood pressure (SBP): control between 120–160 mmHg by fluid resuscitation.
- Blood gases: $PaO_2 > 100$ mmHg, PaO_2/FiO_2 ratio >350, $PaCO_2$ 35 mmHg.
- Urine volume: more than 0.5 ml/kg h^{-1}.
- Serum glucose: 120–140 mg/dl by drip of rapid-action insulin (Humarin R): 50 U diluted with 100 ml saline.
- Serum potassium: control at 3.5–4.5 mEq/l.
- Serum magnesium: control >1.0 mmol/l.
- Serum inorganic phosphate: 2.5–4.5 mg/dl.
- Prolactin: male 2–18 ng/ml, female 2–30 ng/ml.
- T4-throxin: free 0.8–1.8 ng/dl, total 4.5–12 μg/dl.
- Estron: male 29–81 pg/mL, female 40–150 pg/ml.

Stage 6.3.

Intervention:

- Electrical median nerve stimulation for 3 weeks: 10–20 mA, 20 s on, 30 s off, 30 pulse/s, duration time 300 ms.
- Emotional stimulation: music therapy and talking.

Stage 6.4.

Medication:

- Intracerebral dopamine replacement therapy:
  Levodopa (300–400 mg/day)
  Amantadine (100–200 mg/day)
  Parodel (10–15 mg/day).
- Estrogen (Estraderm TTS patch 2 mg/day) patch therapy.
- Antiepileptic therapy.
- Replacement of vitamin B.

Stage 6.5.

Brain monitoring and management:

- CSF neurotransmitter analysis: dopamine, norepinephrine, and serotonin.
- Responsiveness of dopamine A10 nervous system: increasing of CSF dopamine/CSF prolactin ratio after treatment.
- EEG.
- CT.
- MRI.
- Xe-CBF.
- Somatosensory evoked potential (extend N20 position or disappearance of N20).
- Visual evoked potential (extend the P300 300 msec positive wave).

Stage 6.6.

Monitoring and management of systemic homodynamic changes:

- SBP $>$ 100 mmHg, O_2ER 22%–26%.
- Management of cardiac function.
- Electric imbalance: Na, K, Mg, IP, and Ca.
- Neuronal oxygenation:
  $PaO_2/FiO_2 > 300$–350
  Hb $>$ 11 mg/dl
  DPG 12–14 μmol/ml
  inorganic Phosphate $>$3.0 mg/dl.
- Water balance: Ht $<$ 40.
- Laboratory examinations:
  Serum glucose 120–150 mmHg
  Serum albumin $>$3.5 mg/dl
  AT-III $>$ 120%.

Stage 6. Algorithm management

- **Dopamine replacement therapy**: dopamine replacement therapy provider support for the non-functioning dopamine A10 nervous system. The responsiveness of the dopamine A10 nervous system can be diagnosed by the increased CSF dopamine/prolactin ratio even with no neurological response. Our clinical research suggested that the CSF-dopamine/prolactin ratio increased between 3 and 14 days after music emotional stimulation and recorded neuronal recovery from vegetation. No patients recovered from vegetation without response of the CSF dopamine/prolactin ratio. Effective stimulation of the dopamine A10 nervous system includes pharmacological dopamine replacement therapy, estrogen patch therapy, median nerve stimulation, and music therapy. The big responses of the CSF dopamine/prolactin ratio to emotional body contact and music therapy were impressive. However, more effective methods of activation of the dopamine A10 nervous system are still under research.
- **Restoration therapy for vegetation**: in the chronic stage, response of the dopamine A10 nervous system shown as increased of CSF dopamine/prolactin ratio is an essential factor for successful neuronal recovery from vegetation. However, cortical neuronal response is also important for restoration from vegetation. Our preliminary clinical studies of neurotransmitter responsiveness using music therapy suggested that increased CSF epinephrine and homovanillic acid, and small responses of CSF alanine, glutamine, and 5-hydroxyindoleacetic acid suggest good prognosis for recovery from the vegetative state. However, increases of CSF alanine, glutamine, and 5-hydroxyindoleacetic acid are negative indication for vegetation therapy. It was surprising that the release of neurotoxic neurotransmitters was recorded in response to emotional music stimulation in cases of poor prognosis for recovery from vegetation. Response of the dopamine A10 nervous system and dopamine and norepinephrine-releasing neurons, and slight responses of neurotoxic transmitter-releasing neurons are important factors for recovery from vegetation. The mechanism of prolonged brain damage and the responsiveness of neurotoxic transmitter release to emotional stimulation must be considered further. Intracerebral dopamine replacement therapy and suppression of the neuronal activity that releaser glutamate, alanine, and 5-hydroxyindoleacetic acid is an area of future treatment.
- **Neurorehabilitation**: the early planning of neurorehabilitation is very important. However, this book does not discuss neurorehabilitation therapy.

Management of dopamine A10 nervous system in severely brain-injured patients

1. Acute stage: prevent dopamine release and use radical scavengers
   Prevent dopamine release in hypothalamus by administration of metoclopramide
   Brain hypothermia: 32°–34°C, prevent cerebral dopamine release and radical attack to the dopamine A10 nervous system
   Replacement of prolactin and thyroid hormone
   Administration of radical scavengers
2. Chronic stage: activate dopamine A10 nervous system
   Cerebral dopamine replacement therapy
      Pharmacological treatment: Levodopa (300–400 mg/day), Amantadine (100–200 mg/day)
      Uptake of cerebral dopamine: Estrogen (Estraderm TTS Patch 2 mg/day)
      Median nerve stimulation: 10–20 mA 20 s on 30 s off, 30 pulse/s, duration time 30 m/s
   Music therapy

Subject Index